Nature's Healing Practices

A Natural Remedies Encyclopedia

Agatha Thrash, MD

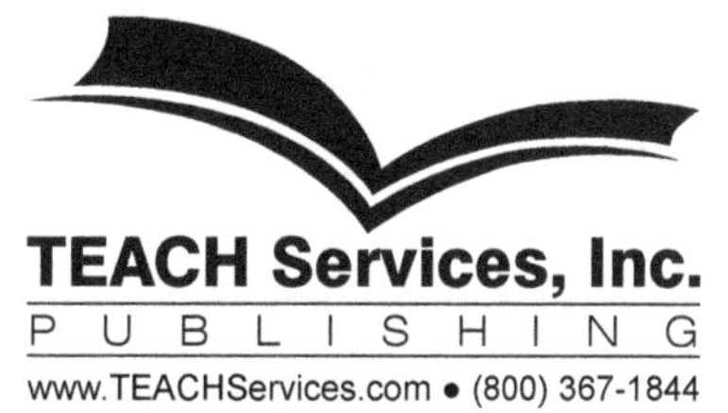
TEACH Services, Inc.
PUBLISHING
www.TEACHServices.com • (800) 367-1844

ISBN-13: 978-1-57258-714-4 (Paperback)
ISBN-13: 978-1-57258-715-1 (Hardback)
ISBN-13: 978-1-57258-716-8 (E-book)
Library of Congress Control Number: 2015908275

Published by

Dedication

We dedicate this book to our heavenly Father whose loving nature provided a remedy for every disease known to humankind. It is His desire that we look for His remedy in every case of sickness. May God bless you with every good blessing.

Also to my two children and three grandchildren who taught me many natural remedies and learned many more.

Carol Ann Thrash-Trumbo
Calvin Lassetter Thrash, III
Christina Cherie' Thrash
Melissa Ann Thrash
Taylor Jonathan Trumbo

Table of Contents

Conditions and Diseases

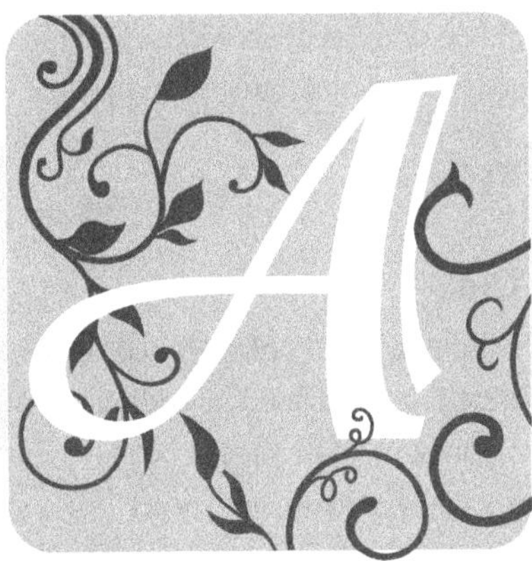

Abdominal Pain

Possible causes of abdominal pain are overeating, eating too fast, foods that don't agree, appendicitis, cancer, colitis, constipation, diarrhea, diverticulitis, food allergies, food poisoning, gas, glandular disorders, hiatal hernia, influenza, irritable bowel syndrome, menstrual problems.

(See also "Abdominal Pain" in the *Home Emergencies* and *Supplemental Information* sections and "Pain Control" in the *Conditions and Diseases* section.)

Abortion, Threatened

(See "Women's Conditions and Diseases" in the *Conditions and Diseases* section.)

Aids and HIV Complex

AIDS (acquired immune deficiency syndrome) is a disease caused by the human immunodeficiency virus (HIV). Because of damage to the immune system, all manner of physical diseases can arise, from minor skin diseases to life-threatening infections and malignancies.

Counsel for HIV Positive Person

- Avoid travel as much as possible. Get regular exercise, maintain a good diet, and avoid stress.
- The plant-based diet is most favorable in HIV complex and full-blown AIDS. This diet strengthens the immune system.
- Avoid pregnancy if you are HIV positive as it often brings on AIDS. There is a 50 percent chance also for the baby to get AIDS.
- Avoid vaccines, cortisone, antibiotics, chemotherapy, stress, and all high-risk sexual behavior.
- Avoid immunosuppressive drugs as well as aspirin, alcohol, tobacco, caffeine drinks, and all illicit drugs; these suppress the immune system.
- Do not donate blood, tissues, or organs; do not share toothbrushes or razors; do not have tattooing or ears pierced.
- Decontaminate surfaces and fabrics contacting your blood. Use bleach, 1 part to 10 parts water.
- Avoid cats. They transmit toxoplasmosis. Avoid close contact with birds. They transmit psittacosis. Avoid other pets and all animal foods. These serious diseases may accompany or precipitate AIDS.

There is currently no effective standard treatment for AIDS, and none anticipated. Therefore, any help for the AIDS patient must come from the application of the laws that govern immunity. These laws should be studied and applied religiously in order to strengthen the immune system.

Family and friends should have regular prayer for a miracle from heaven. Trust God that He is loving, forgiving, healing, and comforting. A strong faith strengthens the immune system. Trust Him that every trial from the evil one can result in a more trusting relationship with God who walks beside us, even when the trial appears to be totally destructive. God has not promised us freedom from trials, but He has promised to be with us. The faith developed by trusting God is itself a miracle. When Jacob wrestled with the angel,

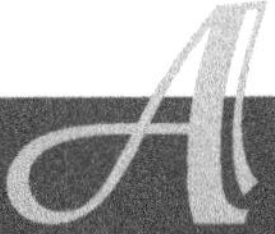

it appeared that having his thigh go out of joint was a terrible calamity that would disqualify him physically from saving himself and his family from the armed men with Esau. But the limp which resulted was partly what stimulated sympathy from his brother Esau and turned away his murderous wrath. Furthermore, trust in God stimulates the endorphin system, strengthening the immune system.

The objectives of our treatments are to improve circulation to tissues and oxygenation and nourishment of the cells, to change the intestinal flora with a high fiber vegetarian diet, to discourage cancer cell growth with hot baths, to stimulate the immune mechanism against cancer and infection, and to combat toxins that cause anemia and loss of appetite.

Case Report

A 34-year-old former homosexual, who had changed his lifestyle, got married and had two children. Eight years after getting married he began to lose weight, followed by pneumonia, swollen lymph nodes, and a sore throat. He was diagnosed with AIDS. We used the treatment routine given below. About the middle of the second series of fever treatments, he began to feel improvement with each new day. He gained weight well, had a reduction in the size of the lymph nodes in his neck, and had a general improvement in his sense of well-being.

At the beginning of the course of treatments, he showed strong signs in his blood cells of AIDS infection, but after 45 fever treatments he showed much improvement. He took 15 treatments in three weeks, skipped a week, and repeated this schedule until he had taken 45 treatments.

Blood Work	Before Treatments	After Treatments
Red blood cells	4.43	4.64
White blood cells	8.7	4.1 (level fell as the infection fell)
Platelets	236	183
Sed rate	66	7
Amino trans sera Antibodies (+ S-Co=Sup.A)	730	15.45

While he remained HIV positive, he gained weight, his pneumonia cleared, his lymph nodes became normal in size, and he was able to return to his job for three or four years. He took a series of 15 hot baths, mouth temperature up to 103°F, every three months for two years, then every six months until he again got an overwhelming case of pneumonia and died of AIDS. (It should be noted that six months before his death he left his wife and children and returned to his former lifestyle.)

Treatment

The Ideal Diet

The diet should be totally plant-based, leaving off all refined fats, all refined sugars, chemical additives, hot spices, and vinegar. The majority of food should be raw with occasional fresh juices, especially carrots and beets. Sick animals lead to diseased meat, which often causes sick people. Fermented foods such as beer, wine, cheeses, breads, sauerkraut, many canned soups, and mushrooms (except for portabellas, reishis, and shiitakis) should all be eliminated. The following principles should also be followed:

- Take two meals, or at most three per day, if weight loss is not a problem. Two meals daily are usually best, breakfast and lunch. Never snack.
- Put five hours between the end of one meal and the beginning of the next.
- Have a set time for meals. Establish regularity and regimentation as far as meals and sleep schedules are concerned. It is ideal to quit work and devote oneself to the treatment process for at least 12 months.
- Read labels for irritants and harmful foods and additives such as vinegar, monosodium glutamate, pepper (black, cayenne, hot), baking powder and soda, animal products, and hot spices.
- Omit one to three meals weekly, unless underweight, to lighten the work of the liver.
- Eat a lot of fruits and vegetables, uncooked or only lightly steamed.
- Eat slowly, chewing food to a cream before swallowing.
- Cook grains and legumes thoroughly. Grain preparations such as those cracked or whole kernel must be boiled gently for three hours at least. Rolled grains need one and a half hours of cooking time. A good slow cooker is useful for this. Set the pot to cook at night, and it is ready for breakfast.
- Enjoy gardening or other outdoor work, but do not work to the point of exhaustion.
- Omit liquid foods at meals except on rare occasions. Liquid foods are sodas, juices, watery soups, and other beverages. If juices are used in greater quantity than eight ounces, make a meal of them only, and sip them slowly, mixing with saliva. Fresh juices and fruits help

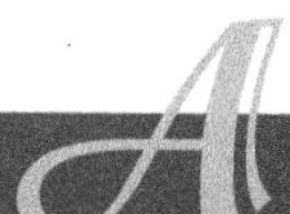

to build the red blood cells and improve the cleansing functions of the glands. Many foods can be taken raw, but those that should be cooked are potatoes, beets, root vegetables (except carrots, rutabagas, turnips, and radishes), grains unless sprouted, eggplant, the winter squash or pumpkin family, and beans.

- Never overeat.
- Exercise out of doors after a meal if possible. A slow outdoor walk for the first 5 to 10 minutes after the meal is beneficial, then continue the walk, picking up the pace to a brisk walk from half an hour to one hour after the meal. Exercise helps digestion.
- Eat only if you are hungry and only at meal times.
- Do not eat when in pain, angry, worried, in emotional states, or tired.
- Keep meals simple; two to three items at a meal.
- Shake dried fruits vigorously for one minute in three rinses of water in a jar to wash off molds and other substances. It is nice to soak dried fruits in pure water overnight in the refrigerator before eating.
- Do not use commercial corn oils, only cold pressed oils or olive oil; never heat oils.
- Eat foods mainly grown in the region where you live.
- Use frozen fruit blended with a little fruit juice, occasionally, as an ice-cream substitute on hot days.
- Shop at health food stores and produce markets that keep fresh food because of a rapid turnover.
- Never use soft drinks, coffees, teas, chocolate, or unproven prescription drugs recently introduced on the market. You may use herb teas.
- Eat fresh carrots, grapes, cabbage, asparagus, Brussels sprouts, beets, broccoli, dark greens, kohlrabi, and cauliflower. Either chew them well or puree fresh fruit and vegetables in a blender or food processor. Eating carrots has been associated with a significant increase in total white cell count. This stimulation to the immune system by carrots was published in the *Journal of Acquired Immune Deficiency Syndrome* (6 [1993]: 272–76). Enough yellow fruits and vegetables should be taken for you to acquire a slightly orange skin color. Do not take both fruits and vegetables at the same meal. If possible, 50 to 80 percent of the meal should be eaten raw. Asparagus and garlic both have antiviral, anticancer, and antifungal qualities.
- Frequently choose cooked grains or vegetables from the following list: potatoes (white or sweet), corn, carrots, oats, buckwheat, wheat, rice, barley, millet, rye. These foods are selected because of their low phenylalanine and lysine content, too much of these two amino acids can cause some degree of suppression of the immune system.
- Use immature legumes such as field peas or green peas no more than twice a week, as they are high in phenylalanine and lysine. Select only one of these at a meal.
- Do not use whole grain cereals or quick breads with sugar, baking powder or soda, or excessive salt.
- Follow a meal plan (see “Health Recovery Program” in the *Supplemental Information* section). Breakfast should consist of simply fruits and whole grains with nuts or seeds. Lunch should feature simply vegetables and whole grains with nuts or seeds. Any supper that is taken should be sparse with fruits and whole grains.
- Selenium and magnesium stimulate the immune system, as do zinc and vitamin C. Animal protein can be toxic to a healing body. Most westerners suffer from protein excesses. No attempt should be made to increase protein in the diet.
- Give a three-week course of zinc supplementation, 15 to 50 milligrams per day.

Hydrotherapy and Massage

Water is a cleanser and a healer, externally and internally. Drink 12 or more cups of water or tea, as pure as possible, between meals each day. (Also, regular bowel movements daily are very important. Two cups of very warm water upon rising in the morning are very helpful for this.)

A daily bath is essential—personal hygiene is a must. Wear a clean change of underclothes daily.

Use fever treatments. The infant under three years of age who has AIDS should have the temperature very carefully controlled, bringing the underarm temperature up to 102°F or rectal temperature up to 103°F, but not holding it there. That may take only five to six minutes for the baby, or less. Do not use a water temperature higher than 106°F. For the newborn up to 6 months 103°F is good.

The treatments are done as follows: let the patient over three years sit and get settled in a tub of water at about 101°F to 102°F, but immediately build up the water temperature to 105°F to 108°F. Obtain 102°F to 104°F orally and maintain it for 5 to 10 minutes, as tolerated. When the oral temperature goes above 100°F or the patient begins to sweat, keep the face and head very cool with cold cloths changed often. Have a small fan for the face if the patient is sitting in water that keeps the shoulders covered. Keep the bath water 105°F to 108°F while the oral temperature is 102°F to 104°F. Do this by draining off some of the cooling water and adding fresh

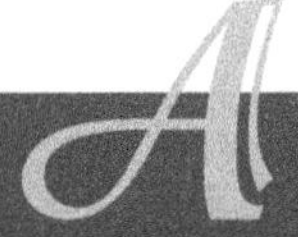

hot water. This treatment should be done only on vigorous patients, and the pulse rate should not be allowed to go above 160. Children under 100 pounds should stay in the hot water only one minute for each year of their age.

End the hot treatment with a cold mitten friction, tepid shower, brisk friction drying, and one hour of bed rest with an ice pack wrapped in a towel on the forehead. The mouth temperature should drop below 100°F before getting up. Prevent chilling after the treatment. Stop the treatment if the heart rate rises above 160 in a person under 50 years of age and above 140 in a person over 50 years of age.

Fifteen fever treatments spread over three weeks constitutes one series of treatments. Give two series of three weeks each, pausing for one week or more after the first three weeks before beginning the second series. There should be five treatments in a week, but not usually more than one fever treatment per day for adults. Interrupt the treatment program every five days with a two-day rest. If the patient responds to the two series of treatments in three months, using the same routine, go through another two series of the fever treatments. Repeat every three months.

Cold mitten friction hydrotherapy treatments can be done several times a day, as often as once an hour, but usually at a rate of twice a day, as the energy of the patient or the availability of time permit. It is a good stimulant of the immune system, and it is especially beneficial if continued indefinitely after the fever series is finished.

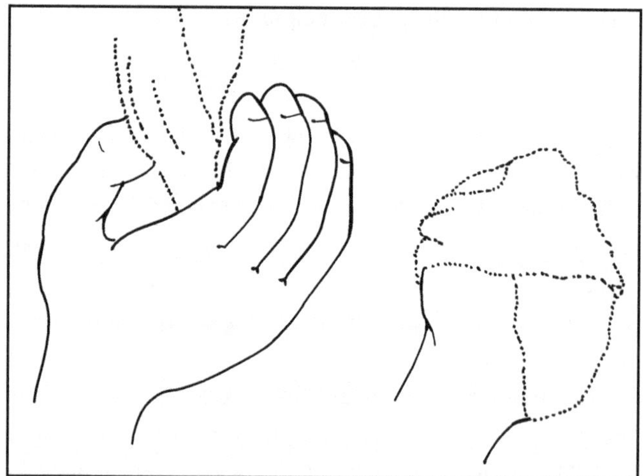

Twice a day have a dry brush massage using gentle short, round strokes all over the body, ending with sweeping strokes over the entire body.

For strengthening the immune system, take hot and cold showers, two to five minutes hot, 10 to 30 seconds cold, alternating, with the force of the water set as high as possible. Finish with a quick brisk rubbing with a coarse towel. Do this treatment twice a day.

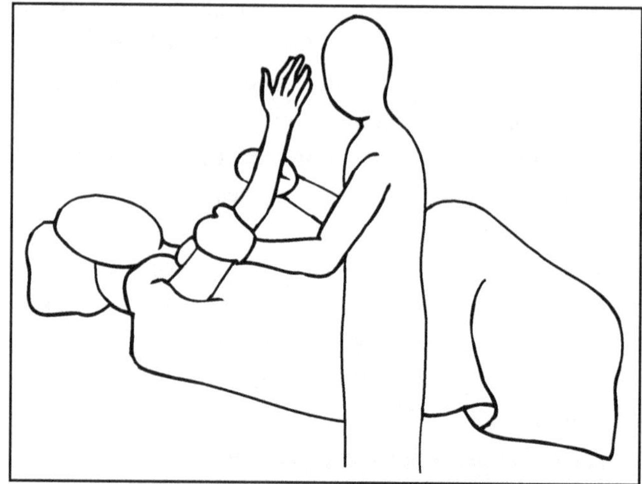

Stimulate the thymus, the source of T-cells, by tapping on the middle of the chest, gently but firmly, pounding rapidly with one fist after the other on the breastbone just below the middle. Do not bruise the tissue. This treatment should be pleasant, not jolting. Do not use this treatment for a patient who has a malignancy in or on the chest.

Adrenal stimulation encourages production of beneficial hormones. Locate the position of the adrenals by putting the right hand on the waist while standing behind the patient. Put the fingertips of your left hand on the lower angle of the right shoulder blade. Then place the thumb of your right hand on a point approximately halfway between the two hands. Then slide the thumb close to the spine. That is the location of the upper pole of the kidney. One fingerbreadth above that is the location of the adrenals. Tap fast and firmly, drumming over the adrenals with the fingertips of alternating hands, like a hammer mill.

Enter a sauna or hot tub at least twice a week. Massage any painful areas of the body while in the sauna. Do not massage malignant tumors. Do not take a cold shower immediately afterward, but rest quietly for at least half an hour, then rinse in lukewarm water, scrubbing the skin again.

(See also "Hydrotherapy" in the *Natural Remedies* section.)

Exercise

Exercise should consist of walking and purposeful outdoor labor as much as possible. Contact with nature is health inducing. Pick fruits, vegetables, and flowers, and walk in the sunshine and fresh air. Take every opportunity to work outdoors, take walks, or just sit outside. Other suggestions for exercise include the following:

- Swim
- Split wood
- Ride a bicycle
- Walk, walk, walk
- Jog on padded surfaces as appropriate
- Use rebounders (small trampolines) and simply bounce if your strength is not sufficient to jump
- Engage in gardening or lawn care

Do exercises daily, progressively, religiously, especially light exercise after meals, which promotes good digestion. Exercise three to four days a week has been associated with slower progression of AIDS (*Clinical Pearls News* 9 [May 1999]: 77).

Get a minimum of 20 minutes and up to 10 miles of walking daily. Exercise produces brain substances (endorphins) that "do good like a medicine." But do not overdo exercise to the point of exhaustion.

If you do not feel like exercising, massage can help as it is passive exercise. Range of motion exercises can also help.

Remember that exhaustion suppresses the immune system and causes physical stress. If you have not recovered from the fatigue of exercise with a night of sleep, do only mild exercise the next day. But gradually increase the amount of exercise as you can tolerate it.

Sunshine

It may be wisest to start sunning only after one week or 10 days into the treatment program, as it produces more T lymphocytes, and it is the hope that the present ones will die or be killed before new uninfected ones are produced.

A 20 to 30 minute sunbath daily would be helpful. All affected parts of the body should be exposed to the sun, including the genitals.

Moderation

God will supply power and help for all your needs once and for all: overeating, snacking between meals, indulgence of unhealthful habits (caffeine, nicotine, and marijuana), prescription or non-prescription drug usage, masturbation or other draining or improper expressions of sexuality.

Air

- Get fresh, outdoor air daily. Avoid cities, smog, motor exhaust, hydrocarbons, tobacco smoke, hair spray, and other toxic substances. Spend more and more time outdoors.
- Keep bedrooms well ventilated, summer and winter, good weather and bad, being careful not to sleep in a draft (a current of air that chills the skin).
- Take 20 deep breaths outdoors or near an open window two to four times per day.
- Blow up two or three balloons each day you cannot be outdoors to encourage oxygenation of tissues.

Rest

Keep the Sabbath holy. God made the Sabbath for humanity, and He especially blesses those who commune with Him that day by spending every possible moment in Bible reading, meditation, prayer, and studying spiritual lessons in nature. You need a day of rest, and you also need the blessing of knowing that particular segment of the week is a memorial of God for creating you. We are that special to God. Rest in that thought.

Try to have one day off each week besides Sabbath. Use this day for personal chores and private projects; this is not selfish. Your first duty to God and to others is that of self-development.

Rise and retire at set times. If you are not sleeping well at night, do not nap during the afternoon. But you may take a short hour or less nap before lunch. If you work afternoon or night shifts, change job assignments if at all possible. Consider stopping work during the two hydrotherapy sessions, and ideally for the first year of treatment.

In addition, consider adopting these other principles:

- Remember that prayer is the breath of the soul. Prioritize your life with much prayer.
- Establish regularity, routine, order and predictability of daily activities.
- Simplicity, quietness of living is the goal.
- Refuse consistent overworking or hectic pacing. Quit your overly stressful job and whittle various involvements out of your life.
- Omit TV, rock music, novels, love stories, idle talk, frivolity, and any other neurologically exciting but depleting activities. Just as things we see can cause profound mental and emotional changes, so can what we hear. Give yourself every advantage.
- Learn to live simply, spending less money on yourself, and more time helping others.
- Refuse to defend yourself, argue, worry, or complain. Learn to be at peace.

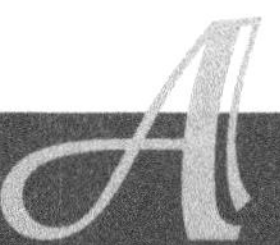

Herbs

Use herbs; avoid drugs as much as possible as they generally weaken the immune system. Take no more than seven herbs at any one time.

- **Detoxification and cleansing:** Echinacea, chickweed, and burdock, as well as a tablespoon of powdered charcoal in a large glass of water four times a day should be taken upon rising, mid-morning, midafternoon, and at bedtime.
- **Healing and antimicrobial:** Golden seal, yellow dock, black walnut, yarrow, Pau d'Arco, licorice root, myrrh, elderberry, and cranberry. Drink four cups of Pau d'Arco tea daily. Make by gently boiling three tablespoons of the herb in four cups water for 15 minutes, then steep for 15 more minutes.
- **Building the immune system:** Chaparral, echinacea, buckthorn, licorice root powder, poke root, red clover, aloe vera, and astragalus.

  Echinacea strengthens the immune system; drink one cup freshly brewed first thing every morning made with two teaspoons of the herb gently simmered for 15 minutes and steeped 15 minutes. Drink three more cups during the day. Make the entire day's supply by using three tablespoons of the herb in one quart of water. Store in refrigerator. After three weeks, take a break for one week, then resume. The break enhances the effectiveness of the echinacea. There is no break time needed for the other herbs. They may be taken continually.

  Drink four cups chaparral tea daily. Make by steeping four teaspoons of leaves per quart of freshly boiled water for 15 minutes. Drink blue violet and red clover tea freely. The herb teas should be continued after the fever treatments stop. Consider these herb teas as part of your daily water intake. Try to drink about 12 glasses of tea or water daily in addition to juices that may be taken; some have suggested up to 25 eight-ounce glasses daily.
- **Herbs that strengthen the glandular system:** Saw palmetto, lobelia, and mullein.
- **Anti-inflammatory herbs:** White willow bark, flaxseed and flaxseed oil, feverfew, boswelia, and hawthorn berry.
- **Endocrine effect:** Evening primrose oil and licorice root powder. Evening primrose oil in large doses incorporates into the viral membrane wall, increasing the susceptibility to the fever treatments. Use up to 12 capsules a day during the fever series. Then it may be discontinued.

Glyke, a substance isolated from the herb Glycyrrhiza uralensis, or licorice root, was tested on 60 HIV positive patients. About 70 percent of the cases improved and three cases were reported to have converted from HIV positive to negative, two of which remained permanently HIV negative. The report was written by Professor Lu Weibo of the Academy of Traditional Chinese Medicine in China, although we have not been able to confirm this report.

Herbs to be taken continually include garlic and aloe vera. Use garlic—four capsules, eight tablets, or two fresh cloves of garlic—taken three times daily at mealtimes. Take also an entire bulb (12 to 15 cloves in a bunch) of briefly baked or steamed garlic with each meal for at least six months. Aloe vera has a carbohydrate that may slow down the reproduction of the HIV retrovirus. Take one or two ounces of juice two or three times daily.

Do not use sweeteners in the teas other than stevia or licorice. Teas are medicinal and, although they may not appeal to your taste, the herbs were given to us by our Creator for healing. Drink them faithfully! You may, however, use one tablespoon more or less of licorice root powder added to the herb mixture before boiling. This herb will sweeten the bitter teas. After three months you may switch to capsules, tinctures, or tablets instead of the teas.

The teas can be prepared at one time first thing each morning for the entire day. Make fresh each day. Boil all the herbs together for 20 minutes, then remove from the heat and add the herbs that are to be only steeped. Let them set all together for 15 more minutes. Strain and drink.

Trust in Divine Power

- Re-evaluate your relationship with God.
- Begin each day and end each day with a quiet hour or so alone with God in prayer and Bible reading.
- Keep your joys, thanks, needs, sorrows, sins, cares, and fears before God.
- Talk to Him all day. Recognize that a divine being, a guardian angel, is always with you.
- Read the following three books by Ellen G. White—*Desire of Ages, Ministry of Healing,* and *Counsels on Diet and Foods*. Take seriously any lessons learned, even if they seem unimportant.

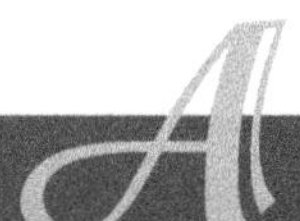

- Participate in morning and evening family devotions. If there is no such gathering in your home, have your own personal devotional time for prayer, singing, and Bible study.
- Become a committed Christian anew every day.
- Accept the circumstances of daily life even if they are not what you may have planned or chosen. Everything God allows to come to you is an education. If accepted graciously, all trials eventually bring joy.
- Pray for God's will to be done, and do not insist on healing. He does not heal everyone in this life, but He desires to save every living soul—all who give their full allegiance to Him. Have faith that God will accomplish the very best thing for your life.
- Be thankful, cheerful, prayerful. These attitudes produce endorphins. These are "merry hormones" and "happy chemicals" that fight disease and promote a sense of well-being.
- Consider being anointed by the church elders. This is a biblical teaching. It is strengthening.
- You will need heavenly grace and power to make these lifestyle changes and to maintain them.

Dress

- Wear simple, modest, healthful, clean, and attractive clothing. Natural fibers and blends are best.
- Never allow the extremities to become chilled. If the skin temperature feels cooler than the temperature of the forehead, you are chilled. Chilling suppresses the immune system.
- Do not have more layers on the trunk than on the arms, feet, and calves.
- Wear no tight bands and restrictive garments, especially around the chest and abdomen.

Alcoholism

If you have a problem with alcohol or any substance abuse, see the "12-Step Program" in the *Supplemental Information* section.

It has been found that 150 milligrams of isoflavones daily per kilogram of body weight suppresses the desire for alcohol. Isoflavones are found in soybeans in high quantities. Kudzu root also is especially high in these nutrients and in phytoestrogens. That means about three to five tablespoons should be the daily intake of kudzu and about one-fourth cup of cooked soybeans daily.

Allergies

An allergy represents an abnormal reaction in the defense we have made against a foreign invader. As an example, a flower pollen (an antigen) sticks to the inside of your nose and threatens to break through the lining. The nose calls for help, and soldiers are sent in the form of white blood cells carrying antibodies (ammunition) against the flower pollen. The battle engages, and every pollen grain is attached and held fast by antibodies. Now the nose feels another problem. Its condition now is worse than in the beginning because its lining is strewn with all these clusters of antigen:antibody clumps that clutter the field. The nose feels irritated by the clumps and reacts by pouring out large amounts of secretions through the lining. Now the nose runs and feels itchy and uncomfortable.

A similar process can occur in the lungs to cause bronchitis or asthma; in the sinuses to cause headaches; and in the joints, intestines, bladder, skin, eyes, or elsewhere to produce what we call an allergy.

Symptoms and signs of disease and possible causes of allergies are air pollution, damp rooms, sick buildings, inherited depressed immune function, malnutrition, poor diet, and vitamin deficiency.

Symptoms

One may experience one or more of the following symptoms:

- Learning disabilities, poor concentration, difficulty keeping organized or focused on a task, overeating, and other neurologic disorders
- Pallor, flushing, dark circles or bags under eyes, acne, eczema, and other types of skin problems or dermatitis
- Respiratory tract symptoms including coughing, sneezing, colds, sore throats, sinusitis, asthma, high pitched or unclear sounding voice, or fever
- Bed wetting (adult and children)
- Cystitis, bladder pain
- Leg aches, growing pains, restless legs
- Backache, painful muscles or other musculoskeletal symptoms, cramps, arthritis, joint pains
- Headache, tinnitus (ringing in the ears), dizziness, blurred vision, stuttering, and poor concentration
- Mouth ulcers (canker sores, aphthous ulcers)
- Indigestion, gas, constipation, food cravings, nausea (especially to milk and dairy products)

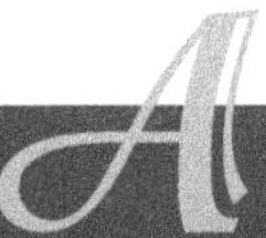

Treatment

Often allergy symptoms can be stopped or even avoided by staying well hydrated. At the first sign of an allergy, drink a glass of water every 10 minutes for an hour, and then continue with an eight-ounce glass every two hours for the rest of the day.

Find and eliminate foods to which you are sensitive by following the "Elimination and Challenge Diet" in the *Dietary Information* section.

Eat the smallest meals while still maintaining weight and strength, and never eat between meals. Chew your food to a cream before swallowing. Thorough and vigorous chewing will stimulate the salivary glands to produce a pint of saliva per meal. Do not drink beverages of any kind with your meals, which cuts down on chewing and dilutes digestive enzymes. With this program your allergies should heal to at least some measure.

Too much food given to small children often sets the stage for lifelong battles with allergies. Failure to breast-feed and introducing solid foods, even strained, before six months promotes allergies for life. The intestinal tract becomes damaged and begins to allow incompletely digested nutrients to pass into the bloodstream, which go to the target areas—nose, lungs, head, joints, etc.—to cause the allergy.

Make your menus simple. For example, select a main dish (an entree consists of rice, beans, root vegetables, such as potatoes and should provide at least 200 to 400 calories), one vegetable, a simple raw dish such as a large wedge of lettuce or a dish of sliced tomatoes (not a mixed salad with five or more items in it), and bread. It is easier for the digestive organs to handle more of one food than to handle less quantity of many different types of foods. This can be compared to a bakery trying to make bread, crackers, and granola in one day. The "personnel" and "equipment" are overtaxed if done this way instead of making bread one day, crackers the next, and granola last.

Rinse the inside of your nose with saline if your symptoms are the result of hay fever. Use a bulb syringe to do the nasal irrigation. If no bulb is available, use a large spoon and sniff one nostril at a time. To make saline, put exactly one teaspoon of salt in exactly one pint (two cups) of water.

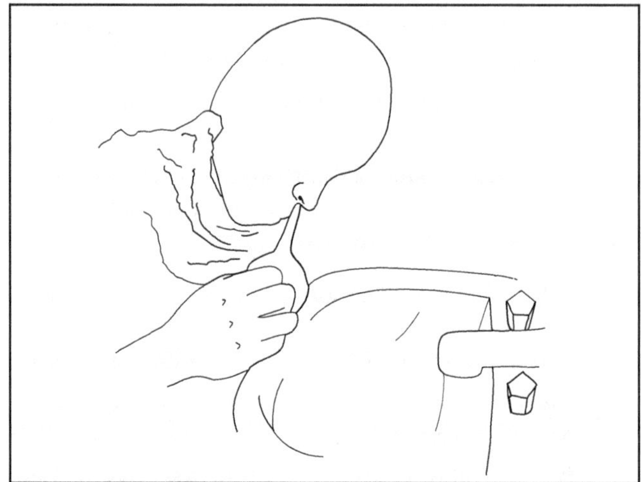

Hay Fever, Sinusitis

The most common symptoms are runny nose, itchy roof of the mouth, eyes and ears, coughing, sneezing, headaches, fatigue, and fever. While avoidance of the thing or things to which one is allergic is still the only known cure, careful attention to the following points will be found helpful.

Treatment

More than 90 percent of individuals with hay fever, chronic cough, and chronic sinusitis will have a complete remission of symptoms after finding the foods to which they are sensitive by following the "Elimination and Challenge Diet" in the *Dietary Information* section. Airborne, waterborne, and other methods of contact with allergens constitute only 10 to 20 percent of allergens.

Avoid as much as possible house dust, mold, pollens of various kinds, and animal dander. Furniture and beds stuffed with horse hair or feathers or covered with plastic (which encourages the growth of mold) should be avoided. A high quality ozone and negative ion generator should be used in houses of allergic patients. Ozone will destroy mold, dust mites, and odors. In excessive amounts ozone is irritating, but it can be easily regulated. Some will need to use a vacuum cleaner for their carpets that has a water trap for dust. Vacuum the entire house or wet mop tile or hardwood floors once or twice a week. Wash all scatter rugs and curtains or other dust catchers once a month. Get rid of figurines, fancy wall hangings, draperies, house plants, and any other object that cannot be dusted easily. The house should be dusted with a damp cloth about once a week.

Keep extremities warm, as chilling causes congestion. Even a minor fall in temperature can turn a simple allergy into a bacterial infection. Dress appropriately for the environmental temperature you are in.

Engage in a regular exercise program to help reduce nasal stuffiness.

Hot foot baths relieve both headaches as well as nasal stuffiness and can reduce fever if it is present. Repeated headaches are most likely because of a food sensitivity. Occasionally airborne pollutants or various fumes such as perfumes, exhaust fumes, and fumes from gas appliances can be a serious problem.

For an acute attack of hay fever, apply ice cold cloths to the nose, face, and forehead, renewing them as soon as they begin to warm up. Continue the treatment for 45 to 60 minutes then stop the treatment for 10 to 15 minutes. Repeat if needed, stopping every 60 minutes for a 10-minute break. For some this will prevent further attacks during that season if also accompanied by dietary measures.

Herbal remedies such as a tea made of nettles with a small amount of ephedra taken three times a day may be helpful. Within one week you should know if nettles are helpful for your case of hay fever. If nettle grows wild in your yard, you may harvest the plant yourself; air dry the plant after rinsing thoroughly. Use one to two teaspoons of the dry, chopped plant in a cup of boiling water. Steep for 30 minutes. Drink four cups daily. Remember that ephedra can raise blood pressure in susceptible persons. While taking the herb, monitor blood pressure. Other herbs useful for allergies include ginkgo, parsley, garlic, feverfew, and boswelia.

We have found that quercetin, a potent bioflavonoid found in onions, selenium found in Brazil nuts, and vitamin E found in whole grains and soy, is useful for prevention during hay fever season. Quercetin is made from blue-green algae but is also present in onions and other vegetables and is available in health food stores. Selenium is a natural mineral and potent antioxidant that should be taken as therapy for allergies. Eat four Brazil nuts daily to give you about 200 micrograms, the therapeutic dose. Vitamin E, another potent, natural antioxidant, may be taken as 200 units of the natural mixed tocopherols twice daily, morning and noon.

One patient reported having her chronic stuffy nose clear up in about an hour after taking two capsules of astragalus as needed each morning.

Bromelain, a digestive enzyme from pineapple, breaks down protein. It works with quercetin, reducing allergic swelling and relieving allergy symptoms. Take the bromelain as a supplement on an empty stomach just before meals.

An allergic headache, or hay fever, can sometimes be dried up by peppermint steam. Simply put a few twigs of fresh peppermint, a teaspoon of the dried leaves, or a few drops of mint oil into a cup of boiling water and breathe the steam.

Apply a fomentation made by soaking a small towel in hot water, squeezing it, and folding it into thirds can be laid on the face from the upper forehead to the end of the nose.

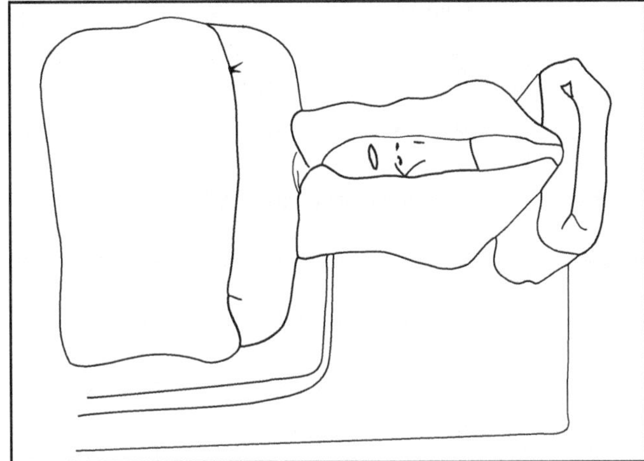

Limiting the number of times one eats to two times within a six-hour period each day, and fasting the other 18 hours would encourage 93 percent fewer cases of allergies and asthma now seen on the present unregulated meal patterns of most people in the Western world. Studies done by Gavin Greenoak and Ray Kearney at Sydney University in Australia produced this striking finding. A controlled eating regimen appears to increase the natural levels of hormones (corticosteroids) that have an anti-inflammatory effect. This effect appears also to reduce the number of cancers and perhaps even collagen diseases according to the researchers.

Eat a totally vegetarian diet. It is the most successful in relieving hay fever on a permanent basis. Even on a healthful vegetarian diet there are certain foods that must be eliminated. Highly allergenic foods include citrus, tomatoes, almonds, peanuts, and strawberries, among many others.

One Month All Vegetable Program

Another restricted regimen, which has been found helpful for allergy sufferers, is the one-month program of all vegetables and a few seeds. Following are some suggestions and dos and don'ts:

- Strive for variety. Eat different grains and vegetables every day, not repeating the same food more often than every third day. Sunday could be rice; Monday, millet; Tuesday, corn; Wednesday, quinoa or buckwheat; Thursday, teff or amaranth; Friday, a leftover repeat from earlier (plan for leftovers to reduce time spent cooking); Saturday an exotic starchy root vegetable

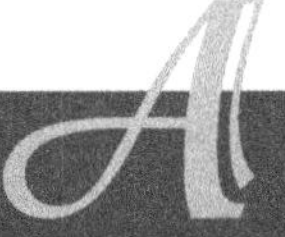

such as jicama or cassava. Following are a variety of options.

- Grains – rice, millet, amaranth, teff, quinoa, sweet rice (no gluten grains: wheat, barley, and rye)
- Beans – black, garbanzo, lentil, pinto, adzuki (the most medicinal)
- Root vegetables – carrots, parsnips, onions, green onions, burdock, daikon, hard winter squashes, radishes, sweet potatoes
- Greens – mustard, kale, collards, broccoli, cauliflower, cabbage, bok choy
- Seaweed – optional, but can add variety to a restricted diet
- Seeds – flax, chia, pumpkin, chestnuts (no fatty nuts or seeds)

- Strive for balance. Try to eat a grain or root with each meal, greens with one meal a day, and beans at least three times a week. You need only about half to one cup of beans per day. Cook grains and beans in a slow cooker overnight for easy carefree preparation. Grains surprisingly require more cooking time than beans to prepare them to be the least allergy-producing. Aim for three to five hours after boiling begins in a slow cooker. Use one cup of rice to two and a third cups of water with a pinch of salt and cook for four hours. Use about the same proportions for millet and corn grits. If you heat the grains in a skillet (called parching or dextrinizing), the consistency and flavor changes.
- Breakfast can be simpler with just a grain, one vegetable, seeds, and seaweed. Seaweeds are unlikely to cause allergies, are very nourishing, and may be eaten with every meal. If possible, a variety of seaweeds should be eaten such as dulse, kelp, alaria, wakame, nori, arame, hijiki, etc. Get these sea vegetables organically grown and not from an ordinary food store, which may be contaminated. Be on the lookout for exotic foods you have not eaten before as allergies develop only to foods you have contacted before.
- Soups can be satisfying. A small bowl of leftover vegetables pureed in the blender can add more interest to your meal. The water from cooking beans can be used for making a cream soup with pureed vegetables. Do not mix more than two vegetables in the puree. The greater the number the more likely you are to have an allergic reaction. Make soup stock from vegetable ends and tops. Boil water, put pieces in, and simmer for 5 to 10 minutes.
- Try to cook vegetables fresh at each meal, except for longer cooking ones like winter squash. Most vegetables can be cut up and steamed in a very short time. Nothing fancy is required, just cut up some carrots and greens and steam. The next day you can cut up some broccoli and a different root, perhaps rutabagas, parsnips, or turnips, and steam.
- Don't use much salt. It can make you tired and irritable and may bring on cravings. You will quickly get used to the simpler tastes of the food and begin to recognize flavors you never tasted before. The seaweeds naturally have salt in them and do not need it added.
- Eat nothing raw for the first week. Raw foods are more likely to cause an allergy. After one week gradually increase the uncooked proportion. Remember to chew thoroughly to promote complete digestion. Eating too fast is one cause of "leaky gut syndrome," which promotes allergies because incompletely digested food particles are absorbed into the bloodstream.
- Don't eat fruit or fatty nuts for one month, then add one kind every five days, observing to see if you get a reaction.
- Don't eat nightshades, such as tomatoes, potatoes, peppers, pimento, paprika, eggplants, for two months. Then add them one by one every five days, watching for a reaction with each food added.
- Be cautious in purchasing market-bought oils. These are usually devoid of nutrients except fats. Omega-3 and omega-6 fatty acids as in flaxseed oil can be allowed, but not for cooking. A small bit of cold-pressed olive or sesame oil may be used on food after cooking if you have a special need for using it based on your weight and strength. Bear in mind that adding fat to food reduces digestibility of the food by coating the food and preventing easy access of the starch digesting juices. Partly digested food encourages allergies.
- The more you cheat, the more you delay healing and pay the consequences. It may be hard at first, but it gets easier, and you'll get used to it. Finally, it becomes a preference if you never cheat. This process takes one to three years.
- Cook up enough grains to last through several days. Cook up your day's supply of vegetables all at once if you need to. Give this program a good try with real commitment, and you will be very pleased with the results.

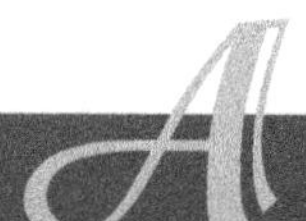

How to Make Your Home Allergen Proof

- Purchase a high efficiency particulate air filter.
- Turn the exhaust fan on any time water is running in the bathroom to discourage mold.
- Check the refrigerator drip pan for mold once a month.
- Install HEPA filters for vacuums and air intake or air conditioner vents. Change or wash filters once a month.
- Install electrostatic filters.
- Get rid of pets and large aquariums, which promote mold. (Small solid glass aquariums are allowable.) Sixty percent of all United States families own pets, and 20 percent of families include members with allergies or asthma aggravated by animals. It may be traumatic to remove a pet from the home, but living with bronchial asthma is even more traumatic.
- Dispose of feather pillows or down comforters and cotton-filled bedding. Use only washable bedding.
- Pillows must be enclosed in allergen proof cases.
- Wash all bed linens once a week. Launder in the hot water cycle to kill dust mites and carpet mites.
- Room air should be filtered.
- Use only throw rugs and curtains that can be laundered about once a month.
- Do not have houseplants or dust catching knick-knacks.
- Use surgeon type face masks when dusting, and irrigate nose with saline when finished.

Pollen Allergies Point to Food Allergies

Persons with a pollen allergy or other airborne allergy almost always have food sensitivities as well, such as to meat, milk, nuts (hazelnuts, walnuts, Brazil nuts, peanuts, and almonds), fruits (apples, citrus, strawberries, and bananas), and vegetables (tomatoes, lettuce, peppers, soy, and potatoes). Of patients with birch pollen allergy, as an example, 70 percent have sensitivities to some of the above listed foods, compared to only 19 percent of persons without birch pollen allergy. Other foods often found in investigation of allergies are as follows: shellfish, eggs, fish, chocolate, coffee, tea, wheat, corn, barley, rye, oats, peanuts, cane sugar, honey, and alcoholic beverages, especially beer (*Allergy,* 37 [1982]: 437–43).

Since it is possible only to cut down on, not eliminate, particles in the air that cause allergy, the most important way to manage your allergies is to control food sensitivities, which are almost always present, even if the person is unaware of them. Upon eliminating a food, sometimes immediately the person is aware that the allergy is better. While the food may not have caused the allergy symptoms at first, removing a part of the load of allergy-producing substances the person is carrying results in improvement or even healing of the primary allergy. Therefore, the most rational treatment of airborne allergy is removing those foods to which one is sensitive.

To do that, see the list of foods in the previous paragraph and in the "Elimination and Challenge Diet" entry in the *Dietary Information* section and eliminate all of them at one time. Some people eliminate only a few at a time, but since many foods have a cross sensitivity, the process is less accurate and takes much longer than to take a plunge and go all the way. After you have eliminated the list, if you are sensitive to any food on the list, your symptoms will improve over the next several weeks. Make preparation for a two-month testing period. But a greater or shorter period may be needed. Some people are free of symptoms in one week, but occasionally a person will require three to six months before the symptoms subside. Not only must the offending substances be evicted from the body, but the tissues must heal themselves, and this may take time, as in arthritis.

When the symptoms are gone or are greatly improved, start adding foods back one at a time every five to seven days. When a food causes a return of symptoms, that food should be written down on a list you are keeping of foods causing a problem. Then do not taste that food for a year. After that you can test yourself slowly with a small amount and see if you have had some healing of the sensitivity. Some people have a complete healing, others can use a small amount infrequently of the food without a return of symptoms. Be careful with the foods to which you are sensitive as an allergy can express itself in a more severe form as exposure continues.

Preventing Allergies in Babies

Babies should be fed nothing but mother's milk until the baby is six months old. A truly herculean effort should be made to maintain breastfeeding until at least one year and preferably longer for the many physical and mental advantages—less allergies, asthma, eczema, digestive upsets, and a higher IQ by about five points. Solid food may be very gradually introduced, about a tablespoonful with the breakfast meal after the sixth month begins if there is good reason to do so, but delaying until 8, 10, or 12 months is also not a bad idea. Watch the child carefully for good growth progress when solid foods are started; watch the child for digestive reactions, allergies, or difficulty breathing.

Because sensitivities are more likely to develop in children, they should not be fed certain foods under the age of one year: oranges, apples, strawberries, wheat, or soft drinks

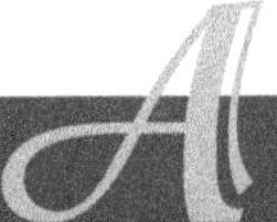

of any kind, and bananas should not be used unless fully ripe and pureed. Certain foods should not be given to children until after the age of two: peanuts, cashews, cow's milk, cheese, and all milk products. Allergies to these foods are more likely to occur the younger in life the child has an exposure to them. Because of diseases in cattle, we do not recommend dairy milk or cheese for anyone, certainly not infants.

Alopecia, Baldness, Hair Loss

(See "Skin Diseases" in the *Conditions and Diseases* section.)

Alzheimer's Disease

More than four million Americans are believed to have Alzheimer's, and a hundred thousand per year die of it. It is estimated that 14 million Americans will have Alzheimer's by the middle of the twenty-first century.

Alzheimer's disease is dementia, usually of the elderly, but it is increasingly found in the young. It is characterized by tangles of the nerve fibers, vacuoles in cells, and amyloid plaques. These changes are found in the hippocampus, an area of the brain having to do with memory. Amyloidosis in the brain is of uncertain origin but may occur because of repeated bouts of acidity caused by reactions to foods or failure to properly de-acidify heavy protein foods such as meat and other animal products or failure to properly digest food because of eating fast.

(See also "Toxic Heavy Metals" in the *Supplemental Information* section.)

Causes

More than 100,000 chemical reactions occur every second in the brain, requiring a large amount of energy, chiefly from glucose. Causes of reduced glucose to the brain include too much insulin from the pancreas (more striking in the afternoon); hypoglycemia in diabetic patients; a sweet tooth with consumption of sugar and refined grains; hurried eating; eating only one very large meal a day; excessive coffee, tea, colas, and chocolate; as well as the use of alcohol and tobacco. Severe dietary restriction can also cause reduced brain fuel.

Factors causing reduced oxygen to the brain include lung and heart disease, smoking, prolonged sleeping, prolonged anesthesia, air travel, spasm of blood vessels occurring during attacks of migraine, and decrease of size or number of cerebral blood vessels. Since migraines are in most cases associated with food sensitivities, any food known to cause sensitivity or an allergy should be avoided.

Some conditions that encourage getting Alzheimer's include about 50 different disorders such as strokes from high blood pressure or cardiovascular disease; infections such as HIV, TB, and syphilis; the use of medications such as those that impair mental functioning—sedatives, sleep medication, and antidepressants—even some antibiotics can produce temporary symptoms of dementia; serious head injuries; brain tumors; low thyroid hormones or vitamin B12 deficiency; depression; and alcohol abuse.

Antihistamines have been shown to be associated with Alzheimer's disease. Several studies of schizophrenics have shown an extremely high prevalence of Alzheimer's disease, apparently because of the drugs taken, some of these being antihistamines such as Chlorpromazine (*Medical Hypotheses* 44 [1995]: 47, 48). Alzheimer's is more than four times as likely to occur in persons with lower serum B12 levels than those with the highest levels (*Loma Linda University Vegetarian Nutrition and Health Letter*, May 2000, 5). B12 should be given as a supplement to persons at high risk and those suspected of developing Alzheimer's.

High levels of the amino acid known as homocysteine, already linked to increased risk of heart disease, is now found to be associated with Alzheimer's disease. Homocysteine levels are significantly higher, and serum folate and B12 levels are lower in groups of patients with Alzheimer's dementia ("Plasma Homocysteine As A Risk Factor For Dementia And Alzheimer's," *New England Journal of Medicine* 346, no. 7 [February 14, 2012]: 476-483.). The way to get the homocysteine level down is through supplementation with folic acid, vitamin B12, and vitamin B6. These may ward off at least some cases of Alzheimer's disease (Ibid.). Homocysteine is elevated if it is over 10. If a high level is discovered, the patient should take 1,000 micrograms of B12 daily, 50 milligrams of B6, and 600 micrograms of folic acid until the level is down. Check the level every six months until it has been below 10 three times.

Also helpful may be high-potency lecithin having at least 50 percent phosphatidyl choline. The dosage is half a teaspoon a day for one week; then half a teaspoon twice a day thereafter until the homocysteine level is down.

A Canadian study showed that occupational exposure to glues, as well as pesticides and fertilizers, was associated with an increased risk for Alzheimer's disease. Those having

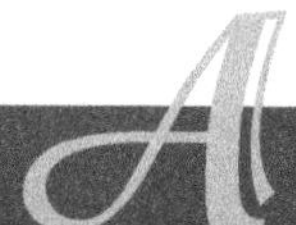

arthritis had a low risk for Alzheimer's disease. Head injuries showed borderline significance for increasing Alzheimer's disease, as well as those with less education (*Neurology* 44 [1994]: 2073).

A study done in St. Louis in about 1994 showed that susceptible people who take zinc supplements may be accelerating the progression of Alzheimer's disease by encouraging amyloid plaques in the brain, the principal suspect for the cause of Alzheimer's disease.

Persons with Alzheimer's disease were found to have increased platelet activity. This condition causes a secretion of the components of the amyloid plaques found in the brains of Alzheimer's patients (*Medical Tribune Neurology,* June 18, 1998, 31). It is known that overeating, the use of free fats in large quantities, such as meats, cheeses, and other animal products, are more likely to activate platelets and cause platelet clumping. Grape juice, turmeric, garlic, and other vegetarian foods are known to reduce platelet aggregation. Lack of exercise and dehydration will also cause platelet stickiness and clumping.

Dysfunction of the blood/brain barrier may be part of the cause of Alzheimer's disease. Leakiness of the blood/brain barrier has been linked to alcoholism and perhaps to inadequately cooked grains (*Neurology* 50 [1998]: 966).

Both chronic and acute stress interfere with memory formation (*The Lancet* 352, no. 9135 [October 10, 1998]: 1201). In addition, memory impairment can occur during extended periods of moderate to severe psychologic stress. This kind of memory deficit is reversible, and when the stress is relieved, the memory returns gradually. A study on long-term drug therapy (from 2 months to 11 years) showed an association with damage to the large nerve cells in the grey matter of certain portions of the brain (caudate nucleus). About 50 percent of cases taking drugs for a long period of time are susceptible to certain neurological problems such as persistent dyskinesia (muscle dysfunction). While the drugs in the study were tranquilizers, they had a much worse effect when mixed with certain other drugs (*Nutrition Health Review*, Winter 1984, 15).

Beta amyloid, a protein that produces fatty deposits of plaque that can clog arteries, is the same protein that deposits in the brain and causes memory cells to cease to function. Calcium enters brain cells with much greater affinity in Alzheimer's disease. Calcium then damages the cell. It is possible that taking calcium supplements may contribute to the increasing development of Alzheimer's seen in recent years. Perhaps the calcium supplementation is part of why women are more likely to get Alzheimer's. Therefore, some investigators believe that Alzheimer's disease and osteoporosis could have a similar origin, as upsetting the delicate balance of calcium in the cell can lead to the formation of tangles in neurons characteristic of Alzheimer's (*Medical News*, January 7, 1985, 3). Use care in mineral supplementation, especially calcium, zinc, and iron.

Alzheimer's rates are increased with the consumption of both total and saturated fats and cholesterol (*Annals of Neurology* 42 [1997]: 776–82). Risks of developing Alzheimer's disease are higher in first-degree relatives of those having Alzheimer's.

Tests for Mental Decline

Some questions to establish whether mental decline is present are found in the following test:

- Have the patient write a short paragraph about the reason they are doing something—going to town, using the mower, etc. Expect accuracy.
- Have the patient draw a simple picture such as a clock or bicycle. The drawing should be comparable to one you can draw.
- Show the patient a picture. Allow one minute for study. A few minutes later ask what was in the picture. Several things should be recalled.
- Ask the patient to read a paragraph. A few minutes later ask the patient what the paragraph was about. The answer should be to your expectation.
- Alzheimer's disease victims have trouble telling time and making change. First, show the patient a clock with a hand set at 11:10 and ask him/her to tell the time. Next ask him/her to select a dollar in change from a mixture of coins (three quarters, seven dimes, and seven nickels). Of 84 patients with age-related forgetfulness who were not demented, 96 percent had no difficulty with this test; however, it was less accurate in establishing the diagnosis of early Alzheimer's disease. When a patient's doctor suspects this condition, more careful testing is required. Nevertheless, this test is a useful, rapid screening test and can help allay the fear of Alzheimer's disease in forgetful, but otherwise mentally normal people (*Geriatrics* 54, no. 3 [1999]: 16).
- Another diagnostic possibility is an increased pupil size or an exaggerated response to the medicine used by eye doctors to dilate the eyes (acetylcholine antagonist). Eighteen out of 19 persons with Alzheimer's showed excessive pupillary dilation with a single drop

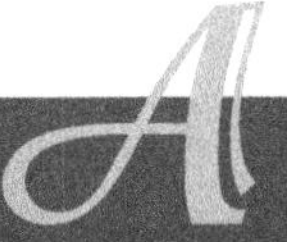

of the medicine (*Science* 266 [November 11,1994]: 51–4).

- Administer the "Orientation, Memory, and Concentration Test." (See Figure 1 on page 23 for a test from the July 17, 2000, issue of *Time*).
- Administer the "Daily-Activities and Social-Independence Test." (See Figure 2 on page 23).

Signs of Alzheimer's Disease

- Recent memory loss that affects job performance such as forgetting things, not remembering important appointments, and often asking the same question.
- Difficulty performing familiar tasks.
- Problems with language such as forgetting words, using inappropriate words, or trouble articulating complex ideas.
- Disorientation of time and place such as getting lost on their own street.
- Poor or decreased judgment such as failing to watch or care for a child left in their keeping.
- Problems with abstract thinking.
- Misplacing things.
- Changes in mood or behavior, loss of emotional control.
- Changes in personality.
- Loss of initiative.
- Craving for sweets.
- Loss of sense of smell.
- Failure to remember the name of a prominent public official such as the president.
- Failure to remember the top news story of the day.
- Continued expressions of concern about the poor memory of the suspected patient by family members or friends.
- Thiamin deficiency may contribute to impaired brain function in Alzheimer's disease. It would be well to test the suspected Alzheimer's patient with a daily supplement of thiamin to see if memory improves in a few weeks. Use a dosage of about 200 to 240 milligrams per day for three months as a test.
- Positron emission tomography (PET) scans, using a radioisotope-tagged sugar that provides nourishment for nerve cells, can reveal a decreased ability to utilize glucose by the brain, particularly the lateral lobes of the brain which are associated with memory, language, and other functions. This test can help to make the diagnosis (*Science News* 147 [1995]: 181).

Treatment

The person with Alzheimer's disease, or one who has a family history of it, should ideally become a vegetarian, abstain from all alcohol and other drugs as much as possible, eliminate all caffeinated drinks, even decaffeinated, and avoid smoking. Cut your calories to the point that you are always able to eat more. When on a low calorie diet, one must be very careful that one rarely take in empty calories such as sugar, alcohol, syrup, molasses, honey, free fats, refined grains, and refined proteins as in the textured vegetarian meat substitutes, etc. Reducing calories lowers body temperature, which is consistent with anti-aging mechanisms in biologic cells (*Proc. Natl. Acad. Sci. USA* 93 [April 1996]: 4159).

A diet containing approximately 15 to 17 percent of calories from monounsaturated fatty acids, such as olive oil, walnuts, sesame seed, palm, corn, and sunflower oils as well as soybean oil, can be helpful to prevent memory loss.

Folic acid may help improve memory in Alzheimer's patients. Good sources of folates are dark green-leafy vegetables, especially spinach, broccoli, and asparagus; also beans, potatoes, kidney beans, lima beans, and whole wheat bread. Reflexes improve and IQ goes up with folate.

It has been postulated that poor cooking of grains or white potatoes could be a factor in Alzheimer's. Because of the size and configuration of the starch granules in these particular foods, inadequate cooking leaves starch particles a little larger than white blood cells but still quite capable of entering the bloodstream, which could then form an embolism to small blood vessels in the brain. The theory is that some of the tiny "lacunar scars" seen by radiologists in the brain are because of these emboli. It has been shown in the study of dogs that embolization of small brain blood vessels would result in softening of the brain tissue followed by "micronecroses and scarring, followed by a reduction in the number of nerve cells capable of sending impulses."

If grains are cooked with too little water, or for too short a time, they will contain many intact starch granules. In one study 200 grams (one cup) of inadequately cooked wheat or rolled oats yielded 60 starch granules in 10 milliliters of venous blood. This represents about 12,000 granules in circulation after an average meal, 15 percent of which goes to the brain. Some have felt that the decline in mental functioning with advancing years may be at least partly because of accumulated starch emboli over a period of many years to small blood vessels of the brain. The micro scars resulting could be related to the loss of brain cells that generally occurs with aging. Some researchers in this field have estimated that a loss

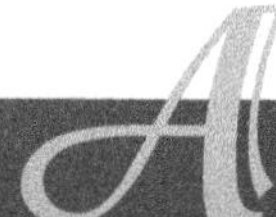

Figure 1 – *Orientation, Memory, and Concentration Test*

Instructions: Score 1 point for each wrong answer, up to the maximum. Multiply the number of mistakes by the value. Then add to get the final score.

Questions:	**Max., no. of Errors When Scoring**	**Errors x Value = Score**		
1. What year is it now?	**1**	______	**x 4 =**	______
2. What month is it now? After you've answered the question repeat after me: John Brown, 42 Market Street, Chicago.	**1**	______	**x 3 =**	______
3. About what time is it? (within 1 hour)	**1**	______	**x 3 =**	______
4. Count backwards 20 to 1.	**2**	______	**x 2 =**	______
5. Say the months in reverse order.	**2**	______	**x 2 =**	______
6. Repeat the memory phrase (John Brown, 42 Market Street, Chicago)	**5**	______	**x 2 =**	______
	Total		=	______

Total score can range from 0 (no mistakes) to 28 (all wrong).

A score **greater than 10** is usually consistent with dementia/Alzheimer's.

Figure 2 – *Daily-Activities and Social-Independence Test*

Explanation: This test measures how functionally dependent someone has become. The higher the number, the more dependent.

How to Score: Select the answer that best describes the current situation and give the following number values:

- 3 points – Dependent
- 2 points – Requires assistance
- 1 point – Does (or could do) by self but with difficulty
- 0 points – Does (or could do) with no difficulty

Activities:

1. Writing checks, paying bills, balancing checkbook
2. Assembling tax records or papers, handling business affairs
3. Shopping alone for clothes, household necessities or groceries
4. Playing game of skill, working on hobby
5. Heating water, making cup of coffee, turning off stove
6. Preparing a balanced meal
7. Keeping track of current events
8. Paying attention to, understanding, discussing TV, book, magazine
9. Remembering appointments, family occasions, holidays, medicines
10. Traveling out of neighborhood, driving, arranging to take bus

Total score ranges from 0 (totally independent) to 30 (totally dependent)

A score **higher than 9** usually indicates dementia/Alzheimer's.

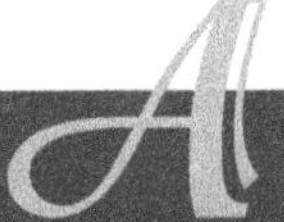

of 100,000 cells per day might occur from this source alone (*Medical Hypotheses* 35 [1991]: 85–7). That would represent as much loss of brain cells as from alcoholism.

A study done in Italy in 1999 showed that in an elderly population with a typical Mediterranean diet, those individuals who had a high intake of monounsaturated fatty acids appeared to be protected against age-related decline in memory, word processing, and other cognitive functions (*Neurology* 52 [1999]: 1563). Apparently the high monounsaturated fatty acid intake helps to maintain the structure of nerve cell membranes in the brain. As the aging process advances, there is an increasing demand for unsaturated fatty acids. It has been shown that a high intake of polyunsaturated fatty acid is more likely associated with impairment of these cognitive functions (*American Journal of Epidemiology* 145 [1997]: 33). Eating a serving of various nuts each day may be very beneficial to the aging brain.

Antioxidants from foods protect against the thinking impairment and memory loss that occurs in old age (*Journal of the American Geriatric Society* 46 [1998]: 1407). Mice normally begin to falter in memory at about 15 months of life, corresponding to about 45 to 50 years of age in humans. Mice who were given either spinach or strawberry extracts daily to raise their blood antioxidant capacity kept their memory throughout their entire lives. Responsiveness of brain cells in the brains of mice that were on the extract as compared to control animals fed a regular diet was twice as high when tested. The antioxidant value of spinach is a little less than that of strawberries, and both values fall with long storage or cooking.

Alzheimer's can be treated with spinach juice or strawberry juice or the purified extract of these juices. These extracts or juices raise the antioxidant level, helping individuals to retain their memory. The highest oxygen radical absorbance capacity (ORAC) goes to prunes, followed by raisins, blueberries, blackberries, cranberries, strawberries, raspberries; then all common melons and fruits. Among the vegetables, kale is highest on the list with spinach second, then followed by all the common vegetables. A normal adult needs from 3,000 to 5,000 ORAC units a day for ideal protection. (See also "Oxygen Radical Absorbent Capacity" in the *Dietary Information* section.)

It is also important for Alzheimer patients to correct any other underlying health conditions. Be certain to maintain a weight that will give you a waist measurement under 35 inches if you are a woman and under 41 inches if you are a man. Waist measurements higher than that indicate a serious risk of weight- related health problems.

By far the most important treatment in preventing or slowing down Alzheimer's is to remain physically fit and mentally active and alert. Since Alzheimer's patients often have as much as a 30 percent reduction in normal blood flow to the brain, any activity keeping the arteries open will be of benefit. This includes plenty of physical and mental exercise, a vegetarian diet low in free fats, salt, and sugars, and keeping blood chemistries in normal range.

Jogging increases the number of cells in the hippocampus in animals. With slowing memory, begin a walking program immediately with the intention of keeping it up every day, rain or shine, good weather or bad, even if one must get a treadmill or stationary bicycle. Such a program will also have very favorable effects on avoiding falls, as both balance and strength improve with physical exercise. Exercise also assists in maintaining proper weight. Stretching exercises help eliminate the accumulated stiffness of a lifetime—usually about 10 minutes three times a week will do wonders for the individual.

Individuals who keep their minds active between 40 to 60 years of age are less likely to develop Alzheimer's disease than those who turn into couch potatoes. Those who watch television from four to six hours a day are more than three times as likely to have Alzheimer's compared to those who are more active ("Effects of educational attainment on the clinical expression of Alzheimer's disease: Results from a research registry," *American Journal of Alzheimer's Disease and Other Dementias* 16 [2001]: 369-376). Higher occupational and educational levels are associated with a decreased risk of developing Alzheimer's. The treatment for Alzheimer's that seems to be the most promising, apart from physical conditioning, is that of keeping the mind active. The more intensely educated the brain, the smaller the likelihood the person will develop Alzheimer's.

Alzheimer's persons having disturbed sleep patterns will sleep better if they are exposed to a bright light early in the morning on a consistent basis. They will also have less behavior disorders (*Acta Psychiatr Scand* 89 [1994]: 1–7). Try shining the light at about the hour when the patient should be getting up.

Dr. Dharma Singh Khalsa, the author of *Brain Longevity*, says that the top brain supplements to prevent deterioration are CoQ10 (100 milligrams or more daily), phosphatidyl serine (100 milligrams twice daily), docosa-hexaenoic acid (50 to 100 milligrams daily) and vitamin E (200 IU daily).

Huperzine A from Huperzia serrata moss blocks the breakdown of acetylcholine. This substance is a neurotransmitter critical in the role of memory. Huperzine A improved

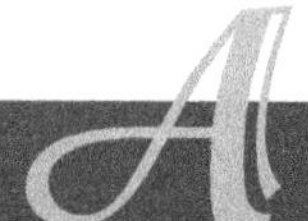

mental function in 58 percent of those who took it as compared to 36 percent of those who took a placebo. It can be purchased over the counter (*Health* 14, no. 1 [January 2000]: 1).

Some studies seem to indicate there is a protective effect from vitamin E and from maintaining mental fitness by leading an intellectually challenging life into old age (perhaps by promoting the growth of additional synapses between nerve cells).

Two studies were published in the year 2000 implicating estrogen supplements as part of the picture of dementia. In one study MRIs showed slightly more brain decay in women on estrogen. The more atrophy, the worse the women performed on mental function tests. The second test also showed that women who take estrogen show "slightly more brain decay." This research was done by Teri Manolio, MD, of The National Heart, Lung, and Blood Institute (*Copyright 200* Healtheon/WebMD). Another study published later showed that estrogen plus progestin supplementation increases the risk of dementia in postmenopausal women ("The Women's Health Initiative Memory Study; A Randomized Controlled Trial," JAMA 289 [May 28, 2003]: 2651–62).

A 15-year study from Loma Linda University revealed that a high calorie intake in elderly individuals resulted in lower mental activity than in those who consumed a diet low in calories.

An extract from periwinkle called vinpocetine has exhibited rather promising results for Alzheimer's patients of mild to moderate degree. Of 203 patients with a variety of neurologic disorders, including Parkinson's, Alzheimer's, after administration of vinpocetine 86 percent of patients improved. Mental function increased 77 percent within three months. Improvement in healthy people without Alzheimer's could be demonstrated within an hour after taking vinpocetine, specifically in short term memory, scoring 50 percent better than those taking the placebo. Vinpocetine enhances blood flow to the brain, raises alertness and increases glucose metabolism. It is believed that it may increase the production of ATP, the energy storage molecule of the body ("Efficacy and Tolerance of Vinpocetine in Ambulant Patients Suffering from Mild to Moderate Psycho Syndromes," *International Clinical Psychopharmacology* 61, no. 1 [1991]: 31–43; *Current Therapeutic Research* 40, no. 4 [1986]: 702–9).

A form of carnitine called acetyl *L-Carnitine* (ALC) shows promise for treating Alzheimer's. It is available over the counter at most health food stores. It is found that the compound slows down the deterioration of mental function in Alzheimer's patients. It apparently protects nerve cells from degenerating by acting as a precursor to the neurotransmitter acetylcholine.

One man reported in 1996 or 1997 that when he put Nicoderm patches on his wife who had advanced Alzheimer's disease she improved markedly, being able to perform certain functions she had previously been unable to perform. He felt that if he had started much earlier in the course of her disease she might have preserved most of her function. The man was a Lake District rancher named Ted Imus from Burns Lake, British Columbia (*Lake District News*, viewpoint column, box 309).

Individuals who work very close to electrical motors, such as seamstresses using sewing machines, and individuals who live within 200 feet of high tension power lines are at three to five times higher risks for getting Alzheimer's (*Your Health*, March 4, 1997, 78). While some researchers believe there is no health hazard to electromagnetic fields, until this matter is clarified, we encourage placing electrical appliances, nightstand electrical equipment, etc., at the greatest distance possible from the head. These fields may have biologic plausibility because of adversely influencing calcium balance, or inappropriately affecting immune system cells such as microglial cells which might initiate some degeneration of nerve cells.

Magnets have been used for Alzheimer's disease, placed at the back of the head, the top of the head, and the side of the head. Strip or sheet magnets are best for this purpose. A disk magnet should also be placed over each eye during sleep, either in the daytime or at night. The negative magnetic field should be placed next to the skin.

Keep a low hematocrit. Donate blood to the Red Cross if you are eligible, keeping your hemoglobin level down below 14.5 for men and 13.5 for women.

The more social and leisure activities an older person engages in, the lower the risk of developing Alzheimer's disease. Encourage participation in such things as church activities, odd jobs, gardening, and charity work. If blood pressure is high at the age of 70, there is a greater risk of developing Alzheimer's disease, possibly because of the drugs taken.

Praying for assistance is not only a comfort, but it also works to make favorable neurohormones in the brain (*Lancet* 349 [May 3, 1997]: 1300). Spirituality has been downplayed for so long that many people have forgotten about its physical benefits. Not only are there direct physical advantages to prayer, but by persistently asking for assistance, the Lord is enabled to do for us through the plan of salvation what He could not do if we did not ask.

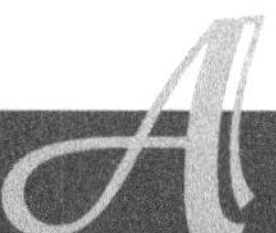

Herbs for Alzheimer's Disease

Certain herbal preparations have been shown to improve blood flow to the brain. Ginkgo biloba extract, 240 milligrams daily in two or three doses, will help to protect the brain from free radical damage. Ginkgo also increases and normalizes serotonin production and also increases the number of serotonin receptors in the brain. It is also effective for treatment of depression in the elderly, which may be a part of Alzheimer's disease. There is less serotonin produced in the brain with aging, and the serotonin receptor sites begin to deteriorate. Thus it is more difficult to fall asleep and stay asleep. Ginkgo reverses that process associated with aging.

Serotonin is an inhibitory neurotransmitter, a chemical that reduces messages between the nerves and the brain. It reduces excess nerve activity at night so one can go to sleep. L-tryptophan converts into serotonin. Bananas contain L-tryptophan. In fact, one banana contains enough to make a difference in serotonin production. Nutmeg, one-half teaspoon stirred into water or juice, also contains sufficient tryptophan to favorably influence serotonin production.

Also, boswellia has been observed clinically to help in the management of Alzheimer's disease. The patient may improve clinically quite a great deal on the boswellia (200 to 400 milligrams of boswellic acid three times a day standardized to about 60 percent boswellic acid).

The common kitchen herb sage may help Alzheimer's sufferers. Sage has long borne a good reputation for improvement of memory. Sage has also been used against cancer and colds.

Asian ginseng (100 milligrams twice daily; a preparation containing 4 to 7 percent ginsenosides) can protect the brain and increase serotonin activity. It increases mental alertness.

Alzheimer's Versus Blood Vessel Disease

The way to distinguish between Alzheimer's disease and loss of memory because of blood vessel disease is by several observations:

1. An abnormal gait. Usually the person with blood vessel disease takes much shorter steps and seems less secure.
2. They are also far more likely to have depression than the person with Alzheimer's disease. If the person has a history of stroke or TIA, it is more likely they have blood vessel disease than Alzheimer's.

Living With an Alzheimer's Patient

Not only must the patient be cared for, but a close watch should also be kept over the patient's primary caregivers. Whenever the healthcare provider sees the caregiver and the patient, an assessment should be made. The following are signs of caregiver stress:

- Denial of stress
- Irritability, anger about small things or about restrictions on life made necessary by the illness
- Social withdrawal, depression
- Anxiety, difficulty concentrating
- Exhaustion, insomnia
- Various physical health problems

The families of individuals with Alzheimer's disease need to learn a number of things that can make it easier to live with Alzheimer's. Since a slow degeneration may last more than a decade, certain provisions need to be made.

Reduce wandering, which is a common problem. A patient may become lost while taking a walk or shopping in a store. A daily vigorous walk with a family member may reduce wandering. Hiding all shoes may also bring an abrupt halt to wandering. For caretakers of persons with Alzheimer's, it would be well to install a motion detector outside the patient's bedroom door with an alarm to awaken the caregiver should the patient start wandering at night (*Geriatrics* 43, no. 3 [1991]: 38).

If the patient talks too much and is disruptive, the caregiver may find that playing music can stop the talking and calm the Alzheimer's patient (*American Journal of Occupational Therapy* 48 [1994]: 883). In addition, seating the patient in front of a mirror can allow the patient to talk with the "person" in the mirror, bringing relief to the caregiver.

Use some memory aids. Write out a list of the day's activities, the phone number where you will be, and instructions about how to do tasks such as getting dressed and eating food. The patient may be able to complete a task if shown how or prompted step by step. Have clocks and calendars in view.

Provide structure and routine for the home environment. This should provide serenity and stability. Reduce noise, the number of new situations, and large groups of people. Soothe the agitated individual by speaking calmly, holding hands, rocking, or gentle patting.

Establish a nighttime ritual. Behavior is often worse at night. Leave lights on to prevent disorientation, but establish

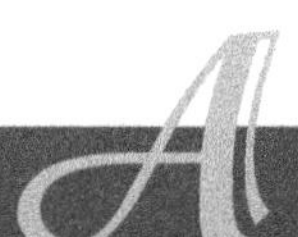

a bedtime ritual. Discourage late afternoon napping. Daytime exercise may prevent nighttime restlessness.

Enhance communication. Use gestures and cues such as pointing to objects. Avoid asking questions or offering difficult choices because they may frustrate the person.

Make a safe environment. Create a familiar home with furniture in the same place and no clutter. Low gloss paints are calming, as are pastel colors. House and yard plants need to be nontoxic. Locks should be kept on all cabinets containing any substance or item that might be dangerous, such as utensils, knives, tools, or chemicals. Set the water heater temperature no higher than 120°F to prevent scalding. Install grab rails to prevent falls. Avoid arguing, but be firm about no driving.

Amyotrophic Lateral Sclerosis

Amyotrophic lateral sclerosis (also known as ALS or Lou Gehrig's Disease) is first recognized by weakness and fatigue. It progresses steadily to involve all voluntary movements.

ALS families have mutations in a gene that results in an under production of SOD, an enzyme called superoxide dismutase. In a healthy person, the enzyme protects cells from free radicals. Therefore, ALS families are believed to be at special risk of free radical and other damage to the neuromuscular system and should make it a practice to severely limit factors producing free radicals—city living, smog, trauma, injury, inflammation, too much ultraviolet light, excessive radiation, too much or too little oxygen for too long, overeating, free fats (especially if rancid), and a high-fat diet. The best sources of beneficial fats are found in beans, whole grain breads, peas, nuts, seeds, olives, and avocados, and certain of these should be eaten daily to provide adequate fatty acids for health.

A number of agricultural workers exposed to agricultural chemicals, particularly pesticides, have been found to have an increased incidence of amyotrophic lateral sclerosis, as well as Parkinson's and other nerve disorders.

Treatments

ALS is very difficult to treat. The best routine includes diet, massage, hydrotherapy, physical therapy, exercise, and perhaps some electrical stimulation in areas where there is weakness or particular disability.

For several nerve disorders, British researchers recently found that sensitivity to gluten grains was a major factor in 53 of 147 patients with undiagnosed nerve disorders. The gluten grains are wheat, rye, and barley. These should be totally eliminated from the diet for six months as a test. If you would like to read more about it, the original article was published in the February 10, 1996, issue of *Lancet* (347: 369–71).

Vitamin E may be beneficial in a certain subgroup of ALS patients, those who have abnormalities in chromosome 21 and SOD abnormality. This abnormality appears in approximately 20 percent of patients with a family history of ALS (*Archives of Neurology* 54 [May 1997]: 527, 528).

Swallowing often becomes difficult and is a particularly serious problem in ALS. Bear in mind that soft foods, rather than liquids or hard foods, can be swallowed most easily. If the patient is not able to chew food very well, it should be blenderized or pureed in some way so that the food can more easily be swallowed. Very small bites can be swallowed easier than large bites.

If the patient has access to saunas or treatment baths, we recommend the baths, raising the mouth temperature to around 101°F. If the patient can no longer get in a tub, fomentations to the spine and chest may be adequate to raise the mouth temperature to 100°F or more. Also a far infrared sauna can be purchased at a reasonable price on the Internet. Artificial fevers up to 101°F can be easily reached using these home saunas. (See "Hydrotherapy" in the *Natural Remedies* section.)

Herbal remedies can be helpful. We recommend ginkgo, cat's claw, and hawthorn berry in routine quantity (four cups of the tea daily or equivalent doses of pills). The first of these three herbs is for general circulation to internal structures; the second a strengthener for the immune system and a general healing herb; and the third has anti-inflammatory properties as well as muscle stimulatory properties. It stimulates the heart and can also stimulate the contraction of the smooth muscles of swallowing.

Dr. Frank Lang treated his wife, Charlotte, with the treatments listed above, and he also gave her 100 milligrams of CoQ10 three times daily. It seemed to slow down the progress of the disease, and perhaps achieve some reversal. He also used NADH or Coenzyme 1 (one tablet per day) and five or six tablets of garlic three or four times daily on the possible chance that both MS and ALS are related to an infectious agent. This idea was based on research done at Vanderbilt. We believe he was able to prolong her life several years with the treatments.

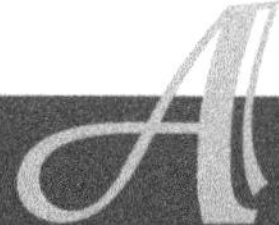

Fifteen patients with ALS were supplemented for one month with five grams of creatine three times daily. The patients showed improved energy on the creatine.

Anemia

There are two to three million red blood cells produced per second in the bone marrow. The definition of anemia is low hemoglobin, the oxygen carrying part of the blood. This means that there are (1) too few red blood cells being produced by the bone marrow, (2) too little iron or other nutrients to make hemoglobin for the cells, or (3) blood is being lost somehow, such as by being broken down too quickly by the body or through bleeding.

Thus, any problem with nutrients, such as an imbalance or deficiency of iron, copper, cobalt, nickel, folic acid, vitamins B6 or B12, or protein; any suppression of production of blood cells as from toxins or cancer; any increase in breakdown as from sickle cells or hemolytic anemia; or prolonged loss of red blood cells such as from bleeding from the uterus, stomach, or bowel can result in anemia.

Symptoms may be nonexistent or may include fatigue, headache, dizziness, unusual ringing in the ears, rapid heart rate, shortness of breath on exertion, cravings for unusual substances (such as starch, clay, or ice), abnormal sensations on the skin (burning, prickling, numbness, tingling), palpitation of the heart, shortness of breath, and sore tongue.

Nutrient deficiencies can occur because of failure to absorb a nutrient, as occurs in malabsorption of iron in rheumatoid arthritis or malabsorption of B12 in pernicious anemia. The diet may contain adequate or even abundant supplies, but the intestines simply fail to take it up.

Chronic blood loss is perhaps the commonest form of iron deficiency anemia in the world, and is often because of menstrual losses, parasites, bleeding peptic ulcers, and drugs such as aspirin and alcohol and irritants such as vinegar and spices. We often find coupled with chronic blood loss an impaired gastrointestinal uptake of iron. Following are three types of anemia: iron deficiency, pernicious anemia, and sickle cell anemia.

Iron Deficiency Anemia

This is the most common form of anemia. Under normal circumstances the body takes up only 5 to 10 percent of the iron in food. In excessive need, 45 to 64 percent may be absorbed. Our food usually contains far more iron than the body can use, or even take in. Iron supplements may be an injury unless there is laboratory proven need for more iron in the blood. Low hemoglobin is far more common in young girls after the onset of menstrual periods. In men the disorder is uncommon and always demands a full hematologic workup. For women the ideal laboratory numbers for hemoglobin range from 10.5 to 12.5 and after menopause up to 13.5; for men 12.5 to 14.5.

A mild case of celiac disease, which is not even recognized, can be a cause of chronic iron-deficiency anemia. (See "Celiac Disease" in the *Conditions and Diseases* section.)

Treatment

Avoid milk, eggs, alcohol, hot or spicy foods, caffeinated and decaffeinated beverages, and high phosphate foods (see "Food Sources High in Certain Nutrients" in the *Dietary Information* section) as these substances all compete with or block absorption of iron. Avoid dairy products as they contain very little iron and tend to bind iron present in other foods.

Avoid drugs as many bind iron, reduce absorption from the small bowel, or depress the activity of the bone marrow. Some drugs tie up nutrients needed to produce blood cells. Avoid all antacids as they tie up iron. Aspirin is the commonest drug causing anemia because it causes a little bleeding with each tablet.

Eat generously of apricots, peaches, prunes (dried or fresh), and oranges as they contain factors favorable for hemoglobin development. Other good foods are raisins, grapes, dried or fresh apples, whole grains cereals (oats, wheat, corn, rye, barley), fresh fruits and vegetables containing high vitamin C content (especially kiwis, tomatoes, potatoes, and green leafy vegetables), wheat germ, beans (including soybeans), and bananas. Vitamin C encourages the absorption of iron. (See also "Food Sources High in Certain Nutrients" in the *Dietary Information* section.)

The use of iron pots for cooking increases the iron content of the diet. Persons whose hemoglobin levels are already high should not cook in iron pots as they can get overloaded with iron. (See also "Polycythemia" in the *Conditions and Diseases* section.)

Drink plenty of water, generally two glasses before breakfast, two in the mid-morning, two again in the midafternoon, and one to two at night.

Regularity in all of one's habits not only stimulates the bone marrow to produce plenty of red blood cells but also stimulates the bone marrow to send signals to absorb iron from food.

Avoid nervous tension. Remember that exercise neutralizes tension. Alternating both exercise and rest stimulates the

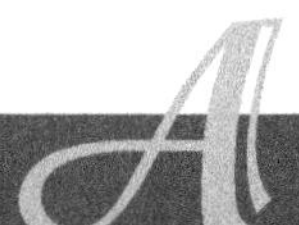

bone marrow to produce blood cells. Get adequate rest for body repair and rebuilding of blood cells. Excessive fatigue causes poor quality blood. Eight hours of sleep each day is about right for most adults. Too much sleep is also suppressive to health.

Fresh air is essential for cleansing the blood. Good posture and deep breathing of pure air are good ways to build blood and to nourish all cells of the body. It is a natural protection against anemia.

Vitamin D developed from an average of only 10 minutes direct sun exposure per day on a patch of skin six inches square, even with the rest of the body fully clothed, stimulates the bone marrow.

Proper clothing of the extremities keeps the circulation equalized between the trunk and extremities. Proper blood building can be accomplished only by healthy bone marrow activity. Habitual chilling of the extremities causes congestion of the blood, forming marrow in the core of the body.

Massage and cold mitten friction are both very effective in quickening the circulation, stimulating blood cell production, and strengthening the immune system.

A short cold bath will stimulate the bone marrow in many people, as will a cool or tepid morning shower followed by a cold mitten friction. These treatments strengthen the immune system. (See "Hydrotherapy" in the *Natural Remedies* section.)

The herb angelica is helpful in anemia to encourage health of the bone marrow and intestinal tract. For iron deficiency anemia you can also use yellow dock root. It may be taken as capsules with or just before meals or drunk as tea between meals.

Pernicious Anemia, Macrocytic Anemia, B12 Deficiency Anemia

Since two to three million red blood cells are being produced per second in the bone marrow, any interference in the long chain of essential steps will cause difficulties in the manufacture of the cells. If B12 is not readily available in proper quantity, a problem can develop at the end of the production line, as revealed by the laboratory reports on the blood cells. With B12 deficiency we see large red blood cells and too little hemoglobin. This less common form of anemia is called pernicious anemia.

Vitamin B12 is definitely a complicated subject. Folic acid deficiency is often confused with B12 deficiency. Ten to 15 percent of normal people in the population have "low B12." This group of normal people do not have increased methylmalonate in blood and urine. Methylmalonate is a chemical giving evidence that B12 is not being supplied in adequate amounts for our body processes. Individuals who have low B12 should be checked not only for methylmalonate but also homocysteine, another chemical that accumulates when B12 is needed in greater supply than is being delivered to the cells. (See also "Heart" in the *Conditions and Diseases* section.)

Pernicious anemia is caused primarily by a stomach disorder in which failure to absorb vitamin B12 is the result. Mainly fair skin blonds suffer from this disease. They are often tall and have premature graying and big ears. Various nerve symptoms may also be experienced such as loss of balance, tingling in the extremities, pain, burning or loss of sensation in hands or feet, etc. These neurologic signs may or may not be prominent. Failure to treat this can result in permanent nerve damage. In infants and children, B12 deficiency is usually recognized by loss of some developmental features they previously had such as talking, walking, turning, paying attention, etc.

Laboratory tests are needed to distinguish this form of anemia from others. Metabolic disease may be confused with B12 deficiency anemia, liver disease, alcoholism, stomach disease, malnutrition, hypothyroidism, low folic acid, megaloblastic anemia, etc.

Treatment

If the hemoglobin is below seven grams, B12 may need to be given by shot until the hemoglobin is above 8 or 10. But then B12 supplements may be quite satisfactory. Start with 1,000 micrograms (one milligram) and then, when the hemoglobin is stable, drop down to a maintenance supplement of 100 to 500 micrograms, or the dosage needed to keep the hemoglobin above 10 for women and above 12 for men.

For folic acid deficiency, which also gives large red blood cells and low hemoglobin, simply supplement with folic acid by mouth. Do not depend on B12 to correct folic acid deficiency, or folic acid to correct B12 deficiency, as the neurologic degeneration may not be corrected by B12 alone.

Sickle Cell Anemia, Sickle Cell Trait

Sickle cell disease, either the trait or the disease, can occur as a genetic mutation. Just as pernicious anemia affects mainly fair skinned blonds, sickle cell anemia affects mainly dark skinned people groups. Sickle cell anemia strikes one in 400 blacks in America. The sickle cell genetic trait is much

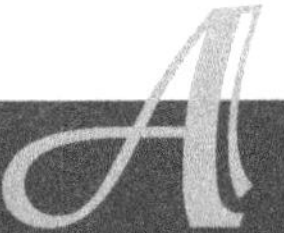

more common. If two individuals both carrying the trait marry, the offspring can have the full-blown disease.

In this disease the red blood cells take on an elongated or quarter moon shape, resembling a sickle because of an abnormal hemoglobin made by these persons. Symptoms during a "sickle cell crisis" include muscle aches, weakness, fever, and yellowing of the skin.

Thalassemia, another form of anemia, which is also genetic like sickle cell anemia, can be treated with natural remedies as with sickle cell disease.

Treatment

Do not use much salt, as even ordinary amounts of salt in the diet can cause the red blood cells of the sickler to be more fragile. Likewise, both free fats and free sugars increase the fragility of the red blood cells. Limit or eliminate margarine, mayonnaise, fried foods, cooking fats and salad oils, sugar, syrup, molasses, honey, and malt.

Dr. Dawud Ujamaa, an Atlanta chef, wrote a book in 1995 titled *Back to Our Roots: Cooking for Control of Sickle Cell Anemia and Cancer Prevention.* This book should be helpful to those suffering from sickle cell anemia.

Drink extra water to keep the red blood cells plumped up. In rare cases the person may need six to eight quarts of water a day. At least 10 glasses daily should be taken. Keep the urine pale.

Exercise is essential for the best of health. Children should be encouraged in vigorous play even though their stamina may be low. Exercising the lungs can help extend their life expectancy, which is 42 years for men and 48 years for women. Many people with sickle cell disease develop lung infections because the pain in their chest muscles prevents them from breathing deeply. A simple breathing device that can be purchased for around $10 is a great incentive to breathe deeply. Asthma sufferers and post-surgery pulmonary patients who use this device help to keep lung infections at bay. It consists of a tube with a ping-pong ball inside. The ping-pong ball must be sucked to a mark on the cylinder by taking deep breaths.

Keep the extremities warm, as chilling causes sickling of red blood cells.

Sleep should be abundant for children and adequate for adults and only in well ventilated bedrooms.

The seeds of *Cajanus cajan* have been observed to have anti-sickling action. It has been used for children under 10 years of age and for adults. In one study there was a significant clinical improvement including absence of sickling crises during the three months of the study and improved sense of well-being with increased physical activity in the participants (*Nutrition Research* 16 [1996]: 1459).

A group of 12 patients with sickle cell anemia were found to have low levels of zinc, copper, and magnesium compared to healthy individuals. It is believed the mineral deficiencies weaken the red blood cell membranes, making them more likely to be damaged from free radicals or any kind of toxins in the system (*Trace Elements and Electrolytes* 12, no. 3 [1995]: 161). It is probable that the same genetic defect that causes the red cell deformity also causes the deficiency of the minerals.

Anesthetics

(See the *Home Emergencies* section.)

Angina

Angina consists of intense discomfort in the chest, described by most people as a viselike tightening to the point of pain. It may be described as pressure, squeezing, choking, heaviness, or smothering. The discomfort is brought on most commonly by physical exercise such as walking uphill or upstairs, being in a hurry, or getting excited. Some people experience angina after a meal, in cold weather, after drinking cold drinks, with any kind of intense emotion, because of stage fright, or while watching TV. Some feel it more when lying in bed.

Men account for 80 percent of cases, and the typical man is 50 to 60 years of age. Angina usually continues until the man begins to experience more serious types of heart disease.

More than 90 percent of cases are because of narrowing of the blood vessels of the heart because of hardening of the arteries. Other causes may be coronary artery spasm, and medicines used for migraines.

Treatment

Since this disorder is usually a lifestyle disease of the same nature as coronary heart disease, the same treatment used for that disorder will also help this one. Almost 100 percent of cases of angina can be cured by following these suggestions.

- A totally vegetarian diet is the most beneficial diet for angina sufferers. Removing all animal protein from the diet (such as meat; milk; eggs; cheese; meat extract such as bouillon; and foods containing animal protein including milk protein such as pastries and bread with whey products or sodium caseinate).

- Free fats of all kinds (both animal and plant origin) must be removed from the diet. These fats are in the form of margarine, mayonnaise, fried foods, cooking fats, salad oils, lard, Crisco, peanut butter, and other nut butters.
- The person with angina must learn to avoid becoming chilled. Avoid extreme cold such as allowing a cold wind to blow on the face or chest, drinking cold drinks, or touching extremely cold items such as car doors with bare hands. Keep the extremities warm as chilled extremities will push blood back into the chest to congest the heart and slow the circulation (*American Heart Journal* 93, no. 6 [June 1977]: 803, 804).
- The angina patient should learn to walk through the angina attack (Ibid.). Walking through the angina attack is done by simply slowing the pace of exercise instead or stopping, sitting, or lying until the angina stops, and then picking up the pace gradually. This procedure is believed to encourage the formation of collateral blood vessels in the heart.
- Take 200 milligrams of a magnesium salt such as magnesium oxide or magnesium sulphate on a daily basis to help prevent angina. The magnesium, when taken with a totally plant-based diet, is often successful in preventing angina as it has blood vessel relaxing properties.
- Bring weight and blood pressure to normal by appropriate measures.
- Never overeat as doing so puts a very heavy load on the heart and lungs from an overfilled stomach, hindering the action of the heart.
- Any condition that would decrease oxygen or increase carbon monoxide or carbon dioxide must be avoided such as smoking, being around a wood fire, being shut up indoors with a gas burning stove, or sleeping or working in a poorly ventilated room, etc.
- For nighttime angina, elevate the head of the bed about six inches on blocks. Be certain to have good ventilation at night and to avoid snoring. Sleeping on the side can help prevent snoring and thus keep the oxygen content of the blood higher.
- Make certain the blood is not too thick. Keep the hematocrit below 40 by frequent donations of blood to the Red Cross (if you are eligible), drinking plenty of water, and getting adequate exercise. Stress also makes the blood thicker. Garlic and onion in large quantities in food, or by supplement, can help normalize the blood thickness. Cilantro is also believed to be effective for normalizing the hematocrit. (See "Blood Viscosity" in the *Supplemental Information* section.)
- CoQ10 used in dosages of 150 to 300 milligrams per day for four to six weeks can cause a significant reduction in attacks of angina (*American Journal of Cardiology* 56 [1985]: 247–51). If it proves to be a benefit, CoQ10 may be continued indefinitely.

Ankylosing Spondylitis

This form of arthritis affects the entire back, often beginning with the joints of the lower back. It may be suspected if the back is sore for a long time, you are very stiff in the morning, and you become unable to touch your toes or twist the trunk to look to the side.

You may be able to get some help for ankylosing spondylitis by treating the intestinal tract for leaky gut syndrome. You can get checked for increased intestinal permeability at a standard laboratory. (See "Leaky Gut Syndrome" in the *Conditions and Diseases* section.)

Treat pain with herbs, massage, and by drinking an abundance of water. Deal with other symptoms as they arise. (See the *Herbal Remedies* section.)

Ant Bites, Spider Bites, Bee Stings

(See the *Home Emergencies* section.)

Anticoagulants

(See "Blood Clotting" in the *Conditions and Diseases* section.)

Anxiety Attacks, Panic Disorders, Agoraphobia

Panic attacks are characterized by anxiety, a feeling of unreality or impending doom, or a sense that you are going crazy or losing control. None of these will happen. They can occur in short attacks or can persist as a chronic response.

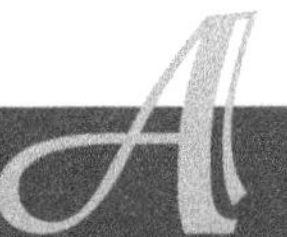

Many people who have both panic disorder and moderate to severe agoraphobia (fear of going out in public) also have balance disorders that cause dizziness and other related symptoms. It would seem wise to treat the person for dizziness if they complain of panic attacks or agoraphobia (*American Journal of Psychiatry* 153 [April 1996]: 503, 513).

These disorders undoubtedly have a metabolic or physiologic component as well as the psychological disorder. Therefore, we should begin by treating the patient physically.

We recommend the following measures:

- If there are any problems with the blood chemistries, these problems should be corrected through the proper measures. Get a battery of laboratory tests such as a complete blood count and a chemistry profile.
- Fast for five days by drinking 10 to 12 glasses of water daily, with added water to make up for any water lost by sweating. Then gradually break the fast with a diet known to be a low-sensitivity diet. We had one patient who had been having anxiety attacks for several years who never had another attack after she went on a five-day fast with water only and then broke her fast very gradually with a gluten-free, plant-based diet. We recommend this approach as a trial. (See "Elimination and Challenge Diet" in the *Dietary Information* section.)
- Anxiety can be caused by a magnesium deficiency. Magnesium deficiency can result from the use of refined carbohydrates, an inherited malabsorption, as well as alcohol use. Food sources of magnesium are found in all nuts, seeds, whole grains, common legumes, carob, greens, beets, and squash.
- Avoid coffee, tea, colas, or chocolate. Avoid caffeine in all its forms which stimulate anxiety. Some people are very sensitive to certain alkaloid compounds in these products and react with anxiety.
- The leaky gut syndrome can cause a wide variety of symptoms, including anxiety. A test for this disorder can be obtained from a clinical laboratory.
- The ears should be examined for an object that may be resting against the eardrum, an infection behind the drum, or some internal ear disorder. One patient had complete clearing of anxiety when an insect was removed from her ear canal where it had crawled against the drum and remained there for several weeks. Another had a single hair that had gotten pushed against the eardrum. When it was removed, the anxiety abated quickly. Irrigation of the ear can remove such foreign objects. A problem with the semicircular canals in the internal ear could cause a fear of heights. A visit to the ear doctor may be rewarding.
- It has been discovered that in persons with anxiety the blood becomes thicker than in normal persons, resulting in a slow-flow condition in the blood vessels, somewhat like honey on a cold morning. It is not known whether the anxiety comes first and causes the thick blood or whether the thick blood comes first and causes the anxiety. We favor the latter position. We believe that too many red blood cells and plasma containing too many nutrients and wastes promotes the development of anxiety (*Blood Viscosity in Heart Disease and Cancer*, eds. L. Dintenfass and G. V. F. Seaman [Pergamon Press, 1981]).
- Persons with generalized anxiety disorders seem more susceptible to upper respiratory tract infections. Therefore, we recommend taking echinacea, which enhances the function of the immune system, on a daily basis as a preventive during cold season.
- An overactive thyroid can be an important cause of anxiety. (See "Thyroid Diseases" in the *Conditions and Diseases* section.)
- Snoring can trigger panic attacks because the brain is alerted that the oxygen level is low. The brain may thus sense danger. A positive pressure respiratory machine may be helpful.

Natural Relief for Anxiety

Try to eliminate sources of anxiety as much as possible. To assist in this, get plenty of outdoor exercise on a daily basis. Exercise out of doors improves symptoms in patients suffering from panic disorders. Try to walk for 30 to 60 minutes or gardem for one to two hours per day. Sunning for even five minutes is calming, and 20 minutes daily is recommended.

Another treatment is a simple breathing exercise that is a specific remedy for this disorder. It takes time to practice it, but the results are worth it. The best position is seated with your back straight.

- Place the tip of your tongue against the ridge of the hard palate just behind your upper front teeth. It should be kept there during the entire exercise, exhaling around your tongue.
- Purse your lips slightly, again keeping them pursed throughout the entire exercise.
- Exhale completely, making a whooshing noise. Do this through the mouth.

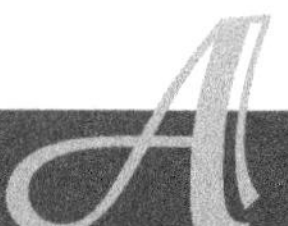

- Inhale quietly through the nose to a relatively slow count of four.
- Hold the breath for a relatively slow count of seven. Hold lips and tongue in same position.
- Again exhale half a breath quickly through the mouth, then try to string it out the rest of the way to a count of eight.
- Repeat the cycle three times for a total of four cycles. This exercise directly affects the autonomic nervous system to create calmness.
- Speed up or slow down as necessary to prevent breathlessness. You will find this exercise will become a natural tranquilizer the more you perform it. It is opposite from drug tranquilizers, which lose their potency over time. Instead, this exercise gains in potency with repetition and practice. At first it should be done at least twice a day. You cannot overdo the exercise. You may become lightheaded during the exercise, which should disappear after a few days of practice.

A simplified version of the above breathing exercise can be done when the condition is in good control:

- Focus attention on breathing.
- Place the hand over the abdomen and push the hand as high as possible by taking a long, slow, even breath to the count of six.
- Hold this breath to the count of three. Exhale through tightly pursed lips to the count of six.
- Repeat this exercise three times.

Abdominal breathing, slowly and steadily, stops the rapid breathing that commonly occurs with a panic attack. Dizziness, a rapid heart rate, lightheadedness, and tingling are also symptoms helped by slow diaphragmatic breathing. Here is the technique:

- Lie on your back with a pillow or towel on your stomach. Time your breathing so that you are taking 8 to 12 breaths a minute, one every five to eight seconds. The pillow will show you the rate you are going.
- Once you have mastered this technique, put the pillow or towel aside and place one hand over your stomach to feel the abdomen rise with each inhalation. This indicates to you that you are indeed doing diaphragmatic breathing rather than chest breathing.
- Once you have mastered the technique, then do it without your hand or a pillow over the stomach. Then try it while slouching on a sofa, while sitting up straight, and then finally while standing. Practice the diaphragmatic breathing five minutes, twice a day. Do not think something bad is going to happen because of your fast heart rate or irregular, labored breathing. Get yourself positioned so that you can do the breathing immediately.

Learn to meditate and pray daily for 20 minutes in a quiet room, relaxed in a chair, with no one to interfere. Precede the practice by Bible readings, which will give you a focus for meditation and prayer. Learn to meditate on heavenly themes.

Learn progressive relaxation by taking one muscle group, such as those of the face and neck, and contracting them as tightly as possible, then relaxing. Then keep that part relaxed throughout the entire relaxation exercise. Next proceed to the hands and arms, and contract all muscles as tightly as possible at one time. Then relax. Move to the muscles of the chest and abdomen and then the hips, thighs, legs, ankles, and feet.

Regular massage can markedly reduce anxiety. It can also improve high blood pressure and immune functioning with an increase in number and activity of natural killer cells (*Journal of Psychosomatic Research* 57, no. 1 [2004]: 45-52; *Journal of Bodywork and Movement Therapies 4 [2000]: 31-38*).

Only 15 minutes of hydrotherapy can have a significant short-term effect on anxiety. Use a hot bath to produce a fever up to 100°F to 102°F, a neutral bath for 20 to 60 minutes, a series of three fomentations, a hot water bottle held against the abdomen for an hour or more, or wet sheet packs for an hour or more, etc. (See "Hydrotherapy" in the *Natural Remedies* section.)

Anxiety can be successfully treated in some individuals by using the same treatment as for depression. (See "Mental Disorders" in the *Conditions and Diseases* section.)

Use certain herbal preparations, especially formulas for sleep or anxiety. One cup twice daily of catnip and valerian root tea (catnip, one teaspoon per cup of boiling water poured over the herb and steeped 20 to 30 minutes; valerian, if powder, one-half teaspoon per cup made similarly to catnip). Also two St. John's wort capsules three times daily can be helpful. (See also the *Herbal Remedies* section.) Other herbs that can be helpful are passionflower, dong quai, licorice root, hops, skullcap, and any other herb that may be useful for correction of psychological problems. California poppy and mistletoe may be useful.

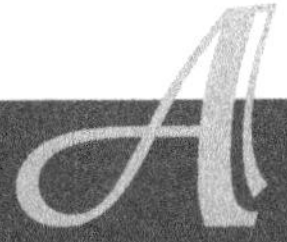

Inositol has been found to decrease depression, panic disorders, and other emotional problems. A trial study of people taking 12 grams per day of inositol resulted in the decline of the frequency and severity of panic attacks and agoraphobia as compared to placebo. Inositol is a nutrient fraction of phytic acid. It is one of the best tranquilizers and sedatives on the market today. It also lowers blood pressure and cholesterol, helps diabetics, provides brain nutrition, and has been used in treatment of obesity and schizophrenia. Some say it can help prevent the loss of hair. There are no known side effects from this nutrient unlike most popular tranquilizers. It is available in health food stores and pharmacies. Inositol is present in many foods such as whole grains, nuts, beans, and fruits, especially cantelope and oranges.

Valerian root, calcium, and magnesium supplements can help to relax nerves and muscles and give a sense of stress reduction. Even though it may take months for the panic attacks to go away, maintain a healthful lifestyle and the breathing exercises, which should be done religiously.

Appendicitis

Appendicitis is an inflammation of the appendix characterized by pain, which often begins all over the abdomen, but after awhile gets more intense in the right lower abdomen. The muscles in the right lower abdomen tighten when pressed in examination. When right lower abdominal quadrant pain begins, it is impossible to determine immediately if it is becuase of gas or solid matter in the first portion of the colon.

After a day or two, the patient gets sicker to the point that coughing or raising the head off the pillow causes intense pain. The patient often walks bent over to try to keep the abdomen more still and avoid stretching the abdominal muscles. The same symptoms can be brought on by many other conditions, and the diagnosis is often very difficult.

The patient usually develops a fever, nausea, and loss of appetite. Additionally, the white blood cell count will usually be elevated above 12,000.

Cause

Most commonly, appendicitis develops when a stone forms in the appendix because of a high-fat, high-sugar diet that causes inflammation or swelling of the appendix as might occur during a virus infection. Since appendicitis almost never occurs in population groups using a very natural diet, the principal cause is probably the use of refined foods, particularly white flour or rice, and mixing sweets such as honey or sugar with a high-fat diet—meats, eggs, dairy products, or free fats (margarine, mayonnaise, fried foods, cooking fats, and salad oil).

People who do not eat meat have a 50 percent lower risk of requiring emergency appendectomy than those who eat meat (*Journal of Epidemiology and Community Health* 49, no. 6 [1995]: 594). Persons who die of cancer, particularly cancer of the colon, breast, ovary, or lymphoma, or leukemia are twice as likely as the normal population to have had an appendectomy as a youth. The lymphoid tissue of the appendix is a part of the immune system. Persons who have had the appendix removed before the age of 30 should be watched more carefully for these cancers (*Medical World News,* March 18, 1966, 108).

Treatment

The first rule in the use of home remedies is to start all treatments with the first symptom. Consider symptoms to be a signal from heaven warning you that tissue damage is about to occur. Any stomachache lasting more than 20 minutes should be treated with simple measures as if you already know the diagnosis is appendicitis. Begin by drinking a glass of water every 10 minutes for an hour, administering a small cold enema (one bulb syringe of cold water), and placing a heating pad over the abdomen.

If early appendicitis is treated while it is still in the inflammatory stage, before it reaches the abscess or ulceration stage, the inflammation often can be scattered and the appendix completely healed. This should always be the objective in treating appendicitis. That the appendix often heals itself of appendicitis is attested to by the many (about 15 to 20 percent) appendices seen by the pathologist that are diagnosed as "fibrotic appendix"—a scar having developed at some time in the past because of appendicitis that healed itself before it could be diagnosed. For advanced appendicitis, an operation to remove the appendix is still the treatment of choice. Only in a field type situation should one elect to use home remedies, and then you should treat the patient diligently, especially being careful to preserve good hydration.

A hot footbath can be done which will relieve congestion in the appendix. Additionally, apply a hot right hip and leg pack with an ice bag over the appendix. Use the ice bag an hour on and 15 minutes off. During those 15 minutes, hot fomentations over the abdomen may be used to good advantage, alternating with cold every three minutes. The effect of the ice bag or the hot water bottle is about the same. Both cause redness of the skin, but either heat or cold is, to

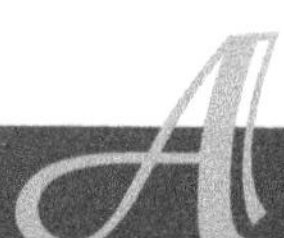

a certain extent, dissipated by the bloodstream and does not penetrate far beneath the surface. The benefit is principally from a reflex action. For most people there is more relief of pain in acute appendicitis from the use of the ice bag than from a hot water bottle.

Charcoal should be taken by mouth as long as bowel movements continue or there is diarrhea. It can also be administered as a poultice. A small charcoal retention enema can be used—eight ounces of tepid water into which a heaping tablespoon of powdered charcoal has been stirred. A poultice of hops or smartweed with charcoal can be effective, both to relieve pain and to scatter inflammation.

Of course, all the known causes for appendicitis should be eliminated. Only juices or pureed fruits or vegetables should be used until the pain and fever are gone. An abundance of water must be taken daily, either by mouth or as a small (eight ounces) lukewarm retention enema of water. Give about eight ounces every two to three hours around the clock for an adult; use correspondingly less for a child.

Castor oil compresses over the appendix are helpful in appendicitis. Make the compress at least six inches square by wetting a cotton cloth with castor oil, laying it on the skin over the appendix, and covering with a plastic or wool piece. It will increase the number of T-cells in the appendix.

Use echinacea and golden seal in maximum doses, either by tea or capsules. Take a dose every two hours around the clock, waking up to take the herbs at night.

Give a dry brush massage twice a day using gentle short round strokes all over the body, ending with gentle, long sweeping strokes. (See also "Hydrotherapy" in the *Natural Remedies* section.)

A full body bath or shower without soap should be used daily if the patient can be moved. Many toxins can be removed from the blood with this measure.

If the patient becomes bedridden, watch the skin over the sacrum for developing pressure dermatitis or bedsores.

Atherosclerosis

(See "Cholesterol" in the *Conditions and Diseases* section.)

Autism

(See "Mental Disorders" in the *Conditions and Diseases* section.)

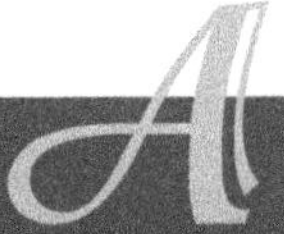

Backache, Back Pain, Low Back Pain

(See "Skeletal Problems" in the *Conditions and Diseases* section.)

Bad Breath

More than 90 percent of cases of bad breath are caused by decaying bits of food that have not been brushed off teeth or dentures or from bacterial growth caused by gum disease.

Bad breath can also be a sign of health problems such as oral candidiasis, mouth and throat cancers, infection of the stomach by Helicobacter pylori, Sjogren's syndrome (dry mouth and eyes), gastric reflux, sinusitis, bronchitis, diabetic acidosis (produces sweet-fruity odor), kidney failure (produces fishy odors), and cirrhosis of the liver (rotten egg odor) to name a few. There are many who have had bad breath all their lives from retaining fecal matter and having a sluggish colon. Many drugs can cause bad breath because of the resulting dryness of the mouth, such as antidepressants, antihistamines, and chemotherapy (*American Family Physician* 53 [March 1996]: 1215).

Treatment

The first objective is removal of all known causes. Bad breath always signals a condition that needs to be investigated and, if possible, eliminated, no matter how small the factor may appear. Since more than 90 percent of bad breath arises in the mouth itself, proper attention to good oral hygiene with dental floss and a soft bristle toothbrush after each meal will go far toward eliminating mouth odors. Even rinsing with water can be helpful.

Brushing the tongue with the toothbrush can reduce bad breath. In one study, brushing just the teeth reduced mouth odor by 25 percent, whereas brushing just the tongue reduced mouth odor by 75 percent. Brushing both brought about a reduction in oral odors of 85 percent.

The use of mouthwash is probably not more useful, and may not be as useful as rinsing the mouth with water or drinking water.

Dehydration either acute or chronic is one of the causes of bad breath, because not enough water is drunk to wash away germs from the mouth through the free flow of saliva. That encourages putrefaction of shedding lining cells of the mouth, as they are not removed by the flow of saliva. Mouth breathing intensifies this condition, accounting for morning bad breath. Smokers have notoriously bad breath; not just from the tobacco smoke and tars but also from heating and drying of the oral cavity, tongue, and pharynx. Speakers have bad breath after lectures if they do not drink sufficient water or if they mouth breathe while talking.

An especially foul smelling breath can occur from a lung abscess, tonsil abscess, acute or chronic sinusitis, abscessed dental cavities, or severe gum disease.

If the above causes are eliminated and the breath still smells bad, consider the following: Some forms of bad breath are caused by food sensitivities. Elimination of a list of foods for five weeks should be tested. (See "Elimination and Challenge Diet" in the *Dietary Information* section.) If certain foods smell bad on the breath, they may not agree with

some other system either, and might lead to some metabolic strain that would develop into a serious condition. Fats, dairy products, and many other foods can be the culprits.

Charcoal taken by mouth can assist in abolishing bad breath caused by bowel odors, constipation, allergies, and food odors excreted through the breath. Rinsing the mouth with powdered charcoal stirred in water will instantly remove all mouth odors, except that caused by onions and garlic.

Chewing parsley, cilantro, or alfalfa after eating onions or garlic may help some persons not to smell strongly of garlic. These same herbs can be helpful in other forms of bad breath.

Baldness, Alopecia, Hair Loss

(See "Skin Diseases" in the *Conditions and Diseases* section.)

Bedsores

A bedsore is a degeneration of skin at a particular spot, which may seem rather insignificant; but to a bed-ridden, paralyzed, or aged person, it is such a troublesome problem that herculean efforts must be made to prevent them. They are much easier to prevent than to cure. Protracted pressure from lying in one position too long is the immediate cause, and this may be prevented by shifting the position in bed about every two hours. If the person is either unable or too weak to turn alone, assistance must be given. Pillows may be used to great advantage.

Wet skin, or even damp skin, is much more easily damaged by friction or pressure than dry skin. So urinary leakage or incontinence must be controlled. Reddening of the skin in one area, which disappears if lightly pressed but returns immediately, is the danger signal warning of a developing bedsore. Such spots should receive prompt attention. Take the pressure off the area by using a rolled towel or specially designed plastic donut, and be conscientious in keeping the patient turned or propped on pillows. At least small changes in position need to be made every two hours.

"Egg crate" foam pads may help, and pneumatic mattresses that inflate different sections in a massaging manner can be rented.

Once a bedsore develops, it must be treated by frequent cleansing and dressing, preferably three or four times a day, using hydrogen peroxide and flooding with water to cleanse away secretions and debris. Odors may be controlled by charcoal, and if necessary the powdered charcoal may be put in a salt shaker and gently sprinkled on. Infection may be controlled by the use of powdered sugar (confectioner's sugar). The sugar is simply sprinkled on the wound from a saltshaker, making a condition in which germs cannot grow. None of the sugar is absorbed into the blood, so diabetics can use this treatment.

Bedsores are difficult to heal, and require persistent determination. In an acute case we had, an ice cube rubbed around the edge and gradually toward the center worked wonders in healing. We were able to apply the ice while the sore was still in the blister stage before the skin broke open. Only twice did we have to apply this treatment before healing occurred.

Bed-Wetting, Enuresis

Urination during sleep after the age of three is defined as bed-wetting, as by that time normal bladder control is ordinarily expected to be established.

In most instances bed-wetting is caused by physical problems such as food sensitivity or sleeping too soundly. It is the rare child, if any, who is trying to punish his parents, as the Freudian psychologists believe. Most children are highly embarrassed by the problem, yet 50 percent of 2-year-olds wet the bed, 15 percent of 4-year-olds, and 5 percent of 12-year-olds. The bladder becomes very sensitive to certain food elements, and bed-wetting occurs because of this irritability of the bladder. If the cause of the irritability is removed, the bed-wetting stops.

Treatment

Determining food sensitivities will find the cause of around 80 percent of bed-wetting. (See "Elimination and Challenge Diet" in the *Dietary Information* section.) Cow's milk and various milk products are the chief offenders, accounting for at least 60 percent of cases.

One doctor reported that a child he was treating for bed-wetting was cured in a week by removing orange juice from his diet (*Lancet*, 2 [December 29, 1962]: 1387).

Anything that irritates the lower colon will also encourage bed-wetting, including pin worms, constipation, spices, and any other thing known to irritate the colon. Vinegar and sauces are also capable of irritating the colon.

Anemia, upper respiratory tract infections, any toxic

condition, chilled extremities, and lack of exercise may all predispose to bed-wetting.

Chronic dehydration results in strong urine, which may irritate the bladder and encourage bed-wetting. Give the child plenty of water during the day, but limit water or other fluid after 5:00 p.m.

Be regular in all habits of life, going to bed four to five hours before midnight so that the most refreshment can be obtained from sleep to enable the person to awaken early enough to empty the bladder before bed-wetting occurs.

Magnesium can cure bed-wetting in some individuals. Use 500 milligrams of a magnesium salt (such as Epsom salts or magnesium citrate) per day (*Natural Health,* January/February 1997, 132).

Bee Stings

(See "Bite Wounds" in the *Home Emergencies* section.)

Bell's Palsy

This condition is a paralysis of one side of the face of unknown origin. It usually comes on suddenly, the patient awakens one morning with the inability to swallow foods properly or to blink tightly. If the palsy involves the entire side of the face, there is a slightly worse prognosis than if the palsy involves only a part of the side of the face or is only a partial paralysis rather than complete. If either taste or smell is impaired, there is a worse prognosis. Most cases occur in persons between 20 and 40 years of age. The younger the patient, the greater the likelihood of complete recovery.

There are several theories as to its origin, but no one knows for certain. Some have felt that a cold draft blowing on the side of the face might be a cause. Others have felt a germ was implicated. It is of interest that Bell's palsy is a fairly common occurrence in Lyme disease patients, and studies should be made to determine if Lyme disease is present. In the early 1940s it was already being reported that there was evidence in support of a viral cause of Bell's palsy. Inflammatory cells had been found infiltrating the facial nerve, and the microscopic appearance of the nerve was similar to that in herpes zoster (shingles) (*Post Graduate Medicine* 90, no. 2 [August 1991]: 115). By the mid 1990s it was stated that the herpes simplex virus (cause of fever blisters) is apparently a cause of Bell's palsy (*Annals of Internal Medicine* 124 [January 1, 1996]: 27).

Treatment

Change the patient's diet to include soft foods, which are usually easier to swallow than liquid foods, and to remove salt, as edema around the nerve may be a part of the picture. Salt encourages swelling.

Since most cases recover without any treatment, no pharmaceutical or surgical treatment should ever be done in the acute stages. If the condition gets progressively worse and lasts for several months or a year or two, it may be because of a tumor. In these cases there is usually a gradual onset of facial paralysis on that side.

We recommend that heat in the form of hot compresses be used to relieve tension or pain. The patient may use adhesive tape to close the eye or lift the lid if the muscles sag much, and the eye should be protected against dust or drying by the use of saline solution periodically dropped into the eye. An eye patch should be used at night. Using a humidifier in the room can be helpful in keeping the eye moist.

As muscle tone begins to return, facial muscles may be exercised as follows: Standing in front of a mirror, wrinkle the forehead, close the affected eye, purse the lips, pull the mouth first to one side and then to the other, make a "silent scream" by contracting every muscle of the face while opening the mouth widely; and finally, try to whistle. Watching the normal side move can sometimes be helpful to make the paralyzed side move.

A charcoal compress worn at night may decrease swelling around the nerve and promote recovery. Avoid getting the affected side of the face chilled, but be certain to get plenty of fresh air in the bedroom at night. Avoid drafts (a current of air that chills the skin).

If dry mouth is a part of the condition, the mouth may be lubricated with lubricating jelly obtained from a pharmacy. Apply several times a day for the comfort of the patient.

Certainly the steroid medications such as prednisone and cortisone should not be used, as there is no indication they help and there are many unwanted side effects.

Calcium deficiency may be expressed as Bell's palsy at times. Every acute case of Bell's palsy should be treated with a trial of 1500 milligrams of calcium daily for five to seven days. Give magnesium also since it works with calcium in muscle function.

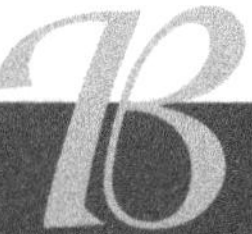

Birth Defects

Neural tube closure defects, such as spina bifida, can be prevented in roughly three-quarters of cases by a diet adequate in folic acid. It is noteworthy that vegetarian diets are rich in folic acid, and neural tube defects are extremely rare among vegetarians. Vegetables and fruits should be eaten generously during pregnancy, as well as beans.

Bite Wounds

(See "Bite Wounds" in the *Home Emergencies* section.)

Bleeding

(See "Hemorrhage" in the *Conditions and Diseases* section.)

Blood Clotting, Anticoagulation, Intravascular Clotting

It is not expected under normal conditions that a clot would ever form inside the blood vessels. There are many conditions and circumstances, however, which promote abnormal blood clotting. These factors must all be identified in the person at risk of intravascular clotting. Even those not understood to be at high risk should learn these factors and work diligently to develop habits of lifestyle to enable them to avoid ever stepping over the line into the high-risk group.

Factors Increasing Probability of Blood Clots and Strokes

People who are at high risk of clotting are those with varicose veins, those recently having had surgery, having atrial fibrillation, those taking birth control pills, pregnant women, the elderly, the obese, the sedentary, the highly-stressed, and anyone with a history of circulatory problems or embolism.

A single high-fat, high-salt meal can cause a serious increase in risk that a clot will form. A customary diet of meat, lard, butter, margarine, pork, etc., forms the basis for many a tragedy because of clotting of the blood (*Haemostasis* 2 [1973]: 21–72). Repeatedly, studies have indicated that the more free fats one eats, the greater the risk of blood clotting. Free fats include margarine, butter, mayonnaise, fried foods, cooking fats, salad oils, and all nut butters.

Eating foods high in sugar increases the content of serotonin in platelets. It is known that platelets with increased quantities of serotonin are more likely to have stickiness. Therefore, it can be concluded that the habit of eating big meals (which increases blood sugar) or large quantities of sugar would increase platelet stickiness and, therefore, increase the likelihood of having intravascular clotting (*Diabetes* 40, suppl. 1 [May 1991]: 588A; *Journal of Internal Medicine* 227 [1990]: 273–78).

In a study done at the University of Georgia at Athens, rats fed a diet high in milk protein were found to have an acceleration of the rate at which they made blood clots. The researchers concluded that the diet high in milk proteins caused sensitizing of the metabolic factors that initiate clotting inside blood vessels (*Journal of Nutrition* 123, no. 6 [1993]: 1010–16).

Guard against overeating as it causes a marked increase in the risk of blood clots. Overeating causes insulin levels to rise, which interferes with the mechanism that keeps fibrinogen levels low. High fibrinogen, an element in clots, encourages clots to form.

Always stay well hydrated. If you allow the blood to become concentrated because of lack of water, you encourage a condition favorable to clotting.

Alcohol damages blood cells as well as platelets and encourages clotting.

As acute stress increases, platelets get stickier. Stress both increases the activity of the clotting mechanism and causes dehydration because of the diuretic action of stress. The extra adrenalin from stress is apparently the culprit. Thus stress must be offset by exercise, a low-fat diet, abundant water, and perhaps an herbal anticoagulant such as garlic, five ounces daily of red or purple grape juice, or red clover tea (*Progress in Clin. and Biol. Res.* 67 [1981]: 361). Hostility, anger, excessive stress, and other tense emotional states cause increased clotting of the blood.

Coffee and its close relatives, tea, colas, and chocolate, are all injurious to blood cells and dehydrate the blood. The dehydration occurs because of their diuretic effect. One cup of coffee per day in the morning increases stress hormones until around 10:00 p.m. and increases the systolic blood pressure by 10 points. Both of these effects may increase the risk of clots.

A sedentary, indoor lifestyle with no sunlight exposure encourages intravascular clotting. When exercise is

consistent, there is round-the-clock protection (*Columbus Ledger*, May 9, 1991, C-3).

Long trips without periods of rest to walk around promote blood clotting. Make it a habit to move at least every 15 minutes when traveling. Every two hours stop the car and walk around for two minutes. On long plane trips, stretch and yawn frequently. You should wear loose clothing not heavy tight belts or waistbands. Do not eat gas-forming foods before or during air travel as gas expands at high altitudes and can put pressure on the large veins returning through the abdomen to the heart. This pressure can cause stagnation of blood in the legs and pelvic veins leading to a clot. Elasticized stockings can help in preventing pooling of blood in the legs.

Smoking (even secondhand) increases platelet stickiness and promotes clotting.

Hormones, including contraceptive pills and testosterone, encourage blood clots.

Fevers, infections, and other sicknesses promote blood clots. Some of the inflammatory diseases such as lupus, Crohn's disease, and ulcerative colitis encourage clots. Allergies can also promote clots.

Persons with high iron content of the blood or a high hemoglobin level have a greatly increased risk of intravascular clotting. It is well to keep these levels down by stress reduction, abundant exercise, and regular donations of blood to the Red Cross. Keep the iron level well below 100 and the hemoglobin below 14.5 for men and 13.5 for women.

High cholesterol levels, triglyceride levels, and homocysteine levels increase the risk of intravascular clots.

Some have observed an increased likelihood of strokes in persons who suffer migraines. While there is some slight evidence of strokes, there does not seem to be an increase in intravascular clotting. Perhaps pooling and congestion or reflexive spasm are at fault.

Atrial fibrillation, an irregularity in the rhythm of the heart, comes on with such factors as old age, hypertension, or overactive thyroid, etc. Because the blood tends to pool in the upper chambers of the heart, the slow moving blood can develop a clot. Persons with atrial fibrillation should take special care not to allow factors that increase the probability of clots to develop.

While anticoagulants have been used for many decades in the treatment of blood clots and to prevent blood clots, all is not entirely well in the field of pharmaceutical anticoagulants. There are some experts in heart attacks, strokes, and arteriosclerosis who feel that anticoagulants may actually increase the risk of strokes in some patients. While anticoagulants may be helpful to prevent a clot that would form on the outside of a plaque, the blood clot that forms on the interior of plaques is probably more common and is caused by hemorrhage within the substance of the plaque itself. The use of anticoagulants increases the likelihood that a hemorrhage will occur within the plaque. Therefore, in a sizable percentage of people using anticoagulants, it could be expected that their cases would be worsened by the use of anticoagulants (*Medical World News,* April 8, 1985, 85). All doctors are very well aware that clots and strokes occur even when a patient is being carefully treated with anticoagulants.

Factors Known to Reduce Blood Clots

The most favorable diet to prevent clots is a completely plant-based cuisine. Meat, milk, and especially cheese increase clotting risks. These food items must be eliminated when one is at high risk for clots.

Free fats such as margarine, mayonnaise, fried foods, cooking fats, salad oils, nut butters, and many other fatty foods increase platelet stickiness and increase risks of clots. One of the most important lifestyle changes one can make to reduce the risk of clotting is to eliminate free fats from the diet.

Antioxidant foods slow blood clotting by the effect they have on platelets which discourages platelet stickiness. Antioxidants are found principally in fruits, vegetables, whole grains, nuts, and seeds. Antioxidants include beta-carotene, vitamins C and E, and selenium. Carrots or other deep yellow or dark green vegetables or fruits feature protective beta-carotenes. All of these are high in plant-based foods and low in foods of animal origin (*Lancet* 342 [1993]: 1007).

Pycnogenol is a complex of antioxidants studied by many groups, notably the American Society for Biochemistry and Molecular Biology. In 1998 at the annual meeting of that group a study was presented in which pycnogenol significantly reduced platelet aggregation. Unlike aspirin, which can increase bleeding time and create stomach problems, including fatal hemorrhages, pycnogenol did not increase bleeding time. While both pycnogenol and aspirin reduce platelet aggregation, a single smaller dose of pycnogenol is as effective as a five times larger dose of aspirin, and it produces its effects within minutes (Ronald Watson, PhD, Professor of Public Health Research at the University of Arizona School of Medicine in Tucson, in a paper published in *Cardiovascular Reviews and Reports,* June 1999). Food sources that contain pycnogenol are the skins, peels, and

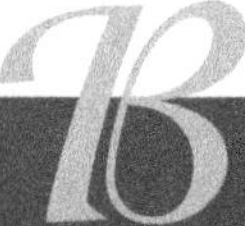

seeds of grapes, blueberries, cherries, and plums. It is also found in filberts, feverfew, and gingko.

Peanuts decrease platelet stickiness and clumping together. The peanuts should be quite fresh, however, as two and three year old peanuts can become very rancid and actually damage the blood vessels (*Revista Clinica Espanola* 165, no. 2 [April 30, 1982]: 85–9).

Soy also inhibits clot formation thereby reducing the risk of stroke and heart attacks. The isoflavones in soybeans are antioxidants, meaning that they slow the aging process. They also reduce platelet stickiness.

Polyunsaturated fatty acids in their natural state help to reduce the likelihood that the blood will clot inside your veins. This reduces the risk of stroke. These fatty acids can be found in whole grains, nuts, freshly ground flaxseed, seeds, legumes, avocados, and olives.

A nutrient formed by heating garlic called ajoene decreases platelet stickiness and inhibits the formation of thromboxane A2, which encourages clot formation (*Prostaglandins, Leukotrienes, and Essential Fatty Acids* 49, no. 2 [August 1993]: 587–95). Garlic is packed with beneficial properties. Its best anticlotting factor is released on gentle heating. More of the ajoene will be formed if one to three cloves are chopped or crushed before steaming, baking, stirring in a dry skillet, or boiling gently three or four minutes with food. If you must meet the public, you may choose to use one of the deodorized kinds of garlic extracts such as Kyolic. Much of the beneficial properties are preserved in these garlic extracts.

A tongue twister found in parsley named polyacetylenes are also anticlotting agents. A medium size sprig eaten daily provides sufficient anticlotting in a high-risk person along with daily exercise and not eating fatty meals.

If you are overweight or have high blood cholesterol, triglycerides, or uric acid, if you have hypertension or hyperthyroid condition, these must be corrected as promptly as possible.

Another essential lifestyle change to make when risks of clotting increase for any reason is drinking plenty of water. After age 60, an average size person should drink around 10 to 12 eight-ounce glasses per day. If you get up at night to use the bathroom, take two or three ounces of water each time. Risk of clotting is reduced more than 60 percent by doing so. Remember that juice, soft drinks, and lemonade are not water, and may actually increase risks of clotting by increasing insulin levels.

Avoid coffee, black, green, and pekoe tea, colas, and chocolate. These dehydrate the blood because of their diuretic action, and they increase platelet stickiness.

Exercise generates endorphins that provide anticlotting activity for days. Some portion of each day should be spent in outdoor exercise. Regular exercise increases the body's production of tissue plasminogen activator, a protein that helps dissolve blood clots should they form.

One study indicated that about 13 men ages 60 to 62 who exercised four to five times a week for six months showed a 39 percent increase in the ability to dissolve blood clots which had already formed. This study was published in a prestigious medical journal named *Circulation.* One of the authors was Dr. Wayne Chandler, a University of Washington scientist. The exercise program consisted of walking, jogging, and cycling for 45 minutes five times a week. An additional interesting finding was that clot dissolving ability is lowest in the early morning and highest in the evening. It is known that more heart attacks occur in the morning than any other time of day. Therefore, the most favorable time to exercise seems to be early in the morning. When exercise is consistent, there is round-the-clock protection from blood clotting inside the veins (*Columbus Ledger-Enquirer*, May 9, 1991, C-3).

Keep the limbs warm. Cool, deoxygenated blood has a greater probability of clotting than warm, properly oxygenated blood.

Work, when it is tense, stressful, or oppressive is quite harmful. Many strokes or heart attacks have their origin in stress.

Since sunshine also decreases clotting it would be well to get an average of at least 10 minutes of daily sunshine. One study of the effect of solar activity on the blood system showed that blood coagulation and anticoagulation systems were affected by both the 11-year solar cycle and other periodic changes in solar activity. We have long believed that failure to have adequate exposure to sunlight causes body systems to be less than optimal in their functioning. It appears from research that the effect of sunlight on the blood coagulation system is favorable. Persons who are at risk of intravascular clotting should be taught that failure to have adequate exposure to sunlight may increase the likelihood of intravascular clots (*Lab Delo,* no. 2 [1983]: 3–6).

Another physician suggests that to prevent blood from clotting inside your veins, take a daily short cold bath at 61°F.

Vitamin E also has an anti-platelet stickiness factor and is best protective at a dosage of around 400 IU.

Coumarins (natural anticlotting factors) have been recognized in clover for several decades. One cup of clover tea taken three times daily, or its equivalent in capsules or tablets, can be effective as an anticlotting agent.

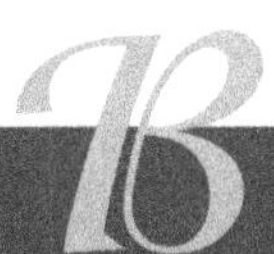

Aspirin does not seem to be very effective at preventing blood clotting in the veins and is used primarily to prevent clots in arteries (*Lancet* 347 [1996]: 1195).

Ginger inhibits platelet aggregation and could be used as an adjunct to anticlotting herbs. The daily dosage is about one-fifth of a teaspoon of the dry powder (*Anesthesia* 46, no. 8 [1991]: 705). Ginger has significant anticoagulation properties because of gingerol (*Eclectic Medical Journal* 56, no. 7 [1896]: 342; *Medical Herbalism* 11, no. 1 [Spring 1999]: 1).

Turmeric with its active agent curcumin, one-half teaspoon two times daily, is also helpful. Mix it with water and drink just at the beginning of a meal along with grape juice.

Other herbs possessing anticlotting properties include flax, ginkgo, hawthorn, angelica, anise, fenugreek, ginkgo, ginseng, meadowsweet, motherwort, myrrh, and astragalus. Several can be used together (two to four or more) at once.

Traveling Advice

For people susceptible to blood clots, it would be well advised to fast before a whole day of traveling. They should also drink a lot of water to keep the blood thin. Take two garlic capsules three times a day. They should also wear loose clothing and move every 15 minutes during periods of long sitting by stretching, yawning, moving the legs, and tightening and relaxing their muscles. Dr. Michael Murray suggests the following formula for high-risk individuals who are traveling on an intercontinental flight or driving a long distance:

- Garlic – take one raw clove with each meal.
- Vitamin E – he suggests 800 IU every day, but we prefer to recommend 400 IU or less daily. High doses of vitamin E may also be associated with excessive hemorrhage in trauma and with thrombophlebitis (*Angiology* 30 [March 1979]: 169–77).
- Flax seed oil – one tablespoon twice a day.
- Ginkgo biloba – take one cup of the ginkgo tea four times a day, or an equivalent dose with tablets or capsules. Ginkgo biloba dilates blood vessels, thins the blood, and has some ability to dissolve blood clots (*Clinical Therapeutics*, 15, no. 3 [1993]: 549).

To test if the formula is working for the person Dr. Murray suggests doing a bleeding time and clotting time. Prothrombin time, the usual test for controlling the commonest drug given to prevent clots, would not be helpful to test the effect of the formula.

Flavanoids and Grape Juice

Red or purple grape juice has a plant nutrient named resveratrol which possesses excellent anticlotting properties. Five ounces more or less taken once or twice daily give more protection from clots than aspirin. Researchers from the University of Wisconsin Medical School, led by Dr. John D. Folts, compared purple and white grape juice, orange juice, grapefruit juice, and aspirin for their anticlotting effects. The purple juice is more potent than any of the other agents tested, even aspirin.

The mechanism of benefit is in the prevention of small blood clots that stick to fatty deposits in the walls of the heart and its arteries, choking off the blood supply. Flavonoids found in different kinds of foods are being investigated now for their ability to prevent clots. About 4,000 flavonoids are found in plants. Seventeen volunteers were studied and both aspirin and red wine slowed the activity of blood platelets by about 45 percent, while purple grape juice slowed the activity by about 75 percent! Folts presented his findings at the Conference of the American College of Cardiology in April 1997 in Anaheim, California.

Both grapefruit and orange juice contain many flavonoids, but they are different from those contained in purple grape juice. The protection from grape juice is around the clock. While Dr. Folts did not recommend that people stop taking aspirin and start drinking grape juice, we very confidently make a recommendation to people to adopt a program that includes grape juice. Five ounces sipped slowly at breakfast time, along with a low-fat and low-salt totally plant-based diet, which includes five to seven servings a day of vegetables, fruits, and juices, an ounce or so of nuts or seeds, and three to four servings per day of whole grains (in the form of breads, rice, cereals), daily exercise outdoors, sunshine, fresh air indoors, adequate sleep, and occasional rest or naps during the day, constitute the best possible program for slowing down the stickiness of platelets and protecting yourself from strokes and heart attacks (*Observer-Reporter* Mar 19, 1997, 5).

Summary of Natural Anticoagulants

- Red or purple grape juice, five ounces once or twice a day
- Parsley, one sprig daily
- Flaxseed, two tablespoons at breakfast or lunch, freshly ground
- Turmeric, one-half to one teaspoon twice a day

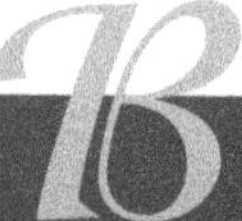

- Ginger, one-fifth teaspoon twice a day
- Garlic, one clove three times a day or Kyolic, two tablets three times a day or one capsule three times a day
- Water, 8 to 10 glasses daily
- Vitamin E, 200 to 400 IU twice daily
- Red clover tea, one cup four times a day, also ginkgo, hawthorn, and astragalus
- Avoid diuretics if possible, including coffee, tea, colas, and chocolate
- Lose weight if necessary
- Keep iron levels in the blood below 80 to 100, and hemoglobin in ideal ranges
- Exercise, one mile or more of walking every day, but avoid over exercising, chilled extremities, or overwork

High Blood Pressure / Hypertension

High blood pressure gives few symptoms, and most people feel healthy during the early stages. Yet if undetected and untreated high blood pressure can be a contributing cause of heart disease, blood vessel disease, and degenerative disease of the kidneys. It is estimated that more than 60 million Americans are suffering from high blood pressure, and as many as half may be unaware they have it. Reaction to various physical, dietary, and emotional influences may cause the blood pressure to rise. These include diet, exercise, cold exposure or chilling, anxiety, guilt, or other emotional or physical stresses. Blood pressure can remain at an unhealthy high, even if it fluctuates up and down for a time.

Since high blood pressure seems to have a definite tendency to be inherited, those who have a family history should be especially careful on all the points given below to prevent, or treat, the disorder. Persons not physically fit are at greater risk of increased blood pressure (*Journal of the American Medical Association* 252 [July 27, 1984]: 487–90).

Prolonged stress causes kidney changes which are reversible. However, those previously stressed are more likely to become highly sensitive to salt and develop salt-sensitive hypertension according to a report in 2008 by Richard Johnson, Department of Nephrology, University of Washington Medical Center, Seattle.

Interestingly, religious people who tune in regularly to broadcast religious programming have higher blood pressure than those who practice their religion in person at least once per week at church, a synagogue, or some other organized forum, a Duke University study says ("Televangelism linked to high blood pressure," United Press International, August 11, 1998).

Dr. Harold Koenig said the diastolic blood pressure was 40 percent lower among those who attended a religious service once a week and prayed or studied the Bible once a day than among those who did so less often.

A study done at the National Institutes of Health by Dr. David B. Larson revealed that churchgoing smokers have lower blood pressures than non-churchgoing smokers (*JAMA. 274 no. 8, [Aug 23-30, 1995]:620-5*).

Treatment of established hypertension with drugs is expensive and does not reduce cardiovascular disease as much as had been originally hoped, and these patients remain at a higher risk of heart disease and strokes than patients without hypertension. Reduction in blood pressure as small as two millimeters can produce a reduction in cardiovascular risks of 6 percent for coronary heart disease and 15 percent for strokes and TIAs (*Archives of Internal Medicine,* 157 [1997]: 596).

Calcium channel blockers, which have been widely used to treat high blood pressure, increase the risk of a heart attack by 60 percent. Six million Americans take these calcium channel blockers, even though national guidelines recommend the use of beta blockers and diuretics to lower high blood pressure (*The Atlanta Journal and Constitution,* March 11, 1995). The names of some calcium channel blockers include nifedipine, diltiazem, and verapamil. Various brand names include Adalat, Calan, Cardizem, Dilacor, Isoptin, Procardia, and Verelan.

Low blood pressure in the very old may be associated with poor functional status, cardiac insufficiency, and difficulty thinking. It could have been anticipated that low blood pressure is indeed associated with increased mortality in the elderly (*Journal of American Geriatric Society,* 45 [1997]: 701–5). Blood pressure medications should not be used to bring the blood pressure to the same low level in the elderly that we would consider to be ideal in a person under 40. If blood pressure drops low by lifestyle changes, the body is in control and knows best.

To prevent damage to the kidneys it is recommended that blood pressure levels be kept below 150/95 unless the person is diabetic, in which case it should be kept below 140/85. This is particularly important for high-risk groups, including those with a family history of hypertension, blacks, older individuals, and persons with serum creatinine levels greater than 1.5 (*Southern Medical Journal* 87 [1994]: 1038).

Having high blood pressure causes one to have lower mental functioning, especially if one is treated with

medications (*Internal Medicine News* 33, no. 3 [February 1, 2000]). We believe the blood pressure medications are largely responsible for this problem.

Cigarette smoking increases blood viscosity as does chronic anxiety (*Blood Viscosity in Heart Disease and Cancer* eds, L. Dintenfass, G.V.F. Seaman, Pergamon Press, 1981). Hypertensives should avoid cold extremities which also makes the blood viscosity increase.

Persons with hypertension will often also show insulin resistance which impairs the ability of the body to control the production of small clots which may be formed inside the bloodstream with the small traumas of life (*American Journal of Hypertension* 9 [1996]: 484).

Long-term use of pharmaceutical diuretics causes an increase in homocysteine in the blood and a reduction in folic acid (a B vitamin). It is probable that the long-term use of diuretics is one of the reasons heart attacks and hardening of the arteries are greater in hypertensives on long-term medication (*Southern Medical Journal,* 92 [1999]: 866).

A high hematocrit, a laboratory test on red blood cells, has been reported as a factor often found in elderly people with hypertension; therefore, an increased hematocrit should be looked for as one of the factors especially involved in diastolic hypertension (*Industrial Health,* 37, no. 1 [1999]: 76). One cause of high hematocrits is chronic dehydration. Another cause is high iron levels, stress, and/or overeating.

Persons with mild elevation of blood pressure had an increase in blood pressure after a few weeks of taking aspirin. In another study, the blood pressure of rats which were repeatedly overfed then underfed increased, whereas rats continuously underfed did not (*J Nutr.* ;138, no. 9 [Sept. 2008]:1622-27).

A neurohormone has been discovered in the brain and other nerve structures, which causes the body to retain salt. Certain people overproduce this neurohormone, and when the salt is retained in muscle cells of blood vessels, the salt attracts water to it, making the muscle cells of the blood vessels swell and contract. Then the heart must pump more strongly to force the blood through the smaller arteries. Thus causing the blood pressure to rise (*Albany Georgia Herald,* February 15, 1984,16-C).

Persons who were overweight as a child, those with a family history of high blood pressure, and those who are underweight at birth all appear to be at increased risk for high blood pressure later in life (*Circulation* 94, no 6 [Sept. 15, 1996]:1310-15; *Pediatrics* 127, no. 5 [May 2011]: e1272–e1279).

Blood pressure is elevated with the drinking of coffee (*Journal of Behavioral Medicine* 19, no. 2 [1996]: 111). Exercise naturally increases blood pressure slightly, and a cup of coffee may cause the blood pressure to surge during exercise. So while coffee is not good for anyone, if you have a tendency to high blood pressure, you especially should stay off the coffee.

Individuals exposed to low levels of lead over a period of time are more likely to have high blood pressure.

Magnesium deficiency is epidemic in the United States because of the use of refined grains and sugary junk foods. Magnesium deficiency is one of the causes of hypertension.

A bad night's sleep may cause your blood pressure to rise. Chronic sleeplessness can result in chronically high blood pressure (*Internal Medicine News* 29, no. 15 [1996]: 44).

A higher white blood cell count is associated with an increased incidence of high blood pressure. Vegetarians generally tend to have lower white blood cell counts. The most favorable diet in hypertension is a plant-based diet. A 50 percent increased risk of hypertension was found over a 10 year follow-up period in men ages 25 to 74 with white blood cell counts greater than 8600 compared to men with white blood cell counts under 6200 (*Journal of Clinical Epidemiology* 47, no. 8 [1994]: 911).

Persons who use non-steroidal anti-inflammatory drugs (NSAIDS) are more likely to have high blood pressure than people not using them (*Drug Saf* 17, no 5 [Nov. 1997]:277-89). NSAIDS include drugs such as acetaminophen and ibuprofen.

Hypothyroidism as well as hyperthyroidism can lead to hypertension. One case showed a nine millimeter drop in diastolic blood pressure resulting from thyroid hormone replacement alone.

Testing

The risk of heart attacks in people with hypertension complicated by thickening of the left ventricular wall (hypertrophy) is three times greater than that of hypertensives who do not have left ventricular hypertrophy (*Journal of the American Medical Association* 273 [1995]: 1592).

Obtain your own blood pressure cuff and stethoscope to check your own blood pressure every six months after the age of 30, and once a year from the age of 10 to 30. The blood pressure should be taken two or three times in a row as the initial reading is always higher than subsequent readings.

Predicting the seriousness of arterial disease in a person may be done with fair accuracy by taking the blood pressure

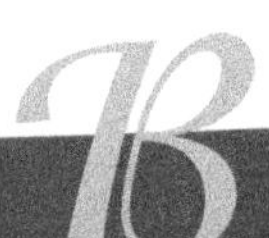

in both the arm and in the ankle. Numbers in normal people are about the same in both the arm and the ankle, varying less than about 10 points on the systolic and three points on the diastolic. In arterial disease, the lower the blood pressure in the legs, the worse the hardening of the arteries. If hardening of the arteries is advanced, the legs will have much less pressure than the arms.

Apparently healthy older women with an ankle/arm index of 0.9 or less were found to be at high risk of death during the next four years. Deaths were from heart disease, other cardiovascular disease, cancer, and several other causes. The method for testing is that of comparing the systolic blood pressure in the arm with that in the leg. Check the leg by listening behind the knee or a tap on the foot with a large cuff placed above the knee. Those with a positive test should be aggressively treated with lifestyle change (*Journal of the American Medical Association* 270 [1993]: 465).

Proper Blood Pressure Readings

After applying the blood pressure cuff and inflating it, place the stethoscope in your ears and the diaphragm on the arm where the artery is located on the inside region just above the bend in the elbow. You can find this pulse with your two fingers. The blood pressure cuff should be applied so the stethoscope can be put directly over the artery. As you begin to release the pressure you will hear the following five phases:

- Phase 1 – faint, clear, tapping sounds that gradually increase in intensity
- Phase 2 – a swishing quality is heard
- Phase 3 – the sounds become crisper and increase in intensity
- Phase 4 – a distinct, abrupt muffling of sound so that a soft blowing quality is heard
- Phase 5 – the point at which sounds disappear completely

The patient ideally should rest 30 minutes without eating, drinking, or smoking beforehand. The cuff should not be placed too tightly or too loosely initially. If you are taking your own blood pressure, do not try to inflate the cuff with the hand on the same side as the arm in which the blood pressure is being recorded. Do not allow the inflation to diminish too rapidly. Be certain the stethoscope earpieces fit properly in your ears or you can block the stethoscope.

These factors influence blood pressure results.

- Exercising before the test; a 10 to 30 minute rest period should intervene before taking the blood pressure reading.
- Emotions such as guilt, anger, worry can skew the test.
- Heavy, rich foods or those that cause allergies, simply overeating good food can create problems.
- Talking or noise in the room where the blood pressure is being tested.
- Drugs, tobacco, and alcohol use in the last few hours.
- Improper blood pressure taking technique.
- There is a variation of more than eight millimeter in the systolic blood pressure between right and left arms of nearly 25 percent of patients, and in one study one case showed a 20 millimeter difference. Therefore, the blood pressure should be measured in both arms (*JAMA* 274, no. 17 [1995]: 1343).
- Blood pressure may vary with different settings. We have long known of "white coat hypertension," abnormal readings occurring only in the doctor's office. The reverse is also true: doctors may not catch a condition of hypertension in the office, but the blood pressure rises or even soars during daily stress. About one in four with normal readings at the doctor's office will have daytime high levels when monitored at home or work.

Tests for Cardiovascular Risks Based on Blood Pressure

Tests to predict the risk of death from a heart attack caused by arterial disease and high blood pressure are as follows:

Exercise Hypertension

1. Rest lying down for five minutes.
2. Record blood pressure after five minutes.
3. Exercise on a stationary bicycle at a vigorous rate.
4. Take blood pressure readings at two minutes, four minutes, and six minutes. You will need an automatic blood pressure reading device for recording during exercise. Obtain from a drug store or department store.
5. If the blood pressure is above 140 while lying down and goes above 200 systolic after exercise, the heart attack risk is 18 percent in the next four years, compared to 9.5 percent if the blood pressure is above 140 while lying down but stays below 200 after six minutes of exercise.

6. Furthermore, the likelihood of dying of the heart attack is 55 percent if the blood pressure goes over 200 compared to 33 percent for the general population.
7. If the blood pressure rises to 200 before six minutes, the condition is even more serious (*Hypertension* 27, part 1 [1996]: 324).

Left Ventricular Hypertrophy

This condition usually results from a long sustained high blood pressure. L-arginine administration can help to reduce the thickness of the left ventricular wall (*Hypertension* 27 [1996]: 14). Reduction of the blood pressure can gradually reduce the thickness of the heart wall. Be persistent and hopeful. It takes time to accomplish the desired result.

Pulse Pressure

Pulse pressure is the difference between the systolic and diastolic readings. Ideal pulse pressure is around 40 as calculated from 120/80. For each 10 millimeter elevation in pulse pressure there is a 14 percent increase in risk of congestive heart failure in a study of 1,621 men and women. Those in the highest third of pulse pressure (greater than 67 millimeter) had a 55 percent increased risk of congestive heart failure compared with those in the lowest quarter (less than 54 millimeter). Pulse pressure was more predictive of congestive heart failure than systolic blood pressure alone and was completely independent of diastolic blood pressure (*Cardiology Today*, June 1999, 16).

Blood Viscosity

An increase in the thickness of the blood can increase the blood pressure. An increase in blood viscosity factors (that means thick blood because of high levels of cells and various chemicals, nutrients, and waste products) increases the likelihood of cardiovascular, hypertensive diseases, and cancer! An elevation of any of the blood viscosity factors should be recognized as a major risk factor. Blood viscosity problems include clumping of red cells, rigidity of red cells, thickening of plasma by increasing levels of various blood chemicals as reported by the laboratory tests, and increased risk of clotting. If the hemoglobin and blood iron go up, there is a probability that the blood pressure will go up also in susceptible individuals (*Hypertension* 5 [1983]: 757). Get a blood test to check the hematocrit.

Treatments

The treatments listed here are so simple most people will consider them to be unnecessary or not helpful. Those who have had experience with them, however, will recognize their usefulness. We encourage your faithful performance of each one on a regular basis. It may take a few weeks to see results, or they may begin overnight.

General and Emotional Factors

During each moment that your mind is not occupied by active labor or social intercourse, practice concentrating on certain virtues (love, joy, peace, patience, goodness, meekness, faith, etc.) and the attributes of God (His eternalness, faithfulness, lovingkindness, intelligence, creativity, self-sacrificing love, etc.). Very religious persons, those who have no mental conflicts, and persons who are happy usually have lower blood pressures than others.

As a tranquilizer take a long walk at a rapid pace to use up excess nervous energy, concentrating on the beauties of nature, the sky and trees, the rocks and flowers, as you walk. The stress of life can be largely eliminated by proper attention to exercise, a non-stimulatory diet, and a proper philosophy of life. Trust in divine power is the mainstay of fighting a disease. A strong religious faith can reduce blood pressure.

High blood pressure can be reduced by ultraviolet light quite markedly. The ultraviolet light promotes the synthesis of vitamin D that regulates calcium levels, which can help regulate hormones that affect blood pressure. Get a minimum of 5 to 10 minutes of exposure to sunlight—hands, face, and arms—two or three times a week. The darker the skin, the more sun exposure needed.

Exposure to competitive mental tasks significantly reduces the output of sodium in the urine, indicating sodium retention in the blood. This is followed by fluid accumulating in the body. These factors then contribute to high blood pressure. A competition at computer games between siblings, husband and wife, employer and employee, or on the golf course, has the same metabolic effect, even if combatants have settled down to a "steady state" of cold war and do not recognize themselves to be in battle.

Feelings of discontent, even in men with treated hypertension, causes an increase in the thickness of the walls of the carotid arteries, those going up to the head (*American Journal of Hypertension* 9 [1996]: 545).

Depression in persons with hypertension, especially in the elderly, is associated with a substantial increase in the risk of heart failure. This association is not caused by myocardial infarction (*Archives of Internal Medicine* 161 [2001]: 1725).

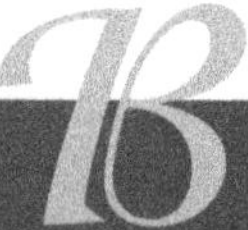

Dietary Factors

Diet control is essential in the treatment of hypertension. Out of 850 patients on hypertensive drugs for five years or more, 97 percent were easily withdrawn from their medication with dietary intervention. The success of withdrawal was dependent on reducing salt intake or losing weight (*Internal Medicine News* 17, no. 5 [March 1984]: 9).

Use a non-stimulatory diet free from caffeine drinks, alcohol, irritating spices, and fermented or aged products. In cheese and other fermented foods, the amino acid tyrosine is broken down by bacterial action into tyramine, a chemical capable of constricting blood vessels and causing headaches or an increase in blood pressure. Avoid food with the faintest taint of spoilage.

Use few concentrated foods (sweeteners, free fats, refined foods, isolated nutrients, etc.), but eat freely of fruits, vegetables, and whole grains—non-concentrated foods. Achieve normal weight.

At the beginning of a program to reduce severely elevated blood pressure, begin with a day of fasting, followed by three days in which only apples are eaten at each of the three meals. Apples have been found by Dr. B. S. Levin to have a curative effect on the blood pressure. After three days of apples, for the next two days eat only fruit of your choice and salt-free whole grain bread or popcorn for breakfast and vegetables and salt-free whole grain bread or popcorn for lunch. Eat only one apple for supper. Graduate to a regular plant-based diet low in free fats, free sugars, and salt; omit supper altogether.

Use no free fats (margarine, fat-containing butters, fried foods, cooking fats, salad oils, or mayonnaise). A low-fat diet will decrease the resistance of blood vessels to the flow of the blood which will lower the blood pressure. Any fat added to food (free fats) should be eliminated. A reduction of dietary fat will lower blood pressure independent of other measures.

Both systolic and diastolic blood pressures were reduced in men and women with normal blood pressure with a low fat, high polyunsaturated to saturated fats ratio (p/s ratio) diet. This was accomplished without any other changes in major factors such as weight loss and reduced sodium intake (*Nutrition News Brief* 4, no. 2 [April 1984]). That means the free fats in the diet should be severely reduced or eliminated and animal fats removed (*New England Journal of Medicine* 336 [1997]: 1117).

Generally vegetarians have lower blood pressures as do those who eat a high fiber diet, weigh less, and avoid tobacco, alcohol, and caffeinated beverages (even when decaffeinated). Pork has been recognized since 1938 as a cause of hypertension, probably because of specific blood vessel sensitivity to some factor in pork.

Garlic reduces blood pressure. Use it liberally on food; a fresh garlic clove may be taken with every meal to good advantage. A very effective smoothie is made from one or two oranges and one or two garlic cloves whizzed in a blender. The smoothie is taken two times daily and is usually very helpful in reducing high blood pressure. The combination is not as bad as it sounds.

To prevent high blood pressure, do not use more than one-half to one teaspoon of salt per day. The food alone contains sufficient salt to supply all the body needs, and adding salt is not actually essential for proper nourishment. All dairy products are naturally high in salt, as are many types of meat. Children of susceptible parents generally tend to develop cravings for salt. Elderly women are more likely to benefit from leaving salt out of their diet, particularly if they have a small waist to hip ratio (*Journal of Hypertension* 11 [1993]: 1387).

Baking soda and baking power are also high in sodium, as well as being unhealthful in other ways. All baked goods using these substances should be avoided. After high blood pressure has developed, salt, baking soda, and baking powder, all soft drinks (they are even named "sodas"), even toothpaste sources of sodium may need to be eliminated for a time until the blood pressure is entirely normal and stable. Do not forget that sodium is in many drugs, both over-the-counter and prescription drugs. Sodium is present in most antacids. Use Dr. Lewis Dahl's guidelines to reduce daily salt intake to less than 1,000 milligrams:

Figure 3

Evaluation	Blood Pressure
Normal	120/80
Mild	130/85
Borderline high blood pressure	140/90
High blood pressure	Over 140/90

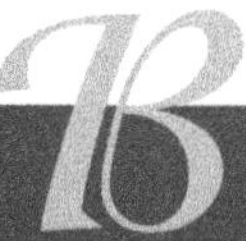

- Never add salt to food in cooking or at the table.
- Avoid milk and all dairy products; they are naturally high in sodium.
- Use no processed foods as they contain salt (meat, baked goods, olives, canned vegetables, and a few frozen; read labels).
- Use no salted foods (nuts, popcorn, etc.).
- Total vegetarians tend to have better blood pressure control. We recommend that all animal products—meat, milk, eggs, and cheese—be eliminated from the diet of the hypertensive.

Calorie restriction reduces blood pressure (*Hypertension* 27, no. 1 [1996]: 408). Calorie restriction is even more important than restriction of sodium (salt) in preventing hypertension (*Archives of Internal Medicine* 155 [1995]: 701). Eat the smallest amount of food you can to maintain strength and weight. Experiment with eating about half the usual quantity for a period of four weeks. You will gradually become accustomed to the smaller quantity and all weakness and hunger will disappear after one to three weeks. Do not overeat even if underweight. Overeating has been shown to raise blood pressure in rats and other animals, particularly if they alternate with periods of under eating. Overeating tends to imbalance nutrients. Specifically for hypertensives, it raises the level of salt, even on salt free diets, since all foods naturally contain some sodium. High blood pressure tends to run in families, and so do habits of overeating. The habits of life must be changed. Never eat between meals, cut down on portion sizes, and cut out all junk foods. Eat more of foods that are not highly concentrated.

In the Ukraine a folk remedy for hypertension is said to be quite effective. The person takes one eight-ounce glass of freshly made beet juice with each of two meals daily. The blood pressure is expected to be in the normal range within two months. When it drops to normal range, the quantity of beet juice can be halved or even quartered for many people.

Eggplant has been used for hypertension. The method for preparing the eggplant is as follows: Use a wide-mouth gallon glass jar or covered glass bowl. Cut a medium-sized, washed but unpeeled eggplant into half-inch cubes and place them in the glass jar. Fill the jar with spring water. It is better not to use tap water. Store in the refrigerator for four days. On the fifth day start drinking one liquid ounce of the preparation a day. Always keep the jar of liquid in the refrigerator. After a few days the eggplant will begin to swell and it can then be removed from the liquid. Continue drinking an ounce daily, checking your blood pressure each day. It may take a week or two to obtain results. When the diastolic drops below 90, begin taking only half an ounce of the liquid daily to keep the blood pressure from going too low. When the blood pressure reaches 80, stop using the liquid. A component in eggplant called scopoletin, which also has anticonvulsive properties and a general calming effect on the nerves, is one of the active ingredients. Another compound in eggplant called scoparone will lower blood cholesterol as it binds to cholesterol in the intestinal tract (*Experimentelle Pathelogie* 10, no. 3,4 [1975]: 167–79).

An Oriental remedy to lower hypertension is four stalks of celery blended daily. Animal studies showed that blood pressure was reduced by an average of 13 percent by this amount of pureed celery, and cholesterol levels were lowered by 7 percent. The compound in celery that lowers blood pressure is 3-n-butyl phthalide. Although there are some 30 other chemical compounds in celery that might be helpful, three to four stalks of celery should provide the therapeutic level that, in laboratory rats, lowered blood pressure and cholesterol.

A high fiber diet can assist in reducing blood pressure. For persons with mild hypertension, that may be enough to eliminate the need for medication (Dr. James Anderson of the University of Kentucky, *The Post*, March 11, 1984, B-11).

Adding garlic or whole grain barley to the diet may assist in reducing both blood pressure and cholesterol levels (*The Post*, September 26, 1982, A-11).

There are some foods that contain high levels of certain amines known as pressor amines that can elevate blood pressure. These amines include serotonin, norepinephrine, thyronine, tryptamine, and dopamine. Fruits including pineapple, banana, plantain, and avocado have fairly high levels of various amines. While these amines have the potential to elevate blood pressure, it would probably be difficult for the person to eat a sufficient quantity to cause an elevation in blood pressure. Nevertheless, individuals who have high blood pressure should check their blood pressure both before and after using these fruits to determine the effect on the blood pressure. Since many other foods contain smaller amounts of nutrients that elevate blood pressure, it may be that the reason overeating causes an elevation in blood pressure rests partly in these amines.

A study done in China on individuals who ate half a cup of oatmeal or half a cup of buckwheat had lower blood cholesterol levels and lower blood pressure than those who did not eat these grains (*American Journal of Clinical Nutrition* 61 [1995]: 366).

One pint daily of freshly squeezed grapefruit juice is helpful in treating high blood pressure.

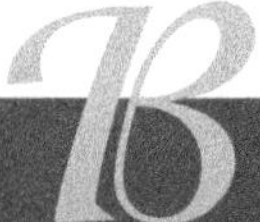

A diet high in vegetables and fruits, containing generous quantities of calcium (high in greens) can reduce blood pressure (*American Journal of Hypertension* 9 [1996]: 144).

It has been found that vitamin C can help to lower blood pressure, especially in African Americans. As vitamin C goes up in the blood, the pulse rate and blood pressure go down. A group of Seventh-day Adventists was studied by Lynn Toohey, a researcher at Colorado State University, who found that around 300 milligrams of vitamin C consumed in foods each day seems to be about the ideal quantity (*Medical Tribune News Service*, February 8, 1996; *Journal of the American College of Nutrition* 11, no. 2 [1992]: 139).

Supplements

Phenylaminoalkyl selenides, a natural compound of selenium, have shown antihypertensive activity possessing remarkable properties. The selenide can be taken orally. Selenium should always be considered for hypertensives. It is naturally found in Brazil nuts and many other foods.

Niacin has been used to control blood pressure and blood cholesterol, but certain persons should not take extra niacin as it can interfere with the body's ability to dispose of sugar and can cause borderline diabetes to turn into the full blown disease. Niacin can also interfere with the control of uric acid bringing on attacks of gout in persons prone to this disease (*Post Graduate Medicine* 89, no. 4 [1991]: 262).

Vitamin B6 supplementation reduces serum norepinephrine as well as systolic and diastolic blood pressure (*Arzneim Forsch* 45 [1995]: 1271–3; *American Journal of Natural Medicine* 3, no. 4 [May 1996]: 16).

L-Carnitine, two grams daily for 22 weeks, showed a very good response in the blood pressure (*Clinica Terapeutica* 144 [1994]: 391).

Potassium supplementation reduces blood pressure substantially in African Americans consuming a diet low in potassium (*Alternative Medicine Review* 1, no. 1 [1996]: 46; *Archives of Internal Medicine* 156 [1996]: 61). You can get potassium from bananas, tomatoes, and most fruits and vegetables.

Coenzyme Q-10 can help to promote a normal thickness of the left ventricular wall and normal diastolic blood pressure in individuals with hypertension. Since a thick left ventricular wall is a precursor of more serious heart disease, CoQ10 can be very helpful in these patients (*Molecular Aspects of Medicine* 15 [1994]: S265).

L-arginine is a precursor of nitric oxide known to decrease blood pressure by dilating blood vessels. Nitrous oxide is produced in the endothelium, the lining tissue of blood vessels and the heart. A vegetarian diet supplies a lot of L-arginine. L-arginine inhibits the renin-angiotensin system.

Magnesium deficiency may play as important a role as sodium overload in causing high blood pressure. Unprocessed grains and legumes are high in magnesium. Diuretics cause a loss of magnesium and can intensify the burden already experienced by the metabolic systems of the body. Since softened water and magnesium deficient soil are more and more common, conditions that increase the likelihood of deficiency, the American public is continually more and more likely to have magnesium deficiencies. In 1900 the average American got 475 milligrams daily of magnesium, whereas today only 245 milligrams.

Magnesium may regulate the sodium-calcium exchange pump of the cells. When sodium levels are high and magnesium is low, the pump is inefficient, cells become loaded with calcium and blood vessels contract. Potassium also has a role in the control of calcium, sodium, and magnesium in the body. The role of each of these is very poorly understood at present (*Science News* 125 [March 24, 1984]: 182). It is known, however, that a totally vegetarian diet of unrefined foods gives the best opportunity to keep these minerals balanced. Taking a supplement of magnesium of 300 to 500 milligrams daily is worthwhile and may significantly reduce blood pressure. Increase the dose as needed, but do not take enough to cause diarrhea. A large overdose causes severe diarrhea, and if continued other signs develop. A determined effort to overdose can cause the other symptoms of magnesium overload which include nausea, vomiting, flushing, slow pulse, irregular heart rhythm, low blood pressure, muscle paralysis, and eventually coma (*Mayo Clinic Proceedings* 70 [1995]: 1091). But diarrhea occurs long before these symptoms appear.

Hydrotherapy

In general, it has been found that hot baths lower blood pressure and cold baths raise it. Steam baths and sweating have a beneficial effect on hypertension with a drop in both systolic and diastolic pressures (*Journal of the American Medical Association* 243, no. 4 [January 25, 1980]: 370). Strasburger found that the results from the use of heat and cold are complicated and that a cold bath may produce an initial rise in blood pressure, followed by a fall and again by a second rise. He noticed, also, that hot baths above 104°F (40°C) often gave a blood pressure above normal. While warm baths are generally associated with a fall of pressure, a neutral bath at 93°F to 95°F (34°C to 35°C) in his study produced no change in blood pressure (*American Journal of Physiology* 70 [October 1924]: 412).

A hot bath for 30 to 60 minutes at 104°F has been shown to have a remarkably calming effect. It will invariably reduce blood pressure after about 20 to 30 minutes. Cool down gradually after the bath while lying well-covered in bed. After 30 minutes, when sweating has stopped, take a regular shower, friction the skin dry with a coarse towel and dress in dry clothing. (See "Hydrotherapy" in the *Natural Remedies* section.)

A hot bath increasing the body temperature to 100.4°F leads to a greater number of significant and favorable metabolic changes in high blood pressure, such as a decrease in blood cell sodium level and plasma and urine cortisol levels. There may be a reduction in diastolic blood pressure lasting two hours or more after the bath. There may be a diuresis of significant degree, losing much excess fluid.

A "neutral bath" for 10 to 30 minutes in a tub of water that feels neither warm nor cool (96°F to 98°F) at the end of the day has been shown to have a distinctly relaxing effect and often lowers blood pressure.

A study done by Dr. Olga Walek and Arlene Lee in 1970 at Loma Linda University for a thesis showed that a neutral bath caused systolic reductions of 14 millimeters, while bed rest only reduced the systolic blood pressure six millimeters. A neutral bath reduced diastolic pressure seven millimeters, and bed rest only half a millimeter. A neutral bath reduced the pulse rate five beats per minute and bed rest two beats per minute. Any kind of activity the patients had such as interacting with other patients or participating in some of the patient activities, such as watching television, increased systolic and diastolic blood pressures as well as heart rate.

A study done on 27 pregnant women showed that a 40 minute bath in water at neutral temperature caused an increase in urine flow, as well as in excretion of salt, potassium, and creatinine. The researchers said the bath had a flushing effect believed to be because of activation of kidney function and mobilizing of tissue fluids (*Zentralbl-Gynakol* 111, no. 13 [1989]: 864–70). Such a reaction should gradually bring the blood pressure down if done on a daily basis for several weeks.

Head-out-of-water immersion results in significant loss of water in the urine as well as sodium and potassium and a suppression of the kidneys in the production of hormones that raise blood pressure. It can be quite helpful for the patient to be immersed in water for half an hour at a water temperature of 93.4°F to which has been added two tablespoons of table salt for every five gallons of water estimated to be used. The loss of sodium and water in this manner helps to lower blood pressure (*IRCS Medical Science* 10 [1982]: 251).

Alternating hot and cold baths for high blood pressure has a decidedly good effect on the blood pressure. The person should sit in a tub of hot water at 110°F, then cold water at 85°F for 30 seconds. Continue alternating back and forth for 20 minutes. This same treatment is good for constipation as well. Two tubs are required.

Exercise

Research shows that physically active men and women have lower average blood pressures and are diagnosed less frequently with hypertension than their sedentary counterparts. The minimum amount of activity associated with lower blood pressure appears to be 30 to 60 minutes per day at a moderate intensity level plus a gradual warm-up and cool down period.

Exercise training studies in people with high-normal blood pressure or "borderline hypertension" have shown that performing moderate-intensity cardiovascular exercise for 45 minutes per day of accumulated time at least three times per week causes a reduction in blood pressure at rest and during moderate exercise. Examples of exercise include brisk walking, jogging, gardening, and housework.

A group of mildly hypertensive patients lowered their blood pressure from 135 to 121 systolic pressure, and from 93 to 83 diastolic pressure in a three-month program of aerobic exercise. "Most hypertensive patients would rather exercise than take a pill … because it feels good and becomes a part of their lifestyle." Compliance to drug routines are not always successful because of unpleasant medication side effects (*Internal Medicine News* 17, no. 5 [March 1984]: 9).

A physically fit person with hypertension has a lower chance of dying from heart and artery disease than does an unfit person with normal blood pressure (*United States News and World Report,* May 4, 1994, 88).

Run in place twice daily for six minutes to reduce blood pressure. Keep the chest high with shoulders back and down.

Certain disorders improve with vigorous exercise, some with moderate-intensity exercise, and some health problems vary from person to person as to the intensity of the exercise. High-intensity exercise is favorably associated with improvements in heart, artery, lung problems, cholesterol, triglycerides, and life expectancy. Low to moderate-intensity exercise is associated with improvements in blood pressure (especially for women), psychological well-being, and less risk of musculoskeletal injury. Low-intensity exercise is better for diabetes and for improving blood clotting properties.

In one study regular exercise reduced not only blood pressure but also left ventricular hypertrophy in African

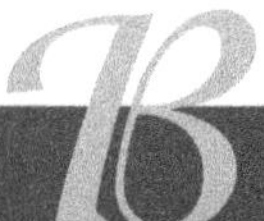

American men with severe hypertension. The men rode bicycles 44 minutes three times a week at 74 percent of the predicted maximum heart rate (*New England Journal of Medicine* 333, no. 22 [November 30, 1995]: 1462–67).

Exercise eases the tensions between the autonomic and somatic divisions of the nervous system and clears the blood of excessive fats, salts, and sugars. The pace should be described as vigorous, though not violent. Outdoor labor is usually more beneficial than indoor labor. Even the sense of satisfaction of work well done is healing. Spend an hour or more every day in outdoor exercise if at all possible.

Dress

Careful attention to proper clothing of the extremities is essential to calm the autonomic nervous system and to equalize the circulation. Cool skin causes an alarm reaction in the autonomic nerves. Chilled tissues cause the blood to shunt from the extremities to the interior of the body where vital organs are congested and their function made less efficient. Keep all of the skin warm except where there is active sweating to cool the body. Check especially the hands and feet, backs of the arms, and the sides of the thighs. These areas should all be as warm as the forehead. Wear loose clothing on all parts of the body. Adaptation to messages from the skin signaling chilling takes a large tax from nerve energy resources, and acclimatizes the person to expect cold temperatures. Therefore, the person allowing the extremities to get chilled in summer in air conditioning will be more likely to suffer excessively during the very hot parts of the day.

A sunbath will lower the blood pressure right away, and dressing the extremities warmly, as warmly as the trunk, will lower both systolic and diastolic blood pressure.

Breathing and Relaxation

Relaxation training can lower blood pressure and keep it down. In their classrooms 62 percent of ninth and tenth graders at high risk for developing hypertension learned relaxation training and lowered their blood pressures below 122, whereas only 24 percent of the control, untrained subjects achieved this (*Internal Medicine News* 17, no. 5 [March 1984]: 9). Starting with the leg muscles, tense the muscles as much as possible and hold for several seconds. Then relax. Next move to the muscles of the thigh, back, abdomen, chest, neck, and face. Repeat the tensing and relaxation process until all tension is gone. Use this routine twice a day.

Poor breathing techniques can contribute to high blood pressure, as shallow breathing decreases the excretion of sodium from the body (*Alternatives* 6, no. 10 [April 1996]: 75–7; *Psychosomatic Medicine* 57, no. 4 [1995]: 373–80). Breathing with the diaphragm from the abdomen rather than from the upper chest allows the lungs to inflate more extensively and has the good side effect of lowering blood pressure and slowing the heart rate. Good posture and training for abdominal breathing will both tend to inflate the lungs more and reduce blood pressure. Lie on a firm surface and place a book or one hand on your abdomen while you concentrate on breathing from the abdomen instead of the chest, watch the upward and downward movement of the book or your hand. When you stand straight, remember to do the abdominal breathing and make certain you breathe several times a day quite deeply from the abdomen to keep yourself reminded to breathe deeply. One way to remember to breathe deeply is to do so every time you pass through a door—car door, house door, room door, or an elevator door. Practice a deep breathing exercise three times daily, consisting of breathing in slowly to the count of four. Hold that breath for a slow count of seven. Then exhale for the slow count of ten. Repeat as many times as necessary to fill up at least five minutes three times a day. This can be done while sitting or driving. It should be repeated at least 10 times, and up to as many as 60 times in one session. This breathing exercise will lower the blood pressure significantly after one month of faithfully performing it.

Singing lessons with an emphasis on warm-up exercises and breath control can also be most helpful.

Massage

Massage in any area (feet, back, full body) will result in a reduction in high blood pressure, sometimes very significantly.

Hot and cold flank fomentations, a wet sheet pack to help relaxation and stress reduction, or a neutral to warm bath followed by a full body massage one to three times a week for one hour, and other days substituted by a mechanical device for relaxation (an ankle shaker or a back massager, or a massage chair, or a foot vibrator) can lower blood pressure after several weeks. Any of these can be helpful in treating hypertension.

Herbs

Garlic, parsley, *Coleus forskohlii*, *Leonurus* (motherwort), *Convallaria majalis*, *Capsicum minimum*, *Sambucus nigra*, celery seed, barberry, buchu, dandelion, dill, fenugreek, ginger, golden seal, juniper, nettle, saffron, sarsaparilla, uva-ursi, corn silk, skullcap, lemon grass, valerian root, black cohosh, etc., can all be helpful herbal remedies

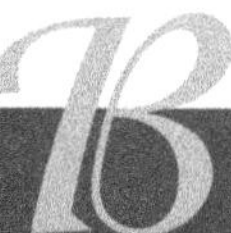

for hypertension. Use the standard dosage of one cup of the tea of each of the herbs four times a day between meals or the equivalent dose of pills or tinctures four times a day. The dosage of garlic is one to three cloves three times daily with meals. More garlic may be needed at first, up to an entire bulb. The garlic should be steamed about eight or nine minutes, enough that it will lose some of the sharp sting to the tongue.

Stevia is very useful in hypertension. Take 250 milligrams of a standard extract four times daily.

Gotu kola helps relieve high blood pressure. Ginkgo biloba protects against strokes and helps to treat strokes. It has good anticoagulant benefits. Ginkgo biloba assists in normalizing conditions of altered production of nitric oxide (*Biochemical and Biophysical Research Communications* 201 [1994]: 748). Nitric oxide plays a part in relaxing the smooth muscle of blood vessels and regulating blood pressure. Nitric oxide is normally produced in artery walls and relaxes arteries. Persons with essential hypertension usually have a reduced quantity of nitric oxide in artery walls, which causes tension in the artery, increasing blood pressure.

Lavender is an herb fragrance that has a relaxing action on blood vessels and nerves, reducing blood pressure. It can be used for depression and headaches. It stimulates thought processes while relaxing emotional tension. It can be taken as a tea or as a glycerine or alcohol extract in a tincture. Use one-half to one teaspoon three times a day. Lavender essential oil relieves anxiety and stress and can relax smooth muscle, a quality that may make it helpful in reducing blood pressure.

A daily dose of three tablespoons ground hawthorn berry, two tablespoons yarrow, one tablespoon mistletoe, and one quart boiling water can be of help. Gently simmer the hawthorn in water for 20 minutes, then add the remaining herbs and steep 30 minutes. The leaves from olive trees will also benefit the heart, retard infections, and lower blood pressure.

High blood pressure may rarely be caused in susceptible persons by ephedra, ginseng, juniper, kelp, kola, licorice, and St. John's wort. Conversely, some of these very herbs can be used to treat high blood pressure.

In the 1800s a tea made from olive leaves was used as a cure for malaria. By the early 1900s olive leaf tea was found to be far superior to quinine for treating malarial infections, but quinine was easier to administer. Therefore, quinine continued to be the treatment of choice. In 1957 oleoropine was isolated from olive leaves as the active ingredient. This same compound was found to lower blood pressure, increase blood flow to the coronary arteries, relieve arrhythmia of the heart, and prevent intestinal spasms.

Hops, peppermint, garlic, and clay internally have been used with success to lower blood pressure. Lemon grass tea, one cup four times a day, will help. *Coleus* has adenyl cyclase activator, a substance that lowers blood pressure. Motherwort is also good for lowering blood pressure. *Capsicum* dilates blood vessels and stimulates the circulation. Valerian, calendula, *Crataegus*, and Ginkgo biloba are also good blood pressure medicines.

Kudzu tea contains puerarin which decreases blood pressure in laboratory animals by 15 percent. It also has 100 times the antioxidant activity of vitamin E. Place two tablespoons of dried kudzu leaves in a quart of water and steep for 30 to 45 minutes daily ("The Green Pharmacy Anti-Aging Prescriptions: Herbs, Foods, and Natural formulas to Keep You Young" *Mother Nature's Medicines* [2001]: 409-410).

An Oriental remedy uses leaves from peanut plants to reduce levels of triglycerides, cholesterol, and blood pressure. Animal experiments using either water or alcohol extracts of the leaves had a sedative, sleep inducing effect. There were no toxic side effects in the animals given a dosage 125 times the amount used to lower blood pressure, cholesterol, and triglycerides (*Chinese Traditional and Herbal Drugs* 18, no. 2 [1987]: 22).

Treatment Summary

The best treatments for high blood pressure are serious, sweeping, and permanent lifestyle changes as described above, as well as a trial of supplements with calcium, magnesium, and potassium; CoQ10; garlic; flax oil; and a large number of herbs, especially ginkgo, Coleus forskohlii, and hawthorn berry or flower. The proper dose of the standardized hawthorn extract is 100 to 250 milligrams three times a day. The extract should be standardized to contain 1.8 percent vitelin-4'-rhamnoside, or 20 percent proanthocyanidins. Side effects are essentially non-existent from any of these measures.

Following is a quick reference guide to the treatments discussed in detail above:

- Sunning
- Drink water – it dilutes the antidiuretic hormone from the posterior pituitary. Fifteen glasses per day are probably ideal for persons with hypertension. Many medications mimic the effects of increased water intake.
- Rest – avoid pain, fear, anger, stress, and noise

- Herbs
  - Hawthorn berry dilates blood vessels, normalizes cardiac output, and increases stroke volume of the heart
  - Valerian contains valerenic acid and valepotriates, enzymes which denature GABA
  - Kudzu contains puerarin
  - Saffron contains crocetin
  - Black cohosh relaxes muscles
  - Cayenne pepper dilates blood vessels
- Diet
  - Fasting
  - Plant-based diet
  - Increase potassium, which decreases sodium
  - Increase magnesium, which is found in leaves, legumes, whole grains, purslane, poppy seeds, carob, string beans, et al. Reduce the ingestion of sodium found in baking soda, soft drinks, saccharine, soy sauce, preservatives, meat tenderizers, water softeners, and dairy products
  - Increase the quantity of garlic, which brings about vasodilation by means of alliin
  - Increase calcium, which can be found in greens, whole wheat, figs, sesame seeds, et al.
  - Grapes contain oligomeric proanthocyanidins, which dilate blood vessels
  - Tomatoes contain GABA (gamma-aminobutyric acid)
  - Four stalks of celery pureed also contain GABA
  - Broccoli contains six separate chemical compounds to reduce blood pressure
  - Similar chemicals are found in fennel (10), oregano (seven), basil and tarragon (six each)
  - Apples contain pectin and other specific blood pressure reducing compounds
  - Vitamins C, E, folic acid, carotenoids, CoQ10, vitamin D, lecithin, bioflavonoids, and taurine
  - Reduce or eliminate free fats
  - Reduce tyrosine and phenylalanine

Drugs for Hypertension

The drugs used to treat hypertension are poisonous, very powerful, and foreign substances to the body. They should be avoided if at all possible. Some drugs can actually make the hypertension worse in certain individuals rather than improve it.

More doctors today are beginning to question the growing popularity of drugs to treat high blood pressure. It is now recognized that many of these drugs increase risks of heart attacks and cancers, and alter metabolism in the liver, kidneys, pancreas (increased risk of diabetes) immune and nervous systems (affecting emotions, behavior, and muscle function). Blood pressure medications cause a number of side effects including loss of memory, dizziness, depression, heart arrhythmias (by Thiazides, a family of diuretic drugs), and many others. Hearing loss has been ascribed to blood pressure medications (*British Medical Journal* 289 [1984]: 1490; *Archives of General Psychiatry* 40 [1983]: 1109; *British Medical Journal* 289 [December 1, 1984]: 1496; *Medical World News,* January 24, 1983, 32).

Other drug side effects are sexual impotence and dysfunction, loss of appetite, nausea, and fatigue. Drug diuretics used for hypertension have been linked to an eleven-fold increase in diabetes (*WDDTY* 5, no. 11 [March 1995]: 1). Furthermore, blood pressure medications are not as effective as could be hoped. Only around 21 percent of patients get their blood pressures reduced to under 140/90.

These facts bring an important focus on natural methods of bringing the blood pressure down. Weight control, exercise, a proper diet, avoidance of smoking, and alcohol consumption, are all features of the natural treatment of hypertension. One of the more serious problems of high blood pressure treated with drugs has also been the associated reduction in mental acuity (*Lancet* 347 [1996]: 1130).

The development of events apparently proceeds first with thickening of blood vessel walls because of elevated blood pressure. Then, if a blood pressure medicine is given and the pressure is driven down, the brain is not perfused properly, and dementia develops (Ibid.: 1141–45).

In some elderly persons, a slightly elevated blood pressure may actually be the optimal level for them. Irregular heartbeats were found to be most common among patients over age 68 whose readings were below 85 on the diastolic reading and whose left ventricle was enlarged. In hypertensives, if the diastolic blood pressure is reduced with medicines below 85, there is evidence that the person may be at increased risk of a heart attack or stroke. Deterioration of mental function also accelerates as the blood pressure falls through the effects of drugs. These problems do not occur with natural means (*Journal of the American Medical Association* 265 [1991]: 489).

Scientists from the National Institutes of Health released the results in September 1982 of a decade-long, nationwide study of 13,000 men. This study revealed an unexpectedly high death rate in those treated with blood pressure drugs. Men with abnormal EKG readings who were treated with drugs had a 65 percent higher rate of mortality than those in a control group who did not receive drugs (*Journal of the American Medical Association* 248 [1982]: 1996–2003).

Case Reports

A 75-year-old man was cured of his hypertension with the following routine: he exercised to his limit, put little salt on anything he ate, and followed a plant-based diet. He took 500 milligrams of calcium with meals three times a day. Of herbal diuretics he used one tablespoon each of any three from the following list—ground watermelon seed, dandelion root, uva ursi, buchu, and corn silk—stirring them into boiling water and immediately setting off to cool. He drank four cups per day. At the beginning his blood pressure was 180/85. Within four months it was 110/78, and it has stayed at that level for four years, even though he no longer takes the herbs.

One 56-year-old white woman came to Uchee Pines Institute complaining of depression, fatigue, and unrelenting hypertension for one year of 240/140, despite her being on Inderal (a beta blocker), Lasix (a diuretic), and Slow-K (potassium supplement because potassium is lost in urine because of the diuretic). Her depression was the most troublesome part of her illness, and she had lost all will to live. She was treated with warm baths, a single day of total fasting with 12 glasses of water, followed by three days of apple fasting with 10 glasses of water, and then a salt-free, oil-free, plant-based diet. Within three weeks her blood pressure, which had baffled her physicians, was down to 195/102. She said several times, "Nobody ever told me how to get my blood pressure down." She was 100 pounds overweight, and in one month she had lost 13 pounds. By one year she had lost 60 pounds, was taking no blood pressure medication, and had a blood pressure reading of 112/72, which she maintained for years. Her depression lifted when she stopped the medications, and her life was transformed. Twenty-four years later she is still alive and well. She is nearly normal in weight and her blood pressure is normal.

Blood Pressure, Postural Hypotension (Low blood pressure)

Some individuals experience a drop in blood pressure when they stand up, sometimes resulting in light-headedness, weakness, impaired concentration, blurring of the vision, tremulousness, and vertigo. Aggravating factors are prolonged standing, exercise, warming by a heater or open fire, and eating. To treat this condition, all lifestyle factors should be evaluated, and corrections made where needed. Licorice root tea may also be quite helpful. Staying well hydrated can also be of great help.

Some women complain of low blood pressure with symptoms, even when the pulse pressure (the difference between the systolic and the diastolic pressures) is greater than 20, which should give them quite an adequate blood circulation. The symptoms may be because of inadequate water intake or inadequate potassium intake. Foods that are high in potassium are generally found in abundant supply in a diet high in fruits, vegetables, whole grains, nuts, and seeds.

Postural hypotension may not be detected in people because the blood pressure is always taken in either the reclining position or the sitting position and not in the standing position. Patients with postural hypotension frequently report weakness across the back and shoulders, especially on the first activity in the morning. Postural hypotension indicates an autonomic nervous system dysfunction such as is present in diabetic patients with neuropathy. Low blood volumes from chronic dehydration or the use of pharmaceutical diuretics can also cause postural hypotension (*Hypertension* 27 [1996]: 408).

There are some individuals who are treated with drugs for high blood pressure who get dangerously low blood pressure. In the elderly, medicines that cause the blood pressure to go quite low when standing can cause dangerously irregular heartbeats, especially if the patient has a thickened heart muscle from high blood pressure. This is called postural hypotension.

Those persons, especially those with diabetic neuropathy who have low blood pressure when they stand up, are in greater risk of dying during the next 10 years than those not having postural hypotension. This may cause them to be weak, dizzy, or even to faint.

Following are ways to control postural hypotension:

- Be aware that the symptoms of hypotension are most severe 30 to 60 minutes after a heavy meal and one to two hours after taking antihypertension medication. Studiously avoid overeating or eating rich or highly concentrated foods.
- Sleep with the head of the bed elevated about 8 to 12 inches.
- Avoid sudden changes in position.
- Never bend down all the way to the floor or stand up too quickly after stooping.
- Postpone activities requiring long standing for at least an hour after rising, such as shaving or fixing hair.
- Wear elastic stockings at night.
- Get out of a hot bath very slowly. Stay bent over or sit while toweling dry.

- Use a rocking chair to improve lower extremity circulation. Women may benefit from wearing elasticized pantyhose from a department store (not the orthopedic devices that require fitting, as they are not usually required for this purpose).
- Do not engage in any strenuous activity that results in holding the breath and bearing down.

Blood Tests, Explanation of Laboratory Reports

(See "Lab Tests" in the *Supplemental Information* section.)

Bone Pain

Bone pain of undetermined origin is often caused by a deficiency of vitamin D. The only remedy usually needed is sunning.

The periosteum (membrane surrounding the bone) can give rise to intense pain and is the cause of much of the localized pain of fractures. Chronic disease affecting the bone marrow such as infection or cancer may result in poorly localized pain having varying degrees of severity.

Intense aching, boring back pain may occur with malignant metastases to the vertebrae in the chest above the waist. Often the pain is referred to the skin zones corresponding to the vertebrae. An X-ray may not locate the lesions, but a bone scan usually will. Hodgkin's disease, lymphosarcoma, and leukemia may all produce pain in the ribs, particularly leukemia in its advanced stages. Point tenderness in the breastbone is often characteristic of these. Multiple myeloma and sarcoma involving the ribs or spine above the waist may cause bone pain.

Botulism

The most severe and dangerous of all food poisonings, botulism occurs as a result of eating canned foods that have been contaminated by the germ Clostridium botulinum, which produces a toxin of extraordinary power. The toxin attacks the nerves, inducing weakness and paralysis, including difficulty swallowing, talking, and seeing. Death, which may quickly follow, results from respiratory failure and has occurred in 65 percent of cases. The danger develops when foods, such as string beans, corn, spinach, asparagus, beets, and apricots, are canned by inadequate heating methods, and the botulism germ survives the processing, grows, and produces its toxin. Sausage, meats, and fish pastes have also produced botulism. The amount of toxin produced depends on the acidity of the food, the presence of sugar, and the length of time heat was applied to the food. The more acid the food, the less likely the germ can grow.

The toxin itself, fortunately, can be rendered harmless by as little as six minutes of boiling. We recommend that all home canned vegetables be boiled 20 minutes to insure adequate heat for destruction of the toxin that might be in them. A pressure canner, using pressures and times as recommended by your Agricultural Extension Service, should always be used for canning vegetables and non-acid fruits such as apricots.

If botulism develops, speed in administering powdered charcoal is a matter of life and death to the victim. Quickly put around four tablespoons into a jar, add water, put the cap on, and shake briefly to dissolve the charcoal. Have the person drink it quickly from the jar. Even if there is a suspicion that botulism might be occurring, only seconds may be allotted you from the first onset of symptoms until death occurs from failure of respiration. The charcoal cannot reverse damage suffered from the toxin, but further progress of the poisoning may be avoided. Administer artificial respiration for hours as long as there is a pulse. One's own tissues will denature the toxin gradually over a matter of hours or days. If the heart action stops, all hope is probably gone for saving the life.

Breast Conditions

The female breasts are composed mainly of fatty tissue, ducts, and glands capable of producing milk. The milk glands empty into small ducts that empty into larger ducts, and finally fuse into the large ducts near the nipple. The male breast is similar except that it lacks glands.

It is not uncommon for one breast to be slightly larger than the other. Nor is it uncommon for the breasts in some women to become tender and engorged just prior to a menstrual period. Pain in breasts which have no lumps or cysts is not uncommon. None of these signs is cause for alarm under all normal circumstances.

Breastfeeding

The longer babies are breast-fed during the first year of life, the greater their chance of being slender later in childhood. A child who is overweight or obese tends to remain overweight throughout life. Major causes of childhood obesity are too much food, fatty foods, snacking between meals, soft drinks, lack of exercise, and a bad example set for them by overweight parents.

Advantages of Breastfeeding to the Baby

- It is the perfect food for the baby, easily digested and has complete nutrition for the baby, at least for the first six months of life. Not even water needs to be added under normal circumstances.
- It provides antibodies to protect the baby from childhood illnesses, including allergies, eczema, and colic. It can help prevent allergies.
- Close contact between the mother and baby brings a bonding relationship.
- Breastfeeding teaches your baby to stop eating on signal of feeling satisfied, as the first milk of each feeding is watery, satisfying thirst and the last milk is rich and fatty, satisfying hunger and appetite. If the infant is wetting or soiling six to eight diapers or more per 24 hours, these are signs of adequate hydration and nourishment.
- Breast-fed babies have a larger thymus, indicating a better immune system (*Acta Paediatrica* 85 [1996]: 1029).
- Three hundred breast-fed children were found to have significantly higher IQs than children who had not been breast-fed (*Lancet* 339 [February 1, 1992]: 261–4).
- Babies who have been breast-fed for six or more months have a reduced likelihood of developing childhood leukemia by 20 percent (*Journal of the National Cancer Institute* 91 [1999]: 1765).
- Your child's academic success may begin with your decision to breastfeed. A study involving 126 siblings from 59 families were studied by the University of Colorado in Denver. They recorded that breast-fed infants get better high school grades and are more likely to go to college than non-breast-fed persons. The breast-fed group's high school grade point averages were higher than their formula-fed siblings.

Advantages of Breastfeeding to the Mother

- It assists the post-delivery uterus to return to a normal size more quickly, a process called involution.
- Breast cancer is lower in women who nurse their babies.
- Breastfeeding serves as a natural contraceptive so that babies are not born too close together.
- Usually the menstrual period does not occur while the mother is breastfeeding.
- Breastfeeding is more economical and convenient than bottle feeding.
- Mothers have a sense of accomplishment with breastfeeding.

Milk Production

When it is desired to increase the production of milk or if a young mother who has stopped breastfeeding for a few weeks wants to begain again, it may be possible to do so with the following regime:

- Mix one tablespoon blessed thistle, one tablespoon milk thistle, and two tablespoons red raspberry leaf with one quart of boiling water and steep for 30 minutes. Strain and drink throughout the morning. Make a second quart and drink throughout the afternoon. Use daily every four hours during the day for six weeks or more while nursing the baby. Always relax in a rocking chair while nursing, concentrating on the baby. Both nipple stimulation from sucking and the mother's thoughts of the baby promote milk production.
- Plenty of outdoor exercise, especially exercise that strengthens the arms and moves them vigorously, such as hanging clothes on the line, using a mop, painting, raking leaves, beating rugs, and hoeing, will assist in milk production.
- Any activity that increases sweating can also boost milk production. This includes warm baths or showers, vigorous exercise, warm clothing, warm bedclothes at night, and sunbathing. Some of the diuretic herbs will also cause sweating, such as watermelon seed tea, corn silk tea, and buchu tea.
- To increase milk production, chew a few caraway seeds two to three times a day.

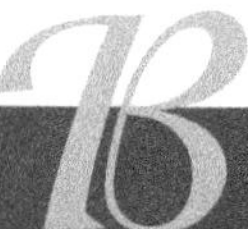

Breast Cancer

Cancer of the breast has several known causes and associations. These should be corrected in every woman's life if possible. The use of saturated (hard) fats in the diet, or the overuse of free fats (margarine, butters, mayonnaise, fried foods, cooking fats, and salad oils) encourages breast cancers. If you have had a first degree relative who has had cancer of the breast, prostate, or colon that increases your likelihood of developing breast cancer, putting a premium on correcting all other possible associations and causes. Diabetes, heart disease, cancer in another organ, and high blood cholesterol all increase the likelihood of developing breast cancer. Breastfeeding has a protective value against breast cancer. Being overweight as a child or teen increases the risk, especially if you are still overweight.

Breast cancer was one of the most rapidly increasing cancers in the 1990s when breast cancer increased from 1 in 12 to 1 in 9 women. At the beginning of 2000 the incidence was 1 in 7. Breast cancer is also associated with having chronically chilled extremities, the heavy use of meat or sugar, any kind of trauma to the breast, including surgery, and deficiencies of iodine, selenium, and B vitamins. The use of rauwolfia or reserpine medications for high blood pressure increase the risk of breast cancer. Some have found an association between the taking of Synthroid for thyroid problems and breast cancer. The earlier in life a little girl begins her menstrual periods and the later she goes through menopause, the greater the likelihood she will develop cancer of the breast. That means the more menstrual cycles a woman has the greater the likelihood of developing breast cancer.

The American Cancer Society reported in April 1994 that 182,000 women are diagnosed with breast cancer in the United States each year, and 46,000 (about 25 percent) die from it. While lifestyle and heredity are closely involved in this increase, the introduction and common use of a variety of chemicals and drugs have been implicated. An increase in the risk of breast cancer has been shown with the use of oral contraceptives (*Cancer Causes and Control* 6 [1995]: 485). There may be a link between environmental pollution and breast cancer according to the New York State Health Department (*Journal of Surgical Oncology* 61 [1996]: 209).

If cancer of the breast has more than 100 blood vessels in a low power microscopic field, it is an indication that there likely will be a recurrence of the cancer within 33 months. By contrast, breast cancer is expected to recur in only 5 percent of women who have 33 or fewer blood vessels per low power microscope field. Since cancers often spread by means of blood vessels, the more blood vessels in a tumor, the greater the likelihood of spreading (*Science News* 142 [1992]: 421). Foods and drugs containing methylxanthines may promote fibrocystic disease, such as asthma medication, Anacin, Dexedrine (an amphetamine), Excedrin, No-Doz, pain relievers, cold and sinus preparations (Dristan), appetite suppressants, and hormones (birth control pills, estrogens, etc.).

Ways to Prevent Breast Cancer

Stress is a big factor in increasing breast cancer risk. An Israeli study published in 2008 showed that women who go through more than one stressful life event in one year, such as losing a spouse, were at greater risk. On the other hand, general feelings of optimism and happiness can stave off cancer.

Various flavonoids, a type of antioxidant, can help to counteract free radical damage that can lead to breast cancer. Emphasizing fruits and vegetables in one's diet, whole grains, nuts, and seeds, will result in 87 percent lower risk of breast cancer than those who rarely or never eat fruits and vegetables.

A small handful of walnuts every day can help prevent breast cancer according to a study from Marshall University School of Medicine. A tumor that may already be growing can be slowed by the walnuts because of the large content of antioxidants, omega-3 fatty acids, and phytosterols which tend to block the estrogen receptors on breast cells.

Chinese women who eat a lot of button mushrooms—at least one tablespoon daily—were 64 percent less likely to develop breast cancer. Researchers say these small mushrooms curb estrogen production while strengthening the immune system.

As little as two ounces of saturated fat-laden red meat a day for seven years gives a woman a 56 percent higher risk of breast cancer than those eating no meat according to a study at the University of Leeds.

A woman drinking just one or two alcohol beverage per day can increase her risk of breast tumors by at least one-third. One of the reasons this occurs is that alcohol is toxic to glandular tissue. As alcoholic consumption increases so does the risk of breast cancer. Of course factors such as smoking and obesity should be eliminated from any women's life.

There are certain pesticides with a molecular structure that mimics estrogen which gains entrance to breast cell hormone receptors and stimulates the breast to produce cancer. A Mayo Clinic report showed that the higher the pesticide level in breast tissue the greater the cancer risk. We should watch out for pesticides around and in our homes as well as on and in our fruits and vegetables.

Radiation exposure to the chest, especially during puberty, increases the risk of cancer. This risk begins about 10 years after the treatment and lasts as long as the person lives. A study published in the *International Journal of Cancer* in 2007 revealed that women given diagnostic chest X-rays before age 20 for pneumonia had twice the normal risk for breast cancer than those who received no diagnostic X-rays before the age of 20. Even radiation for acne or other skin conditions increases risks to develop breast cancer.

Women who are younger than age 40 and are black American are more likely than white Americans to get breast cancer. However, white women over the age of 40 are more likely to get breast cancer than African American women.

Treatment for Breast Cancer

Five treatments per week consisting of fever treatments given on alternate days, preceded with ice compresses for 3 to 10 minutes to get the tumor as cold as possible, and alternating and followed immediately with hot compresses to get the tumor as hot as possible, have been used in some studies with beneficial results. This routine can be used for three weeks, skip a week, and repeat the series twice more. Repeat the routine every three months for the first year, and every six months the second year, and annually after that. (See "Hydrotherapy" in the *Natural Remedies* section.)

It is important in dealing with cancer of the breast that the cancer not be rubbed vigorously, pushed strongly, or pressed firmly. Observations made in the 1970s and 1980s on women who were given the classic vigorous surgical scrub using large sponge forceps, rapidly and vigorously rubbing, shaking, and scrubbing the breast containing cancer, revealed that they suffered more recurrences and metastases than did women who had a gentle surgical scrub, consisting mainly of anointing the skin with the medicines.

Treatment for cancer of the breast should always include a great increase in outdoor exercise. It has been shown that the spread of the cancer is reduced in physically fit women. Bear in mind that exercise can itself be stressful if it is overdone or violent. Stress weakens the immune system against cancer. The vitamin D levels should rise when a woman exercises outside. Studies show that women with breast cancer have lower vitamin D levels than those not having breast cancer.

Certain herbal teas have been used in cancer: red clover, blue violet, chaparral, and Pau d'Arco. Garlic, two to four uncooked cloves three times a day for two months, is a time honored cancer remedy. We also recommend a complete clove lighty steamed with each meal.

Men rarely develop breast cancer. If any lump should develop in the adult male breast, it should be promptly and carefully studied. Breast cancers are more aggressive in men as a general rule. Fortunately, they can usually be discovered more easily as the breasts are small.

(See also "Clay Bath, Mud Bath" in the *Natural Remedies* section.)

Breast Self Examination

By all means a woman should examine the breasts at least as often as once a quarter. An easy way to remember is to schedule self examination on the first day of the change of seasons (first day of spring, summer, fall, and winter) to ensure that no lump has developed without her notice. Breast lumps are found in 80 percent of cases by the woman herself.

Follow these steps to conduct a self examination:

- *Inspection*: First stand before a mirror with a light coming down from one side or the other, not directly in front of you. With the arms raised over the head, observe the breasts for symmetry and for highlights or shadows that might indicate the presence of a lump in the breasts.
- *Armpits:* Often the armpit can be examined easier in a shower than when the fingers are dry. Soap the hands a bit and get them wet and then feel in the armpits to make certain there are no lumps. Hold the arm down toward the side but lifted far enough away from the body for the fingers of the opposite hand to easily reach into the armpit.
- *Flat Hand Exam:* With the flat of the hand, run your hand over the breast in a massaging manner, using a light touch. Look for a lump as you would look for a marble under a blanket.
- *Fingertip Exam:* While lying down with one hand behind the head, use the other hand to examine the breast on the raised-arm side. Systematically go over every inch of the breast from collarbone to the rib under the breast, and from the breastbone all the way out to the outer edge of the breast. A light touch is more conducive to finding lumps than a hard touch. Small breasts are easier to examine than large ones. Discovery of tumors can be enhanced in some cases by examining the breast through a very thin fabric such as a nylon slip (doctors call this the "towel trick").

  One can tell the difference between suspicious lesions and benign lesions in many cases by simply noting the difference in the consistency and whether

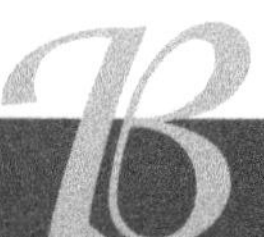

Breast Self-Examination

1. Lie down and put your left arm under your head. Use your right hand to examine your left breast. With your 3 middle fingers flat, move gently in small circular motions over the entire breast, checking for any lump, hard knot, or thickening. Use different levels of pressure - light, medium, and firm - over each area of your breast. Check the whole breast down to the ribs below your breast. Switch arms and repeat on the other breast.

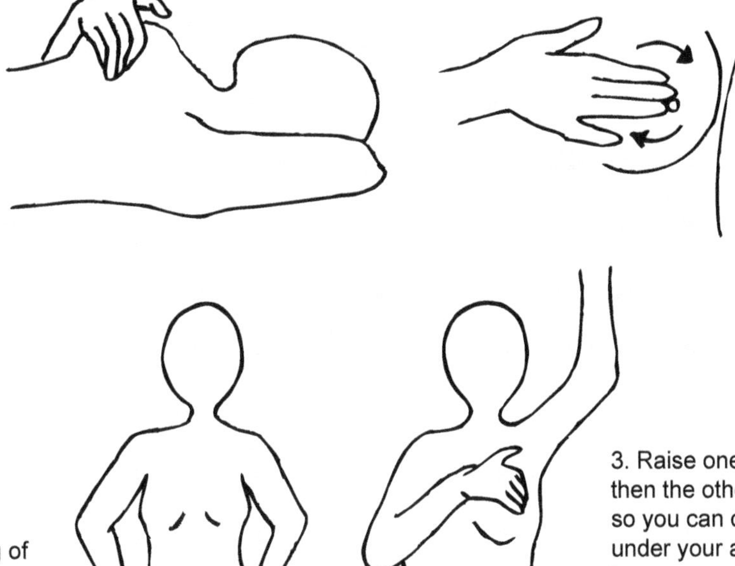

2. Look at your breasts while standing in front of a mirror with your hands on your hips. Look for lumps, new differences in size and shape, and swelling or dimpling of the skin.

3. Raise one arm, then the other, so you can check under your arms for lumps.

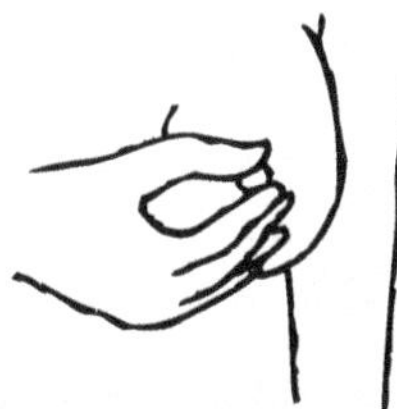

4. Squeeze the nipple of each breast gently between your thumb and index finger. Report to your healthcare provider right away any discharge or fluid from the nipples or any lumps or changes in your breast.

or not the lesion is attached to the tissue of the breast or skids around freely in the breast tissue. To get an idea how a malignant tumor of the breast feels, project the tongue to the side between the teeth out into the cheek. Feel of this through the skin with the fingertips while the tongue is relaxed, a benign consistency. Then stick the tongue firmly into the cheek, contracting the tongue to make the tongue feel hard. The hard tongue is the suspicious feel. Bear in mind that fluid filled benign cysts can also feel hard. The outline of a cyst, however, is rounded and easily moves in the breast.

- *Nipple Exam*: About one-fourth of all women have irregular areas in their breasts at some time. Just before menstruation, irregularities may occur. These feel grainy or finely lumpy and usually occur in the upper quadrants. Some women have persistently irregular breast tissue that feels shot-like or plaque-like even between periods. Such irregularities are not true tumors and are usually bilateral and do not increase in size, or consolidate into a lump. On the other hand, true tumors do not vary in size and are usually unilateral. Cancers persistently grow larger, and are not expected to diminish in size.

After the inspection of the breasts has been completed, the nipples should be squeezed to see if a drop of secretion can be expressed from the nipple. To do this, grasp the nipple back a way and then strip it out to see if you can express a small drop. The presence of milk usually means nothing, but can represent an overactive endocrine system. If there is blood in the secretion, consult a physician. If both nipples present clear or non-bloody secretions, there is usually nothing to worry about. One-sided secretion could mean a tiny polyp inside a duct, usually benign.

If a breast lump is discovered, a physician should be consulted concerning its significance. Most lumps in the breast are not cancer but are small cysts which accumulate fluid,

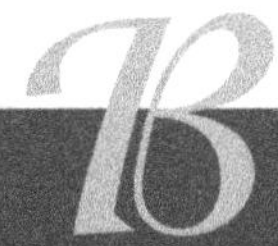

may become inflamed, and cause a firm area to develop. A localized area of bruising will sometimes occur in the breast because of some trauma, a bump, a fall, leaning against a sharp or blunt object, or the blockage of a duct from compression by her bra or her position in sleep.

Breast Lumps or Fibrocystic Breast Disease

Lumpiness or discreet lumps in the breast are usually fibrocystic breast disease as this is the commonest form of breast disease. A woman should learn to examine herself for lumps and to distinguish clearly between benign and suspicious lumps.

Breast cysts are often caused by a sensitivity to substances (methylxanthines) found in coffee, tea, colas, and chocolate. Vitamin E can cause breast cysts and tenderness in some women, but in others vitamin E may help to resolve fibrocystic disease. Drugs containing methylxanthines—asthma medications, Anacin, Midol, Dristan, Excedrin, No-Doz, many pain relievers, cold and sinus preparations, appetite suppressants, and hormones (birth control pills, estrogens, etc.), caffeine, theophylline, and theobromine—may promote fibrocystic disease. The same things that cause acne can cause breast cysts, such as food sensitivities and eating foods containing mixtures of free fats and free sugars.

Treatment

Treatment of benign lumps may cause them to disappear in a few weeks.

Begin by simplifying your diet. The most favorable diet is the plant-based diet, leaving off any substance known to increase the risk of breast disease such as methylxanthines (caffeine, theophylline, and theobromine found in coffee, colas, tea, and chocolate). Milk and dairy products have high estrogen levels that can increase the risk for both fibrocystic disease and breast cancer. Dairy products should be eliminated even in cooking. For resistant cases or multiple lumps, you may wish to try the same diet and general program we use for acne as the conditions have similarities. Free fats (margarine, mayonnaise, fried foods, cooking fats, salad oils) are known to increase the risk of breast disease, particularly animal fats.

Women in a study done in India had a reduction in pain and in the size of breast lumps in 12 of 17 women on a diet low in free fats (*National Medical Journal of India* 7, no. 2 [March-April 1994]: 60 to 2).

Allergies and food sensitivities represent one of the important causes of fibrocystic breast disease. These foods should be discovered and then eliminated indefinitely. (See "Elimination and Challenge Diet" in the *Dietary Information* section.)

Keep well hydrated so that normal breast secretions are thin and easily expelled.

Keep weight as low as is feasible since large breasts are more likely to develop cancer, and in a large breast it is also more difficult to find a small lump. Research indicates that women who weigh less than 140 have fewer cancers and less breast disease than women who weigh more than 140. It is of interest that women who are less than 5 feet 6 inches in height also have less tendency to breast malignancy.

A warm trunk but chilled extremities promotes breast disease by causing congestion and stagnation of blood circulation of the breasts. Wearing vests, lined jumpers, sleeveless garments, or shorts promotes overheating the breasts, but at the same time weakens the effectiveness of the immune system through chilled extremities.

Apply fomentations daily, a series of four alternating every four minutes with a cold compress. (See "Hydrotherapy" in the *Natural Remedies* section.)

If tenderness is present, wear a charcoal compress every night. (See "Charcoal Compress" in the *Natural Remedies* section.)

If the lesion is a cyst, it can be emptied usually with a vacuum tube setup such as is used for drawing blood from the arm. Enlist the help of someone trained in drawing blood using a syringe or a vacuum tube.

Inositol, 500 milligrams daily, can be helpful for women who suffer from fibrocystic breast disease.

Symptoms of fibrocystic disease can be reduced by increasing iodine intake. This procedure was discovered because of the use of caseinated iodine in animal husbandry to increase milk production in cattle. Probably 10 mgs daily of iodine for a month or two followed by that much per week for several months would be sufficient to improve both pain as well as lumpiness (*Oncology Times* 1, no. 1 [January 1984]: 12, 34).

Iodine has been established as a requirement for normal breast tissue, and deficiency results in atypical cell formation in rodents and severe hyperplasia and fibrocystic disease in women. These lesions are considered as slightly prone to be precancerous and can often be reversed by giving iodine therapy (*Biological Trace Element Research* 5: 399–412). Lugol's iodine is available in nearly all drug stores. Use three to eight drops in a glass of water daily, depending on the severity of the problem. Evening primrose oil, two grams (about two-fifths of a teaspoon) twice daily, can also help

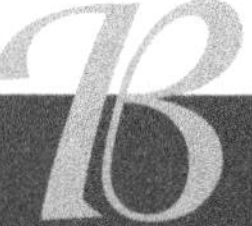

fibrocystic breast disease. When the fibrocystic breast disease improves both the iodine as well as the evening primrose oil can be reduced, but they should be taken in small quantities indefinitely.

For fibrocystic breast disease a diuretic tea can be successfully used to reduce engorgement of the breasts in the premenstrual phase. Doctor Torri Hudson uses Taraxacum leaf as a choice to reduce fluid engorgement of the breasts. Estrogenic effects are observed from the following herbs—foeniculum, angelica, red raspberries, red clover, and Arctium; and a progesterone effect has been observed in glycyrrhiza (licorice), Dioscorea, and smilax. These herbs can help to balance estrogen and progesterone in women who are imbalanced.

Nicotine stimulates the growth of breast tissues and should not be taken in any form.

Mastitis

Mastitis is an inflammation of the breast. It generally occurs between the fifth day postpartum to the second or third week, and is usually limited to one breast. Stasis of milk is an important factor in the development of mastitis. Symptoms include inflammation, redness, pain, fever, chills, and headache. Mastitis should be treated promptly to prevent abscess development. If treated within three to 18 hours of the first symptoms, abscesses are generally avoided. The cause is usually a blocked duct or ducts or an overfilled breast because of a greater milk supply than demand by the baby. It develops much like an acne pimple.

Treatment

Cold compresses can be used to reduce pain and promote healing. The inflammation should not be considered to be an infection as germs are rarely involved at the beginning of the problem, but it may develop after several days of untreated mastitis. The fever results from milk seepage into the tissues and bloodstream. In the blood, milk acts as a foreign protein and causes an intense fever if present in significant amounts.

Have the baby nurse the affected breast as soon as the mastitis is recognized. Nursing the infant from the affected breast as soon as tenderness is noted will often stop the process. By all means do not follow the old-fashioned advice to stop nursing as studies reveal mothers recover in an average of three days if they continue nursing. A control group of 30 women stopped nursing, and some of them had persistent inflammation with infections for an average of two months. Half of them had to have drainage of one or more abscesses. Infants do not have an ill effect from nursing the breast when it has mastitis.

Apply alternating hot and cold compresses three or four times a day, three minutes hot and one minute cold, for four exchanges. If the heat increases discomfort, use only cold compresses, twenty minutes at a time, changing the cold compress every two minutes, or using an ice bag over the compress to keep it cold. Repeat the treatment four times or more daily. A hot footbath may be used with either kind of treatment to reduce engorgement and congestion.

Support the breasts with a nursing bra, and nurse the affected breast twice as often, but for shorter periods of time. Try to keep the affected breast emptied.

Feeding the baby before the breasts become so enlarged that the infant has difficulty grasping the nipple is recommended. Since over-distended breasts are difficult for the baby to grasp, pulling the nipple out with the fingers, putting pressure on the breast behind the nipple to try to reduce engorgement, or expressing or pumping milk from the breasts may be helpful.

Apply comfrey poultices twice daily to the hard, painful area between the application of hot or cold treatments.

The mother should be careful to obtain plenty of rest throughout the treatment period. Frequent naps and rest periods during the day are recommended.

(See also "Clay Bath, Mud Bath" in the *Natural Remedies* section.)

Cracked Nipples

Mothers nursing their first baby are particularly susceptible to this distressing and intensely painful condition.

A small amount of breast milk expressed, rubbed on the nipple, and allowed to dry thoroughly in the air has good antibacterial components, a lubricating fat, and shows excellent healing rates based on studies.

If the nipple soreness is because of thrush in the baby's mouth, the application of vinegar to the nipples just after nursing can be very helpful. If vinegar stings too severely, try a paste of baking soda mixed with a little water or breast milk spread on the nipples and allowed to dry. As soon as the vinegar can be tolerated, it may speed healing more than the baking soda.

If the nipples become sore, an application of cold tea, which contains tannic acid, can promote healing. Ordinary pekoe tea from the grocery store or a preparation from the health food store such as witch hazel is satisfactory for this use. Moisten a folded facial tissue in the tea, lay it over the nipple for 20 minutes, dry, and expose to air for an additional 20 minutes. Rinse nipple before the next nursing.

If the infant is not permitted to nurse too long at one breast, the possibility of fissures of the nipple decrease. Some physicians limit feeding periods to five minutes on each breast for the first few days.

If the mother inserts a portion of the areola (the brown portion around the nipple) into the infant's mouth, his jaws will compress the milk pockets instead of merely the tip of the nipple; this will prevent much nipple soreness. Rubbing the nipple a bit will encourage it to become firm and stand out so the infant more readily grasps it. Pinching up the areola flattens the nipple to fit the infant's mouth better. At the end of feeding, to disengage the infant, place a finger inside the corner of the infant's mouth to allow air to enter the mouth and break the vacuum. After each nursing period it is very important that the nipples be washed with water to remove all saliva, as it contains an enzyme that will soften the skin. Water, vinegar, or alcohol applied to the nipples will toughen the skin and assist in preventing soreness.

The nipples should be checked daily, and if they are sore or cracked, treatment should begin promptly. This is important. Do not wait until the condition is well developed to begin treatment.

Exposing the breasts to the air for 20 minutes at a time, two or three times a day is helpful. The nipples may also be exposed to an ordinary lamp with a 40-watt bulb for 15 to 20 minutes, held one to two inches away from the breasts. This promotes healing. Even better than the light bulb is a 10 minute period of sunning daily.

Mothers should not use soap on the breasts as it is excessively drying without conditioning the skin, or it may cause sensitivity and may lead to cracking.

Plastic liners in the bra should be removed as they hold in moisture and keep the skin of the nipples soft and thin and more subject to cracking. If troubled with breast leakage, mother should use something absorbent such as a folded handkerchief or soft paper towel to absorb the moisture, changing it frequently as it becomes damp.

Changing nursing positions for each feeding assures that different areas of the nipple are subjected to equal stress from sucking.

If the baby is fed before he is overly hungry, he will not suckle the nipple too vigorously. Do not allow the infant to chew and macerate the nipple, opening the way for bacteria.

Breast Pain, Mastodynia

Pain in one or both breasts is most commonly an unexplained benign breast pain called mastodynia, which is caused by contraction or dilation of ducts and glandular tissue of the breast without disease being present. Benign breast tumors, breast cysts, inflamed fibrocystic disease, and even breast cancer may also cause pain. The pain of mastodynia is almost always worsened by the menstrual cycle or chronic fibrocystic disease. It can occasionally occur in postmenopausal women. It most frequently involves the upper outer quadrant that becomes slightly more firm, thick, and tender.

Breast pain may be localized in the breast, may radiate up the breast toward the anterior axillary line, proceed down the back of the arm, even down to the back of the hand. Breast pain may radiate from the breast directly in a horizontal path around behind the chest. Breast pain may radiate from the breast up the front of the chest wall to involve the neck on that side and even the front part of the shoulder on that side.

A large number of drugs will enlarge the breasts and make them tender both in men and women: Digitalis, Digitoxin, Digoxin, Aldomet, and other blood pressure drugs, Aldactone and other diuretics, Inderal and other beta blockers, Chlorpromazine and many mood altering medications, and estrogens. Sometimes female hormones or the use of vitamin E oil, either internally or rubbed on the skin, can cause breast pain.

Shingles can cause pain in only one breast. Early pregnancy may cause pain in one or both breasts, as can milk engorgement after childbirth. Liver damage caused by alcoholism can cause enlargement and pain both in men and women.

Causes of ductal pain may be developmental, related to habitually chilled extremities in childhood and youth, or to over-clothing the chest or breast area by vests, pinafores, heavy jumpers, padded bras, or overly sensitive ducts that dilate in response to a number of stimuli.

Treatment

1. Eliminate chocolate and other brown drinks from the diet
2. Same treatment as for acne
3. Hydrotherapy, such as fomentations
4. Cold compresses
5. Charcoal compresses

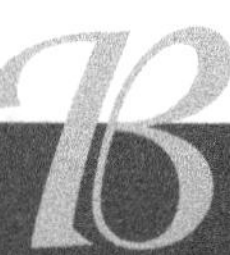

Gynecomastia

The newborn male or female infant may have a swelling under the nipple at birth because of the mother's pregnancy hormones. Boys at puberty sometimes develop hard lumps under the nipple, which usually disappear spontaneously after puberty. This condition is known as gynecomastia. It is entirely benign and requires no treatment, as it will go away in a few months or years without causing either physical or emotional damage. Fatty deposits in the breasts of some men at any age, because of obesity, alcohol abuse, liver damage, or sometimes as a result of body-building hormones, also imitate this disorder. Tenderness may or may not be present.

Bronchiectasis

This disease is a chronic and permanent enlargement of major or minor air passages, which produces an accumulation of mucus and chronic infection, resulting in violent coughing with pus filled sputum, anemia, offensive breath, fever, weight loss, night sweats, and coughing up blood.

It is the result of such diseases as whooping cough, asthma, tuberculosis, pneumonia, or aspiration of foreign bodies that leave partial destruction and permanent dilation and chronic infection of several bronchi and air sacs in a cluster. Diagnosis is by X-ray or other imaging studies.

Treatment

Rest, proper food, fresh air (both day and night, good weather and bad), and sunshine are the usual fundamentals of treatment.

Good hydration is at a premium in these individuals to keep the secretions thin and easy to cough up. The patient should cough in a succession of small coughs and then a forceful cough after deeply inhaling to induce a strong cough reflex.

Tight clothing around the chest or abdomen should be avoided, as should gas forming foods, all of which reduce breathing capacity.

The extremities should be kept well clothed, and the person should avoid crowds, poorly ventilated rooms containing smoke fumes or dust, drafts, and those who are sick with respiratory illnesses. At the first sign of sickness, treatment should be instituted with determination and persistence.

Oral hygiene should be scrupulous, as transfer of germs to the lungs is more common with poor oral hygiene.

If secretions tend to accumulate, the patient should use a slant board or hang the head and shoulders down from a table for twenty minutes twice daily. Elderly persons should avoid this postural drainage to keep from increasing the pressure in the arteries in the head. For them, the foot of their beds may be elevated six to eight inches to encourage drainage.

A vaporizer used at night or in dry weather may assist in keeping secretions thin, maintaining 30 to 50 percent humidity or more. Cough medications and antihistamines should be avoided.

Learn to wear a mask during pollen season or while sweeping and dusting.

The antibacterial herbs may be of real value, especially during acute flare-ups (see the *Herbal Remedies* section). Use garlic, which may be steamed if desired, four to six cloves a day, or use a good quality dehydrated or cold-aged garlic such as Kyolic tablets or liquid. A tea or tincture made of echinacea and golden seal is quite helpful for acute flare-ups. Use a cup of the tea every two hours or a teaspoon of the tincture.

Some form of surgery is sometimes necessary if the person cannot accomplish proper control of the symptoms of coughing and fever by the modalities mentioned. The affected area or lobe of the lung may have to be removed, provided the disease is confined to a relatively small area. If it is generalized, surgery is not possible.

Bronchitis

(See "Coughs" and "Pneumonia" in the *Conditions and Diseases* section.)

Bronchopneumonia

This is a type of inflammation of the lungs. This type of pneumonia may not start as abruptly as other types of pneumonia. Symptoms such as fever, coughing, and shortness of breath gradually become worse. It may run its course in 5 to 10 days, or may require weeks to recover. The temperature gets lower step by step with recovery. (See "Pneumonia" in the *Conditions and Diseases* section for treatment options.)

Bruxism

(See "Dental Care" in the *Conditions and Diseases* section.)

Buerger's Disease

Thromboangiitis obliterans (Buerger's disease) has the highest incidence in Jews but may occur also in some Asians, beginning most frequently between the ages of 20 and 45, and involving 75 men to one woman. The walls of the blood vessels are thickened and scarred, and may eventually close off entirely, especially in the feet.

Buerger's disease may start with pain in one leg, and later spread to the other. The legs may become cold, and spasms of the blood vessels can occur. Swelling, ulceration, and gangrene may ensue. Buerger's disease involves the legs more often than any other part of the body, sometimes spreading to the arms and heart. One of the most important aspects of Buerger's disease is its relationship to smoking. For years it has been recognized that smoking could make it worse, or even cause Buerger's disease. Patients having Buerger's disease may become intensely addicted to tobacco. We have seen tobacco get such a hold on a person that even with all four extremities amputated, they would still demand that an attendant hold a cigarette to the lips, eventually dying of a heart attack.

The disease often starts with persistent chilliness of the extremities with numbness, tingling, blueness, and aching. The legs may diminish in size, the skin may lose its hair, and the person may experience lameness or pain with walking.

Treatment

Discover any food sensitivities. (See "Elimination and Challenge Diet" in the *Dietary Information* section.)

Avoid all free fats such as margarine, mayonnaise, fried foods, cooking fats, and salad oils. Free fats can cause sluggish blood flow through small blood vessels and increase the likelihood of clotting.

Avoid tobacco, even secondhand smoke. Tobacco causes blood vessels to constrict and blood to become more likely to clot inside the blood vessels.

Make certain that the extremities are always well clothed, as chilling increases tightening of blood vessels and clotting potential of the blood. Especially clothe the arms and thighs well to ensure warm hands and feet.

Nothing should be allowed to constrict circulation such as girdles, tight shoes, belts, chairs that put pressure on the thighs, crossing the knees, etc.

Because of the danger of gangrene, people with this condition are urged to take good care of their feet. Keep the toenails trimmed, wear properly fitting shoes, take care of any injury or breaks in the skin immediately to avoid infection. Even very minor scratches can result in gangrene in a Buerger's patient.

Combat tension with exercise. Guard against injury to the extremities as injuries may take a long time to heal. Exercise can assist in sprouting new blood vessels to help supply blood to areas that may have gotten closed off.

Perform the Buerger exercises listed here.

- Lie flat in bed with both legs elevated above the level of the heart for two or three minutes.
- Sit on the edge of the bed with the legs dependent for three minutes.
- Exercise the feet and toes by moving them up, down, inward, outward, and around.
- Return to the first position and hold it for about five minutes.

Repeat these exercises several times during one exercise period and perform periodically throughout the day.

Have a 20-minute massage of the arms and legs three times per week.

Take niacin as a trial to see if it can be of help. Use only 50 to 100 milligrams taken just after meals to minimize the unpleasant flush. Do not use sustained action niacin as it may damage the liver.

Take ginkgo tea, one cup four times a day; or two capsules four times daily. Hawthorn berry tea also has a beneficial effect on heart and blood vessels. One cup three or four times a day may be mixed with ginkgo if taken as tea or may be taken as a tincture, 30 to 40 drops four times daily.

Bulimia and Anorexia

Bulimia is defined as recurring binge eating with a minimum of two binge episodes a week for at least three months and a feeling of uncontrollable eating during the binges. The person will have the regular use of one or more of the following factors to prevent weight gain: self-induced vomiting after binging, use of laxatives or diuretics, strict dieting or fasting when not binging, or vigorous exercise. There may also be excessive concern with body shape and weight.

Between 1985 and 1995 the number of cases of bulimia doubled in the United States. The same can be said for anorexia, which is pathological under-eating resulting in weight loss of at least 15 percent below the normal range.

Bulimia is not as easily detected as anorexia, and bulimics can go for years without revealing their disease. Those

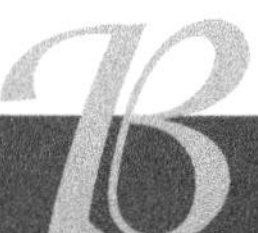

suffering from eating disorders have an excellent chance for complete recovery if they will remain connected to others. The treatment of an eating disorder is also the treatment of an entire family.

More people recover from bulimia than anorexia, as more than 80 percent of patients recover. The complications of bulimia are usually related to the method of purging—self-induced vomiting creates problems in the mouth or with the teeth and sometimes in the esophagus; and the abuse of diuretics and laxatives may produce intestinal, metabolic, and systemic effects. The teeth may become quite eroded from stomach acid, which bathes the teeth during vomiting.

Dr. Alexander Schauss says that bulimia includes an obsessive-compulsive component that involves food and problems of excess weight loss or gain which threaten health. With bulimia some patients consume as much as 20,000 calories at one sitting—not one day, but one sitting. Anorexia affects women at about the rate of 25 for every one man affected. For bulimia the rate is about 85 percent female and 15 percent male. Anorexia generally begins at about the age of 12 to 14, and bulimia usually begins between 15 to 25, but no age is exempt. Bulimics may also be depressed. Antidepressant drugs are frequently found in the history of a person with bulimia.

Test for Bulimia Using a Zinc Supplement

Since zinc is an essential part of a key molecule to produce the sensation of taste, a solution of a zinc tablet to a normal individual "tastes terrible." For the person with bulimia, the zinc solution has no taste at all, or very little. Zinc sulphate at a concentration of 1 milligrams of zinc per cubic centimeter of fluid is most commonly used for this test. Tablets can be obtained in most natural food stores. Make up the solution by crushing a zinc tablet in water. The proper concentration is adjusted to 15 milligrams per tablespoon of water. If the zinc tablets are 50 milligrams in size, crush it in three tablespoons plus one teaspoon of water. Use one teaspoon of the solution for the test.

Treatment

Both anorexia and bulimia can be treated with zinc, about 50 milligrams per day. The symptoms usually improve before the taste test does. Expect to engage in treatment for three to six months or more.

Tryptophan, which is converted to serotonin in the brain and other nerve tissues, can be used to treat bulimia. If vitamin B6 is given with the tryptophan, it increases the conversion of tryptophan to serotonin. In eleven patients given three grams per day for one month, significant improvements in eating behavior were noted. No side effects were reported ("L-tryptophan as an Adjunct to Treatment of Bulimia Nervosa," *Lancet* 2 [1989]: pp. 1162, 1163).

It is good for the bulimic person to have a close companion of the same sex, but it can be someone of the opposite sex if someone, who can watch the bulimic carefully for weeks until the old habits are broken and new habits are well established.

Case Report

We had a 22-year-old nursing student who came to our center for bulimia. Shortly after she arrived we had an elderly retired military chaplain to arrive with his daughter who had Down's syndrome. The elderly chaplain had had skin cancer (melanoma) removed a few weeks before and came for a postoperative boost to his immune system. The young bulimic became friends with the chaplain and his daughter. We asked him if he and his daughter could watch over the girl and help her recover.

For the next five weeks the three of them walked up and down a broad highway near Uchee Pines Institute about eight miles a day. They prayed together several times daily, and they studied the Bible morning and evening. The woman with Down's slept in the same room with the young nurse. She was rarely out of sight of either the father or the Down's woman. Not one binging episode occurred. She felt strong enough to ask for a volunteer job with the institute. Her position was in the office, far removed from food. She was assigned to live and take her meals with a single woman on campus who watched her food expenditures closely and gave little opportunity for sneak binging. For the last eight years she has lived alone but has had almost unbroken victory over binging. Her last binge was a short, single episode lasting only a few hours about six years after her visit to the institute.

Burning Feet

Burning feet is a sensation that your feet are painfully hot, and the problem can be mild or severe. In some cases, burning feet may be so painful that it interferes with sleep.

Some causes of burning feet include fatigue, infections such as athlete's foot, or nerve damage because of diabetes or exposure to toxins. Chemotherapy for cancer is prone to cause burning feet.

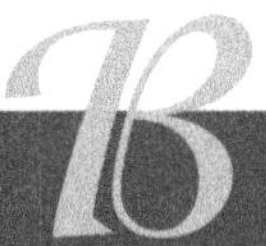

A woman in her early fifties reported that she started taking 1200 units of vitamin E daily (400 units three times a day) and that her restless leg problem along with burning feet went away. The restless legs were completely healed in about three weeks of beginning taking the large dose of vitamin E.

Rub castor oil generously into the areas of burning, massaging the oil into the skin of the feet for about five minutes. Castor oil increases the number of T-cells under the skin of the area where it is used, therefore, increasing the immune system capabilities. Cover with a bread bag slipped over the feet, over which socks are rolled to hold the bread bags in place. If castor oil alone does not alleviate the problem, soak the feet in warm Epsom salt water (one-fourth cup per gallon of water) for 30 minutes, then rub castor oil into the feet and proceed as described. One patient received benefit from taking 1200 IU of vitamin D every day. Try some detoxifying herbs such as milk thistle and St. John's wort.

Burning feet has been associated with thallium excess. Other symptoms of thallium excess are muscle cramps, numbness in the fingers and toes, intestinal problems, heart rhythm problems, and hair loss. Any or all of these symptoms may be attributed to thallium excess. Sources of thallium have been found in air and soil near toxic waste dumps, near cement plants, smelting plants, and wherever thallium compounds are processed. Food grown on these soils even years after the contamination has been removed or cleaned up may represent a major source of exposure. Water and inhalation are other sources. Smokers have twice as much thallium as nonsmokers. Colloidal minerals may indicate levels of thallium on the label. A hair analysis is a reliable indicator for thallium excess.

Treatment of thallium excess can be with activated charcoal or Prussian blue, or both, which interrupts the enterohepatic cycling of thallium, encouraging fecal elimination of the metal. The method of treating cesium contamination with Prussian blue is the same as for thallium excess. Give three grams by mouth three times for 30 to 60 days. Then drop down to one or two grams of Prussian blue daily until the thallium level falls. Brewer's yeast and foods high in potassium are also very helpful to prevent thallium-induced toxicity and to increase renal excretion of thallium (*Great Smokies Diagnostic Laboratory*, Asheville, NC, 1998). Cilantro and spirulina are able to assist in the excretion of heavy metals and may be of help in the thallium excretion. (See "Food Sources High in Certain Nutrients" in the *Dietary Information* section.)

Garlic in large quantities daily can assist in the elimination of thallium from the body. Use from one to three fresh cloves three times a day with food, or as much as a whole globe of garlic steamed or baked, two or three times a day with meals. It is well worth a try.

Burns

(See "Burns" in the *Home Emergencies* section.)

Bursitis

Bursae are small, flat, fluid-filled sacs near the shoulders, elbows, hips, knees, and ankles. They assist in smooth and easy movements of these structures by cushioning and aiding muscles and tendons to glide past each other. Bursitis is an inflammation of this small sac. After middle age the tendons are prone to degenerative changes, and these sacs may begin to have calcium deposited in the area of the degenerating tendons, causing inflammation.

Bursitis often develops in people who have been cutting hedges, moving furniture, shoveling snow, or shopping and carrying heavy bags with one hand or by shoulder bags. The pain begins as an uneasy feeling about the shoulder which progresses to considerable pain within 6 to 12 hours. There may be a bit of swelling at the tip of the shoulder, which is the most common place for bursitis. It may also occur over the hip, in the foot, or in the arms.

Women are more prone to develop bursitis than men because their shoulders slope more sharply. The sloping causes increased pressure on the bursae. Weight lifters and sedentary workers are also very prone to bursitis.

Prevention

Avoid injury to the joints that are especially vulnerable to bursitis. A strain, a direct blow, the stress of overweight, unusual shoulder or knee motions such as from painting, swimming, lifting heavy objects at arm's length, etc., may precipitate bursitis.

Allergies and infections in the body elsewhere may precipitate bursitis. Live at a high level of health to avoid bursitis.

Do not allow excessive fatigue to develop while doing an unusual motion to which you are unaccustomed. When carrying heavy objects like boxes for some distance, the best position is in front of one, using both hands, holding the object somewhat like a tray.

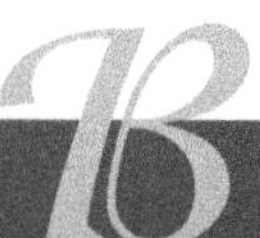

Do not allow chilling of the extremities, as that puts tension on muscles surrounding the inflamed bursae, particularly the shoulders, which are especially vulnerable at night. Be careful to wear warm sleepwear.

Drink plenty of water to minimize your risks for any skeletal problems including bursitis, backache, strains, and fatigue.

Treatment

Initially, apply ice applications by means of packs or an ice massage. (See "Hydrotherapy" in the *Natural Remedies* section.) The packs are applied for 30 minutes every two to three hours. The ice massage is done by rubbing the area with ice for 12 to 15 minutes. It may be repeated three times or more every day.

As pain begins to decrease after a few days, hot applications can begin. After 45 to 60 minutes of the application of heat, the range of motion exercises should begin. These may be either actively done by the patient or passively done by a helper, or by swinging a limp extremity as described below.

Watch out for chilling during the night while sleeping.

Do not allow injury of the painful area, and do not repeat the activity that caused the inflammation.

Never begin heavy work until you have "warmed up" by doing some light work.

There are certain exercises for bursitis in the shoulder that increase blood circulation and prevent freezing or fixation of the bursae. Use after any hot or cold treatment:

- Face the wall at arm's length and lean into your hands, which should be placed against the wall. Starting slightly above the level of the waist, walk hand over hand as high as you can reach without pain. As you make progress bounce a bit to alternate hands, and reach higher with each bounce before pain or tightness stops you. Repeat the exercise four times daily.

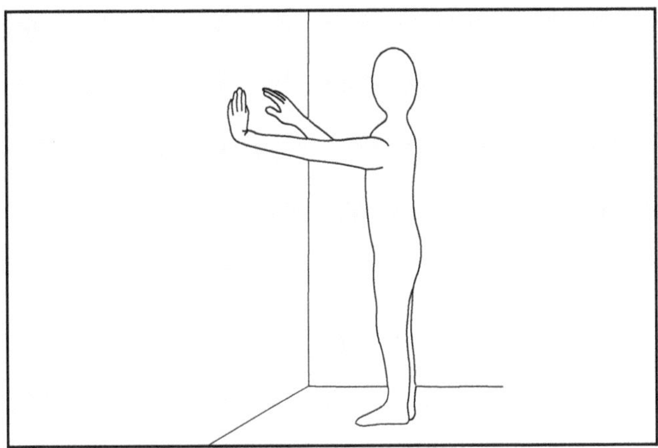

- A small pulley rigged up over the head with a two to five pound weight attached is helpful after the acute phase is over. Pull the arm down by the side and let the weight pull the arm over the head. Start with 5 to 10 pulls and work up to 50 pulls three times a day.

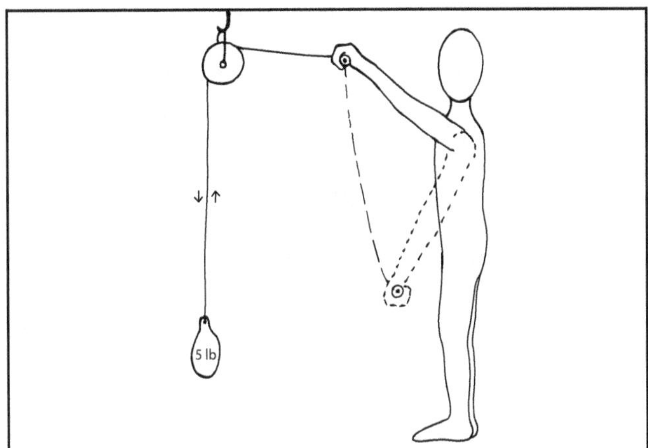

- A bicycle wheel with a small handle attached and mounted shoulder-high to an outside wall or tree can be used to good advantage to get a good range of motion of the shoulder, avoiding a "frozen shoulder."

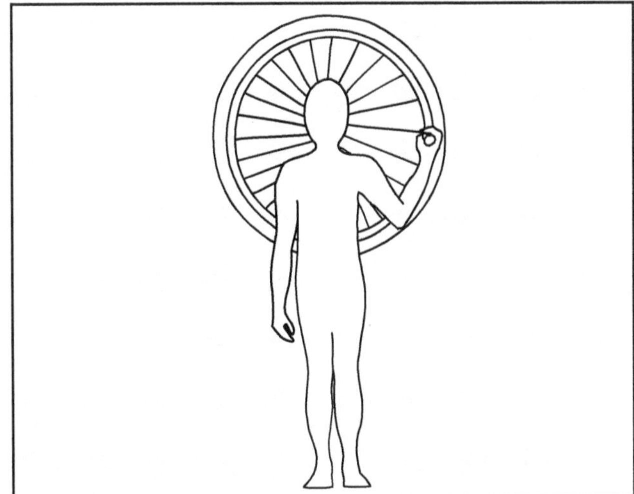

- We do not recommend heavy massage, but we find a light finger massage with aloe vera cream or arnica may promote healing. Following hot or cold applications (choose the one the patient finds most soothing), a very light rubbing of the area, not firm enough to cause major displacement of the tissues or compression of the inflamed bursae, can be very helpful.
- Make a circle with the hand and arm dangling loosely while bending over at the waist until the chest is parallel with the floor. This exercise can be done better if the unaffected arm is used to support the person while

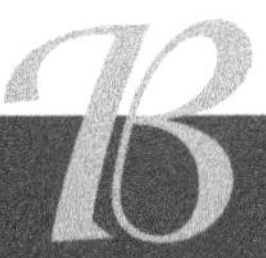

bending over. Grasp the edge of a table or lean the elbow on the table while trying to swing the arm and hand in a circle using a motion of the trunk, not the arm muscles. Increase the size of the circle from day to day making 15 to 20 complete circles.

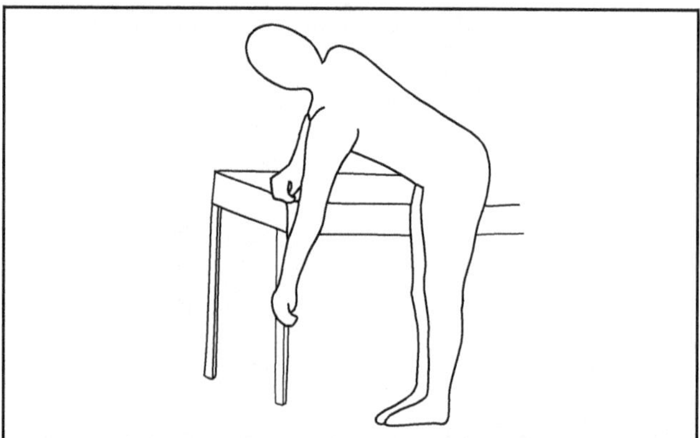

- Slowly extend the affected arm back and up, then front and up. Raise it outward and up. Repeat this exercise for 10 minutes, using the opposite hand and arm as a symmetrical balance.

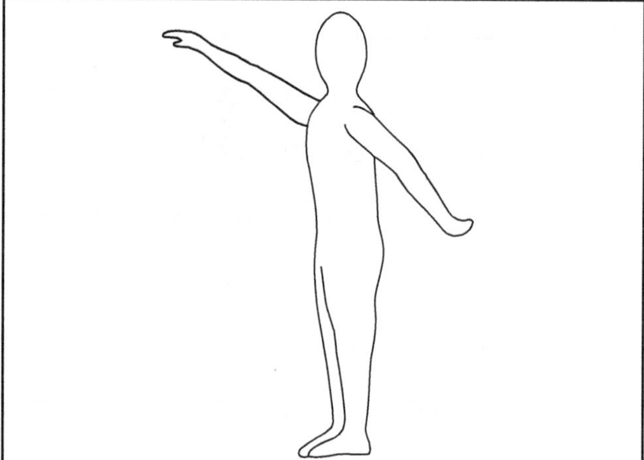

- Continue the usual, accustomed activities as permitted by the pain or stiffness.

Heat applications may relieve pain, but sometimes make it worse. If heat is unpleasant, use ice.

Ice packs to the painful area, especially in the acute phase, may relieve pain. Keep the ice on for about five to seven minutes. Remove for one minute, and repeat three times.

Three minutes of hot compresses as hot as can be tolerated, followed immediately by 20 seconds of ice water compresses, repeated four times, three to four times daily will often help.

A short period of complete rest for the part may decrease the inflammation. A sling may be worn with much comfort. Do not prolong the period of inactivity beyond one week as stiffness may result.

Cancer

This serious disease comes in many stages. Long before a cancer is detectable, it has had its initiating stages. In these stages the cancer is the most curable with simple home remedies. Once it is visible, or palpable, the next best course is usually surgery.

Cancer is one of the more serious and upsetting diagnoses one can get. Often the costs of cancer are high; and the level of disability can be great. Therefore, it is desirable to do whatever is possible to reduce one's risks for cancer. We should start with trying to understand the known causes and methods of prevention of cancer.

Causes and Prevention

About 5 to 10 percent of cancers are linked to inherited faulty genes.

Abdominal fat and upper body fat predominating over hip and thigh fat indicates a genetic pattern that helps predict breast cancer risks (*Cancer Detection and Prevention* 17, no. 1 [1993]: 283–382). Simply stated, it is better to be pear shaped than apple shaped.

Apparently using water from a municipal water supply increases one's risk of cancer. Tap water from a municipal water supply or well water in a farming community can be loaded with toxins; use a water filter if necessary ("Nine Ways to Reduce the Risk of Breast Cancer," *Naturalnews.com*, October 23, 2009). Distilled water may be your best option.

Exposure to herbicides and pesticides increases risk of developing cancer (*Am J Ind Med 39, no. 1 [Jan. 2001]:92-9*).

Asbestos powder, both in buildings and in dusting powders, increases risk of ovarian cancer (when powder is used on the private areas) and mesotheliomas.

Blood transfusions increase the risk of lymphomas and kidney cancer (*British Journal of Cancer* 73 [1996]: 1148).

Testicular cancer in men increases with exposure to xenoestrogens in the environment such as found in dental sealants for children, estrogens fed to cattle, and many agricultural products.

The *Helicobacter pylori* infection of the stomach, which produces gastric and peptic ulcers, increases risk of stomach cancer and B-cell lymphoma (*Journal of the American Medical Association* 275 [1996]: 937–39).

Electromagnetic fields pose a hazard for childhood leukemia, and brain and lung cancers (*American Journal of Epidemiology* 144 [1996]: 150; 134, no. 9 [1991]: 923; 137 [1993]: 609; 144 [1996]: 1107; *Postgraduate Medicine* 100, no. 2 [1996]: 183). Included in this potential risk are electric blankets, diagnostic imaging procedures (especially CT scans, mammograms, MRIs, and X-rays for trauma).

Poultry and dairy farmers are more likely to get multiple myeloma and leukemia than city dwellers (*Science* 213 [Aug. 1981]: 1014).

Using black or brown hair coloring products increases the risk of non-Hodgkin's lymphoma and multiple myeloma.

Many cholesterol reducing drugs cause cancer in rodents, and the use of these drugs in humans should be seriously questioned. However, reducing blood cholesterol naturally through diet and exercise also reduces the risk of certain cancers (*Journal of the American Medical Association.* 275 [1996]: 55).

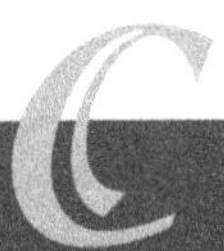

Animals such as monkeys, chickens, cats, dogs, horses, and cattle have all been implicated as cancer virus carriers. We recommend that these animals, if kept at all, be separated some distance from the house and have their own housing. Hands should be washed after touching or feeding them. Be careful with sick animals, especially pets. Sick pets are not for petting. Childhood leukemia has been postulated to be a zoonosis (a disease from animals) (*Journal of Cancer Research and Clinical Oncology* 121 [1995]: S12).

A strong link exists between the use of pharmaceutical diuretics and the occurrence of kidney cancer in both men and women (*Journal of the National Cancer Institute* 77 [1986]: 351; *American Journal of Epidemiology* 140 [1994]: 792–804). Aspirin, diuretics, immunosuppressants, Tolbutamide, Tofranil, and Tapazole (for lowering cholesterol) have all been associated with cancer. Amphetamines have shown an association with the development of Hodgkin's disease. It can easily be seen that drugs of all kinds may be a hazard so far as increasing one's risk for getting cancer. A range of top-selling drugs used to treat high blood pressure has been linked with an increased risk of cancer. Calcium channel blockers are found to be twice as likely to be associated with cancer as are other antihypertensive drugs. Antidepressants (Prozac), antihistamines (Claritin, Benadryl), and senna, an irritating herb found in such products as Senokot, may have mutagenic effects. Nonhormonal drugs (meaning drugs of any kind other than hormones) account for a certain proportion of all human cancers (*Journal of the National Cancer Institute* 86 [1994]: 770; *Cancer Research* 52 [1994]: 3796; *Environmental Health Perspectives* 103, no. S8 [1995]: 191).

Stresses of life and bleak expectations about oneself with a sense of hopelessness increase the risk of both heart disease and cancer (*Science News* 149 [1996]: 230). There is an increased risk of getting lung cancer among persons with a depressed mood (*American Journal of Epidemiology* 144 [1996]: 1096). A chronic irritation or infection, any viral illness, early in life sexual activities, or a kidney transplant all increase one's risk of cancer. Excessive sexual activities increase both cervical and foreskin cancer and possibly prostate cancer.

An association exists between cancer and certain diseases such as diabetes, obesity, and high blood cholesterol. Diabetics have more cancer of all kinds. A lifestyle that encourages diabetes will also encourage cancer. The weakening of the immune system from these diseases may open the door for cancer.

Treatment for Cancer

Despite CT scans, nuclear scans, ultrasound scans, new techniques for surgery, new machines to deliver radiation, and new drugs for chemotherapy, cancer survival statistics are no better than they were in the 1960s. Nobody on earth at this time has discovered a cure for cancer. While it is true that we often see a treatment produce what appears to be a cure, most cancers, treated in any way known, have a great likelihood of recurring. There are certain factors which can aid in treating cancer, regardless of the basic method used.

Self-control in all aspects of lifestyle is very important to the overall health of an individual fighting cancer. This includes total avoidance of tobacco, alcohol, and recreational drugs. This also includes avoidance of the "brown drinks"—coffee, tea, colas, and probably chocolate—as these have been associated with an increase in certain cancers, notably cancer of the ovaries, breast, bladder, pancreas, prostate, and certain gastrointestinal cancers. Besides dispensing with harmful substances, practicing abstemiousness also includes the moderate and judicious use of those things which are good for us. For example, nutritious food is not only good for us, but vital to life; however, if eaten in excess, it saps the very life force it was designed to strengthen. Natural killer cells increase in number and ability to fight cancer cells in animals that are restricted in their food to approximately 60 percent. Food restricted mice have strong anticancer immunity and, as a result, cancer growth is suppressed and survival time prolonged in these mice (*Journal of Nutrition* 130 [2000]: 111).

God will supply power and help to overcome once and for all health-destroying practices. A few of theses are overeating, snacking between meals, use of harmful food items or overuse of marginal items (such as commercial fruit juices, white rice, margarine), purging, indulgence of unhealthful habits such as the use of caffeine, nicotine, alcohol; prescription or nonprescription drug usage, and all improper expressions of sexuality, overworking, television viewing, and late bedtimes.

Often those with cancer have a compromised respiratory system and thus need some outside assistance. There are various products on the market that will increase oxygen delivery to the cells. Some of these, such as CoQ10, magnesium, dimethyl glycine, niacin, Panax ginseng, and thiamine have been recommended as quite beneficial in such cases. L-arginine, 1,000 milligrams on an empty stomach, relaxes arterioles and increases blood flow. Sources of negative air ions include the following: evergreen trees, beach surf,

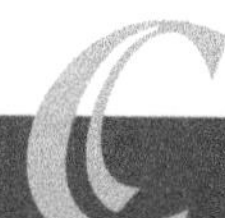

thunderstorms, and natural outdoor environments. Early morning air has more negative ions than later in the day.

The human body rebuilds itself during the hours of darkness and while the person is asleep. It has been shown that every hour before midnight is twice as effectual in this respect as the hours after midnight. A person with cancer needs this healing and rebuilding time. Ben Franklin was right when he said. "Early to bed, early to rise, makes a man healthy, wealthy, and wise."

A special way of treating the body is through fasting. Omitting one to three meals weekly, unless underweight, can do much good. This means taking no food or juice, only pure water. When a person fasts, the energy normally used to digest food is available to fight cancer. Fasting is not, however, recommended in all cases. Insulin-dependent diabetics, those with gout, and those having poor nutrient reserves should not fast. A 10-day fast can be safely self-administered in a normal person. When breaking this fast, take only tiny amounts of food three times daily, gradually increasing the quantity day by day. The principle of breaking a fast is to spend as much time breaking it as you spent on it, gradually increasing the quantity of food meal by meal for the number of days in the fast.

For many people, much of the day's activity is centered around looking for misplaced things, picking up mislaid articles, rearranging items, and catching up on forgotten chores. Such people need to adopt a lifestyle of regularity, routine, order, and predictability of daily activities. Such a lifestyle will create peaceful islands of rest in an otherwise restless sea of activity. Cancer patients must have these islands of refuge. Simplicity and quietness of living should be the goal.

Create a daily schedule. Eat meals at the same time every day within half an hour or so. Rise and retire at set times. If you are not sleeping well at night, do not nap during the afternoon. Arise on schedule. Do not sleep late and take breakfast off schedule. A nap before lunch can be taken instead.

Keep the Sabbath holy. You need this special day of rest. God made the Sabbath for man's body, soul, and spirit. He especially blesses those who commune with Him on that day by spending every possible moment in Bible reading, meditation, prayer, study of spiritual lessons in nature, and family time together. Always maintain a restful state of mind every day. Refuse to defend yourself or to argue, worry, or complain.

Especially when done in the open air and sunshine, exercise can increase the endorphins which do "good like a medicine" and increase white blood cell activity, lower stress, and greatly improve circulation. In cancer, as in all diseases, circulation is paramount. Without good circulation, one cannot enjoy good health. And without exercise, one cannot enjoy good circulation. Try not to miss any exercise periods! Work up to a progressively more vigorous program. Twenty minutes per day is minimal. One hour daily is better, but on certain days three to five hours may be needed. Gradually build to a good exercise level without ever developing sore muscles. And for those weekend exercisers, those who save it all up for a few hours of furious activity; such exercise is viewed by the body as stress. Spread it out over the week and get a week's worth of benefit rather than a day's worth of stress. Gardening and walking may be the best forms of exercise. Do gentle exercise after meals for a few minutes. An easy walk or light gardening is beneficial. Exercise has been shown to increase the number of specific receptors on the surface of monocytes, a form of immune cell in the body. This process is equivalent to increasing the number of guns on the cell so that it can be more active in destroying cancer cells (*Anticancer Research* 15 [1995]: 175).

Sunlight increases the production of lymphocytes. The lymphocyte is also capable of producing a substance called interferon, which is effective against several different kinds of cancer, including carcinoma, sarcoma, and leukemia. Take a 20 to 60 minute sunbath daily. One does not need to expose the entire body all the time, but especially the face and arms. Sunshine furnishes vitamin D for strengthening normal tissue cells against invasion by cancer.

The best food for humans was prescribed in Eden six thousand years ago and that was before cancer ever reared its ugly head. People who adhere to this diet, such as Seventh-day Adventists as reported in the *Saturday Evening Post* of March 1984 and the *National Geographic* cover story of November 2005 enjoy healthier and happier lives and have less cancer than other persons. How much more in this age of cancer should we be following the perfect diet designed for a perfect people? It has been statistically proven that those who most closely adhere to this diet have a much lower incidence of cancer as well as all other diseases. So what is this diet? Fruits, vegetables, whole grains, legumes, nuts, and seeds.

Try to eat 50 to 80 percent of the meal raw for the first three months of the treatment period for cancer. Even when foods are cooked they should not be overdone, and it is vital that you avoid scorched foods which are in themselves carcinogenic. Put at least five hours between the end of one meal and the beginning of the next. Eat a substantial breakfast and lunch; supper should be omitted unless you are underweight, and if eaten, it should be only whole grains or fruit. A two meal plan allows the body the greatest opportunity

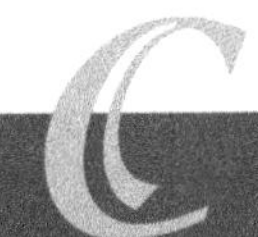

for recovery. While one is chewing food, digestive enzymes, secreted by the salivary glands, are beginning the work of digestion right there in the mouth. Basically, our food should be chewed to a creamy consistency before it is swallowed. Finally, you can and should, with assurance, bow your head and ask God to bless your food.

Foods as Anticancer Agents

There are many foods containing properties or nutrients that help fight cancer in one way or another. Some act as carcinogen inhibitors, some as direct anticancer nutrients, and some inhibit blood vessel growth into the growing cancer while some interfere in enzyme systems needed to grow the cells. We will now consider a few of these anticancer properties of foods.

Antioxidants are plentiful in fruits, vegetables, whole grains, legumes, nuts, and seeds. Many micronutrients such as the carotenoids, vitamin E, selenium, and vitamin C protect the body against free radicals. Selenium in particular seems to have a protective role against the development of ovarian cancer (*Journal of the National Cancer Institute* 88 [1996]: 32) and certain cancers in various parts of the body (*Alternative Therapies in Health and Medicine* 2, no. 4 [1996]: 59; *Cancer Epidemiology, Biomarkers and Prevention* 5 [March 1996]: 233). Selenium is found in whole grain wheat, brown rice, rye, corn, oats and oatmeal, nuts, seeds, and all vegetables. One Brazil nut contains 50 to 60 micrograms of selenium, 70 to 80 micrograms being the daily requirement.

Low levels of vitamins A, C, and E in the blood give one a greater chance of coming down with cancer (*J Natl Cancer Inst 91, no. 6 [Mar 17, 1999]:547-56*), especially lung cancer and prostate cancer. Vitamin E comes from beans, nuts, avocado, olives, seeds, and whole grains (*International Journal of Cancer* 66 [1996]: 145). Other foods containing powerful anticancer properties include grapes, lemons, carrots, asparagus, broccoli and all its relatives, tomatoes, garlic, all berries, onions, apples, and especially whole unprocessed soybeans. Phytosterols decrease cancer risks (*Linus Pauline Institute Research Newsletter* [Spring/Summer 2008]: 4). Sitosterol, a phytosterol, increases apoptosis (spontaneous death) in cancer cells (prostate, breast, colon).

Restricted eating, that is limiting the times one eats to two meals taken during a six hour period each day, and fasting the other 18 hours has been shown to reduce the number of cancer in a population group. In animal studies there were 93 percent fewer cancers than on an on-demand meal pattern such as most people in the western world take. Studies done by Gavin Greenoak and Ray Kearney at Sydney University in Australia produced this striking finding.

Foods and Food Characteristics Promoting Cancer

One must be particular to avoid fermented foods, which contain toxic amines as products of the fermentation process. That includes a number of foods usually considered to be healthful. Scorched foods should also be avoided as they contain advanced glycation end products, which are carcinogenic. Rancid or aged fats act as pro-oxidants and counteract the good a person could get from antioxidants. Chips, toasted nuts, and packaged foods containing oils or eggs are more likely to become rancid before the product is used. The consumption of cured meats, most notably bacon, increases one's risk of getting cancer as it increases the dietary sources of certain nitrogen based compounds that are precursors of nitrosamines, cancer producing chemicals.

There are at least seven cancers that are associated with a high fat intake. These include cancer of the skin, prostate, breast, colon, pancreas, liver, and endometrium. That other cancers may be involved with a diet high in free fats seems unquestionable. Dietary fish oil increases risk for pancreatic cancer. Saturated animal fat increases risks of several cancers such as bowel, lung, endometrium, and prostate (*Oncology* 52 [1995]: 265).

An increase in blood viscosity (that means heavy blood because of high levels of cells, minerals, proteins, various chemicals, nutrients, supplements, and waste products, as well as low water intake) increases the likelihood of cardiovascular, hypertensive diseases, and cancer. A persistent elevation of any of the factors which can increase blood viscosity should be recognized as a major risk factor, and efforts should be made to bring viscosity down (*Blood Viscosity in Heart Disease and Cancer,* eds. L Dintenfass, G. V. F. Seaman [Pergamon Press, 1981).

Donate blood to the Red Cross. Drink at least eight glasses of water daily. Cut down on your food intake. Do not use nutrient supplements.

Therapeutic Plants

Many medicinal herbs and other common plants have strong anticancer properties. In the last hundred years much study has been given to the properties of herbs. Dr. James Duke has spent much time studying plants of the Amazon region. His research has resulted in a marvelous database on the properties of herbs. This database is available online. Those

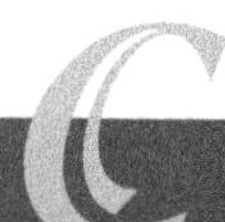

who wish to take more responsibility for their own health would do well to become familiar with this database and refer to it or some similar database.

Some herbs recognized as having anticancer activity include ginseng, which inhibits cancer invasion. Boswellia, pokeroot, mistletoe, chaparral, and sage have all been used against cancer. Pau d'Arco, golden seal and echinacea, red clover, blue violet, and garlic all have excellent anticancer uses. Graviola is a natural product obtained from the rain forests of South America. It has been shown to be effective to kill malignant cells of several different types including colon, breast, prostate, lung, and pancreatic cancers. It is stronger than Adriamycin, a commonly used chemotherapeutic drug used for colon cancer, and it works only on cancer cells without harming healthy cells, which is very unlike chemotherapy.

There are food enhancers such as rosemary, turmeric, and ginger, which are reported to block or inhibit cancer formation or growth. The fiber in whole grains contains phytates which yield IP-6 (inositol hexaphosphate). IP-6 has a strong action on cancer cells to turn off their growth stimulus. When levels of IP-6 are low as in a low fiber diet, the cancer cells are more able to replicate themselves and get out of control. Persons who limit their grains to the whole grain variety definitely have a distinct advantage in preventing cancer.

Garlic contains 50 or more medicinal compounds active in reversing cancer development (*Nutritional Cancer* 14, no. 34 [1990]: 183–93, 297–317). The quantity to take daily is about the equivalent of 15 cloves, whether it is taken raw, steamed, baked, in dry powder form, or the deodorized extract. Pineapple contains bromelain, which is believed by some to break the membranes of cancer cells. Aloe vera was shown to benefit cats suffering from leukemia. Flaxseed lignins, a type of fiber, have been associated with a variety of anticancer actions (*Your Health,* June 11, 1996, 23). A protein source rich in the sulfur amino acids (for example soybeans) is quite useful in most cancers.

Types of Cancer

Breast Cancer

(See "Breast Conditions" in the *Conditions and Diseases* section.)

Cervical Cancer

HPV has been recognized as a cause of cervical cancer as well as genital warts. About 13,500 new cases of cervical cancer are discovered each year in the United States and 6,000 women die of it annually (*Am Fam Physician 45, no. 1 [Jan. 1992]: 143-50*). Women who have had 10 or more sexual partners were found to be 11 times more likely to be infected with human papilloma virus (HPV) than women who were monogamous.

Colon Cancer

If there were ever a premium on prevention, it would begin here. This is the third most common cancer ending in death in the United States. It is largely caused by factors in the American diet. In countries where plant-based diets are the rule, cancer of the colon is rare. This statement can be made of several cancers and other diseases with certainty.

Melanoma

Melanomas are usually hairless moles that spread by invading blood vessels and lymph nodes. In 15 percent of cases they have already metastasized by the time of diagnosis. Lesions less than 1.5 centimeters have a very good prognosis, while ones greater than 1.5 to 4 centimeters have no reliable indicator of how frequently metastasis may occur. Some will metastasize, some will not. Patients 60 years and over have a better prognosis. The peak incidence is 35 to 50 years of age, with men and women being equally vulnerable. In women 71 percent of melanomas occur in the lower extremities (perhaps because of the custom of exposing their legs), whereas 63 percent of melanomas in men occur on the upper extremities or back (perhaps as a result of going shirtless in the sun).

Ovarian Cancer

Cancer of the ovaries is the fourth to fifth leading cause of death in American women. You can get a good bit of useful information from the National Ovarian Cancer Coalition. Some recognized lifestyle factors promoting ovarian cancer include taking Valium and other tricyclic antidepressants, low vitamin D levels, the use of dairy products, exposure to a wide range of industrial chemicals, a low fiber diet, and estrogen therapy (*Medical Tribune for the Family Physician* 36 [April 20, 1995]: 8; *Lancet* 2, no. 8654 [1989]: 66–71; *Journal of the National Cancer Institute* 88 [1996]: 32–7; *Journal of Occupational and Environmental Medicine* 40 [1998]: 632).

Prostate Cancer

Among the most well-known causes of prostate cancer are a diet high in meat, milk, eggs, and cheese, and the use of a high-fat diet. Animal fat, especially fat from red meat and dairy butter, are implicated in an elevated risk of advanced prostate cancer. There is a 50 percent increased risk with the

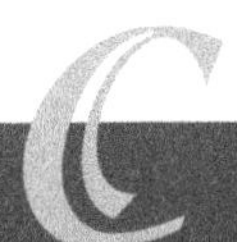

daily use of milk as compared to the rare use of milk (*Cancer Causes and Control* 9 [1998]: 559).

Lack of exercise has been associated with increased mortality from prostate cancer. Being physically fit can protect one against the development of prostate cancer (*Medicine and Science in Sports and Exercise* 28 [1996]: 97). Related to this, a high level of recreational exercise was associated with a low level of testicular cancer (*Cancer Causes and Control* 6 [1995]: 398).

Other factors known or suspected to be involved in some way with prostate cancer are a sedentary occupation like truck driving, an overactive sex life, genetic influences, the use of recreational alcohol, smoking, and occupational exposure to asbestos, steel, dyes and lacquers, bitumen pitch, iron nickel, lead, fertilizer, and certain other agents (*British Journal of Cancer* 74 [1996]: 1682; *Cancer* 77 [1996]: 138; *American Journal of Epidemiology* 143 [1996]: 692).

Cancer of the prostate is also associated with the use of diuretics (*International Agency for Research on Cancer* 50 [1990]: 299).

Candida

Candida problems, both infections and allergic reactions, are becoming more frequent. Many books and large numbers of products are commercially available to deal with various allergy problems. Candida is a form of fungus that readily inhabits humans in many locations, incluing the vagina, esophagus, penis (under the foreskin), feet, skin in general, and the intestinal tract. Candida can grow in any body opening, but especially in the vagina and intestinal tracts. When candida overgrows the flora of the intestinal tract, a natural treatment plan can transform the bowel to a more normal flora.

Treating Candida With Diet

In order to prepare the bowel for treatment, eliminate all heavy refined starches (sugar, honey, or syrup) and sweetened foods and stomach irritating foods such as fermented foods, coffee, cigarettes, alcohol, vinegar, and hot spices such as ginger, cinnamon, nutmeg, cloves, and black or red pepper.

Once these foods have been eliminated, the diet should contain the following:

- About 75 percent high fiber vegetables such as broccoli, celery, radishes, asparagus or cabbage, prepared by steaming or taken raw
- About 10 percent high protein foods such as nuts, seeds, legumes, or peanuts
- Approximately 10 percent complex carbohydrates such as rice, millet, amaranth, quinoa, buckwheat, etc.
- About 5 percent fruits such as papaya, grapefruit, and all types of berries, especially blueberries

Garlic and aloe vera assist in the cleansing process and grapefruit seed extract will also greatly help both in the cleansing process as well as in the treatment of candida. The grapefruit seed extract should be taken between meals. An average-sized person of about 150 pounds on days one to three takes 10 drops twice daily in vegetable or diluted fruit juice or one 125 milligram capsule twice daily. On days four to 15 take 15 drops twice daily or one capsule three times daily or four tablespoons four times daily. On days 16 to 28 take 15 drops three times daily or two capsules two or three times daily or four tablespoons four times daily.

Some persons may be unable to increase to the greater concentration and dosage schedule, but most people will be able to tolerate this much grapefruit seed extract without difficulty. Some people get a stomachache from too much. Once satisfactory improvement is noted, even if it is only two or three weeks into the program, the grapefruit seed extract dosage should be gradually reduced. If symptoms reappear, then return to a higher dosage. For some people, a four-week treatment period may not be sufficient, and long-standing cases may require four to six months of constant treatment.

Instead of the commercial product, you can make your own grapefruit seed extract by scrubbing a grapefruit, quartering it, simmering gently for 20 minutes and pouring the liquid into a jar to be refrigerated. Take two to four tablespoons four times daily.

Avoid all yeast products, including food yeast and brewer's yeast. All fermented foods and soured milk products must also be eliminated. Avoiding all yeast products is quite a challenge, since all bread is raised with yeast. Unleavened bread is all right. Of course, only whole grain breads should be used. Many vegetarian cheeses are flavored with food yeasts which may give a cross reaction with candida.

Anything of a fermented nature should be avoided, particularly alcoholic beverages, vinegar, catsup, pickles, or bread made with vinegar, mayonnaise, soy sauce, sauerkraut, kimchi, and seasoning yeast. These must be avoided.

Many fruit juices are manufactured by using a mold digestion step in extraction of the juice from the fruit pulp. Eliminate all commercial fruit juice. Even dried fruits may have small amounts of mold on them and may cause trouble.

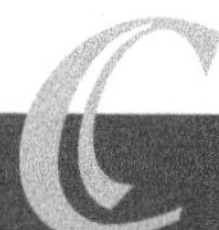

Don't eat any refined carbohydrates. This means no white flour, white rice, white pastas, white or brown sugar or foods or drinks containing these.

Emphasize especially garlic, onions, and fresh green leafy vegetables as they contain antifungal properties. Some find avoiding fruits for one to three months to be helpful.

A total vegetarian diet is the most favorable with strict avoidance of milk and all milk products—whey, sodium caseinate and lactate, yogurt, cheese, etc. Read labels to discover any of these articles of food in lists of ingredients. All cheeses are likely to have mold in them. Cheese is also a common offender.

Eat a couple of tablespoons of pumpkin seeds and sunflower seeds with each meal.

For those having a severe problem, a two-meal plan using only vegetables, whole grains, and seeds may be remarkably helpful. A person can do quite well on two vegetable meals a day, along with the whole grains and nuts. It has been shown that fruits can stimulate the growth of candida in the bowels of some people. After several weeks of improvement, a person may start adding the less sweet fruits carefully, and if they experience no problem, gradually continue with other fruits. Use this plan (breakfast and lunch) if your weight does not drop to the point that you are weak. If you become too thin, also eat a light supper.

About 10 minutes *before* each meal take:

- One-fourth cup aloe vera juice three times per day, 10 minutes before each meal.
- Four capsules (500 milligrams) evening primrose oil two times per day with meals, *or* four tablespoons ground flaxseed two times per day with meals, or flaxseed oil, one teaspoon three or four times a day. Oil of primrose capsules may be of value in supplying some of the essential fatty acids; however, flaxseed oil may be just as effective and is much less expensive than primrose oil.
- One-fourth glass of carrot juice per day, optional.

A patient wrote that she got rid of her candida infection when she began taking digestive enzymes. Whether the digestive enzymes are helpful is not proven, but we thought the association in her case was worthy of mention. Select the preparation of your choice at a health food store.

Medications

Avoid all drugs that promote growth of candida; i.e. antibiotics, birth control, anti-inflammatory drugs such as Cortisone and Prednisone, and immunosuppressive drugs such as Imuran. Eliminate asprin and all other drugs that are considered stomach irritants.

For vaginal yeast infections use an ichthammol and glycerine mixture. Put the material on tampons. (See "Woman's Conditions and Disease" in the *Conditions and Diseases* section.)

Botanicals

Drink four cups of Pau d'Arco (taheebo) tea daily as part of your water intake. Place one teaspoon per eight-ounce cup. Simmer in boiling water for 30 minutes. The taheebo tincture is much more potent, and we have seen several people who seem to have trouble tolerating it. We have not seen anyone have trouble with the Pau d'Arco bark as it is used to make tea, even using it double strength, that is, two teaspoons per cup. A person should generally start with one teaspoon per cup of water and, if necessary, increase it to double strength.

Licorice root contains 25 antifungal compounds. See the *Herbal Remedies* section for instructions on its use.

Cammomile is especially good against candida. Make a strong tea of three or four teaspoons.

Anticandida Supplements

Eat one to three medium cloves of garlic two to three times per day or take four capsules three times per day with meals. Garlic is a strong antifungal agent. You may be able to purchase fresh dehydrated garlic powder in a grocery store. Take one to two tablespoons per day. Kyolic liquid can be used and is more effective than other garlic supplements. Take one teaspoon three times a day. Instead of the liquid form, you may use fresh garlic (one or two cloves) blenderized with water, a citrus smoothie, or a green smoothie. You may also bake or steam from one clove up to one entire bulb and eat it three times daily.

Grapefruit seed extract, made by washing a whole grapefruit, quartering it, and simmering gently for half an hour, may be taken as two tablespoons every two hours for two days, then every four hours during the day for up to two months.

Natural vitamin C with bioflavonoids (500 milligrams two times per day) may be taken with meals for a month or so.

You may wish to try Lactobacillus acidophilus. Some have had a benefit from it. Find a preparation not having traces of milk. Use care reading labels of the preparations sold in health food stores as they could be out of date or are not potent enough to be of any value. Since the germs are

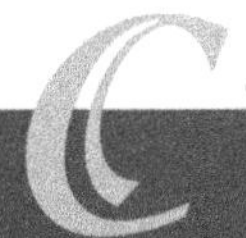

cultured on whey, they may have tiny amounts of milk protein attached to them. If you know you have a milk allergy, it would be well to proceed very carefully. There are sources of acidophilus without the milk traces, but they are often not really potent enough to help much.

Diet is probably the most important factor, but supplements seem to be helpful for many people. If a person has longstanding or severe symptoms, they should probably use all the supplements listed.

Apparently candida is very prone to recur. If one is careful with the diet and is doing well, after three or four months start to taper off the supplements and observe your symptoms and be guided by them.

There is a premium on strictly obeying all the eight laws of health, being especially careful to get 20 to 30 minutes of sunning every day the sun shines and at least eight glasses of water daily. Sleep on a regular schedule in a room with fresh air. (See "Eight (Natural) Laws of Heath" in the *Natural Remedies* section.)

Canker Sores, Mouth Ulcers, Aphthous Ulcers

These small round whitish ulcers surrounded by an area of redness occur on the soft parts of the inner surfaces of the mouth, gums, tongue, and insides of the lips and cheeks. The cause is unknown, although many things have been implicated, such as food sensitivities, dehydration, allergies, stress, hormone imbalances, viral infections,vitamin deficiencies, and endocrine imbalance. Stomach ailments are often listed as potential causes. They tend to occur from the ages of about 15 to 40 years, are of equal frequency in males and females, and are more likely to be milder and fewer in number as the person gets older. They heal spontaneously in one to two weeks but some people are never free of them; as one heals, others occur. They may appear singly or in crops. Canker sores are very painful. They may occur in up to 40 percent of the population. Offspring of parents with frequent mouth ulcers are at a greater risk of also developing them.

Prevention

At the first symptom in a person who is prone to get canker sores, drink an eight-ounce glass of water every 10 minutes for an hour, and in most instances the canker sore will not develop. Usually, if you can start the water drinking within 20 minutes of feeling the first sign of a canker sore, you can prevent its development.

Canker sores may be the result of a food sensitivity, but it is often difficult to discover those foods to which you are sensitive. Follow the guidelines in the "Elimination and Challenge Diet" in the *Dietary Information* section. In one study 56 percent of persons with food allergies were found to have canker sores. Some are unaware of their food sensitivities until investigated.

Highly seasoned or tart foods, citrus fruits, chewing gum, chocolate, alcoholic beverages, and throat lozenges should all be avoided.

Canker sores are made worse by hot foods, biting the inside of the mouth, spices, and other irritating foods.

Drinking tea or colas has been associated in some individuals with outbreaks of mouth ulcers.

Do not smoke or chew tobacco.

Stop using toothpaste with sodium lauryl sulphate in it, as people who use toothpaste containing this detergent are more likely to get canker sores. Do not use dentifrices or mouthwashes, but brush the teeth with plain water, or baking soda, or charcoal powder, until the canker sores cease appearing.

Avoid any kind of trauma to the lining of the mouth by using a soft bristle toothbrush, no sharp instruments to clean the teeth, avoiding or using care with rough foods, such as zwieback, taking small bites and chewing thoroughly, and avoiding hot foods or drinks. Avoid biting the tongue or cheek, which is best done by staying well hydrated so the surfaces of the mouth can slip out of the way of the teeth. Do not talk while chewing, and avoid turning the head to one side while chewing, as the pull on the muscles of the neck and mouth may promote accidental biting of the tongue or cheek.

Avoid vaccines and antibiotics, which are sometimes used in treatment, as they are not beneficial and may be harmful.

Treatment

Stay well hydrated. Drinking 10 to 12 glasses of water daily will help the ulcers to heal more quickly.

A prolonged mouthwash with very warm water, very warm witch hazel tea, or plain saline may be helpful to relieve pain and to promote healing.

A silver nitrate stick or chromic acid applied topically may give temporary relief but may eventually delay healing, enlarge the ulcers, and cause scarring.

Golden seal tea may be used as a mouthwash. The golden seal powder may be sprinkled directly into a mouth ulcer for pain relief. A used golden seal tea bag (fresh ones are too bitter to be tolerated for long and will banish sleep) may be

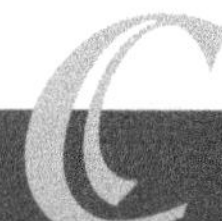

applied directly to the ulcer and left overnight. It promotes healing and may bring rapid relief of pain.

Make a tincture of calendula using one pint of grain alcohol or vodka (not rubbing alcohol) and two ounces of calendula flowers. Soak these together for two weeks, agitating every day. Then strain the mixture and save the alcohol. Moisten a cotton ball with the calendula tincture and put it on a canker sore at the very first indication it is beginning. Hold it there for three minutes. There may be a slight stinging, but it won't be truly painful. This treatment can work literally overnight to reduce or even heal a canker sore. Tea Tree (Melaleuca) oil applied with a cotton swab to beginning canker sores may speed healing.

Carpal Tunnel Syndrome

(See "Skeletal Problems" in the *Conditions and Diseases* section.)

Cataracts

A cataract is a cloudy or opaque area in the lens of the eye that results in failing vision, hazy, fuzzy, or blurred vision, change in the color of the pupil, seeing better without glasses, and the need for frequent changes in eyeglass prescriptions. There may be a sense of a film over the eyes or seeing rings or halos around lights. Cataracts usually begin after the age of 50. Half of people between the ages of 65 and 75 will develop cataracts, and 75 percent of those over age 75.

When a cataract is detected, surgery is not immediately necessary in most instances. One man had his cataracts diagnosed at age 63, but it was not until he was age 85 that his cataracts were operated on. At first he had no symptoms, but by the time the operation occurred everything "was getting pretty foggy." Microsurgery, laser surgery, easily implanted plastic replacement lenses, and other techniques have made this once risky operation almost routine. Clear artificial lenses replace virtually all of the lenses removed.

Sometimes people's cataracts never worsen beyond when they are first detected; therefore, it is best to wait until symptoms make surgery a requirement. Waiting will not affect the outcome of surgery. Risks of surgery are rare, but can include loss of an eye or blindness. Occasionally, the eye may become infected and the retina detached. There is also a slight risk of developing a drooping eyelid, bleeding inside the eye, or high pressure (glaucoma) inside the eye.

Cause and Prevention

Chronic dehydration can result in cataract formation. A typical scenario is this: A person takes a vacation in a foreign country. While there the person develops the traveler's diarrhea, loses a lot of fluid, cannot obtain appropriate drinking water, and returns home in a state of chronic dehydration. The kidneys have accepted the lower water level as being normal and no longer demand larger quantities of water. The appetite for water falls precipitously. Before long the visual signs begin in the eyes. To correct chronic dehydration the person must learn to sip water throughout the day in the quantities of 10 to 12 eight-ounce glasses per day. At the same time less concentrated foods should be taken such as simple fruits and vegetables, small amounts of grains, and only one ounce or two of nuts or seeds. The diet should be ideally totally vegetarian, omitting all free fats and free sugars. Salt should not be added to the food during the rehydration process, which may take as long as two months.

A high sodium content in the diet increases the risk of getting cataracts. A study was done in 2,100 subjects. Those having the highest soft drink intake (because of the high sodium content of "sodas") were approximately twice as likely to develop cataracts as those having the lowest salt intake. We can understand from these studies that a low sodium diet may help prevent cataracts, especially in elderly people (*American Journal of Epidemiology* 151 [2000]: 624).

Taurine strengthens the eye against getting cataracts as well as glaucoma and dry eye syndromes. Taurine is found in legumes, particularly beans and carob, also in food yeast, nuts and seeds, and virtually all foods that are high in protein. Taurine is especially found in breast milk. Cows milk by contrast has very little or no taurine.

Factors that promote cataracts are low levels of certain vitamins and minerals that normally help protect the eye from cataract formation and macular degeneration. Vitamins C, E, beta-carotene, selenium, and all antioxidants appear to be the most significant. The more one eats fruits and vegetables, the more antioxidant nutrients consumed, the lower the incidence of cataracts. Proper selenium levels in the blood are essential to prevent cataracts (*Arch. Ophthalmol. Scand.* 73 [1995]: 329–32). In one study women who used vitamin C supplements for more than 10 years had a 77 percent lower prevalence of early opacities and an 83 percent lower prevalence of moderate opacities (*Invest Ophthalmol Vis Sci 39 no 9 [Aug. 1998]: 1531-1534*).

Dietary choices affect your probability of developing a cataract. If you eat a lot of foods rich in lutein and zeaxanthin,

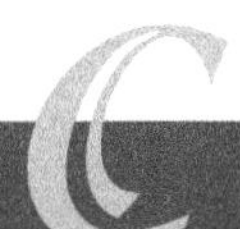

two compounds related to beta-carotene, you are much less likely to get cataracts. Foods that are high in these substances are mostly dark green leafy vegetables, winter squash, corn, carrots, and peppers. About three servings of leafy green vegetables per week are protective. Sweet potatoes and pumpkin are also high in protective compounds (*Tuft's Health and Nutrition Letter* 17, no. 10 [1999]: 1).

A host of other antioxidants are found in fruits, vegetables, soybeans, nuts, seeds, and other plant products. The antioxidants attach the hazardous oxygen fragments known as free radicals, and thus prevent damage to crucial parts of the eyes. Taking antioxidant supplements has not been found as helpful to lower rates of early cataracts compared with taking the whole foods, which are more important in preventing cataracts than taking nutrient supplements, according to researchers at the University of Wisconsin Medical School. Therefore, do not depend on taking vitamin and mineral pills to protect against cataracts, but instead use whole foods, especially fruits and vegetables for their disease-fighting compounds. Dr. Julie Mares-Perlman says, "Focus on eating nutritious foods in and of themselves, rather than specific nutrients," as we do not know for certain what food chemical is actually providing the benefit. Green vegetables were found in one study to have the greatest cataract protection value (*Internal Medicine World Report* 10, no. 7 [April 1–14, 1995]: 8, 9).

Persons prone to cataracts should avoid tobacco (even secondhand smoke), foods containing galactose (dairy products), refined sugars, white rice and white bread, and a high-fat diet. These are all known to promote cataracts.

Bilberry, antioxidants in fruits and vegetables, vitamin B2 (riboflavin), as well as zinc (nuts, seeds, and whole grains), and quercetin (apples and onions) can help prevent cataracts.

The exposure that many people have to milk with its lactose and galactose ingestion can cause a sizable group of our population to have an increased risk of cataracts. This increased risk appears to be because of a genetic deficiency in the galactose metabolic pathway, causing galactose to be handled improperly, resulting in irritation and damage to lenses (*Journal of the American College of Nutrition* 10, no. 1 [1991]: 79–86). The proportion of people in a population with cataracts increases as dairy milk intake increases (*Dyn. Nutr. Res. Basel, Karger* 3 [1993]: 40). The digestion of milk produces galactose from the lactose in milk. Galactose is four times more effective in causing cataracts in animals than is glucose. High levels of dietary sugar, table sugar, fructose, glucose, or xylose have also been associated with the production of cataracts. Therefore, persons with a family history of diabetes are more likely to get cataracts.

In persons aged 65 to 74 who received supplements of riboflavin and niacin the incidence of cataracts was reduced by 44 percent, as compared with persons not taking these vitamins. A group of researchers concluded that taking supplements of riboflavin and niacin could decrease the risk of cataracts. Getting these cataract-protection nutrients directly from whole grains, nuts, fruits, vegetables, and lycopene, found in tomatoes and other fruits and vegetables having a red color, can help prevent cataracts (*Archives of Ophthalmology* 111 [1993]: 1246–53; *American Journal of Epidemiology* 141 [1995]: 322).

Everything should be done to avoid high blood pressure as it apparently increases cataract formation, although some have believed it is the medicines used for hypertension that cause the cataracts. Get plenty of garlic and foods that are rich in pectin (blueberries, apples, etc.) that help to remove a variety of toxic substances including mercury, which may damage the lenses.

Persons wanting to prevent or treat cataracts should avoid lying down after meals and should do deep breathing exercises to stimulate circulation. Being physically fit can prolong the time before cataracts would develop in susceptible persons.

Overweight individuals are much more likely to develop cataracts than those who are lean. Calorie restriction has been shown to slow the development of cataracts (*Archives of Ophthalmology* 113 [September 1995]: 1131–7). Cataracts in women are more likely to occur in those who are currently overweight or even those having a history of being overweight or diabetes, hypertension, and increased cholesterol or triglycerides (*Annals of Epidemiology* 5, no. 3 [1995]: 234–8).

Smoking 20 cigarettes a day doubles the risk of cataracts. Moderate to heavy alcohol drinking increases the risk by four times (*Cigarettes: What the Warning Label Doesn't Tell You*" *2003,. 127;* "Clinical Practice in Small Incision Cataract Surgery, " *Phaco Manual [*2004]: 30-31).

Perform some exercises for the eyes such as tight squinting for 10 seconds three times a day; secondly, turning the eyes to the far right, the far left, as high as you can, as low as you can, and in each of the four quadrants; and thirdly, open the eyelids as widely as possible in a startled stare for 10 seconds. Repeat these exercises frequently when doing close work about once an hour. The exercises improve circulation to the eyes and encourage good eye health.

Another cause of cataracts is bright sunlight or other bright lights shining directly into the eyes. Protect the eyes with a broad brim sun hat when doing work outside, and wear sunglasses at other times. Do not allow bright lights to shine directly into the eyes for long periods (*Arch. Ophthalmol* 109 [1991]: 196, 197).

Excessive stress should be avoided, as under laboratory conditions guinea pigs under stress developed cataracts. Stress can result from chilling of the body, biochemical imbalances, such as might be brought on by overeating, drugs, tobacco, alcohol, any kind of disease, as well as from emotional factors.

Anorexia nervosa, frequent exposure to x-radiation or other kinds of radiation, and high blood levels of phospholipids such as lecithin used in many home recipes, and a lot of commercial products manufactured from eggs and soybeans, all increase cataract risk (*American Journal of Public Health* 83, no. 4 [1993]: 588).

If the environmental temperature is customarily higher, there is a greater risk of developing cataracts (*Transactions of the American Ophthalmological Society* 78 [1980]: 255–64).

A variety of drugs are known to cause cataracts, including barbiturates, drugs for hypertension, oral antidiabetic agents, monoamine oxidase inhibitors, tricyclic antidepressants, phenothiazines, allopurinol, tetracycline and other broad spectrum antibiotics, sulfonamides, antihistamines, pilocarpine, anticholinesterase agents, myleran, oral contraceptives, pontocaine, ergot, the morphine group of narcotics, streptozotocin, paradichlorobenzol (used in deodorants, moth repellents, and insecticides), and many other drugs. Other factors causing cataracts include chronic exposure to mothballs, hair dyes, chronic allergies, chronic stress, and methylmercury exposure (found in sea foods, especially salt water fish and shellfish) (*Ophthalmology* 88 [1981]: 117–24).

Patients who used tranquilizers had a higher risk of cataracts in a study done by Dr. Collman of the National Institute of Environmental Health Sciences in Research Triangle Park, North Carolina (*Science News* 134 [1988]: 318).

The increase in mouth bacteria caused by, as well as causing, cavities may encourage cataracts. Even though these are "friendly bacteria" they may do damage to the body and accelerate aging. A 25 to 50 percent decrease in cavities in mice and rat studies slowed the age-related development of a number of diseases, including cataracts (C. E. Finch and L. Hayflick, *Handbook of the Biology of Aging* [New York: Reinhold, 1977]: 582). (See also "Dental Care" in the *Conditions and Diseases* section for treatment.)

People who suffer from allergies exhibit a greater frequency and an earlier age of onset of cataracts than do nonallergic persons. It seems reasonable that if one is aware of an allergy to a certain substance all efforts should be made to avoid contact with that substance in an effort to protect all the organs of the body, not just the specific target area such as the nose or skin.

Cataracts and glaucoma have both been found to be increased in incidence by the use of corticosteroid ointments (*Lancet* 345 [1995]: 330). Any steroids used repeatedly or on a long-term basis increase the risk of cataracts.

Studies published as far back as 1997 and 1998 suggest that curcumin from turmeric can help prevent cataracts. Take one-half teaspoon twice a day to keep early cataracts from progressing. *Nutrition Research*, Volume 20, Issue 4, Pages 515 to 526, 2004.

Treatment

In early-stage cataracts, vision improved in 60 to 90 percent of cases taking five or more servings daily of food high in vitamin C. Improvement became noticeable in two to eight weeks. It is important to begin treating cataracts when they first begin.

Vitamin E is promoted as a way to prevent cataracts. The authors also mention vitamins C, A, and beta-carotene, but say that supplements are not actually needed, only a well-balanced diet. Nuts, whole wheat, and sunflower seeds are all good sources of vitamin E (*Epidemiology* 4, no. 3 [1993]: 191). Taking zinc and vitamin C has been reported by veterinarians to clear cataracts in animals, particularly dogs (*Let's Live*, March 1986, 69).

Thirty milligrams of zinc daily should give noticeable improvements in early cataracts within six weeks with improvement continuing up to a year or longer. Whole grains, nuts, and seeds, especially pumpkin seeds, are high in zinc. Vitamin B2 (riboflavin) has been found to be deficient in some cataract patients; therefore, it would seem wise to eat a diet high in vitamin B2. It is recommended to take foods sufficient to supply 15 milligrams daily. Within 48 hours improvement may be noticeable and should continue for nine months or longer (*Women's Health* 5, no. 6 [June 1996]: 1). Legumes, green leafy vegetables, whole grain breads, nuts, peanuts, dried fruits, and peanut butter are all good sources of riboflavin. It is suggested that the cataractogenic effect of galactose (a sugar naturally occurring in milk) might be inhibited by plenty of riboflavin in the diet (*Science* 195 [1977]: 205; *Metabolic and Pediatric Ophthalmology* 5 [1981]: 17–20).

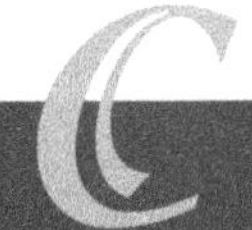

Feeding rats curcumin (in turmeric) at a dose of 75 milligrams per kilogram was compared to feeding rats corn oil for a test period of 14 days. Five days after the feeding phase ended, the lenses of the rats were exposed to a cataract-inducing agent for 72 hours. Then, using a special microscope, the lenses were studied to determine whether cataracts clouded the lenses or not. The curcumin-treated rats had significantly less cataract formation compared to rats fed on the corn oil (*American Journal of Clinical Nutrition* 64 [1996]: 761). The dose for humans would be about one teaspoon of turmeric twice a day. Stir it in water and drink it 10 to 20 minutes before or after meals.

A treatment for cataracts reported in the *Journal of Electrotherapeutics and Radiology* suggested that hydrotherapy for the eyes, a continuous bathing of the eyes for 10 minutes in hot water three times a day, would prevent the growth of cataracts and could be a remedy for many with cataracts (34 [1916]: 419).

Some have said a teaspoon of powdered garlic a day, or a quarter cup of lemon juice a day, or four cups of eyebright a day will all cure cataracts. We have not personally seen any cures. Our hope has been improvement and to halt or slow the progress of cataract development. Certainly no harm could come from trying these healthful foods.

Castor oil has been used for anointing the upper and lower eyelids for cataracts. It could be rubbed on the eyelids at night in much the same way a lotion is applied. It could also be applied to a small piece of cloth and laid on the eyelids as a poultice or compress. Castor oil increases the number of T-cells in the skin under the compress and may be helpful in cataracts or conjunctivitis.

Celiac Disease

(See also "Gluten Sensitivity" in the *Conditions and Diseases* section.)

There are many physical signs and symptoms associated with celiac disease including a small spleen, dermatitis herpetiformis, mouth ulcers, cow's milk intolerance in about 10 percent, a history of a first degree relative with celiac disease, autoimmune diseases, diabetes, and sometimes certain types of lung diseases.

Celiac disease is associated with sensitivity to gluten, a protein present in wheat, rye, barley, and possibly oats. In susceptible individuals, gluten causes the small intestinal villi to flatten and atrophy which produces malabsorption and subsequent diarrhea. The stools may be pale, loose, and of very foul odor.

The gluten molecule consists of at least six components that vary with the different species of wheat, barley, or rye; therefore, some types of wheat cause more severe symptoms than other types, but all appear to be harmful in celiac disease. It is of interest that in 1992 it was discovered in Mexico that mushrooms would cause small intestinal damage characterized by flattening of the mucosa, fusing of villi, and other alterations in the cells of the absorptive intestinal surface. These injuries are sufficient to cause permanent abnormalities of absorption in those who have eaten the mushrooms similar to that seen in celiac sprue, mineral or fat malabsorption, leaky gut syndrome, allergies, etc.

Gluten is composed of gliadin compounds. Some 18 or more different gliadin-associated medical and mental conditions have been identified. They include dermatitis herpetiformis, rosacea, celiac disease, autism and pervasive developmental disorders, some forms of epilepsy, brain atrophy, intellectual deterioration, some forms of chronic schizophrenia, chronic neurologic disorders of unknown cause (ataxias and peripheral neuropathies), dental enamel defects, low bone mineral density, recurring aphthous ulcers (mouth ulcers or canker sores), small bowel lymphomas, arthritis and other joint symptoms, loss of fertility and menstrual periods, as well as miscarriages in women and infertility in men. Gluten sensitivity can cause or worsen certain autoimmune diseases, thyroid diseases, some forms of insulin-dependent diabetes (2 to 4 percent of insulin dependant diabetics), and iron-deficiency anemia in infants and children, abnormally elevated liver enzymes (alkaline phosphatase, etc.), and abnormal intestinal permeability (*Lancet* 349 [1997]: 1755).

Gluten should be removed from the diet as soon as the diagnosis is made to minimize permanent damage to the intestinal tract. Among grains, only rice, millet, corn, and sometimes oats can be used by the celiac patient. These should be cooked for two to three hours if boiling is the form of preparation, and if the grains are baked, they should be browned thoroughly.

The condition is a permanent condition, occurring in families. First degree relatives of adult celiac disease patients are more likely than others to have allergic disorders. A gluten-free diet results in complete restoration in children, but incomplete restoration will occur if the diet is not prescribed before adulthood and irreversible damage may then occur to the small bowel. If gluten is reintroduced at a later date, the damage to the small bowel will recur. There are many symptoms of the disease and these will be summarized in

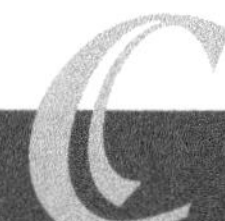

the following table, beginning with the most common and progressing to the least common. There may be many other symptoms than those listed.

Symptoms

- Anemia (megaloblastic or large red blood cells often associated with vitamin B12 or folic acid deficiency)
- Malabsorption of nutrients
- Poor appetite
- Diarrhea
- Fatigue
- Large, foul-smelling stools
- Weight loss
- Irritability
- Osteoporosis
- Acne rosacea
- Small stature
- Delayed puberty
- Poor health in childhood
- Constant abdominal pain
- Colic with vomiting
- Mouth ulcers
- Constipation or loose stools
- Headaches
- Iron deficiency
- Bleeding from various tissues or organs
- Protruding abdomen with bloating
- Rectal prolapse
- Emaciation

Treatment

The major method to treat this disease is to strictly remove gluten from the diet. The person should be impressed with the necessity to be strict since damage can become permanent and irreversible.

Osteoporosis (thinning of the bones) can be treated only in those who have a strictly gluten-free diet. Exercise along with a completely vegetarian diet give the most effective way to prevent further osteoporosis.

Avoid cow's milk as it often increases the sensitivity. Use various vegetarian milks available in health food stores or make your own sunflower seed or nut milk.

Very ripe bananas and garlic can be helpful. Garlic, about half to one teaspoon of dried garlic powder, may be sprinkled on the food to good advantage. Ripe bananas or carob are tolerated well and may assist in the control of diarrhea. Carob paste may be eaten (one to three tablespoons of carob powder in a little water), or a carob milkshake, or a carob-soy milk-banana smoothie may be prepared using one tablespoon of carob blended with a few nuts, water, fruit, or fruit juice to make a nice smoothie to assist in the control of diarrhea because of the high pectin content in carob.

Any food high in pectin (apples, blueberries, peaches, etc.) soothes and heals the bowels.

Other foods usually easily tolerated, which are like grains in their function in the meal, include quinoa, buckwheat, cassava root, amaranth, jicama, rice noodles, jautia (malanga), etc. These foods should all be rotated to keep an allergy from developing. Try not to use a food more frequently than every three days to reduce the likelihood of developing food sensitivities.

If the patient gets well with the diet, it may be considered adequate, but no matter how carefully gluten free the diet, if it does not control the symptoms, additional effort must be made to discover foods to which the patient has become sensitive, and remove them from the diet. Nuts, seeds, tofu, plant gelatins, may be used, but all free fats and free sugars will usually work against the person with celiac disease.

The following list of commercial foods will need to be eliminated as they often contain at least traces of gluten: malt, coffee substitutes, commercial breads, bread mixes, crackers, muffins, cupcakes, rolls, Rye-Krisp, pretzels, puddings, cakes, candies, cookies, ice cream, sherbets, salad dressings, breaded meats, luncheon meats, frankfurters, canned chili, macaroni, noodles, spaghetti, all pastas and pizzas, bread stuffings, commercial soups, cream sauces, bottled meat sauces, condiments, flavorings, syrups, gravies, sauces, cocoa mixes, desserts. Fortunately commercial substitutes, which are gluten free, can now be found for breads, pastas, and many other foods, which make meals more enjoyable.

The person suffering from celiac disease may use any kind of product made from soybeans, potato starch, rice, corn, or millet, although there have at times traces of gluten in corn and millet. All fruits and vegetables are accepted, as are all nuts and seeds. Delaying the diet can result in permanent damage of the intestinal lining. Once on the diet, improvements should be noticeable in a short amount of time.

Chapped Skin, Winter Itch

This condition features a roughened, reddened, irritated skin caused by loss of the natural oils. It occurs especially in winter and is sometimes called the "winter itch." Irritants such as harsh soap, hot water, or dry hot air can cause chapping.

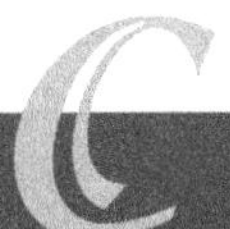

Chapped skin can be minimized if the home is properly heated, avoiding overheating and excessive dryness of the air.

Treatment

1. Stay well hydrated, drinking 10 to 12 glasses of water daily.
2. Avoid soap and hot water as much as possible, using non-water cleansers as needed or plain cold water for washing hands.
3. Use protective rubber gloves for tasks that soil or wet the hands.
4. Avoid hot-air blowers.
5. Keep a fresh application of some kind of moisturizer on the skin at all times.
6. Use tea tree oil or aloe vera cream or gel on the chapped areas. Another alternative is using "petroleum jelly milk." After the hands have been washed in plain water, do not dry. Instead, take a lump of petroleum jelly about the size of a bean and rub vigorously between the palms. The water remaining on the hands, plus the petroleum jelly will make a milky emulsion that can be smoothed gently over the chapped areas.
7. Avoid scratching itchy skin at all costs! It will damage the skin and result in uncontrollable itching. The use of aloe vera gel and/or the "petroleum jelly milk," smoothed on while the skin is still moist from washing hands or showering, will usually control itching. Avoid woolen or scratchy trousers.
8. Some individuals have had good result from washing with lemon or lime juice and then rinsing or by applying a small amount of lemon or lime to the wet skin after washing, with or without rinsing. Lemon and lime are acidic and make the skin smooth They are also keratinolytic (which softens or dissolves the scale on the skin) and antibacterial.
9. Use an anti-itch cream made of one tablespoon of tincture of Tradescantia extract (an herb), one-fourth cup hand lotion, one-fourth cup aloe vera gel, one teaspoon clove oil, and two tablespoons water. This lotion is very effective for almost any kind of itch.

Chicken Pox

Chicken pox is one of the most contagious childhood diseases and is more likely to occur between the ages of two and eight. The disease is more prevalent in the winter and spring. Chicken pox is communicable from one to two days before the rash appears until all the blisters have crusted (usually five or six days). It begins 14 to 21 days after exposure to someone who has chicken pox. The child starts with a low-grade fever, small blisters, and generally feels bad. Once the lesions begin, you can expect several crops to occur for about six days, which may involve the mouth, vagina, eyes, and throat. Adults can also contract chicken pox, and they are often sicker than children. Rarely, chicken pox pneumonia can occur, which is sometimes fatal in infants under six months.

Treatment

At the beginning of the illness, a deep, warm bath for 15 minutes brings out the pox faster but makes the lesions get smaller and fade faster. Use a spinal pack or warm bath daily to stimulate the circulation and white blood cell activity and to soothe the patient. It is not necessary to keep the patient bedfast, but the patient should be kept sheltered and quiet. Protect from chilling. Also, prevent children from scratching the lesions by having them wear gloves or mittens, giving them warm baths, and applying ice or pressure to the itchy areas. DO NOT USE ASPIRIN! as Reye's disease could follow. Do not use Tylenol as it might prolong the illness or result in liver damage. (See also "Itching" in the *Conditions and Diseases* section.)

Watch the pox for secondary infection. Should it occur, combat infection in the pox in the same manner as for impetigo. One may use an oatmeal bath or a warm bath for soothing the lesions and stopping the itch. Be sure to keep the head cool during the warm baths.

Avoid antibiotics and cortisone-like drugs, as these powerful and potentially toxic medicines are not needed in the treatment of this mild, self-limited disease.

The diet should be light, principally of fruits, vegetables, and whole grains, free from concentrated sugars and free fats. If the mouth and throat get sore, use one teaspoon of salt to one pint (two cups) of water to make a saline solution. Gargle or wash the mouth with the saline for soothing and healing.

Chiggers, Mites

(See "Chiggers, Mites" in the *Home Emergencies* section.)

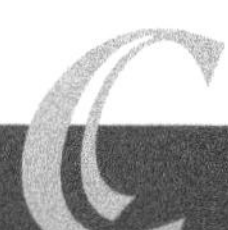

Chloasma, Excessive Facial Pigmentation

During pregnancy a woman is at risk of getting excessive pigmentation of her face. Vinegar can be spread full strength on a section of the face covered by excessive pigmentation to test if it will help in reducing the pigmentation. Apply it every night, and leave it on during the night. In the morning it can be applied along with any face cream or lotion that is normally used. Simply take the amount of lotion you intend to use, then drop approximately four to eight drops of vinegar into your palm with the lotion, mix them by rubbing together, then spread evenly over the face. You may also use the juice of lemons or limes as a skin lightener.

Some individuals have had good results from washing with lemon or lime juice and then rinsing or by applying a small amount of lemon or lime to the wet skin after washing and rinsing as above. Lemons and limes are acidic and make the skin smooth. They are also keratinolytic (softens or dissolves the scale on the skin), a natural lightener, and antimicrobial.

Cholecystitis

(See "Gallbladder" in the *Conditions and Diseases* section.)

Cholera

This disease is caused by cholera vibrio, a germ capable of causing severe diarrhea. Cholera travels around the world, having made this global circuit seven times since 1817. Its last circuit around the globe began in Indonesia in 1961, and at the turn of the century had completed its passage (*Science News* 149 [1996]: 404).

Treatment

There are two objectives in the treatment of cholera: (1) fluid and mineral replacement, and (2) detoxification. Drink one to four heaping tablespoons or more of powdered charcoal stirred into water every one to two hours during the heaviest diarrhea as this will help check the diarrhea. Be prepared to use generous quantities. It is *urgent* to stay ahead of water losses by copious drinking, retention enemas, intravenous administration, or subcutaneous injections.

To prevent potassium depletion, use six to eight ounces of green coconut water per liter (about five cups) of stool produced. If green coconut water is not available, an equal quantity of tomato juice, pureed spinach, turnips, cabbage, Brussels sprouts, broccoli, blackberries (especially good), grape juice, all citrus fruits and juices, bananas, prunes, reconstituted dried barley greens, peaches, or watermelon juice should be used.

Cholera patients can usually take fluids by mouth. Keep a careful chart of the measurement of the quantity of the diarrheic stool, and replace that quantity, plus the natural loses of fluid from urine, skin, and lungs. Frequent fomentations to the abdomen can be helpful. Death is much more likely to occur from water and mineral losses than from toxicity.

One important way to treat cholera is with bromelain, the enzyme from pineapples. It has been shown that bromelain slows down intestinal fluid secretion caused by the cholera germ. The loss of fluid from the intestinal tract is the principal cause of death in persons with cholera dysentery. In areas where cholera is currently in epidemic proportions, pineapples should be kept in good supply, and the enzyme should be taken by capsule as well by all individuals developing diarrhea.

Brewers yeast tablets, three tablets or one tablespoon of flakes, six times a day, can often help the diarrhea within three days (*Lancet* 343 [January 15, 1994]: 171, 172).

Berberine, one of the alkaloids in golden seal, has been reported to be quite effective against the cholera germ. Give large quantities of golden seal tea made double strength, up to one cup per hour. (See the *Herbal Remedies* section.)

Give large quantities of garlic from the first sign of cholera. I suggest two or three cloves whizzed in a blender with tomato juice or other juice and sipped slowly so it can be retained and not vomited. Repeat the dose four to six times a day.

The use of coconut water from immature coconuts as an IV infusion fluid has been reported several times in medical literature. A case of cholera was reported of an adult male in his 40s who was admitted to a hospital in the Solomon Islands where there was no intravenous fluid available. Members of the family climbed coconut trees and got coconuts at the appropriate stage of immaturity and brought them to the hospital for husking and puncturing by administration with a blood infusion set. The man received an estimated 1,200 cc per day for two days. Three days after receiving the intravenous coconut water, he was discharged and returned home. Coconut water is high in potassium and should not be given to patients with kidney failure or who have extensive third degree burns

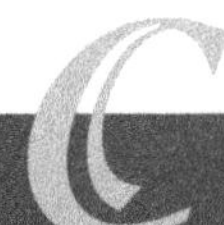

or severe and extensive bruising of muscles. Since coconut is slightly on the acidic side, it should be used sparingly with patients who have diabetic ketosis or other types of metabolic acidosis (*American Journal of Emergency Medicine* 18 [May 2000]: 108).

Cholesterol

Heavy proteins in the diet increase the likelihood of developing high blood cholesterol and hardening of the arteries. Several proteins were studied for their ability to cause these disorders in the blood and arteries. In order of their undesired ability to produce these disorders, purified soy protein was at the bottom of the list, next up from the bottom came wheat gluten, then pork, beef, lactalbumin (from milk), skim milk, and whole eggs (the worst).

There are fats naturally occurring in the blood, principally triglycerides and cholesterol that can cause serious health concerns when present in high levels. To properly control these fats is important. The optimal level of total cholesterol is around 100 plus your age, give or take 10 to15 points. The HDL ("good cholesterol") is optimal from 45 or 50 on the low side, to around 90 to100 on the high side. Higher than 100 increases risk of hardening of the arteries, just as LDL ("bad cholesterol") does. The optimal triglyceride level is about the same as your age, and since it goes up with intake of either fats, or of refined carbohydrates (sweets, alcohol, or refined grains). Triglycerides also cause hardening of the arteries.

The high cholesterol level caused by saturated fats can also be caused by trans fats. These trans fats are formed when manufacturers process oils, as in hydrogenated vegetable oils. The product can be labeled without cholesterol, but it still stimulates the liver to produce cholesterol in excess. Check your commercial foods such as cookies, crackers, canned soups, dry foods, and even cereals for hydrogenated fats, and eliminate trans fats. Fast foods such as French fries, onion rings, fried chicken, doughnuts, and so forth, along with vegetable shortening and margarine usually contain trans fats. Human breast milk is often a very rich source of trans fats because of the mother's use of trans fats in her foods (*New England Journal of Medicine* 341 [1999]: 1396).

Almost 120,000 doctors, dentists, and nurses completed a questionnaire every 24 months over an eight to fourteen year time period. Harvard University conducted the study and found that, for diabetics in the study, eating an egg a day doubled the risk for coronary heart disease and stroke. We recommend that those who are genetically predisposed to high cholesterol that all animal products be removed from the diet. Even animal protein has a deleterious effect on blood cholesterol (*Journal of the American Medical Association* 281 [1999]: 1387).

Both iron and copper have been found in trace amounts in atherosclerotic plaques. It may be that the high iron content of certain animal products, or supplemental iron, accounts for some portion of hardening of the arteries. Many metals are becoming linked with disease such as the link suspected between aluminum and zinc and Alzheimer's disease, and the link between high iron and Parkinson's disease. High iron levels have also been linked to bowel cancer and fatal coronary heart disease (*Atherosclerosis* 140, no. 1 [Sept. 1998]: 105-12). It is not advisable to take supplements containing iron unless your hemoglobin is under 10 grams or your serum iron is under 20.

One meat meal per month keeps the liver turned up to produce an increased quantity of cholesterol. The person who wishes to reduce cholesterol must be off all animal products.

The release of insulin is controlled to a large degree by the type of protein one eats. With plant protein the release of insulin goes down, but with animal protein the release of insulin goes up. Of course, this reflects the release of glucose as it is on the same control system as insulin. The level of insulin in the blood, just as the cholesterol level, is a predictor for cardiovascular disease, hypertension, diabetes, obesity, and cancer, independent of all other factors.

Improving the thyroid function can help remarkably with high cholesterol when low thyroid is a factor. It may be that hypothyroidism is more undiagnosed than we have previously thought. The symptoms include fatigue, depression, cold extremities, dry skin, fluid retention, hair loss, constipation, difficulty concentrating, infertility, menstrual irregularities, high serum cholesterol, and poor resistance to infection. (See "Thyroid Disease" in the *Conditions and Diseases* section.)

Certain prescription drugs such as Dilantin can cause an increase in serum cholesterol, which increases risks of coronary heart disease (*British Medical Journal* 4 [1975]: 85). Serum cholesterol levels were found to be 6 to 48 percent higher during the first three months of treatment with Dilantin, and remained high through the treatment period. The mechanism for this increase is probably through damage to the liver.

Prunes help reduce cholesterol. A University of Minnesota study found that eating 12 prunes a day (about three ounces) helped reduce blood cholesterol levels in 41 men with elevated levels of LDL. Three ounces of prunes

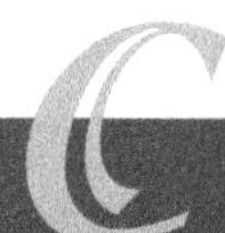

contain 239 calories, 7 grams of fiber, and 745 milligrams of potassium—more than a banana. Prunes are high in iron and are a good source of beta-carotene. Prune paste can replace high-fat shortening in a variety of baked goods, including brownies and bran muffins. Prune paste is made of pitted prunes, vanilla, and water. You can make your own by blending one cup of pitted prunes with six tablespoons of water and one to two teaspoons of vanilla for about two minutes until fluffy. It can be kept in the refrigerator for several days. When substituted for shortening in baked goods, prune paste reduces the fat in the recipe by at least 75 percent (*Br J Nutr* 101, no. 2 [Jan 2009]: 233-9).

Resveratrol, a nutrient found in purple grapes and purple grape juice, lowers cholesterol in rats. It is present also in raisins. A five-ounce glass of grape juice is sufficient, once or twice daily.

Women who ate enough avocado to comprise around 30 percent of their calories had a significant drop of 10 percent in both total and LDL cholesterol, with no change in HDL.

Citrus fruits and juices given to rabbits caused a reduction in LDL cholesterol. In the drinking water of the rabbits either orange juice or grapefruit juice was added, which reduced LDL cholesterol by 43 percent and 32 percent respectively (*Nutrition Research* 20 [2000]: 121).

Try eating a grapefruit twice a day, peeled, de-seeded, and blended in a blender. Continue this practice as long as the cholesterol is elevated. Reports show that pectin in grapefruit can reduce cholesterol by 7 to 20 percent, a better record than most drugs! (*Science News* July 25, 1987, 63). Cholesterol-lowering drugs work by their toxic effect on the liver's ability to make cholesterol. It is this feature that causes liver cancer or hepatitis, which has been reported because of Mevacor or Pravachol; further, about 15 percent is the maximum expected drop in cholesterol, certainly not more than with grapefruit, and probably less. Not worth taking its risks (*Modern Medicine*, 60, no. 6 [1992]: 70, 92).

Use amaranth, the ancient Aztec grain that was lost for many centuries, but has now been found. It contains a form of vitamin E and is able to reduce cholesterol substantially. It can be used as a breakfast cereal or to make vegetarian roasts. The flour can also be used in waffles.

Chromium picolinate, 400 milligrams daily, has been shown to be quite effective in the treatment of high cholesterol and triglycerides. It also decreases high insulin levels in insulin resistant persons (*Health Letter on Current Research on Nutrition and Preventive Medicine* 9, no. 1 [January 1999]: 16).

A 500-milligram inositol supplement is effective in bringing cholesterol down. It is best taken with choline. It is also helpful as a stress neutralizer and to bring blood pressure down.

Heart and blood vessel disease, producing such conditions as angina and hypertension, metabolic disorders such as diabetes and hypoglycemia, and many other ailments are recognized as sedentary lifestyle diseases in those who consume a rich and unwholesome diet. The diet in technologically advanced countries has an average fat content of 30 to 50 percent of the calories consumed. The diet is also very high in refined carbohydrates. An especially damaging food combination is refined fats and refined sugars. Investigators have found that in countries where people eat 20 percent or less of total calories in fat, where the diet consists mainly of unrefined carbohydrates such as whole grains, fruits, and vegetables, these diseases are almost nonexistent. The more fat and refined carbohydrates eaten, the more degenerative diseases are found.

Soybeans cause a reduction in cholesterol. Soybeans contain isoflavones that have a very marked influence on reducing high blood cholesterol, yet it does not reduce HDL (*Health Letter on Current Research on Nutrition and Preventive Medicine* 9, no. 1 [1999]: 9). A daily serving of one-half cup of soybeans reduces LDL cholesterol an average of 10 percent in about four months.

A diet high in soluble fibers (oat bran and beans) will lower cholesterol significantly. Insoluble fiber (wheat bran) is not so effective. Extra water, at least two eight-ounce glasses a day, should also be taken with the soluble dietary fiber as that will increase the effectiveness of the fiber. If gas or flatulence is a problem from the extra fiber, the use of digestive enzymes such as papaya, bromelain, etc. can be very helpful (*American Family Physician* 51 [1995]: 419).

Phytosterols inhibit the intestinal absorption of cholesterol and lower the serum LDL (*Am J Med* 107, no. 6 [Dec. 1999]: 588-94).

Take red yeast rice (Monascus purpureus). The starting dose is 600 milligrams twice a day with meals, with the maximum dosage being 2400 milligrams a day. Liver enzymes can be altered by red yeast rice.

Certain mushrooms contain lovastatin. Red yeast that grows on rice produces a family of 10 different statin compounds, lovastatin among them. Statin drugs to lower cholesterol can injure the liver and disturb muscle function in some people, sometimes seriously. CoQ10 has been shown to protect and enhance muscle metabolism including that of the heart. Statins inhibit synthesis of CoQ10.

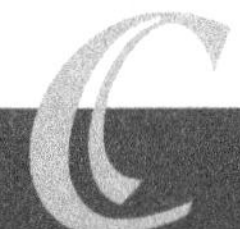

Lose any extra weight, even 5 to 10 pounds. The following rule of thumb will help you determine a good weight. Calculate 100 pounds for your first five feet, and for women, five pounds per inch thereafter. Allow six to seven pounds per inch for men, depending on how muscular he is. Example: If you are a 5'5" woman, you could weigh as much as 125, but no more unless your cholesterol and triglycerides are quite low. To help lose weight, be careful with your eating habits. Eat meals at a specific time, and don't overeat.

Do not allow yourself to get stressed. We have a heavenly Father who can give us peace. Forgive your insults from the past. Face squarely those things that trouble you and deal with each one dispassionately, patiently, and kindly. Do not watch TV or engage in games that will add stress to your life.

You can also reduce stress or neutralize it by lots of exercise. This is probably the single most beneficial thing for the majority of people. Make exercise a top priority every day. This is medicine for you, and can be a recreation if you pick an exercise you truly enjoy. Walking is easy to do, and you should do it as frequently as possible. Get a buddy who exercises with you so you will have no excuse not to get moving.

A large vital capacity also helps bring down cholesterol. This is the amount of air blown out after a full inspiration. The more air we can take in, the more oxygen in the blood, and the less likely we are to damage our blood vessels to start the process of atherosclerosis. Smoking, poor posture, and a sedentary lifestyle decrease the vital capacity, whereas exercise increases vital capacity.

A breathing exercise may be very helpful. One can be done by breathing in to the count of four, holding it to the count of seven and breathing out to the count of nine. You should do this exercise slowly enough that it will reduce your breathing to perhaps six times a minute or less. Continue this breathing exercise for five minutes and repeat three times a day for one month.

Increase omega-3 fatty acids by using walnuts, flax seeds, chia seeds, and almonds. Get plenty of soluble fiber, which is found in oatmeal, kidney beans, bananas, apples, pears, psyllium seeds, lemons, kiwis, barley, prunes, and blueberries.

Oat bran is known as the "king of cholesterol-lowering foods." Also, guggal, a resin from an Indian tree, is very helpful in reducing cholesterol.

Not only cholesterol but homocysteine needs to be reduced. There are factors known to be associated with an elevated homocysteine level including increased clotting time inside your blood vessels, myocardial infarction, stroke, and Alzheimer's disease.

Polycosinol from the wax of the cortex of sugar cane is very helpful. Take a dose of 10 milligrams per day.

An Oriental remedy uses leaves from peanut plants to reduce levels of triglycerides, cholesterol, and blood pressure. Animal experiments using either water or alcohol extracts of the leaves had a sedative, sleep inducing effect. There were no toxic side effects in the animals given a dosage 125 times the amount used to lower blood pressure, cholesterol, and triglycerides (*Chinese Traditional and Herbal Drugs* 18, no. 2 [1987]: 22).

Even as far back as 1962, and especially more recently, garlic has been shown to inhibit the synthesis of lipids in the liver and to increase the utilization of serum insulin, benefiting both heart disease and diabetes (*Medical Science Research* 20 [1962]: 729–731). In a study on the effects of garlic to lower cholesterol and triglycerides, 20 healthy volunteers were fed garlic oil (0.25/mg/kg per day in two divided doses) for six months (*The Lawrence Review of Natural Products* [April 1994]). The treatment significantly lowered average cholesterol and triglyceride levels while raising HDL levels, the good cholesterol.

In a separate study 62 patients with coronary artery disease and elevated cholesterol levels were assigned to two subgroups: one group was fed garlic for 10 months and the second group served as the untreated control. Garlic decreased the cholesterol, triglycerides, and LDL cholesterol, while increasing the HDL. The anticoagulant properties, cholesterol-lowering properties, blood pressure-reducing properties, and most others are not lost when cooking garlic, although they may be slightly reduced. (See "Garlic" in the *Herbal Remedies* section.)

A study conducted by Tulane University revealed that total cholesterol levels in those taking garlic tablets dropped by 6 percent and LDL cholesterol was reduced by 11 percent. Researchers at the University of Kansas discovered that garlic tablets reduced the susceptibility of LDL oxidation by 34 percent compared to the placebo group.

Walnuts and flaxseed have a more favorable ratio of total to saturated fatty acids than any other foods. A couple of tablespoons of walnuts or flaxseed taken daily can be an important factor in controlling cholesterol. The total cholesterol to HDL ratio considered by many to be the most accurate measure of heart attack risk dropped from 4.0 to 3.7 for 31,000 Seventh-day Adventists taking nuts at least five times a week, and they had half the risk of fatal heart attacks of those who had nuts less than once a week. Even in as short a time as two months the difference can be seen. Volunteers took a diet containing 20 percent of calories from

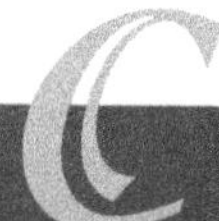

walnuts, as compared to a diet entirely nut free: the no-nuts volunteers had a 6 percent reduction in cholesterol, and an additional 12 percent when they switched to the walnut diet for two months. Walnuts contain omega-3 fatty acids which have a cholesterol lowering effect ("Walnuts Lower Lipids," *New England Journal of Medicine* 329, no. 5 [July 29, 1993]: 358-360). Eating walnuts can increase the HDL cholesterol level. Flaxseed often can be purchased at a fraction of the cost of walnuts, and it is just as effective.

The ideal diet for those with high cholesterol is a completely plant-based diet with no exceptions. The *occasional* use of foods high in saturated fats causes a much higher level of cholesterol than is expected from only a rare exposure.

Breakfast eaters have lower blood cholesterol readings than persons who do not eat breakfast. It was found that children who consistently skipped breakfast had significantly higher blood cholesterol levels. The national average for cholesterol in students ages nine to 19 is 165. Students who eat breakfast as a routine have cholesterol levels from 140 to 150. Those who regularly skip breakfast average about 172, according to a study by Dr. Ken Resnicow that was reported in the March 18, 1991, issue of *USA Today*.

High cholesterol has long been blamed for heart disease and hardening of the arteries. It is now recognized that it is possible that very low cholesterol levels are associated with special features of mental processing. Two hundred seventy-nine students were measured in relation to the speed and accuracy of making choices in tasks that were timed. Female subjects with low plasma cholesterol levels were less impulsive, had slower movement times, and more deliberate decision times. It may be that some factors associated with high cholesterol may make women more bold or less cautious. Additional studies have been planned (*Psychosomatic Medicine* 57 [January 1995]: 50).

The pineal gland and its melatonin secretion is associated with the control of levels of cholesterol. It may be that very high and difficult cholesterol levels which are not brought down by ordinary means might respond to a trial of sun baths four or five days a week for 20 minutes each time, along with an early bedtime in a dark room, or if all else fails, melatonin administration (*International Journal of Neuroscience* 76 [1994]: 81).

The best level for triglycerides is surely below 140, and probably below 100 is safer. Many people can achieve an enviable triglyceride level around the same as their age, which is ideal. The heart attack rate is two times higher if the triglyceride level is above 250 as compared to below 170. Ninety percent of overweight people have increased triglycerides. Other causes of increased triglycerides are alcohol, sugar, the type of fats in dairy products and refined carbohydrates such as white bread, white rice, white flour products, white pastries, and white starch. Even large quantities of fruit juices or very sweet or dried fruits (dates, raisins, and figs) may increase triglycerides in some people.

One way to raise the HDL cholesterol is with the juice of one white or yellow onion a day. The HDL cholesterol will rise by 30 percent in three to four months. Onions are also remedial in stimulating a weak heart, but the benefit is in the bite. Mild onions lack the HDL-elevating effect.

Activated charcoal has also been used to lower cholesterol. (See "Charcoal" in the *Natural Remedies* section.)

Helpful Foods

- Fruit – All fruit, including olives and avocados; two or more servings daily.
- Vegetables – All vegetables, greens and herbs; two or more servings daily of green or yellow vegetables.
- Legumes – All peas, beans, lentils, and garbanzos; at least one serving of these daily.
- Tubers – Yams, potatoes, beets, carrots, radishes, etc.; use as needed in place of vegetables or grains or to increase the total number of calories if needed.
- Cereals – All whole grains; two or more servings of whole grains, varied from time to time.
- Nuts and Seeds – Walnuts, almonds, some peanuts and cashews, pecans, all seeds; one ounce of any, which is roughly two tablespoons.

Note: The whole fruit or vegetable has 6 to 10 times as much fiber as the juice. Fiber attaches to cholesterol and takes it out of the body.

Harmful Foods

- Sugar, syrup, honey, molasses
- Oil, margarine, shortening, peanut butter, other nut butters
- Animal products, including animal protein extracts
- Alcohol and caffeinated beverages
- Strong spices and salt

Herbs to Lower Cholesterol

Cholesterol can be helped by a number of herbs: fresh ginger root, hawthorn berry, myrrh, psyllium, and turmeric.

A tea made from one teaspoon of powdered myrrh steeped for 10 minutes in boiling water is reported to bring cholesterol down. Use two cups per day.

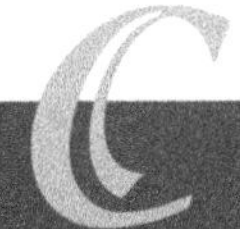

Another tea can be made from one tablespoon of powdered hawthorn berries, with or without one tablespoon of powdered turmeric, and/or one tablespoon of powdered ginger root boiled gently in one quart of water for 10 minutes. Strain if desired and drink the entire quantity in one day. Use daily for three months, and continue if needed to keep cholesterol down.

Chia seed or psyllium seed, one to three teaspoons stirred into a glass of water two or three times daily, has a cholesterol lowering effect and also helps prevent cancer of the colon. The cost of these treatments is one-tenth that of cholesterol lowering drugs, and yet just as effective, or more, without any of the serious side effects seen with the drugs (*Washington Drug Letter* 44, no. 10 [March 5, 2012]). Milk thistle can also be helpful to bring cholesterol down. Take the standard dosage.

(See also "Cholesterol" in the *Supplemental Information* section for more information.)

Chorea, St. Vitus Dance, Sydenham's Chorea

This neurologic disorder is far less common now than formerly, just as are the related diseases of rheumatic fever and Bright's disease (acute glomerulonephritis), because of the natural waxing and waning of disease. About one to six weeks following a streptococcal infection such as "strep throat" or streptococcal impetigo, there is sometimes the onset of a secondary illness that may manifest itself in one of three ways: acute glomerulonephritis (Bright's disease), rheumatic fever with or without heart involvement, or a neurological disorder called chorea. The latter is recognized by inappropriate movements of the extremities or head. It is almost always seen only in individuals before the age of 20. A child may jump from his chair or make writhing movements with his hands and arms while exhibiting involuntary tic-like movements of the head.

Fever therapy is the most effective way of controlling an attack of chorea. Raise the oral temperature to 101°F to 103°F and maintain this level from 30 minutes up to four hours each day for one week, the higher the temperature the shorter the time. Also, the younger the child the shorter the time. If the child is too young to hold a thermometer in the mouth, or if you do not have an electronic rectal thermometer, this method of treatment is not applicable. The choreiform movements should diminish daily.

Two studies are related here to illustrate the management in the 1920s and 1930s when this disease was prevalent. In a two year study, 45 patients with Sydenham's chorea were treated with artificial fever sessions of 105°F to 105.4°F (rectal), each lasting for two and a half hours. The average number of treatments was 12.6, the average number of hours being 32.9, and average time under treatment 22.3 days. Excellent recovery was seen in the majority of cases. There were only four recurrences during the next two years. There was an incidence of prior carditis in 42.4 percent, but this condition did not interfere with the treatments, and the majority of the patients were benefited. Associated delirious episodes were infrequent during the treatments. The delirium is because of the high temperature with associated dozing while still attempting to talk.

The second study had 99 children in the treated groups. They were given fever therapy for chorea and compared with 60 patients who did not receive this treatment. For 48 of the treated patients the observation period was one to three years. For 51 of the treated patients the observation period was four to six years. The most striking finding was the higher incidence of polyarthritis and deaths from heart disease in both observation periods among the untreated cases. None of the treated cases observed from one to three years had aortic lesions; whereas one of the untreated patients did. Aortic disease developed in one patient in the second treated group (observed from four to six years); whereas six in the untreated group (37 patients observed four to six years) had organic heart disease. In the treated group 6.6 percent developed heart disease, whereas 46 percent of the untreated group developed heart disease.

Chronic Obstructive Pulmonary Disease

Chronic obstructive pulmonary disease (COPD) is one of the most common lung diseases that causes extreme breathing difficulty in patients. There are two main forms: chronic bronchitis, which is characterized by a long-term cough with mucus; and emphysema, which is actual destruction of lung tissue, usually occurring over a period of time. Most people have a combination of both conditions.

Symptoms include cough with mucus, shortness of breath, fatigue, frequent respiratory infections, wheezing, and other noises with breathing.

A 20-year study of diet and its effect on COPD showed that there is a protective effect of fruit and possibly vitamin E

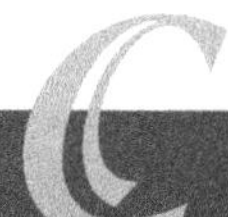

intake against the disease. The most favorable diet in COPD is a low-fat, plant-based diet. The reason for this is the greater ease of pulmonary circulation with this low-fat diet.

Claudication

(See "Lameness" in the *Conditions and Diseases* section.)

Cleansing Program

(See "Cleansing Program" in the *Supplemental Information* section.)

Clotting

(See "Blood Clotting" in the *Conditions and Diseases* section.)

Cold Sores

(See "Fever Blisters, Cold Sores, Herpes I" in the *Conditions and Diseases* section.)

Colds

This is the commonest viral affliction in humans. The average person has two to four colds per year. It is caused primarily by rhinoviruses and coronaviruses. Common symptoms include a sore throat, runny nose, and sometimes a fever. While there is not a cure, there are treatments that make the disease run a shorter course and make the symptoms easier to bear.

(See also "Immune System, How to Strengthen" in the *Conditions and Diseases* section.)

Prevention

Eat a well balanced diet. Never eat purchased fruit and vegetables without first washing them. Several methods of cleaning fruits and vegetables are acceptable. One way is with liquid detergent, dissolving the detergent in the water and plunging the fruit up and down, rinsing three times for grapes and other fruits with edible skins. Soaking in a sink of water to which has been added 20 to 50 drops of concentrated grapefruit seed extract is also helpful. Rinse well while gently rubbing. Another method of cleaning is a spray on product which can be purchased at a health food store for this purpose. Rub a bit if possible and rinse well in running water or by sousing up and down in water.

Forty-five minutes or more of moderately intense exercise, such as walking or cycling in the sunshine, a day will enhance your resistance. If a person walks briskly five days a week during winter, it reduces the number of days suffered from colds and flu by half. But overly strenuous exercise can run down your immunity. If you are an athlete undergoing hard physical training several times a week, you can run your immunity back up again by backing off the strenuous exercise.

Keep the extremities warm, being certain to stay unusually warm when colds are going around. Body temperature often falls a degree or so one to two days just before you get a cold.

A disciplined regimen of cool baths each day raises the number of white blood cells that fight off viruses by significant amounts. We recommend regular bathing in cool water to fortify against colds.

Nasal irrigation protects one against developing colds. Administer nasal irrigation on a daily basis during cold season.

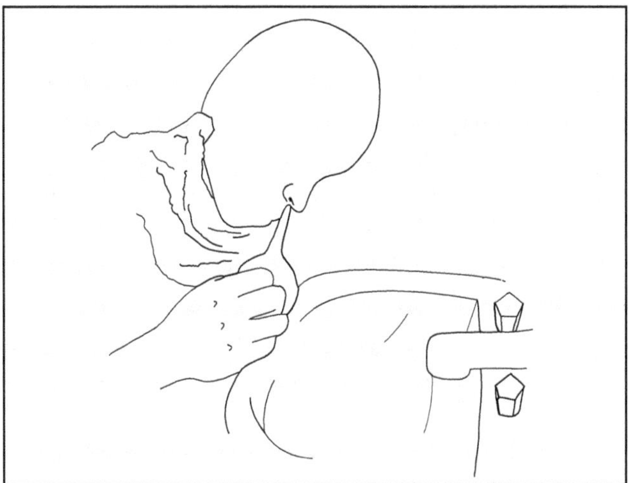

Wash your hands often, and keep your fingers away from your eyes and nose and mouth. This has been proven to greatly reduce the number of colds one acquires.

Sponges and dish rags provide the warm moist environment where cold germs thrive. Put these items in the clothes washer with bleach after a day or two of use.

Keep at least three feet away from coughers and sneezers.

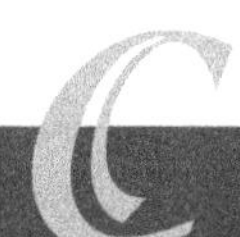

If you must spend time in enclosed spaces with low humidity, such as airplanes and poorly ventilated offices, make sure you stay well hydrated by drinking a glass of water every two hours. Try to wear a surgeon's mask for your protection.

Get a good night's sleep every night. When one gets only four hours of sleep overnight, there is a 30 percent drop in natural killer cells, as well as a decrease in other immune cells such as T-lymphocytes.

Taking drugs promotes colds. Aspirin and Tylenol and many other drugs weaken the immune system.

Treatment

The first objective in the treatment of a cold is to prevent its entrenchment by early therapy. When symptoms are first noted, engage in a deep breathing exercise. Inhale deeply and hold the breath for a slow count of 20. Exhale deeply and hold it for a slow count of 10. Repeat 40 to 50 times while at work or in the car. This will often head off a cold.

Within 10 or 20 minutes of the first symptoms, get the extremities warm. You may put the feet in hot water, kept continually hot for 20 minutes then go to bed for half an hour. If you are away from home, you may only be able to stand close to a source of heat until you are thoroughly warmed up; but, one way or another, get warm.

Keep the bowels open. An enema taken at the first hint of the onset of symptoms will often prevent the development of a cold.

Get plenty of vigorous exercise. The question is often asked, "Is it safe to exercise when you feel sick with a cold?" If your symptoms are above the neck—stuffy nose, sneezing, sore throat, headache—exercise is safe. Just start slowly and stop if you feel ill. It is probably best to avoid intense activity if you have below the neck symptoms such as muscle aches, cough, chills, diarrhea, vomiting, or fever over 100°F (*Physician and Sports Medicine* 24 [January 1996]: 55). Some say it is hard on the heart to exercise vigorously with below the neck symptoms, but others say exercise is no problem in a viral infection.

Drink plenty of water, enough to keep the urine pale yellow to clear in color.

Eat sparingly and only on the usual meal-time schedule. Take no juice between meals. Use no free fats, sugar or honey. Eat whole grain breads and cereals. Eliminate all free fats: margarine, mayonnaise, salad oils, cooking fats, and fried foods, as fats make the circulation sluggish.

Take six charcoal tablets three times daily between meals. If the throat is sore, or there are mouth ulcers, allow the charcoal to dissolve in the mouth to constantly bathe the inflamed areas.

Take a hot nasal irrigation at 110°F to 115°F for 20 minutes. (See "Irrigation Fluids" in the *Natural Remedies* section.) It will often cure a cold if taken early.

Use a hot water gargle for 10 minutes four times daily if needed for sore throat or earache. The ears can be treated through the throat by reflex action.

Take a 15 minute hot bath, followed by a cold shower for 10 to 30 seconds and skin friction with a dry towel for general symptoms of muscle and joint aches.

Apply a sinus pack for sinus congestion or runny nose. (See "Hydrotherapy" in the *Natural Remedies* section.)

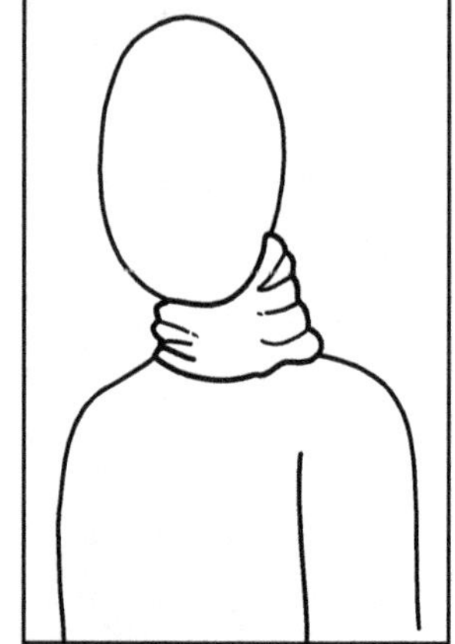

Apply a heating compress to the throat or chest as needed for sore throat or cough. (See "Hydrotherapy" in the *Conditions and Diseases* section.)

Keep the feet, hands, neck and ears warmly clothed both day and night. Chilled body parts weaken the immune system.

Rub the feet with Vicks salve to treat a sore throat. It will miraculously open up the nose and sinuses.

Keep the bedroom at 65°F to 68°F. Have circulating fresh air in the bedroom as a healing agency.

Put one quarter teaspoon of salt and one quarter teaspoon of baking soda in eight ounces of water to be used as a nasal spray to break up and dry the runny nose of a cold. Do not use antihistamines or commercial nose drops or inhalers as they give a rebound effect and eventually increase the symptoms.

Foods high in zinc can help to shorten the length of time spent with a cold. These foods include cereals, beans, nuts, pumpkin seed, and popcorn. Use a zinc lozenge at the first sign of a sore throat. Do not use lozenges with sugar.

Garlic is also quite helpful as it has antiviral and antifungal properties. Grind together in a blender one clove of raw garlic, one fresh tomato (or three-fourth cup of canned tomatoes), one teaspoon of olive oil, and one teaspoon of dried oregano. Take a tablespoonful into the mouth and hold. Swallow a little slowly. This mixture is good for colds and sore throats. Inhaling misted colloidal silver through the nose may reverse the progress of a cold.

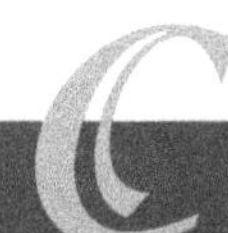

The following herbal remedies are helpful:

- Take echinacea to boost the immune system.
- Take golden seal as an antiviral, antibacterial agent.
- Take grapefruit seed extract and elderberry extract. Both have remarkable antiviral properties when begun at the very first signs of a cold or flu.
- Take astragalus for its antiviral effect. One of the herbal remedies used for viral diseases in animals is astragalus. One study showed that mice injected with a lethal number of Japanese encephalitis viruses after having received an initial dosing of astragalus were compared to mice receiving no astragalus. Twenty-five days later only 20 percent of the control mice were still alive compared to 40 percent in the treatment group. Furthermore, the mice treated with astragalus extract that finally died, stayed alive quite a lot longer than the control mice, indicating the protective effect of astragalus. The protective benefits of astragalus began before the body mounted its own defense through the production of antibodies (*Biol Pharm Bull* 19 [1996]: 1106–9).
- Use the herbs boneset, mint, and sage for specific treatment for colds, taking one cup of one or more four times a day until the cold is gone.
- Place eucalyptus oil in boiling water to make an air humidifier to soothe and heal the nose.
- Drink one cup of hot yarrow tea four times a day.
- For a deluxe treatment of head colds, put six to eight drops of cinnamon oil in a warm bath and sit in the tub 20 minutes or more. Rub some of the undiluted oil into the temples, sinus areas, and chest four times a day. This treatment is also good for the flu. If the skin is irritated by the oil, dilute it half and half with olive or corn oil.
- Place four drops of lemon oil in a cup of hot water and use as a gargle to treat a head cold, a sore throat, or bleeding gums. Repeat up to four to six times a day, tapering off as the infection goes away.
- Beta 1, 3/1, 6-D Glucan is as much as ten times more effective as an immune booster than echinacea alone.

Colic, Infantile

Colic is a word used to signify forceful contractions with pain of a hollow organ such as the bile ducts, tubes of the kidney, or more frequently the intestinal tract. Kidney or gallbladder colic may be caused by stones or inflammation. Intestinal colic may be caused by a simple chill, spoiled food, a nervous condition, stress, or most commonly a food sensitivity. Gas may be associated with the condition.

A fussy baby with inconsolable crying day after day may be suffering from colic. It is more common in the newborn or up to four weeks of age, and usually stops by about the fourth month. Some babies continue to have colic for eight or nine months. The mother of a colicky baby should be given relief from constant care so that she can have an opportunity to get away from the crying for a few hours. She may approach the care of the baby with an altogether different attitude with regular relief of this kind.

Treatment

The first thing is to stop using cow's milk if the baby is on formula. In breast fed babies remove milk from the mother's diet, as even breast fed babies can receive a sensitivity to cow's milk by their mother's milk drinking. The breastfeeding mother should stop using foods to which she knows she is sensitive. These can be discovered by very strict application of an "Elimination and Challenge Diet," which is found in the *Dietary Information* section. In most cases when the problematic food is eliminated, the colic disappears immediately.

Other foods that may need to be removed are chocolate, bananas, apples, oranges and other citrus, strawberries, coffee, nuts, shellfish, eggs, beef, veal, potatoes, sugar and honey, wheat, beans, celery, corn, tomatoes, onions, legumes, and sweet potatoes. All animal products are suspect for causing colic.

In one of our cases, the baby cried most of the day and for long periods at night. When we eliminated the 2:00 a.m. feeding, he was fussy for about 30 to 45 minutes, but he was given a little water and soon went back to sleep. The next day he hardly cried at all. Soon he slept through the entire night. We concluded he was being overfed and his intestinal tract was protesting with colic.

Tight clothing around the waist, leaving red marks on the skin, chilled hands or feet (indicated in some babies by a mottled color of the skin), and overfeeding even a small amount should be corrected. The tiny abdomen can get overcrowded with even a tablespoon more added to its already limited space. A tight diaper or waist band on a garment can constrict the abdomen and cause pain.

Repetitive motion can soothe the baby such as rocking, swinging, and singing to the baby. A battery operated rocking cradle, an automobile ride, or fastening the baby in an infant seat secured on top of a washing machine or dryer while doing a load of laundry may help soothe the child.

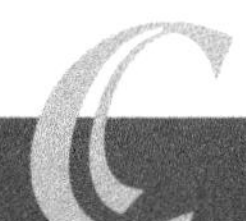

The use of pacifiers, feeding the baby in a sitting position, and frequent burping can be helpful. After feeding, let the infant lie on the right side with a loosely filled hot water bottle. Be very careful with the temperature of the bottle.

If gas is obvious, slowly insert your little finger, coated thickly with a lubricant, into the rectum, to aid the passage of flatus. A teaspoon of charcoal in a small amount of water to make a thin paste will also help gas pains. Put the thin paste in a nursing bottle or hypodermic syringe (no needles); insert it in the corner of the baby's mouth and gently inject the paste into the mouth. You are certain to drop some of the charcoal paste, so put on a large apron and do the procedure in the bathroom with the baby undressed.

A tablespoon of catnip or peppermint tea by mouth as often as needed may be helpful. Other herb teas that may be used include bay leaf (boil one leaf in one cup of water for 15 minutes), chamomile, garlic, thyme, or anise seed.

One or two ounces of very cold water as an enema can stimulate the passage of gas or stool.

Colitis, Crohn's Disease, Ulcerative Colitis, Regional Enteritis

Colitis

Colitis is an inflammation of the colon. It may be a simple irritation or it may be a more serious form called ulcerative colitis, or Crohn's disease, characterized by actual ulceration of the lining of the colon. In these cases, symptoms range from painless excretion of blood in the stools to constant, painful diarrhea, or painful, bloody diarrhea.

Symptoms are diarrhea and pain, but fever, weight loss, and abdominal masses may also be present. Abdominal pain may be made worse by eating and is improved by fasting, rest, and local heat. Diarrhea is generally no more than four or five stools daily but up to 20 or more stools may occasionally be passed. Weight loss is common. There may be tenderness in the right lower abdominal quadrant and even a palpable mass in that region. There is often a history of mouth ulcers.

In the average case the disease continues, periods of being better will be followed by periods of being worse. In the most severe cases, the entire length of the colon becomes scarred and thickened with ulcerations. Perforation of the bowel, fistulae, malignant bowel tumor, nutritional deficiency, and intestinal obstruction, may occur.

Crohn's Disease

There are many hidden triggers that can initiate a flare-up of Crohn's or can be a part of the inception of the disease. Ulcerative colitis occurs about twice as often worldwide as does Crohn's disease, but the incidence of Crohn's disease is rising while that of ulcerative colitis appears to be remaining stable, especially among children (*Canada Health Rep.* 71 [1990]: 343). Crohn's disease is believed to be autoimmune in nature and involves all layers of the bowel. It can also affect any part of the gastrointestinal tract from the mouth to the anus. Ulcerative colitis more often affects only the colon and rectum. Many illnesses can be mistaken for Crohn's disease including intestinal tuberculosis, inflammatory bowel disease, ulcerative colitis, irritable bowel syndrome, infectious diarrhea, and others.

History and Suspected Causes

Crohn's disease, like ulcerative colitis, is more common in the United States and northern Europe, less frequent in central Europe and the Middle East, and infrequent in Africa and Asia. Crohn's disease tends to run in families and to involve Jewish men six times more than non-Jews, beginning most often between 10 and 20 years of age. Blacks and American Indians are at low risk. Somewhere between 5,000 and 10,000 new cases are diagnosed each year in the United States.

Persons with Crohn's disease who smoke are likely to have a more serious case than those who do not smoke. More immunosuppressive medication and more relapses of their disease are likely to accompany the smoking Crohn's patients. Furthermore, individuals who do not have Crohn's are more likely to develop the condition if they smoke (*Gastroenterology.* 117 [1999]: 877).

Several causes of these intestinal diseases have been postulated, including infection, parasites, environmental toxins, food sensitivity, gluten sensitivity, autoimmune disease, and toothpaste. Crohn's disease was first described in the twentieth century at the same time toothpaste was just coming into common usage. While it may be a coincidence, some authorities feel it should be investigated (*Lancet* 336 [1990]: 1096).

Crohn's disease may be caused by antibiotics. It is true that Crohn's disease was a rare condition prior to 1950, and since this time there has been a rapid climb in all developed countries, particularly the United States where it is presently at epidemic proportions. Penicillin and tetracycline have been

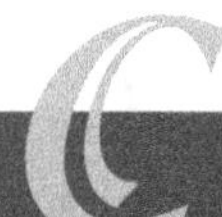

available in oral form since 1953. The increased number of prescribed antibiotics per year and the increased annual incidence of Crohn's disease are parallel (*Hepato-Gastroenterol* 41 [1994]: 549–51). Some believe the antibiotics may play a role.

Large studies have shown that there is an increasing incidence of Crohn's disease in Japan as the westernized diet has been introduced with its increase in total fat and protein, particularly animal fat and milk protein, which strongly correlate with increases in Crohn's disease. Vegetables and fruit intake actually reduce the risk of Crohn's. Earlier studies have related high refined sugar use to an increased risk of Crohn's disease (*American Journal of Clinical Nutrition* 63 [1996]: 741–5).

There are other disorders that often accompany bowel diseases of the kind usually diagnosed as ulcerative colitis or Crohn's disease. These include arthritis, ankylosing spondylitis, low back pain and stiffness, mouth ulcers, thrombophlebitis, finger clubbing, iritis and uveitis, gallstones, kidney stones, and in children, failure to thrive.

Treatment

There is no known medical cure for Crohn's disease and treatment is directed toward relieving the symptoms and healing the bowel lesions by physiologic remedies. Avoid steroids (ACTH, Prednisone, Prednisolone, Aldactone, cortisone, etc.) as dependency on them develops quickly and can lead to other problems. Also, avoid surgery if at all possible unless there is a disabling or life-threatening complication—bowel perforation or major hemorrhage—as complications are usually worse after treatment. Osteoporosis, hypoglycemia, peptic ulcers, cataracts, pancreatitis, and a host of other diseases are known to follow the steroid-type drugs. (See "Adverse Effects of Cortisone or Prednisone" in the *Supplemental Information* section.)

Carefully determining the foods to which the person exhibits sensitivities will help in controlling the disease. Cow's milk is always suspect, including all foods containing any fraction of milk, such as whey products, caseinates, lactates, and milk solids. Sauces, gravies, and all ready-prepared foods must be scrutinized for ingredients from cow's milk. Even tiny traces must be avoided by very sensitive persons. Eggs, tomatoes, beef, coffee, condiments, spinach, citrus, soups, foods having "natural flavors or colors" which could come from tomatoes and apples are most frequently listed as troublesome in ulcerative colitis. But each individual is different; therefore, a very careful search must be made. (See "Elimination and Challenge Diet" in the *Dietary Information* section).

A trial on a gluten free diet is essential. The gluten grains are wheat, rye, barley, and, by contamination from processing plants, oats. Buckwheat is not a grain but the seed of another plant and may be used along with millet, rice, and sometimes corn. Quinoa, amaranth, and cassava root may be used as high carbohydrate sources instead of grains.

It has been found that most ulcerative colitis patients were given cow's milk as infants, and not breast fed. This is another of the many reasons to promote breastfeeding of infants. The patient should become a pure vegetarian, as all animal products tend to putrefy in the colon. A diet high in fiber from fruits and vegetables and moderate amounts of whole grains, legumes, and nuts represents the best diet. Do not use free sugars, as only natural and unprocessed foods, avoiding vitamin and mineral supplements, are the best defense against bowel disease. Some studies have shown an association between the use of large quantities of refined foods in childhood and subsequent development of chronic intestinal disease (*British Medical Journal* 2 [1979]: 762–4). Patients with Crohn's utilize fats poorly and do not tolerate high-fat diets well. A diet not containing free fats (margarine, mayonnaise, fried foods, salad oils, and cooking fats) may greatly improve diarrhea.

Any food having a high pectin content can be very helpful, These foods include carob, carrots, apples, bananas, blueberries, and other fruits. In addition to that, the patient should take one heaping tablespoon of pectin three times daily at mealtime. Pectin is the main raw material for making short chain fatty acids such as butyrate, which are the major nutrient source for the mucous membrane of the bowel.

Hot or cold foods or beverages may stimulate peristalsis, and thereby irritate the inflamed colon. Of course, irritants such as coffee, tea, and all their relatives, vinegar, "food additives," spices (ginger, cinnamon, nutmeg, cloves, horseradish, black and red pepper), alcohol, laxative or gas-forming foods, and carbonated beverages should all be avoided as they may irritate the colon.

Small bites, thorough chewing, and slow eating should characterize the person with Crohn's or ulcerative colitis. This cannot be overemphasized. Overeating or compulsive eating and eating between meals or late at night must always be avoided. Use only two or three foods at a meal.The more nutrients that are mixed together internally increases the likelihood of forming unfavorable chemical compounds resulting in an internal war.

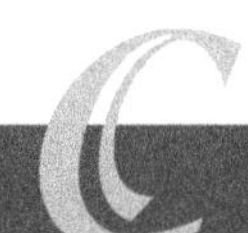

A two meal schedule, breakfast and lunch, may be possible, but in very thin individuals a light and early third meal may be essential. The simpler the meals and the fewer meals taken, the better rest and recovery the digestive system can make. If a meal is going to be served off schedule by more than one hour, it is often best to fast during that meal.

One of the most helpful remedies we have found is charcoal. Take one to four tablespoons three to four times a day between meals. Stir the powdered charcoal into a glass of water and drink the water. If the powder itself gives you pain, let it settle to the bottom of the glass and drink the overlying water. Persons with Crohn's disease should be very careful to stay well hydrated, as dehydration irritates the bowel.

An eight-ounce glass of freshly made cabbage juice given about 10 minutes before meals has a healing effect. It can be mixed with carrot juice for improved flavor.

The water used from cooking one cup of rice in a gallon of water for 90 minutes and then pressed through a strainer, will assist in the control of diarrhea.

Switching from tap water to distilled water has been found helpful to many. If distilled water is not available, one may use the water from a charcoal slurry. Stir a tablespoon of charcoal into a quart of water and allow to settle; use the water off the top.

Regularity in all things is essential. Make regularity the study of your life to capitalize on the natural circadian rhythms.

The out of doors is a great friend to the person with colitis. After each meal engage in some light exercise, such as walking, and enjoy as much additional exercise in the out of doors as possible. Sun baths, even while fully clothed, will promote immune system functioning and reduce susceptibility to infections.

Some patients profit from artificial fever treatments. (See "Hydrotherapy" in the *Natural Remedies* section.)

Enemas can often be helpful. Use either retention or irrigation enemas depending on the patient's need. If dehydrated, use the retention enema; if constipated or toxic, use the irrigation. (See "Hydrotherapy" in the *Natural Remedies* section.)

To decrease or halt bloody diarrhea, a 15 to 30 minute cold sitz bath with a hot foot bath may be helpful. If you need to, you may use a number 2 washtub purchased from a hardware store into which you put four to six inches of water at 92°F to 94°F for the sitz, and a foot tub for the hot water at 108°F to 112°F.

Very hot compresses over the abdomen at 118°F to 120°F for two minutes at most (timing is crucial. It should be for only as long as it takes to stop the bleeding.), can reflexively stop bleeding and should be attempted before the hot enema. To stop bleeding, hot enemas at 115°F to 118°F, and held for one minute only before discharging will usually cause immediate constriction of blood vessels. It should be noted that hot water at lower temperatures, between 104°F to 108°F can be used to decrease pain and improve the circulation, but not only will water at cooler temperatures not stop bleeding, but may actually cause it to increase by dilating blood vessels. Very hot water constricts blood vessels if left in contact for less than three minutes.

Charcoal compresses made with charcoal powder and strong hops tea and applied at bedtime have been used for over a century for bowel inflammation. It is a good treatment.

Stress, anxiety, and worry, as well as competitive games and excessive social activity, all make Crohn's disease worse. Fresh air and sunshine assist in the improvement of generalized immunity. Be regular in all your habits, and avoid any kind of medications other than those remedies which nature provides.

Country living and a low stress, low emotional tension environment, in addition to drinking well water, may be the most helpful program for some patients.

Aloe vera gel or juice has antibacterial and anti-inflammatory factors; use one to two ounces four times a day taken approximately 10 minutes before meals and at bedtime. Garlic has an antimicrobial quality as well, and may be tolerated. Use one to three cloves with each meal, minced finely. If necessary, to make the garlic tolerated by the patient, the cloves can be lightly steamed beforehand. Use more garlic if steaming is necessary.

Also, cold compresses made by wringing large towels from ice water applied to the abdomen for one to five minutes have been helpful for some. Hot compresses may also be helpful, using a simultaneous hot foot bath for the relief of pain. Both types of compresses should be tried.

Certain herbal teas may be helpful. For infection and tissue healing, the best combination is echinacea and golden seal or chaparral. The first boosts the immune system, and the other two have antibacterial, antiviral, and healing properties. If you have an acute flare-up, use the tincture if you can obtain it (otherwise use the tea); take one teaspoon every hour the first day for an acute infection, dropping down to one teaspoon six times a day the second day, waking the patient during the night for evening doses. This program should be continued for 10 days.

For chronic infection the tea may be used; boil one tablespoon of echinacea and one tablespoon of golden seal

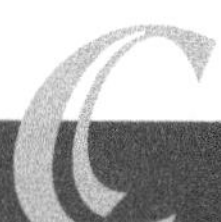

or chaparral in one quart of water for 20 minutes. Use one to four cups a day. One teaspoon of licorice root powder in a cup of hot water taken twice daily can also be very helpful. Licorice has similar effects to anti-inflammatory properties of steroids. Peppermint, astragalus, and slippery elm tea have healing and soothing properties as well. Catnip tea will often quiet bowel action. A retention enema of lukewarm golden seal tea will help heal and soothe the rectum. (See "Hydotherapy" in the *Natural Remedies* section.)

One may also try turmeric, starting with one-half teaspoon in one cup of hot water three times a day and increasing it to one teaspoon in a cup of hot water three times a day. Capsules of turmeric and golden seal may be substituted for the teas if absolutely intolerable because of taste. Use two capsules in place of one cup of tea. The tea is more effective in the acute stages. Turmeric can cause a stomachache in larger quantities and should be discontinued if a stomachache develops.

Other useful teas are chaparral and juniper berries. Generally, no more than seven herbs should be used at one time.

Collagen Diseases

Collagen disease is a disorder of the connective tissue in which collagen, a type of connective tissue in the body, deteriorates and becomes inflamed. It is generally believed that the immune system becomes confused so that normal body cells are mistaken for invaders and are attacked. Several diseases in this group will be discussed, and treatment for all will be given after the section on lupus unless some treatment is specific for a certain type of collagen disease.

Silicone gel breast implants have been accused as one of the causes of autoimmune diseases such as lupus, rheumatoid arthritis, and scleroderma (*Lancet* [November 28, 1992]: 1304; *Science News* 142 [Dec. 12, 1992]: 414). Whether it be that the silicone gel actually causes or whether it simply hastens the onset of symptoms among women already developing an autoimmune disease has not been determined.

Dermatomyositis

This disorder involves the skin and muscles, affecting people of all races and colors and both sexes. It is most common between the ages of 10 and 50. The symptoms include difficulties with vision, tender muscles, swallowing, breathing, speech, etc. These symptoms are accompanied by weakness and loss of weight.

Polyarteritis Nodosa

This is a disease producing nodules along the course of the blood vessels. It may occur in any part of the body. The condition affects men four times as often as women, and mostly those between the ages of 20 and 40. Arthritis and other signs of hypersensitivity are observed in this disease. There may be widespread serious damage to blood vessels, which may eventually cause death.

Scleroderma

This disease hardens the connective tissue principally in the skin. It occurs in women chiefly between the ages of 30 and 50. The swelling of the skin may be followed by calcification. The disease comes on slowly and insidiously. As it progresses changes occur in the skin of the face, neck, and arms. The skin looks waxy and tight, and it loses its color and hair. It may occasionally progress to the point that the extremities become contracted and useless by the tightly stretched skin. When the face is involved, there may be difficulty in moving the jaw. The esophagus and bowel may become involved, creating a more serious situation of difficulty swallowing or digesting food. It is not a common disease, and not generally as serious as polyarteritis nodosa or lupus. Rarely does it progress to be life threatening.

Heavy metals, particularly copper and iron, in abnormal amounts were found to be associated with scleroderma in some people. It is postulated that this increase in these heavy metals causes malfunctioning at a cellular level. Heavy metals have been shown to be decreased in tissues by the use of garlic in significant quantities—more than one clove per day—and cilantro, a kitchen herb. Use two or three sprigs or more once or twice daily. Modified citrus pectin can be used also. These foods increase the rate of heavy metal excretion.

Dimethylsulfoxide (DMSO) is a solvent that readily penetrates the skin and can soften the skin. It can be used in scleroderma. The part to which DMSO will be applied should be washed with clear water and dried thoroughly prior to application, as DMSO tends to unite with any substance on the skin and carry it with it into the skin. If possible keep the part uncovered for about 30 minutes until the DMSO has penetrated completely. Give three treatments a day for three months, until softness and range of motion return to normal. Then cut down the number of treatments to two per day, and finally to one a day. Some patients will go into remission, most will receive some benefit, but some patients may receive no benefit. DMSO can give a garlic odor to the breath.

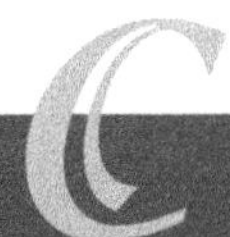

In those receiving no benefit, their sessions were changed to involve immersion of the hands in 50 percent DMSO for 5 to 10 minutes twice a day. Side effects may be brief periods of redness, burning, or sharp prickling sensations, which subsides in about a week. Some researchers have felt that DMSO could alleviate all symptoms of scleroderma. It is certainly worth a try.

GLA (gamma-linolenic acid) is converted to prostaglandin E1, a potent anti-inflammatory hormone-like fatty acid. Some have felt that both scleroderma and Sjogren's syndrome are because of a lack of synthesis of prostaglandin E1. GLA has also been helpful in rheumatoid arthritis. It can be found in evening primrose oil, borage oil, or black currant seed oil. Borage oil is the most concentrated and economical source. Flaxseed oil, one to two tablespoons once or twice a day, can also be helpful in scleroderma.

Other things known to be helpful in scleroderma include all known antioxidants, boswellia (150 milligrams of standardized extract three times a day), five ounces of purple grape juice daily, and careful attention to natural laws of health—nutrition, exercise, water, sunshine, temperance, pure air, rest and adequate naps, and trust in divine power.

Lupus Erythematosus

Disseminated or systemic lupus is a chronic, usually severe disorder occurring more often in females ages 15 to 40. Lupus strikes about one in one thousand white women and one in five hundred black women worldwide. Men are about one-tenth as likely to get the disease. A characteristic butterfly-shaped rash or inflammation may occur over the nose, cheeks, forehead, and chin. Other parts of the face may be free from inflammation. Frequently there are additional symptoms that involve the joints, kidneys, lungs, heart, blood vessels, red blood cells, white blood cells, or platelets. A common sign of lupus is mouth ulcers lasting longer than two weeks. The disease can involve any one or any combination of organ systems. Chronic systemic lupus has been shown to be associated with a family history of autoimmune diseases, a history of shingles, and a history of allergies (*American Journal of Epidemiology* 140 [1994]: 632-42).

Persons who own dogs having immune system disorders may be likely to suffer from similar defects. Former President George W. Bush, Barbara Bush, and their dog, Millie, all suffered from immune system illnesses (Graves' disease). A study compared the immune system of 15 dogs of lupus sufferers, nine dogs of healthy people, and 10 dogs known to suffer from lupus. The dogs of lupus patients had antibodies against their own cells, similar to the conditions suffered by their owners. Immune cells of these dogs were significantly different from dogs of healthy people, and similar to dogs suffering from lupus.

Treatment

Avoid direct sunlight. If you are out in the sun, make sure you are fully covered with clothing, wear a broad brimmed, protective hat, or use an umbrella. While not all patients with collagen diseases are sensitive to sun, heavy sunning has been found to reduce the sensitivity of the immune system. Therefore, before engaging in prolonged sunning, be certain you are not so sensitive. However, get plenty of sunshine in your home, every room being open to the sun during some part of the day.

Exercise has been shown to be an excellent treatment for persons with lupus. Exercise out of doors in the early morning is the most advantageous. Exercise is essential to keep the immune system healthy and to avoid depression, fatigue, and physical degeneration. Early morning air contains more negative air ions.

Fever treatments should be given three to five times a week until 15 treatments have been received. The mouth temperature should be raised to 102°F to 103°F if the general condition of the patient will allow it, but as little as 100°F mouth temperature is beneficial. Keep the temperature elevated for 20 to 30 minutes, using care to keep the head cool with cloths wrung from ice water. If the patient does not tolerate heat treatments, use the short cold bath, filling the bathtub with water from 60°F to 90°F, the colder the better, and soaking for one to three minutes. The physiologic effects are similar to the longer heat treatments for collagen disease patients. (See "Hydrotherapy" in the *Conditions and Diseases* section for information about fever and cold treatments.)

Warm clay baths have been used at temperatures about 102°F, more or less, with the patient remaining in the tub for three or four hours. We have taken an old bathtub, lined it with a plastic liner, and made the soupy clay paste in a protected outdoor area to facilitate disposal of the clay after the bath. The plastic liner is optional.

Echinacea tea will boost the normal functioning of the immune system and inhibit the abnormal. Add one tablespoon to a quart of water and gently boil for 10 to 15 minutes. Drink the entire amount throughout the day for 21 days.

The use of drugs should be carefully avoided. Contraceptive pills, penicillin and sulfonamides, cimetidine, and corticosteroids should all be avoided. If you are currently taking any cortisone-like medications, do not discontinue without the help of a professional.

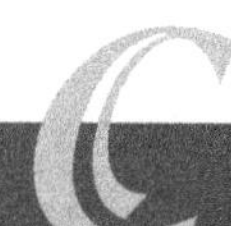

There is no alteration in the course of the disease with the use of steroid drugs, only in the symptoms. These drugs should be avoided if at all possible as the side effects are serious, and dependency develops easily. (See "Adverse Effects of Cortisone or Prednisone" in the *Supplemental Information* section.)

Also avoid hair coloring agents, hair sprays, cosmetics to which the person is sensitive, perfumes, and cleaning agents that may cause sensitivities.

The diet should be free from all animal products, especially dairy. Persons with collagen diseases do much better on a plant-based diet. Those with arthritic symptoms should avoid members of the nightshade family (tomatoes, potatoes, eggplant, peppers, paprika, pimento, and tobacco). Determining food allergies and eliminating those foods has been beneficial to some lupus patients (*Journal of the American Dietetic Association* 95 [1995]: A-31). (See "Elimination and Challenge Diet" in the *Dietary Information* section.)

There are certain dietary substances known to either aggravate or relieve lupus symptoms. Aggravating substances include L-canavanine found in some alfalfa tablets and immature alfalfa sprouts younger than five days old. These should be strictly avoided by collagen disease sufferers. Dietary measures found to relieve lupus symptoms include reducing the total number of calories and making the diet low in protein while increasing foods that contain vitamin E and vitamin A, as well as foods containing selenium and omega-3 fatty acids.

The diet is best when free from refined sugars, free fats, and all irritating spices. A trial diet of foods high in natural plant sterols may be useful. These foods are listed in our discussion of menopause. (See "Menopause" in the *Conditions and Diseases* section.) Some of these foods, although high in plant sterols, may be foods to which you have a food sensitivity. If so, simply omit those and use others on the list. There are beneficial effects from reducing the intake of visible or free polyunsaturated fatty acids in the diet for one year in patients with lupus (*Annuals of the Rheumatic Diseases* 49, no. 2 [February 1990]: 134). These include margarine, mayonnaise, fried foods, salad oils, and cooking fats.

Food should be taken in small bites and chewed to a cream. Eat slowly. It may be that the "leaky gut" syndrome may be a part of the cause of collagen diseases. Care should be taken to eat at regular times and avoid complex mixtures in salads and casseroles. Avoid too great a variety of food at a meal. The menu should contain a simple main dish, a cooked fruit or vegetable, an uncooked fruit or vegetable, and bread and spread. The smorgasbord menu is unhealthy.

Charcoal taken by mouth may help remove toxins from the body. One teaspoon of the powder stirred into a glass of water taken four times daily may be the appropriate dosage.

Bee venom has been found to be anti-inflammatory for lupus. Three stings three times weekly have been used with very good success by some naturopaths. I would certainly try it if I had a collagen disease, as it is harmless if you are not sensitive to bees. Some persons with lupus and rheumatoid arthritis have even used six bee stings per week for six months to good effect.

Nephritis from lupus can be benefited by the high lignin content of flaxseed. It is recommended for its anti-inflammatory properties. For those who suffer from nephritis take two to four tablespoons of flaxseed, freshly ground, each day on cereal or in juice (*Clinical and Investigative Medicine* 17, no. 4 [August 1994]: B97, 98). It has also been shown that soy protein is healing for the kidneys. A small serving (one quarter cup more or less) daily is beneficial.

Whole body heating, such as in a hot tub bath, causes the body to increase the production of soluble necrosis factor receptors that are helpful to persons suffering from a variety of rheumatic diseases. Whole body heating produces endorphins that provide some relief of pain as well as an increased rate of healing (*Journal of Rheumatology* 26 [1999]: 2513).

A group of researchers believes that, under appropriate conditions of family susceptibility, dental fillings may contribute to immunologic aberrations that could lead to autoimmune diseases (*FASEB Journal* 8, no. 14 [1994]: 1183; *Toxicology and Applied Pharmacology* 132, no. 2 [1995]: 299). Silver fillings, which contain mercury and other metals, should probably be avoided until this matter can be clarified.

To produce more platelets, take folic acid. Cat's claw, which in Latin is *Uncaria tomentosa*, has been shown to stimulate the bone marrow. It might be good to use some of that as well.

One young lady with lupus began to take a silver solution. Within weeks her lupus had cleared up which she had had for eight years. This is another harmless treatment I would try if I had a collagen disease. Silver 100 is one such product.

Sjogren's Syndrome, Dry Eyes

This collagen disease is unique in that it attacks certain glands causing dry eyes, nose, and mouth and can involve many organs. It is slowly progressive, attacking primarily women age 50 and over. The cause is unknown, and there

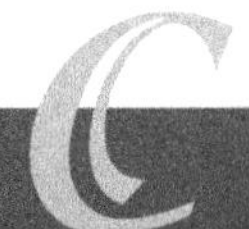

is no known cure, but there are several treatments. About 50 percent of the time, people with Sjogren's syndrome also have lupus, rheumatoid arthritis, or some other connective tissue disease.

Tears are produced in adequate quantities in most people to keep the eyes nicely lubricated so that blinking the eyes causes no discomfort. In some persons tears dry up and an uncomfortable sensation is felt each time the eyes are blinked. The problem may be severe enough that upon blinking, the lids refuse to cover the eyes, getting stuck on the eyeballs.

Symptoms of dryness, grittiness, soreness, sensation of a foreign body in the eye, scratchiness, unusual sensitivity to air conditioning, reddening, and burning are the most common symptoms of dry eye syndrome.

Treatment

Eat a diet low in protein, salt, and fat, as each of these requires extra water to maintain the fluid equilibrium. White sugar and all refined carbohydrates similarly cause a drying up of body fluids.

Since constipation alternating with diarrhea may characterize Sjogren's syndrome, daily or near daily abdominal massage, moving in a clockwise pattern, can be helpful. A supplement of magnesium may help both the dry eyes and the constipation.

These patients may be very sensitive to heat and cold. Regulate room temperature as needed. During cold weather a heating pad can be placed in the chair and turned on low for the patient who may be sensitive to cold. After the chair is warmed, the heating pad can be unplugged if desired. A heating pad can also be used in bed to warm the bed or to be used for the feet. In summer the appropriate use of electric fans can accomplish much in keeping the patient comfortable.

At any time the humidity in a room is below 40 percent, it is important to have some source of added humidity, a humidifier, a crock pot containing water and left uncovered, or a kettle on a stove.

Chronic dehydration is a part of the syndrome in some patients. Stay well hydrated by drinking 8 to 12 glasses of water per day, keeping the urine quite pale. The quantity of water should be measured out in the morning and drunk before going to bed that night.

Just prior to bedtime, apply hot compresses to painful joints or muscles for 10 minutes, ending with one minute of cold.

For dry eyes put one teaspoon of salt and one teaspoon of charcoal in a quart jar. Pour two cups of boiling water into the jar. Let it cool a little, strain through a coffee filter, use as artificial tears instilled with a dropper into the eyes. You can also wet pieces of gauze in the solution and lay them over the eyes at night. The fluid should be stored in the refrigerator with only a small amount taken out at a time.

A gentle massage that leads to relaxation reduces tension and can counteract fatigue. Avoid any technique that causes pain. Following the massage the patient should rest in bed for at least 30 minutes.

The eyes can be gently massaged by repeatedly squeezing the eyelids tightly shut. While the eyelids are squinted shut, move the eyes from side to side or up and down. This procedure will often provide a little secretion of tears to relieve the dryness for a short time. You can also massage the eyelids using tiny rotary strokes and progressing from the lower inner portions of the eyelids around the eyes to the upper inner portion of the eyelids. This will often stimulate the tear glands to produce sufficient tears to lubricate the eyes.

Exercise should be selected carefully and should be described as vigorous but not violent. When tissues are inflamed, too much exercise can be harmful, but when things are going quite well, as much exercise as can be tolerated should be used.

Reduce stress with neutral baths, herbal teas, exercise, massage, and trust in divine power. Since individuals with chronic illnesses tend to stay at home, getting out of the house constitutes a mini-vacation. Daily excursions from the house should be planned, even if only as far as the yard or garden. Seek from God the grace to overcome temptations to vent angry feelings, to feel hopeless, to be depressed, etc. Select someone in your community who needs some kind of benevolent work done for them that you would be able to do. It may be a babysitting job or transportation to the grocery store or simply a telephone call for prayer and encouragement.

Taurine, a nutrient present in food yeast, beans, or carob, is good for dry eye syndrome. If the uric acid in the blood is not high, take two teaspoons of food yeast daily. One can also get a good quantity from a fourth to one-half cup serving of beans daily or from one serving of carob powder, about one tablespoon.

GLA, gamma linolenic acid, is also beneficial in dry eye syndrome. The best source is borage oil, but GLA is also present in flaxseed oil, black currant seed oil, and evening primrose oil. The dosage for flaxseed oil is one tablespoon once or twice per day. The whole flaxseed may be used instead of the oil, and may be about equivalent if you use two tablespoons with each meal. Grind the seed freshly with each meal as the fat in already ground flaxseed meal deteriorates quickly.

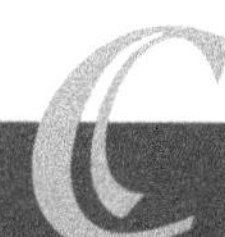

Boswellia oil or licorice root may be taken as tea or pills, one dose four times daily. Hot teas of chamomile, elder flowers, lime blossoms, cleavers, and burdock may be taken two to four times daily.

Fifteen milligrams of zinc taken daily may help to increase saliva and tears, as will large doses of vitamin B6 (500 milligrams daily).

Five ounces of purple grape juice daily may be very helpful for dry eye syndrome.

A localized water deficiency in the tear ducts and a mucin deficiency can be at the basis of dry eye syndrome. Additionally, the conjunctiva may be maturing its superficial cells in an abnormal way. Therefore, the use of vitamin A as a maturing agent for conjunctiva, for a stimulus to mucin production, and as an antioxidant can assist remarkably in treatment of dry eyes. One company produces a liquid containing vitamin A named Viva-Drops. Doctors who have used this treatment report impressive clinical results. Unlike other dry eye preparations that are merely wetting agents, the underlying cellular changes causing dry eyes are reversed by topical vitamin A (*Practical Optometry* 4 [1993]: 163–5; *Contact Lens Journal* 19 [1989]: 165–73).

Compulsions

(See "Mental Disorders" in the *Conditions and Diseases* section.)

Conjunctivitis, Pink Eye, Sore Eyes

Sore eyes, characterized by redness, swelling, tears, and a discharge of watery or stringy white or yellowish material can be treated quite successfully by hourly irrigations with saline in a syringe, catching the runoff over a sink or with a small basin or bowl. Make the saline by mixing one teaspoon of table salt into one pint of water. If the discharge is thin and watery, it is more likely to be an allergy or a virus; if thick and yellowish, it is probably a bacterial infection.

Treatment

If the conjunctivitis is because of an allergy, the person may need to avoid pollens, molds, house dust, animal dander, chemicals, drugs, and cosmetics. Even foods can cause chronic conjunctivitis. Rinsing with a drop or so of saline every couple of hours during the worst part of the allergy season may completely control symptoms. Allergies to foods can usually be controlled. (See "Elimination and Challenge Diet" in the *Dietary Information* section.)

Cold compresses to the eyes are very helpful to relieve congestion and discomfort in acute conjunctivitis. Use small, ice cold compresses every two or three minutes for half an hour, discontinue for 30 to 60 minutes and reapply for half an hour.

A derivative effect to relieve discomfort may be achieved by applying heat to the sides of the face, chin, and mouth. Use very hot applications every two to four hours, wringing a washcloth from hot water and applying it to the eyes for two minutes, alternating with ice cold applications for 30 seconds and continuing for 20 to 30 minutes.

If the eyes are itchy, tightly squinting the eyelids together and rotating the eyes in all quadrants can relieve the itchiness. The eyes should not be rubbed except with the lightest fingertip massage and freshly washed hands.

Frequently wash the hands carefully to avoid spreading to the other eye or other individuals.

If you have a bacterial infection, do not put patches on the eyes overnight as some bacteria may overgrow and the condition worsen. You may use comfrey compresses for viral infections or allergies. Charcoal compresses are quite good for allergic conjunctivitis, and may also help viral conjunctivitis, but may or may not help bacterial conjunctivitis.

The following compress may be used for bacterial conjunctivitis: one-half cup boiled water, one-half teaspoon golden seal powder, and one teaspoon eyebright, heaping. Stir to wet herbs. Let it sit for 30 minutes. Strain it through a muslin strainer or coffee filter to get all particles of powder out of the fluid. Make the tea fresh daily. Use an eye cup (purchased from a pharmacy) filled with the fluid six to eight times daily. Bend over the cup, put your eye into the liquid, and blink your eyes repeatedly while bending over the cup. Even in chronic cases, a bacterial infection should be well within three weeks.

The best way to use charcoal for conjunctivitis is to stir two or three tablespoons of charcoal powder into a pint of saline (one teaspoon of salt per pint of purified water), let the black part settle, and use the top part with a syringe or an eyedropper, for irrigations. Irrigate the eyes with this or some other fluid every hour or two until the inflammation is cleared. Other irrigation fluids include saline or boric acid (made with one teaspoon of boric acid to a pint of warm tap water). There should not be very noticeable burning from the solution or your measurements may not be accurate.

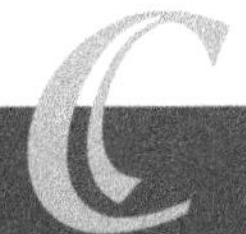

Constipation

Evacuation of the bowel ordinarily occurs once or twice every 24 hours; failure to do so is called constipation. Constipation may be caused by insufficient intake of water or underfeeding or overfeeding, especially of fat or refined foods. Tight waist bands, recent enemas, inadequate exercise, the laxative habit, and many other factors cause constipation. Nervous tension or an overly busy schedule can also cause one to ignore the first signals to empty the bowel until they are no longer felt.

Treatment

Try taking magnesium citrate for about six weeks to see if that will make your bowels less sluggish. Take the maximum dose you can without causing diarrhea, which is usually twice the recommended dosage on the container. Sometimes people who have low functioning thyroid or tendency to have diabetes also have magnesium deficiency. Use magnesium high foods for maintenance of magnesium levels. (See "Food Sources High in Certain Nutrients" in the *Dietary Information* section.)

We have found not only prunes but also other dried fruits to be especially helpful in relieving constipation. Foods known to have a laxative action include apples, figs, strawberries, bananas, peaches, soybean sprouts, and raw spinach. Four to six olives eaten with each meal will cure constipation in many cases. Pears, both fresh and dried, have the ability to help sluggish bowels.

A diet low in vegetable fiber and high in meats, sugar, cheese, and other dairy products promotes constipation. The diet should be corrected by eliminating animal products and refined foods and increasing the intake of fruits, vegetables, whole grains, and a few nuts. Fruits are especially helpful to overcome constipation. A meal composed entirely of fruits of all forms (dried, fresh, canned, stewed, etc.) will be found corrective for most cases of acute constipation.

Eliminating all grains for a few days will help some people improve the tone of the intestinal tract. Eat plenty of fruits and fresh vegetables to supply calories.

Eat meals at the same time every day, and chew the food to a cream before it is swallowed. The act of chewing produces dopamine, a neurotransmitter in the brain. The act of swallowing also regulates to some degree the activity of the colon. Therefore, small bites that are chewed longer increase the number of bowel movements per day and decrease constipation. Hurried and irregular meals may induce constipation and should be avoided.

Certain seeds are effective. Take two tablespoons of flaxseed ground fresh daily on food or in juice, one teaspoon or more of psyllium seed, or two or more tablespoons of pumpkin seed. Agar, wheat, rice, or oat bran, and slippery elm are all useful. An excellent recipe is one tablespoon of finely ground flax seed and one tablespoon of wheat or oat bran with cereal each morning. Chia seeds are also helpful for constipation.

Overeating may cause either constipation or diarrhea, whether or not it has resulted in overweight, but overweight is certainly a cause of sluggish bowel action in many people.

An adequate intake of water is essential for prevention or treatment. Eight to 10 glasses of water daily are recommended. Some who have moist skin may need as much as two additional glasses. Do not use coffee or tea as they induce constipation.

Decongestants and antihistamines, diet pills, pain killers, amphetamines, cough preparations, and many other drugs may cause constipation.

Exercising, particularly a brisk walk before breakfast and a small moderate walk after each meal, can assist in developing bowel tone.

No band should constrict the abdomen. It is wisest at night to have the abdomen entirely free, even of underwear bands or pajama bands, and even if the clothing does not seem constricting. One woman reported that any band that hugged her skin while sleeping, no matter how lightly, could cause constipation for her.

Proper positioning on the toilet can assist in bowel evacuation. Use a small stool for the feet, bringing the thighs up against the abdomen while leaning forward slightly.

We have found that if the person who suffers from constipation will kneel, bending over a low table such as a coffee table, for about 15 or 20 minutes, this often stimulates the bowel to produce easy bowel movements. While kneeling, massage the abdomen with the fist pressed and rotated in an inching advance from right to left side, following the path of the colon.

Wear a heating compress on the abdomen each night. (See "Hydrotherapy" in the *Natural Remedies* section.)

Get an infant syringe from a pharmacy, about three to four ounce size, fill it with cold water and give yourself a small cold enema at the time you expect a bowel movement. Hold the cold water for one minute, expel it, and usually a bowel movement will ensue in about one minute. Do not take an enema (one to two quarts of very warm water or solution) as that can paralyze the bowel for several days, making it impossible for you to have another bowel movement.

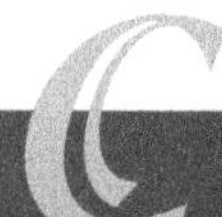

An abdominal massage is helpful. A rocking motion of the abdomen achieved while lying on the back and pressing into the sides of the waist with a fist on either side, bouncing the abdomen back and forth somewhat like bouncing a ball, can encourage the passage of gas or the elimination of a constipated stool.

There are many herbal remedies that can be most effective. Licorice root, one to three teaspoons of the powder stirred in cold water or made into a tea, may be effective. With the tea you may discard the sediment or drink it if you like. Other herbs good for constipation are senna and cascara. Commercial laxatives should not be used routinely, as they are usually counter productive in the long run. Do not use licorice root on a long term basis, as it may lead to sodium retention.

Contact Dermatitis

(See "Skin Diseases" in the *Conditions and Diseases* section.)

Convulsions, Epilepsy

A grand mal seizure is an involuntary generalized attack of muscle contractions. Before the muscle contractions begin, the person may experience an aura in which lights or sounds or odors may be experienced. The second portion of the attack is the muscle contraction occurring without relaxation while the person loses consciousness and is in a stiffened position—the tonic convulsion. The skin may turn blue because of lack of oxygen. This part may start with a high pitched scream caused by contraction of the diaphragm forcing air past the larynx, which is also tightly contracted. The person may foam at the mouth, lose bladder or bowel control, or vomit.

This is followed by the clonic phase which is alternating contractions of opposing groups of muscles and results in generalized jerking. During this phase some breathing begins and the blue color lessens. This phase lasts about 10 to 90 seconds. The last phase begins relaxation, unconsciousness continues, and then sleep. It may last for a few seconds or up to a day. It is usually best to let the person sleep.

Convulsions are usually frightening to bystanders, but if the patient is protected from injury during the convulsion, and no force is used, it is relatively harmless to the victim. Major injuries result from falling in such a way as to get hurt, vomiting and breathing in the vomitus, or damage done to the teeth by trying to force a hard piece of material between the teeth in the false hope that it will help prevent injury to the tongue. If anything is introduced between the teeth, it should be something like a folded handkerchief. But generally it is best to leave the mouth alone until the jerking has stopped. Injury to teeth by ill advised attempts to pry open the jaw are much more of a problem than a chewed tongue. To prevent aspiration of vomitus, the patient should be merely turned on one side with the head slightly down.

In the case of fever convulsions, do not give medications to prevent seizures to a child as this does not decrease the risk of later development of epilepsy. Half the children given these medications have at least one serious adverse effect. It is generally recognized among pediatricians that medication given in this condition is to treat the parent and not the child!

Febrile seizures often occur as the temperature is rising rapidly, rather than after a long period of fever. A slow rise, even to a higher degree, is less likely to induce a fever convulsion. Artificial fevers brought on by hot air or hot water do not cause seizures. The quality of the toxin causing the fever and the rapidity of rise are more instrumental in bringing on a fever convulsion than the height of the temperature. The major objective with convulsions in children from fevers is that of comforting the distraught parents. They should be reassured that a single convulsion does not mean their child has epilepsy or that any brain or other damage has occurred.

The fear that grand mal seizures will progressively increase both as to duration of the seizure as well as a reduction in the time between seizures should not be used as an argument in favor of early drug treatment for children with epilepsy. Apparently there is not a progressive deterioration of the condition with delay in starting medication—unless the number of seizures exceed 20 (*British Medical Journal* 314 [February 8, 1997]: 401). Bear in mind that the anti-epilepsy medication may be more harmful than a seizure.

With a comprehensive approach, epilepsy can usually be helped and sometimes treated quite effectively without the use of medication.

Causes

There are several widely-used medicines that can set off seizures, even in people who have never had a seizure before. While convulsions are more likely to occur from medications if the person has had some kind of seizure previously, drugs that act primarily upon the brain such as tranquilizers, antidepressants, and antipsychotics are the ones most likely to set off seizures. Another class of drugs commonly used for relief

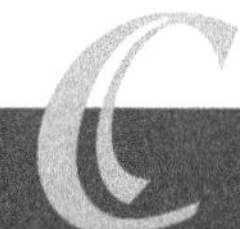

of respiratory tract illnesses such as coughs, colds, hay fever, allergies, and asthma, even many of the over-the-counter drugs, can cause seizures. The third class of drugs much less commonly causing seizures are some antibiotics (penicillin, erythromycin, and metronidazole) (*Post Graduate Medicine* 201, no. 1 [1997]: 165).

Some foods and drinks may at times trigger seizures in sensitive persons. Usually these foods or drinks are found to contain trace amounts of fungicides or pesticides. Apples, oranges, lemons, and grapes are the most common offenders in this regard. Salmon can sometimes cause a problem because the salmon eat from ponds and tanks that have been treated with herbicides to prevent parasite infestation of the fish. Sometimes tap water can trigger seizures in the susceptible person as it also may contain traces of pesticides. It can be very difficult to trace the cause if there is a delay of 24 to 48 hours between ingesting the food or water contaminated with a pesticide or fungicide and the time the seizure occurs (*Journal of the Royal Society of Medicine* 90, no. 7 [1997]: 413).

Treatment

Diet and Supplements

The most favorable diet for an epileptic is a totally plant-based diet from which all sugar and other refined carbohydrates have been eliminated and protein levels are kept relatively low. Use an oil-free, salt-free diet unless you are testing the oil formula given in the next paragraph.

A very high fat, moderate protein, and low carbohydrate diet has been shown for several decades to give improvements in seizure control in about 70 to 75 percent of patients, eliminating seizures in 50 percent of patients who stay firmly on the diet (*Journal of American Dietetic Association* 95 [1995]: 59). But this diet is not as healthful, and not well balanced for long-term use, and we prefer to try other methods before trying this diet. It may eventually be necessary to use it, but reserve it until later. In children with complex partial epilepsy, significant abnormalities were found in spinal fluid such as low blood lactate and alanine, low spinal fluid ketones, and low spinal fluid-to-blood ratio for ketones (*Epilepsy Research* 21 [January 1995]). Administering a mix of beneficial oils such as flaxseed oil (three or four parts), evening primrose oil (one part), and olive oil (two parts) may be helpful. Give one to two tablespoons of the mixture two to four times a day for one month, depending on the age of the patient, then drop down to one tablespoon three times a day (*Epilepsy Research* 21, no. 1 [May 1995]: 59-63).

In another study, calorie restriction reduced the number of seizures and the length of individual seizures (*Epilepsia* 42, no. 11 [Novemer 2001]: 1371).

Food allergies can cause seizures. Peanuts, cashews, almonds, and other tree nuts are perhaps the worst offenders for this. These should be removed from the diet on a trial basis. Any food known to make the person have a sensitivity should be identified and eliminated. One person with epilepsy following a stroke became seizure free when she eliminated caffeine from her diet (*Prevention,* July 1995, 12). Remove any toxins on food by thorough washing. (See "Colds" in the *Conditions and Diseases* section.)

Eggplant contains active ingredients having anticonvulsive properties. The method for preparing the eggplant is as follows: Use a wide-mouth gallon glass jar. Cut a medium-sized, washed but unpeeled eggplant into half-inch cubes and place them in the glass jar. Fill the jar with spring water. It is better not to use tap or distilled water. Store in the refrigerator for four days. On the fifth day start drinking one liquid ounce of the preparation each day. Always keep the jar of liquid in the refrigerator. After a few days the eggplant will begin to swell and it can then be removed from the liquid. Continue drinking one ounce of the liquid each day. It may take a week or two to obtain results. After two weeks, begin taking only half an ounce of the liquid daily. Check the blood pressure to make certain it is not going too low. A component in eggplant called scopoletin, which has anticonvulsive properties and a general calming effect on the nerves, is one of the active ingredients. (*Experimentelle Pathelogie* 10, nos. 3, 4 [1975]: 167–79).

Two cases of epilepsy in which celiac disease was diagnosed, and a folic acid deficiency was discovered, were successfully treated with a gluten-free diet and supplementation with folic acid. A diet containing large amounts of green leafy vegetables should also be give for its high folic acid content. The diet led to complete EEG normalization and cessation of seizures in one case and significant improvement in the other (*Acta Paediatrica Scandanavia* 80, no. 5 [1991]: 559). In patients with epilepsy a search should be made for celiac disease, particularly if there are gastrointestinal symptoms or calcifications in the brain. At any rate, a gluten free diet is worthwhile to try as a test.

Since 70 percent or more of epileptics have abnormal glucose tolerance tests, and constant or periodic low fasting blood sugar levels, close attention to the control of calories and the glycemic index of foods may be helpful in epilepsy. It may be that one of the reasons the "ketogenic diet" has been

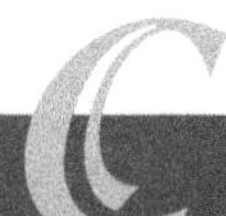

shown to be beneficial in epilepsy is because of its stabilizing effect on the blood sugar.

Some epilepsy patients have benefitted from enriching the diet with omega-3 fatty acids (*Epilepsia* 43, no. 1 [2002]:103).

Epileptics have significantly lower blood magnesium levels than controls. A deficiency of magnesium increases muscle tone, muscle tremors, and convulsive seizures. A group of 30 epileptics were able to control seizure activity when supplemented with 450 milligrams of magnesium daily. If manganese levels are low, supplements of this mineral should also be taken; the dosage is 10 milligrams three times a day. Children with epilepsy may also be deficient in zinc. Its role in brain metabolism is not clearly understood, but may inhibit the neurotransmitter GABA. A dose of 25 milligrams daily for children may be helpful. Supplemental vitamin E (400 IU daily) significantly reduced seizures in 10 of the 12 children tested. Vitamin E and selenium work together to reduce seizures. The dosage of selenium is 100 micrograms daily. One Brazil nut contains about 55 micrograms of selenium. Make certain to chew the nuts thoroughly.

Low iron in the body appears to decrease the risk of both febrile and post traumatic seizures (*Journal of Child Neurology* 10 [1995]: 105–9). Iron tends to collect in sites of brain injury and contributes to seizures. Seizures in response to fever have been shown to be related to a family history of epilepsy (*Epilepsia* 36, no. 3 [1995]: 224). Never give iron supplements to an epileptic. The hemoglobin should be kept under 13 grams and the serum iron under 80 milligrams percent by blood donations if eligible, or therapeutic phlebotomies for those not meeting the Red Cross criteria.

Taurine, one of the most abundant amino acids in the brain, has significant anticonvulsive activity. Taurine increases levels of GABA. Epileptics have significantly lower levels of taurine in platelets than controls, and it may be assumed that they have a reduction in taurine in the brain. One study of patients who were unresponsive to anticonvulsant drugs had a 30 percent reduction in the number of seizures by taking 500 milligrams of taurine three times a day. Taurine is an antioxidant, and it has been shown to greatly help some cases of epilepsy and macular degeneration. Taurine may be used separately, two capsules (approximately 500 milligrams in each capsule) two hours after supper and at bedtime. If necessary, increase the taurine to four times a day, taking it 30 to 45 minutes before meals. You can increase to three capsules each time if necessary.

The following supplements and herbs have been found to be helpful in some cases. Take vitamin B6 up to 50 milligrams per day. You can also try tryptophan, up to 1000 milligrams two hours before a meal and again at bedtime. Taurine, up to 1000 milligrams, may be taken between the two doses of tryptophan. As needed, the tryptophan dose can be given on awaking in the morning and before lunch if an approaching seizure is suspected.

Food sources of tryptophan include pumpkin seeds, almonds, collards. Bear in mind that almonds may promote seizures in certain susceptible persons and should be given only if they have been determined by testing not to be a cause of seizures. Test them by omitting them from the diet for two months. Then reintroduce into the diet and see if a seizure occurs.

Take two tablets of magnesium oxide, which is found in health food stores, three times a day, or one-half teaspoon Epsom salts (magnesium sulfate) twice daily or more (increase gradually until you begin to get diarrhea, then reduce the dose slightly until there is no more diarrhea).

Magnesium citrate may be better absorbed. Try taking one ounce three times daily for epilepsy. If diarrhea occurs, reduce the dosage.

Persons with epilepsy produce more melatonin than others, and there is a difference in the time of day when melatonin is produced in the epileptic as compared to the normal subject. Daily work in the sun from sunrise to 10:00 or 11:00 a.m., and making the sleeping room dark by 9:00 p.m. may help adjust the melatonin production.

For all epileptics eliminate certain compounds known to irritate the nervous system: isoniazid, dopamine, oral contraceptives, alcohol, and hydrazine dyes (FD & C yellow #5).

Some physicians believe that epilepsy should not be treated with drugs unless the patient has had more than 10 seizures. Not until the number of seizures prior to beginning drug treatment for epilepsy exceeds 20 is all question that the epilepsy may not be as easily controlled without drugs or put into remission (*Neurology* 46 [1996]: 41). But giving drugs too quickly after only a few seizures may cause many to be treated with drugs who could be controlled by lifestyle changes and a few simple treatments.

Exercise

Some forms of epileptic seizures can be helped by a breathing technique with relaxation. Begin the breathing exercise when conditions seem favorable for a seizure or if the person has an aura indicating the approach of a seizure. The following exercises are suggested and should be performed five or six times twice a day and at the first sign of a seizure. Standing tall with shoulders back and breathing deeply will

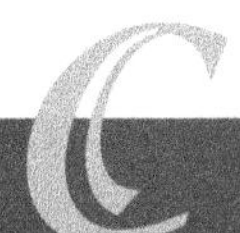

develop proper breathing techniques as you exercise. (See also "Exercise" in the *Supplemental Information* section.)

1. Stand tall with your hands on your shoulders, and elbows together in front of you. Breathe in deeply while stretching the elbows out to the side, returning them to the center as you exhale.
2. Stand straight with one arm at the side of your body and the other curved up over your head. Breathe in while sliding the arm at the side of the body down the leg, and back up as you exhale. Reverse arm positions, and repeat the procedure.
3. Vertical stretch and lifting of the rib cage may be achieved by kneeling so that you sit back on your legs. While breathing in, stretch both hands up as you come up straight on your knees; breathe out while sitting back on your legs and lowering your arms.
4. Lying on your stomach, clasp your hands together over your hips. Lift your head and shoulders while breathing in, relaxing as you exhale.
5. Turn over on your back with your arms above your head. Breathe in as you lift both legs; lower them as you breathe out. This gives abdominal muscle control.
6. Still laying on your back, bend your knees up and place feet flat on the floor. Lift your hips off the floor as you breathe in, lower them as you breathe out.
7. Lie on your back with arms at your side and your feet slightly apart. Breathe in as you lift your arms up and back over your head; breathe out as you sit up to reach for your toes. Breathe in while lying back, and breathe out as you relax.
8. Lie flat on a firm surface with the knees bent. Slowly raise the right knee to the chest while breathing out and tensing the abdominal muscles; lower the right leg, inhale and relax the abdominal muscles. Repeat the procedure with the left leg.
9. For 10 minutes, and at the first sign of a seizure, sit up straight in a chair. Inhale through your nose, and exhale forcefully through tightly pursed lips. Pursing the lips assists in opening the bronchial tubes.

Herbs

Coleus forskohlii has been shown to increase brain enzyme activity by more than 500 percent. This is the greatest increase in activity found in 100 plants studied. The enzymes slow down brain activity and reduce the likelihood of a seizure. Use 5 to 10 milligrams of *Coleus forskohlii* two to three times daily.

Valerian root, two capsules four times a day, may be helpful to control seizures, as may passion flower, hyssop, and skullcap prepared as follows. Stir two tablespoons each of passion flower, hyssop, and skullcap into a quart to a quart-and-a-half of boiling water. Then immediately set off the heat and steep for half an hour. Drink a cup of this tea four to six times a day, evenly distributed in time. Make up fresh every day. Half the quantity can be given to a child. More may be used for adults if necessary.

The Chinese herbal medicine combination called Saiko-keishi-to (SK) has demonstrated a dramatic therapeutic effectiveness with difficult cases of epilepsy that have long been unsuccessfully treated with standard anticonvulsive drugs. As many as one in four epileptics may have a reduction in seizures using this product. SK is a combination of nine botanicals. This herbal treatment works by slowing down transmitter activity from one nerve cell to another, thus decreasing seizure activity.

A decoction of the root of *Afrormosia laxiflora (leguminosae)* is beneficial in epilepsy in that it can reduce the duration of convulsive symptoms and increase the time between seizures (*Phytotherapy Research.* 14, no. 1 [2000]: 57–9).

Use golden seal and St. John's wort for epilepsy on a long term basis.

Other Treatments

Dr. William Philpott, of Oklahoma, a neurologist and a psychiatrist, used magnets to help epileptics. He moved the magnets to various places over the scalp until he found the focus of the abnormal activity in the brain. It was at that point that a one-and-a-fourth inch magnet of 3,150 gauss was attached externally to the scalp, the north-seeking side next to the skin. Dr. Philpott said he had success in treating epileptics in this way. It may be worth a trial as it might divert some abnormal activity toward the magnet.

Cooling of the brain in one study on rats using a thermal electric device (Peltier) shortened the duration of seizures from 104.3 to 8.4 seconds. Even when the brain was allowed to re-warm after prior cooling, there was still a marked reduction in the length of seizures. No damage to the brain was demonstrated (*Annals of Neurology* 49, no. 6 [2001]: 721).

Corns

(See "Skin Diseases" in the *Conditions and Diseases* section.)

Coronary Thrombosis, Heart Attack

A heart attack is often called a "coronary" because the coronary arteries that ordinarily feed the heart are blocked somewhere in the system. It is usually caused by atherosclerosis and associated with high blood cholesterol, high C-reactive protein level, or a high homocysteine level. (See "Cholesterol" in the *Conditions and Diseases* section.)

The first symptom may be severe pain in the chest. The blood pressure may not be altered, but the pulse rate may be 80 or below. The pain sometimes is referred down the left arm to the jaw, neck, or left shoulder. It is often described as a severe pressure just beneath the "breastbone" (sternum). Sometimes it is only felt in the shoulder, jaw, neck, or elbow with little or no sensation in the chest. The "pain" may be felt as a great need to belch which cannot be relieved. It is nearly always accompanied by sweating and weakness. Occasionally vomiting and shock associated with low blood pressure may be seen.

In giving first aid, the first thing to do is to have the person sit in a chair and relax, preferably the chair should be one that can recline very slightly. Place the feet in hot water. Keep a current of cool, but not cold, air circulating, and keep all persons who are merely curious out of the room or away from the person to provide for more oxygen and less commotion. The victim should not be required to talk with anyone, especially anxious ones, but should be kept as quiet and calm as possible. A cool compress (not cold) should be placed over the chest. The hands may also be placed in warm or hot water.

As soon as the chest pain begins to abate somewhat or to stabilize, the patient may be transferred to a bed if desired, preferably by being lifted by several people, preventing any exertion by the person until the most critical period has passed, which is about six hours. The patient usually feels best being slightly propped up in bed. A straight chair can be turned upside down in the bed so that the front legs are touching the headboard, and the top of the back of the chair becomes a slant board.

Cushions can be put on the back of the chair to make a slanting surface for a semi-upright position. Make certain the extremities are kept quite warm, as even the slightest degree of chilling can cause congestion in the heart with an added burden on the heart. Also, shivering is worse for the muscles and taxes the heart to supply blood.

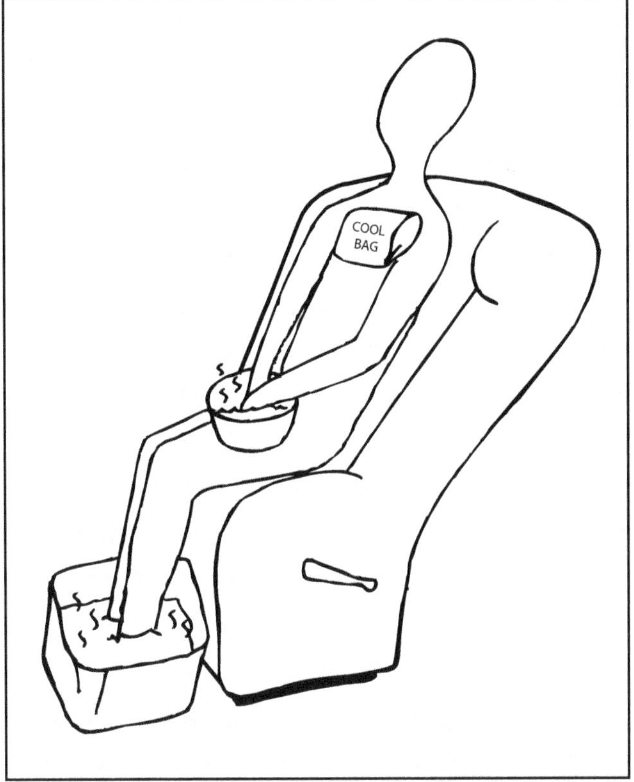

Several herbal teas may be used in the acute phase, such as hawthorn berry tea, ginkgo, and the mildly sedative teas such as catnip, hops, valerian, and skullcap.

Traditional medical care demands that the coronary victim be transferred immediately to a hospital with a coronary care unit. A few innovative physicians have been experimenting with keeping their patients out of CCU's, such as Dr. Demetrio Sodi Pallares of Mexico City, who will not allow his patients inside the CCU. He feels that the atmosphere is so strong and frightening to the patient that any benefit is far outweighed by the anxiety it produces. A few physicians are keeping their patients at home, under close surveillance with intelligent and caring attendants, and the results have been good. With our present lawsuit prone society, however, we would have to recommend that suspected heart attack patients be sent to a hospital as soon as possible, unless you or a member of your family are the victim and can choose. It is mainly for nursing care that a hospital would be chosen. If nursing care can be done at home, you will probably be better treated at home.

As soon after the heart attack as it can be prepared, take a cup of hawthorn berry tea followed immediately by a glass of cool (not cold) water containing some form of magnesium and

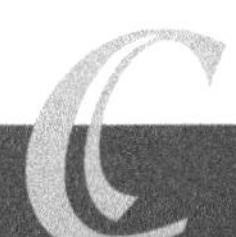

potassium. Magnesium sulfate (Epsom salts) stirred into water from boiling a scrubbed and quartered potato (unpeeled) for 10 to 15 minutes will create magnesium/potassium broth. The broth can be drunk every 15 minutes. Give a light diet for a few days. The patient can get up for a bedside commode after six hours, and for the bathroom and meals after one day. Then light strolling on the level until full activity can be resumed when the patient feels good, the fever is down, CPK, CRP and WBC have returned to normal. Get these tests by sending blood to a laboratory on the first day of the heart attack.

Coughs, Bronchitis

(See also "Pneumonia" in the *Conditions and Diseases* section.)

Bronchitis is an inflammation of the bronchi and can be caused by viruses, chemical agents, or airborne pollutants such as fumes, smoke, dust, and so forth. Coughing is the commonest symptom, but there may also be fever, hoarseness, and discomfort in the throat. Bronchitis may be acute or chronic. The acute form is quite common with "chest colds" or with the other causes noted. Continued infection or irritation, such as is seen in the smoker, will cause chronic bronchitis, which may last for years and may become quite disabling. It can also promote emphysema.

Adults who have the recent onset of a troublesome chronic cough lasting more than three weeks should consider getting themselves tested for whooping cough. In adults with whooping cough there is a greater likelihood that after a bout of coughing the person will get choked rather than having a whoop. Adults are more likely to experience sinus pain and headaches with whooping cough. They may also have sudden sweating attacks.

Treatment

If a cough lasts more than a week after a cold, begin to suspect that an allergy may have developed. Start testing for an allergy by removing milk from the diet and following the "Elimination and Challenge Diet" in the *Dietary Information* section.

Treat a cough by avoiding fumes, smoke, dust, animal dander, and pollens. Wood stoves or gas stoves for cooking or heating increase the incidence of coughs. Some perfumes can cause bronchitis in chemically sensitive persons.

Avoid cough suppressants and commercial expectorants, but anise or fenugreek tea and sips of almond milk have all been reported helpful in bronchitis, as has garlic tea, hot drinks to produce coughing up dried secretions, and the use of a vaporizer. The very best cough medicine we have found is water. A glass of water every 10 minutes for an hour will do wonders for a nagging cough. Good hydration is essential to treating bronchitis. If coughing occurs at night, a large swallow of water should be taken with each cough.

The extremities must be kept warm. Walking barefoot or with very thinly clad feet on a cold floor will prolong symptoms. Cool arms are notorious for provoking coughing in bronchitis.

Any kind of exercise is beneficial in chronic bronchitis, and a deep breathing exercise will assist in the removal of mucus, especially if accompanied by drinking plenty of water. With the deep breath make a light cough once every minute.

Use a heating compress to the chest each night until the cough is entirely gone. Fomentations to the chest once or twice daily, using a thick stationary fomentation to the back, and three exchanges to the front of the chest will often break up a cough within five to seven days, even if it has lasted for several weeks. A simultaneous hot foot bath is very good to break up a cough and pull excessive blood from a congested area. Place the small tub in the bed and keep the water as hot as easily tolerated. (See "Hydrotherapy" in the *Natural Remedies* section.)

An excellent cough medicine for the hacking cough can be made from honey and eucalyptus oil (available from most health food stores and pharmacies). Bring a cup of honey to a boil to thin it. Add six drops of the eucalyptus oil to the honey, and stir well. Sip it from the edge of a spoon as needed.

Herbs that can be used for coughs include the following: anise, slippery elm, fenugreek, licorice, mullein, oregano, thyme, and wild cherry. Horehound, bee propolis, colt's foot, and garlic can also be taken to good advantage.

Combine four buds of cloves, one teaspoon of coriander seeds, a few slices of fresh ginger root, half a lemon, one pint of honey. Bring all to a boil in a double boiler for one hour. Strain and store in a dark bottle. Use a few drops as needed for a cough. Chewing a few caraway seeds as needed also works well for coughs.

Pour one can of asparagus into a blender. Liquify and refrigerate. Drink a fourth cup every morning and evening. Add hot water to make a hot drink if desired. You should notice quite an improvement in chronic bronchitis in a few days or weeks (Jude C. Williams, *Jude's Herbal Home Remedies* [St. Paul, MN: Llewellyn Publications, 1996]).

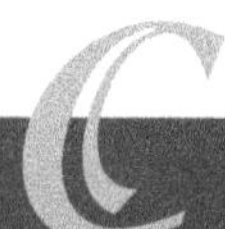

Any object next to the eardrum can cause a chronic cough: a wad of earwax, a bean, a hair. While it is rare, it does sometimes happen. Irrigate the ears with lukewarm water in any case of unexplained chronic cough (*Cleveland Clinic Journal of Medicine* 56 [1989]: 273).

Deep seated coughs and respiratory infections are often well treated with an onion poultice. It helps to loosen mucus and improve circulation. In a medium sized pan, sauté an onion in a little oil at medium heat. When the onion pieces become translucent add just enough vinegar so that it covers the onions. Stir in enough corn meal to thicken the mixture to the consistency of thick oatmeal. Remove from heat and spread the mixture about one-half inch thick onto a paper towel placed atop a piece of plastic wrap about an inch bigger than the paper towel. Leave a one inch border around the edge of the paper towel. Fold a second paper towel over the first paper towel. Seal the edges with masking tape to prevent leakage. Place the poultice, wet side against the skin and the plastic side out, on the affected area (chest, neck, behind the ears, etc.). Cover the poultice with a towel and a small blanket. Leave the poultice in place for 30 to 60 minutes, making certain the skin does not become irritated. Remove the poultice and discard. Wipe the skin with a mixture of half water and half vinegar at room temperature. Repeat the poultice every few hours if necessary. Keep the skin warm after removal of a poultice. The chopped, heated onion without vinegar or oil may also be used.

Bronchitis in nursing babies can be treated by having the mother take three cloves of raw garlic with her food three times daily. That would mean nine cloves of garlic in one day. The garlic is excreted in the milk, and the baby receives remarkable benefit sometimes overnight. Interestingly, babies usually like breast milk better when mom has eaten garlic. A garlic smoothie can be prepared in a blender from three cloves of garlic and two or three oranges. Blend until smooth.

Coughing Blood, Hemoptysis

(See "Hemorrhage" in the *Conditions and Diseases* section.)

Cradle Cap

A scaly, thick, yellowish, or crusty lesion on a newborn's scalp, but may also appear on the eyelids, ears, and the fold between the nose and the cheek. This may be associated with food or environmental allergies, inadequate scalp hygiene, or wearing a cap too long without a change.

Foods commonly observed to cause cradle cap are milk, any flesh foods, wheat, eggs, oranges, beans, peas, and sometimes oatmeal. If cradle cap does not clear up entirely with treatment, try omitting those foods, even from the mother's diet in a breast fed baby.

Shampooing the hair daily or twice daily with plain water and rubbing some olive oil into the scalp will generally eliminate cradle cap in a few days. Do not be fearful of the soft spot on the baby's head, as it is quite tough and will not tear or puncture with ordinary handling.

The objective is the removal of scales and the treatment of the inflamed skin beneath the scales. If the scalp beneath the scales is moist and weeping, treat using cornstarch or the frequent applications of a wet dressing (see "Hydrotherapy" in the *Natural Remedies* section). If the inflamed area is dry, use a little olive oil to keep it soft.

Cramps of Legs and Other Muscles

These are sudden involuntary contractions of muscles, which most often occur in the calves. However, they may occur in any muscle. They often occur when sleeping, sitting for a long period of time, driving, or upon getting chilled.

The cause of muscle cramps also may be a result of overstretching, overuse, or under-use of the muscle. Occasionally a mineral imbalance such as a magnesium or sodium deficiency may cause cramps, but these are not the usual cause.

Treatment

To get rid of an acute cramp, the muscle should be vigorously rubbed and the area forcibly extended so the muscle contracture can be released. One special form of muscle cramping is that caused by hyperventilation. This can be stopped almost instantly by rebreathing one's own breath in a paper or plastic bag.

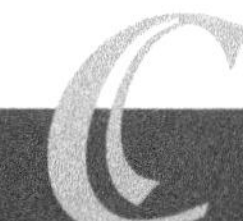

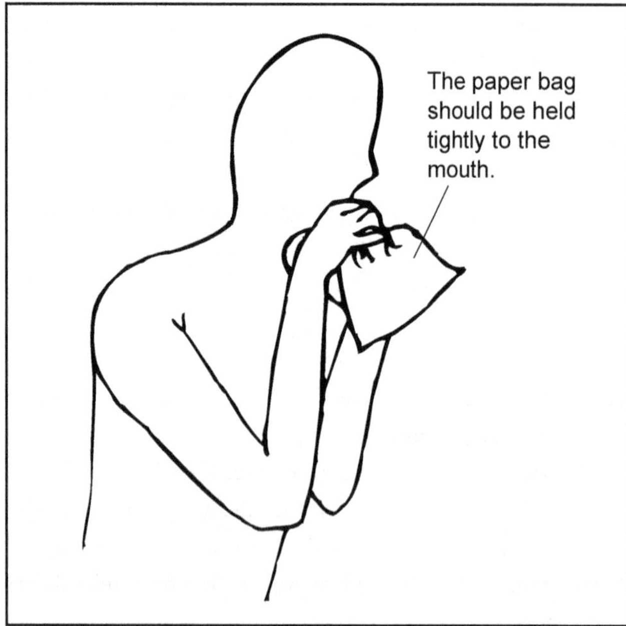

Night cramps in the calves are often associated with getting chilled. There are three things to do to prevent leg cramps.

- Exercise to strengthen the feet and legs.
- Stretch by standing and facing a wall with your toes about two feet from the wall. Place your hands on the wall at shoulder height and lean your chest into the wall while keeping your heels flat on the floor. Hold that position for 10 seconds, push away from the wall for five seconds, then lean in again for 10 more seconds. Repeat the series of exercises three times a day for 30 days, then only once a week thereafter to keep your muscles stretched so they will not be so likely to cramp.

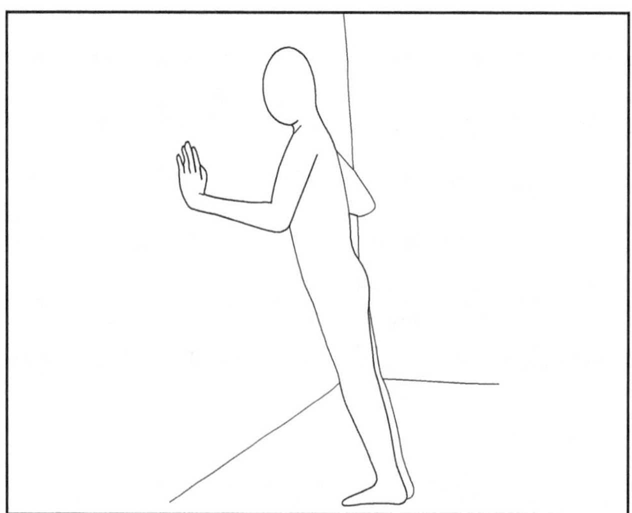

- Keep the feet and legs warm during the night by the use of warm wool socks. Feet drop in temperature more than other parts of the body, and the muscles automatically tighten. With a further drop in temperature, the muscles draw up in a cramp.

Cramps in the abdomen, neck, or back are more painful than leg cramps. The application of heat is often beneficial. Abdominal pain may be because of improper digestion or an inflammation of the intestinal tract or stomach. This can often be relieved by a heaping tablespoon of activated charcoal powder stirred in water.

A "sure cure" for cramps is to pinch very firmly the upper lip just at the junction with the nose. At the same time push upward toward the nostrils and hold for one minute. It should be painful, but some say it will invariably relax the cramp if held long enough.

Gingko biloba can be very helpful with leg cramps, but it is not as good as exercise. In patients who are unable to exercise, gingko may form an important part of their treatment. Black cohosh is another muscle relaxant.

Creutzfeldt-Jakob's Disease

This is a type of subacute spongiform encephalopathy (vacant spaces in the brain). This is similar to mad cow disease in cattle and is caused by a transmissible agent termed a prion. Mainly older adults are affected, characterized by progressive loss of the mind, some jerking of the muscles, and some difficulty in speaking, which progresses rather rapidly to death, usually within about a year. The diagnosis can be made by an EEG. There is no known treatment, but I should think fever baths and an emphasis on all the eight natural laws of health would be a good place to start and may slow down the progress of the disease.

Some say a super charged silver solution may be helpful—one teaspoon of the liquid taken every three hours while awake. This solution is different from colloidal silver and may be more effective. Silver 100 is one such type.

Cricks, Neck and Back

A crick is usually discovered when you first wake up after a long sleep. You find you cannot move your neck, or back, without pain. Holding your head in an awkward

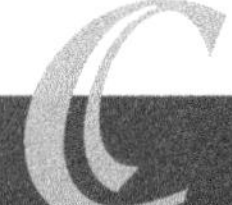

position helps to avoid the pain. About 75 percent of "cricks in the neck" are because of myositis, an inflammation of the muscle tissue. Other causes include arthritis, trigger points, and disk related pain.

The treatment of choice is a fever treatment in a bathtub, bringing the mouth temperature up to 101°F for about 10 to 20 minutes. Then spend an hour in bed under a warm blanket. Finish off the hot treatment if you wish with a brief cold mitten friction or cool shower. The cold portion of the remedy is not essential for cricks.

Massage the neck and shoulders to well below the bottom edge of the shoulder blades and far out on the sides with firm but gentle upward strokes until the pain and muscle spasm are gone. Spastic muscles are recognized because they are tighter than nearby muscles and have a "mass-of-tight-cords" consistency.

Some cricks can be relieved by finding trigger points and holding firm pressure on the tight, swollen muscle for 7 to 10 seconds. Then the thumb is moved the width of the thumb to an adjacent area, and again pressure is held for 7 to 10 seconds. Surround the first trigger point by pressing out satellite trigger points in a circle around the first one, and a second circle around the first circle. In this way all the trigger points and satellite trigger points will be pressed out, which often initiates healing.

Simple stroking of the muscle across its fibers, not length-wise, for 10 minutes can start the healing process.

Crohn's Disease

(See "Colitis" in the *Conditions and Diseases* section.)

Croup

Croup is recognized by a harsh, barking cough, hoarseness, low grade fever, harsh high-pitched respiratory sounds, and almost invariably a history of a cold preceding it for a day or so. Infants from three months to three years are typically affected.

Treatment

Make certain the child takes plenty of water which will loosen secretions.

Avoid milk and sweet drinks as they promote mucus formation. So does wheat in many children.

The child may seem anxious and want to be held. Holding the child should not be denied as both mother and infant will feel reassured.

Keep the child dressed warmly to avoid chilling, but use care to avoid sweating.

Use a vaporizer or humidifier at night, even an old-fashioned tea kettle or a steam tent.

The hot bath is the treatment of choice, using three minutes for children age three and under, and one minute for each year of the child's age thereafter. (See "Hydrotherapy" in the Natural Remedies section.)

The child should be given a heating compress to the chest even for tiny infants. (See "Hydrotherapy" in the Natural Remedies section.)

Avoid cough syrups and antibiotics as these are of no value in viral croup and tend to dry and thicken secretions. You may use the honey and eucalyptus mixture described under coughs.

Recurrent croup may be because of an allergy, and common food allergens, dust, animal dander, smoke, and pollens should be banished from the home. Do an Elimination and Challenge Diet. Following the "Elimination and Challenge Diet" in the *Dietary Information* section is a must.

If the patient becomes short of breath or cannot be comforted by the mother, go promptly to the emergency room at your local hospital.

Cystic Fibrosis

This is a chronic disease beginning in childhood and involving the glands of several internal organs, as well as skin glands. Cystic fibrosis is a cruel and deadly disease affecting the respiratory system, the digestive system (both pancreas and liver), endocrine system, sweat glands, and reproductive system. Individuals with this disease have an uncertain life span. It is hereditary and often fatal unless diagnosed early and appropriate treatment instituted.

Treatment

We advise to keep the relative humidity in the air at above 80 percent. When any sickness arises in the person with cystic fibrosis, the relative humidity should approach 98 percent in the house. One of the first things to be achieved is that of proper hydration. At no time should a person with cystic fibrosis be allowed to become dehydrated. An appropriate quantity of water should be given commensurate with

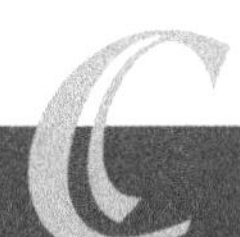

the age, and it should be measured out daily and drunk before going to bed.

The second thing is to avoid free sugars and fats in the diet as these foods tend to dehydrate the blood and body secretions. Eliminate sugars, syrup, honey, molasses, all vitamin and mineral preparations, margarine, mayonnaise, fried foods, cooking fats, salad oils, oil extractions, and nut butters. You may make nut butters in a blender by a method using just nuts and water that does not extract the oils. Make the diet as simple, unmixed, and natural as possible. Some persons with cystic fibrosis lose excessive quantities of salt through the skin and need extra salt added to the diet to prevent low blood sodium (which gives a sense of weakness). The person usually knows how much to add by the craving.

A good vegetarian cookbook will be invaluable. The most favorable diet is a plant-based diet. While many foods are removed from the diet, there is still more variety than can ever be sampled, even during a lifetime. Make an effort to discover foods that are nourishing, will be relished, and will fit into the cuisine your family prefers, whether it be American, Oriental, Italian, Mexican, Middle-Eastern, etc.

The third matter is that of keeping the child in tiptop physical fitness by regular exercise, fresh air, sunshine, and adherence to the other natural health laws. Attention to detail may be what determines success or failure.

One researcher suggested soy oil for cystic fibrosis. Take one tablespoon twice daily for an adult and half that amount for a child. Watch the child carefully, and if there seems to be an increase in coughing, the oil should be discontinued.

CoQ-10 from a drug store or health food store may assist in the management of cystic fibrosis. It should be given on a one-month trial basis at 300 to 400 milligrams per day. Mix the powder with a little coconut oil for best absorption.

Many antioxidants, proanthocyanidins, and amino acid therapies have proven to be helpful in managing the disease (*Alternative Medicine Review* 2 [1997]: 104). Look for preparations of these in health food stores. (See the *Dietary Information* section for foods high in these areas.)

Boston researchers discovered that most persons who have cystic fibrosis are deficient in omega-3 fatty acid and DHA (docosahexaenoic acid). Trial studies are being conducted with persons with cystic fibrosis using a dietary supplement of DHA (*Science News*. 16, no. 19 [1999]: 303). (See the *Dietary Information* section for foods high in omega-3 fatty acid.)

A gluten-free diet should be tested for these individuals as there is often a sensitivity to gluten. Garlic should be used rather heavily in foods, and garlic as a medicine should also be used with any lung illness. Garlic is secreted through the lungs and as it is secreted it loosens secretions and increases the fluid content of the secretions.

Herbs that are helpful include mullein, colts foot, wild cherry, and thyme.

Cystitis

Cystitis is an inflammation in the bladder that may give symptoms of frequency and urgency in urination. Women and little boys are especially subject to cystitis. Sometimes pus or even blood may be found in the urine. Occasionally the patient may experience chills and fever, an increased pulse, and urinary retention. Painful urination is another sign of cystitis. If the pain occurs before urination begins while the bladder is stretched, a bladder ulcer is a likely cause, but if the pain occurs at the end of urination when the bladder is contracting, it is more likely merely an inflammation of the floor or lining of the bladder. Generalized symptoms may occur with a fever up to 101°F or above, nausea, vomiting, and a sense of feeling poorly.

About 15 percent of women have recurrent bladder infections at one time or another. Some of the treatments many women receive on a regular basis, such as dilation of the urethra, irrigation of the bladder, cystoscopy, etc., are unneeded and can lead to permanent injury to the bladder neck and sphincter of the urethra and a prolongation of the very symptoms for which she sought help. Women often need only to correct conditions of chronic dehydration and food sensitivity and the discomforts and symptoms will disappear over a few weeks. To discover food sensitivities, see the "Elimination and Challenge Diet" in the *Dietary Information* section.

Calcium supplements increase the risk of getting a urinary tract infection. Apparently calcium in the urine increases the ability of germs to stick to the bladder lining (*Clinical Research* 40, no. 2 [1992]: 562A).

Trauma from marital relations, wearing heavy sanitary napkins, the use of tampons, history of multiple cystoscopies and/or dilations, certain athletic activities, and any other trauma to the opening of the urinary tract can result in an increased number of bacteria growing at the first part of the urinary tract. Germs from the outside, however, are not the most important cause of cystitis. A weakening of the bladder lining because of allergy, overwork, stress, etc., is the most common cause.

Dehydration, which causes a concentration of urine; the presence of irritating substances from the diet; or foods to

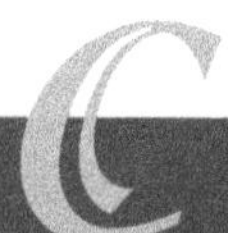

which one is sensitive, which leave a residue in the urine, are all far more common in the cause of cystitis than are bacteria. Generally, bacteria will not attack the urinary tract if it is healthy. It is the weakening of the lining of the urinary tract by allergy or irritation that enables germs to gain access.

Treatments

Try to start treatment within the very first 20 minutes of feeling the symptoms. Start by drinking either a glass of water every 10 minutes for an hour or a cup of one of the herbal teas mentioned below. Then drink 8 to 10 glasses daily of pure water or herb teas made from pure water. Do not use tap water as it may contain irritating chemicals. Since chronic dehydration can occur, and in fact, involves more than 60 percent of Americans, it is well to take measures to correct chronic dehydration if one has a bout of cystitis.

The diet should be carefully controlled. Sugar or other concentrated sweeteners; oil; caffeine or other methylxanthines found in coffee, tea, colas, and chocolate; spices such as black or red pepper, ginger, cinnamon, cloves, nutmeg; alcohol; or baking soda or baking powder products should be avoided. The individual should take only two meals daily, breakfast and a midday meal. Do not eat or drink between meals, except taking plenty of water and clear herb teas. Avoid the use of animal products. Milk or other animal products may also be the culprit. All dairy products must be eliminated, including whey products and sodium caseinate and sodium lactate ingredients.

Persons taking cranberry juice showed a reduced frequency of germs and pus in the urine, particularly in older women (*Journal of the American Medical Association* 271 [1994]: 751-4). Other members of the *Vaccinium* family, such as bilberry leaves and blueberries, may be suitable alternatives to the commercial cranberry juice. Cranberries and blueberries both contain proanthocyanidins, which cause bacteria to be unable to anchor themselves in the bladder.

Much of repeated cystitis or chronic or interstitial cystitis is simply allergic in origin, and the the "Elimination and Challenge Diet" in the *Dietary Information* section must be used to discover which foods are involved. In our experience, eggs are frequently the culprit. Cystitis usually clears up within a few days or weeks of leaving off all eggs from the diet. Even egg whites can irritate such individuals.

Use hot compresses alone or alternate with brief cold compresses accompanied by much friction. Cover the lower abdomen and upper thighs with the fomentation, keeping it hot continuously for eight minutes, then 20 to 30 seconds of cold with friction. Repeat three or four times. A hot sitz bath may be substituted.

A heating pad or heat lamp centered over the suprapubic area may be used continuously between other treatments to control pain or other discomfort.

Always wash the perineum before sexual activity with plain water, no soap. This same treatment should be done each time the bathroom is used during the day. The method is to pour hot water or quite cold, if preferred, but not lukewarm. The idea is to create a marked change in temperature, which encourages a heavier blood flow to the pubic area and encourage its flowing into the folds of all the perineal area. Wash and blot with a tissue, moving from front to back, but never from back to front, as germs from the rectal area can be transferred forward. After marital relations always urinate to assist in flushing out bacteria. This has been found helpful, especially in "honeymoon cystitis."

Do not use birth control pills or spermicides, as they encourage cystitis.

Be especially careful of hygiene in menstruation as bacteria may grow more prolifically. Avoid using tampons, tub baths, bubble baths, bath oils, soap, or any kind of chemicals on the perineal area. Plain water can bathe the area adequately.

Use only natural fiber panties—cotton or silk. Underwear washed with laundry soap can promote cystitis. It is usually necessary to rinse underwear a second time in a soap-free cycle until the problem gets under control.

The extremities must be kept constantly warm. In Germany doctors characterize this disease as "cold foot cystitis."

When emptying the bladder, relax the sphincter for a sufficient length of time at the end of the passage of urine, even using a little bearing down action to fully empty the bladder. The last few seconds of voiding represent a cleansing of the bladder by squeezing. and cellular debris are removed at that time.

Give cleavers, burdock, corn silk, watermelon seed, barberry, dill, echinacea, horsetail, or other diuretic healing and soothing herbal teas. Use one cup per hour during the acute phase until symptoms subside (usually about four to five hours), then one cup four times a day for three to five days. If symptoms persist, continue the teas for 30 days. For each tea, use one teaspoon of the herb per cup of water. Leaves, silks, and flowers are steeped for 30 minutes, all other parts of plants are gently simmered for 20 minutes, less if they have been powdered. Then strain and drink when cool. One

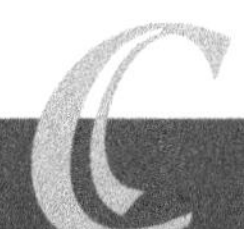

day's supply can be made at a time. As many as five to seven herbs can be mixed in one tea.

Blood in the Urine

Some common causes of blood in the urine include anticoagulant therapy, food sensitivity, aspirin, polycythemia vera, coagulation factor disturbances, hemophilia, hyperglobulinemia syndromes, generalized blood vessel bleeding, scurvy, and sickle cell disease. The presence of red blood cells in the urine is spoken of as hematuria.

Cystitis, Interstitial

A noninfectious form of chronic cystitis is called interstitial cystitis. It is characterized by pelvic pain or an ache just above the pubic bone or in the low abdomen. It may start in the same way acute cystitis does, except that it is more likely in middle-age women.

Avoid all bladder irritants such as alcohol, caffeine, sodas, citrus juices, chocolate, spices, including black and red pepper, and any food to which you may be allergic. We have found eggs in our experience to be a likely irritant.

Since certain inflammatory components, which are not well understood, are present in interstitial cystitis, it would be well to take some anti-inflammatory agents such as marshmallow root, celery seed, uva ursi, buchu, licorice root, golden seal, kava kava, dandelion leaf, cranberry, turmeric, corn silk, and especially white willow bark, flax seed oil, and hawthorn berry. Any seven of these can be mixed into one formula, but two or three are also effective.

Interstitial cystitis symptoms can be made worse by tight belts or bands around the waist. Even the elastic of panties, tights or long underwear can cause trouble.

Cystocele

A cystocele is essentially a herniation of the bladder through the front wall of the vagina, causing an easily compressible bulge into the vagina next to the opening for urination. This condition may cause discomfort and problems with emptying the bladder. It is usually caused by the trauma of childbirth.

Be very careful not to wear any tight bands around the waist, including panties and panty hose. All garments worn around the waist should be loose enough so as not to leave a red mark on the skin when they are removed. If necessary, clothing can be pinned to an undershirt to hold them in place, rather than wearing tight elastic bands around the waist.

Use Kegel exercises, shutting off the urine in midstream. Each time you pass urine it should be stopped in midstream to strengthen the muscles of the floor of the pelvis. Additionally, never allow urine to drip before being seated on the toilet, but by sheer determination prevent any leakage. The same muscles used to stop the urine should be contracted 80 to 100 times daily for three seconds each time. A schedule of 10 times a day, 8 to 10 repetitions each time, should be followed. After three months the muscles of the pelvic floor will reach their maximum strength. These muscles can be kept strong by 25 contractions daily two to three seconds each. These exercises may stop the advance of the hernia and prevent an operation.

Lose weight if any excess fat can be pinched up over the abdomen (the fat fold while standing erect should not exceed one and a half inches in thickness). Sometimes a woman can be quite thin in other areas but carry a little excess fat in the abdomen, which increases discomfort from a cystocele by bulging the hernia into the vagina.

Be certain there is no inflammation or infection in the bladder. To add to a weakness of the bladder wall, an urgency to urinate caused by an irritated or infected bladder can lead to accidents in holding urine. Buchu tea, using one teaspoon per cup of boiling water, steeped for 20 to 30 minutes, can do wonders in keeping the bladder free from irritation.

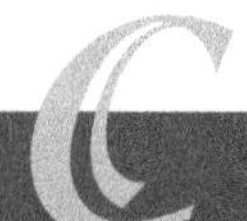

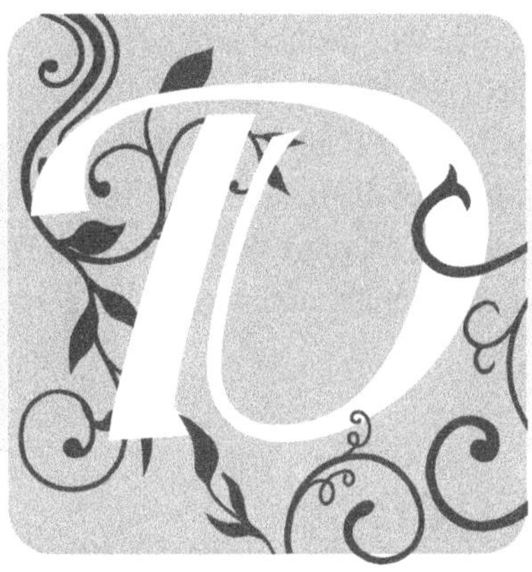

Deafness

Babies are often born hearing impaired because of loud noises from machinery or other noisy sources experienced during the prenatal time. Sounds of greater than 85 decibels intensity reaching the fetus through the mother's abdomen may not only damage the ears but can cause growth retardation and prematurity. Machinery noise is most often to blame, but the average city bus emits about 80 decibels, just under the safe upper limit, whereas a moving subway train is about 100 decibels, which is well above it. The mother's voice is the sound most often reaching the fetus, and when she is speaking loudly its intensity in the uterus is just under 85 decibels because of the better transmission through the mother's tissues than through air. Just after birth, during the first few days, babies may be injured by noise of only 45 decibels intensity.

Various drugs may damage the hearing—aspirin, antibiotics, and certain chemotherapy drugs. Temporary hearing loss can result from allergies, colds, or ear infections. One may hear the heartbeat or one's own voice in one or both ears during dehydration because of the collapse of the eustacian tube. Any factor that reduces circulation can cause a decline in hearing: high cholesterol, high salt diet, low thyroid function, arthritis, nicotine, caffeine, etc. Some of the causes may result in permanent loss.

Treatment

The basic natural laws of health should be applied with dedication, and pray for the Lord's blessing on these simple health practices.

Remove free fats (margarine, butter, mayonnaise, fried foods, cooking fats, salad oils, and peanut butter) and free sugars (honey, sugar, malt, syrups, and molasses) from the diet for six weeks as they tend to cut down on the oxygen content of blood and alter the metabolism of nerves and brain tissue.

Do not eat too much as overeating produces certain quantities of alcohols and other reducing substances that can damage the delicate sensory organs of the head.

Certain herbal remedies may be helpful. These include ginkgo, black cohosh, and skullcap. The way to make tea is to boil one quart of water, add one-half tablespoon of black cohosh, and simmer gently for half an hour. Then add three heaping tablespoons of the ginkgo and skullcap. The quart should be taken in four doses, one cup every four to five hours during one day. The tea should be made up fresh every day.

During the six-week period you are taking the herbs, you should apply hydrotherapy to your ears. The best way is to apply hot compresses to the ears for three to six minutes, then apply an ice cold compress for 30 to 60 seconds. Alternate back and forth for four to six changes, ending with the cold. Do the treatment at least once a day for the entire time.

A zinc supplement may help. Take 15 to 50 milligrams per day for 30 days.

Dehydration

Signs of dehydration in a child may be difficult to detect. One sign is that the lips may be shriveled or cracked or a dehydration headache may occur. Other signs are irritability, lethargy, fainting, dizziness, chapped lips, dry mouth and skin, cough, fast pulse, acting spacey, or poor appetite. For a

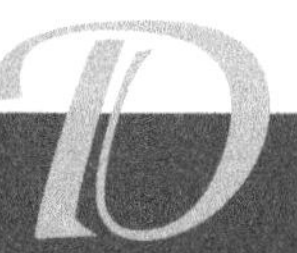

child who is prone to constipation or urinary tract infections, dehydration may be the source of these problems.

Of course, you expect dehydration if a child has a high fever, diarrhea or vomiting, or is playing a lot in hot weather. The child may become weak, dizzy, nauseated, irritable, or tired. The child may lose appetite altogether or complain of a dry mouth or have thick, stringy saliva. The eyes may look sunken and tearless. Urine may look dark yellow and may smell strong. For a small infant, the soft spot on the head may be sunken.

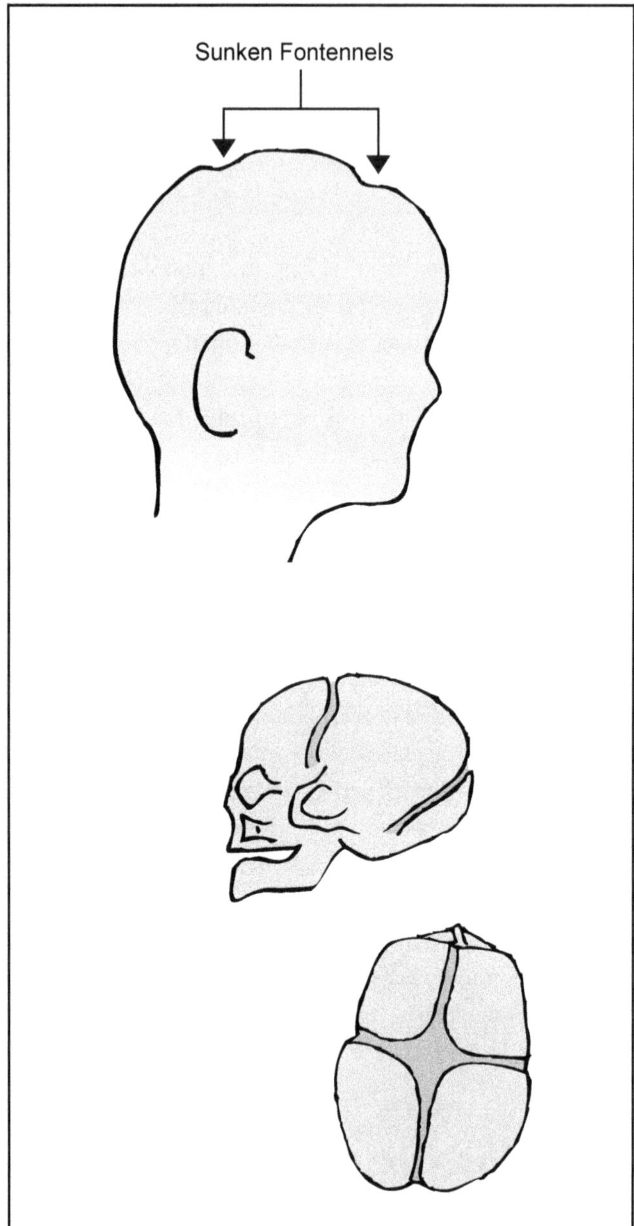

If the person is able to take oral fluids, this is the easiest, safest, and cheapest way to rehydrate someone. The next most convenient and comfortable is the retention enema. (See "Hydrotherapy" in the *Natural Remedies* section.) The next best way is to give saline or glucose for injection as a subcutaneous push-in. This method requires only a syringe and not an IV setup. Use about two quarts of water per 24 hours for an adult, unless there are other fluid losses such as from sweating, vomiting, or diarrhea. If there is a fever, or if heating treatments are given, more fluid is needed. Weeping skin lesions or tears all require more fluid to be given to prevent dehydration.

Delinquency

(See "Mental Disorders" in the *Conditions and Diseases* section.)

Dental Care

Abscessed tooth

A tooth abscess should be treated both locally as well as systemically.

Local Treatments

If a cracked filling is involved, the filling should be removed in order that the tooth can drain through the opening to the nerve space. Select a dentist who is willing to cooperate with your desires.

Local treatments should include charcoal compresses to the tooth whenever possible, but at least at night. If the person must get up during the night, the old compress should be removed, the mouth rinsed, herbal remedies taken, and a fresh charcoal compress applied. Make a thick paste of charcoal and water, put the paste on a one inch square of paper towel and lay it in a spoon. Carefully insert the spoon in the mouth and bite down on the compress. Keep it there several hours.

Following each meal the tooth should be thoroughly cleaned. Any food packed into the cavity should be carefully removed with a water pick or syringe, making certain no impacted food remains in the cavity. Floss thoroughly and brush with a soft bristle brush to remove any particles that might lodge between the gum margin and the tooth.

If it becomes desirable to prevent food, fluids, or medicines from touching the nerve space, the tooth cavity can be filled with bee propolis, covered with wax such as Gulf wax used in canning, or with the cotton removed from the end of a cotton applicator tip, packed into the tooth cavity with a toothpick.

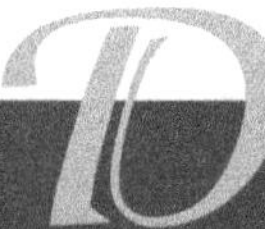

A tea of golden seal and echinacea should be prepared and the mouth rinsed frequently, preferably every half an hour, but at least every two to three hours. Instead of tea a solution of grapefruit seed extract in water can be used—about 20 drops of the extract per cup. Swish about one tablespoon or so around approximately every half an hour. The solution should be swallowed whether it is the herbs or the grapefruit seed extract.

The mouth should be rinsed with hydrogen peroxide at least three times a day. Use one tablespoon of standard commercial hydrogen peroxide, which is about 3 percent. Do not swallow.

Tea tree oil should be applied with a cotton applicator to the gums around the affected tooth. The cotton tip should be wet with the oil, removed from the stick, and packed into the tooth cavity.

Hot mouthwashes should be done as frequently as possible, but at least four times a day. To a glass of hot water you may add two teaspoons of salt or two teaspoons of turmeric powder, or you may use a glass of hot golden seal and echinacea tea. Except for the salt and about one quarter only of the turmeric, the solution should be swallowed.

Systemic Treatments

Systemic treatments should consist of antimicrobial herbs such as golden seal, myrrh, echinacea, garlic, grapefruit seed extract, bee propolis, etc. Tinctures of mixed golden seal, echinacea, and propolis can be obtained and should be taken in the quantity of about one teaspoon every two hours around the clock until the acute phase is over and healing is well underway. Then cut back to every four hours. The first three herbs listed are usually most effective.

Fever treatments may be taken, bringing the mouth temperature up to 101°F or 102°F. (See "Hydrotherapy" in the *Natural Remedies* section.)

A daily exercise program should be followed to keep the immune system strong, the circulation brisk, and the defenses high.

Anti-inflammatory herbs may be quite helpful such as flaxseed oil (one tablespoon three times daily), white willow bark tea (one cup of tea four times daily, or the equivalent in capsules or tablets), or turmeric (one teaspoon twice a day) stirred in water and swished before swallowing. Licorice root is very helpful. Make a tea, swish, and swallow. Take up to six cups daily.

To control pain, an ice pack can be used on the jaw outside the abscessed tooth, or clove oil can be put on the tooth or on the gum adjacent to the tooth to reduce pain. White willow bark is very effective. Do not use hot mouthwashes if doing so makes pain worse.

It should be understood that weeks or even months of treatment may be involved, as the tooth must make its own root canal by scarring. The cavity where germs can get into the nerve space must be closed up by fibrous tissue (scarring), which the tooth itself can produce. The abscess may appear to be almost entirely well, then return because of a reinfection. For this reason, the treatment should not be cut short.

Case Report

A first molar, filled with composite about six years ago, chipped on one side after about four years. Every effort was made to keep the tooth clean by brushing and flossing after each meal and never eating between meals. Nevertheless, about two or three years after the filling chipped, pain began to develop when chewing. Then the pain spread to the surrounding gum, indicating a beginning abscess. Then a toothache began to be constant.

A dentist removed the composite and various home remedies were instituted in an effort to heal the abscess without a root canal. The dentist predicted that the abscess would never heal and that the constant packing of food into the cavity from eating would cause a continued source of infection, making it impossible to heal the abscess that would develop. The dentist was faithful to his training and warned the patient that there is the rare possibility that an abscess from an upper tooth could come to a head in a sinus or inside the skull and result in a brain abscess.

Natural treatments from the above list were successful to bring the abscess to a head inside the mouth, adjacent to the tooth. This process took about three weeks. The abscess head ruptured after about two more weeks. Then began the long process of healing. Close attention and unwearied persistence are required. It must be noted that if one decides to treat an upper tooth abscess oneself, one should be aware that a long-continued untreated abscess could lead to erosion of bone of the floor of the skull and result in a brain abscess.

A woman from North Carolina shared the following experience in a letter dated November 9, 1999. "Last spring I had a toothache; I realized after several days of suffering I needed to go to the dentist. His diagnosis: I had an infected tooth. He said a root canal was needed, and maybe they could save the tooth. He did not do root canals. A specialist was needed. This tooth was one of two that a four-tooth

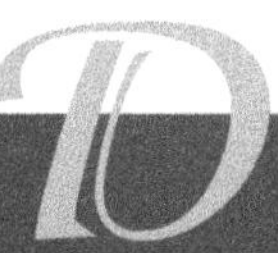

bridge was secured to. Since I had a lot of aching and pain, and tenderness with chewing, I went to the specialist. He said he would try to save the tooth, but he could not guarantee it. Antibiotic shots would be needed over a period of four weeks, costing approximately $500. He made it very plain it was only a chance he could save the tooth. He told me he thought I should talk it over with my husband, thinking maybe I would go ahead and have the tooth pulled and then go through all the other weeks involved in whatever needed to be done in regard to the four-tooth bridge. I paid the office fee, went home, told my husband and then my daughter and son-in-law.

A preventive medicine doctor of my acquaintance suggested I apply charcoal poultices, day and night, changing as often as every three hours during the day; taking garlic as an antimicrobial and echinacea to build up my immune system. He made a small poultice, 1" x 2" gauze, put a thick charcoal paste on it, folded it up small, and I put it up on the tooth (upper left in the back). I did this for two months all told, several times daily. I had a small pus bump come to the surface, which I lanced myself. And finally the pain was totally gone. I could chew normally. By October, my husband and I went to our dentist to have our yearly cleaning. He was amazed I had that tooth and X-rays showed it had cleared up completely. God is so good!"

Bruxism, Teeth Grinding

This symptom occurs at night and is characterized by the grinding of the teeth together, which results in a fairly loud noise that cannot be duplicated except during sleep. The teeth may become grooved or ground down by the process. This condition may be seen in children or adults.

It is almost always associated with allergies, and discovery of food sensitivities will result in a cure in most cases. A carefully performed "Elimination and Challenge Diet" found in the *Dietary Information* section will usually result in the discovery of foods causing the teeth grinding.

Cavities

It is now believed that tooth decay is a bacterial disease affecting all the layers of the tooth. Cavities are very much influenced by lifestyle. When the mouth becomes too acidic, calcium and phosphate are lost from the enamel. Further, a bacterium often found in the mouth called *Streptococcus mutans* and other germs produce acids and toxins from sugars eaten. These substances further remove calcium from the enamel, which leads to cavities. The more sugar and refined carbohydrates eaten, the greater the chances of cavity formation. The first sign of a cavity is a white spot on the tooth.

Natural remedies for cavities include changing the hygiene of the mouth, flossing and brushing after each eating experience. Eating between meals encourages the formation of cavities, especially if the food sticks to the teeth, as with sticky candy, dried fruit, etc.

Prepare chamomile tea and drink two to three cups daily as a mouthwash, swallowing the tea after it has washed across the teeth. Golden seal and echinacea tea are also effective as a mouthwash. These have antimicrobial and anti-inflammatory properties.

Licorice root tea specifically inhibits the growth of *streptococcus*, which is the principal cause of cavities. Put a teaspoon of licorice root powder in a quart of water and bring it to a boil. Swish the mouth frequently throughout the day and swallow the tea, using the entire quart during the day.

Cranberry juice not only blocks bacteria from adhering to the interior of the urinary bladder, but it also blocks the adherence of plaque-forming bacteria to the teeth (*Journal of the American Dental Association* [December 1998]).

Denture Adhesive

Powdered apple pectin used in a shaker, such as a saltshaker or an empty plastic bottle filled with pectin, can serve very well as an adhesive for false teeth. Wet the dentures first and then put a little of the powdered apple pectin on the dentures in the same way one would for commercial denture adhesives.

Mercury Amalgam

Amalgam contains approximately 50 percent metallic mercury, 35 percent silver, 9 percent tin, 6 percent copper, and a trace of zinc.

For more than 160 years dentists have used "silver amalgam" for filling teeth, containing approximately 50 percent mercury metal. Mercury is continuously released as vapor into the mouth. When it is inhaled it is absorbed into body tissues, oxidized to ionic mercury, and finally bound to proteins in the cells. Fillings are the major source of mercury for humans. At the present time, current research does not support the idea that amalgam fillings are safe. Research is now focused on the immune system, the kidneys, bacteria in the mouth and intestinal tract, the reproductive system, and the central nervous system (*FASEB Journal* 9, no. 7 [1995]: 504).

Eleven manic depressed persons had their amalgams removed, and nine subjects with amalgams were given a placebo or a sealant. Depression and hypomania scores improved

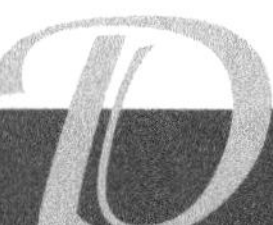

significantly as did anxiety, anger, schizophrenia, paranoia, and many others with amalgam removal, compared to the sealant-placebo group. There was a 42 percent decrease in the number of physical health problems after amalgam removal compared to an 8 percent increase in physical symptoms in the placebo-sealant group (*Journal of Ortho-molecular Medicine* 13, no. 1 [1998]: 31–41).

There are mixed reports on amalgam fillings as we could expect. Another study was undertaken to answer the question if enough mercury is absorbed from dental amalgam fillings to produce kidney damage. One hundred patients were selected ages 18 to 44 and divided into a group having fillings and a group not having fillings. No mention is made in the study of how many fillings those having fillings had, but only a very small increase in urinary mercury absorption was found from the fillings. It was believed by the researchers that the dose of mercury absorbed from the amalgam fillings was too little to be injurious to the kidneys (*Pharmacology and Toxicology* 76, no. 1 [1995]: 47).

A study done on 108 children ages one day to five years showed an unexpected high level of mercury of older infants from mothers with higher numbers of amalgam fillings. The researchers in this study felt that unrestricted amalgam fillings in women before and during the child bearing age should be reconsidered as the mercury was a threat to the health of the offspring (*European Journal of Pediatrics* 153, no. 8 [1994]: 607).

Another group of researchers believes that, under appropriate conditions of family susceptibility, dental fillings may contribute to immunologic aberrations that could lead to autoimmune diseases (*FASEB Journal* 8, no. 14 [1994]: 1183; *Toxicology and Applied Pharmacology* 132, no. 2 [1995]: 299).

Not all is smooth sailing with the principle alternative to amalgam. Cis-phenol ACS, a component of composite fillings, can have a continuous out-gassing of toxic substances. Studies have not yet been done to determine if these toxic substances actually cause significant problems or are even absorbed by the body. (See also "Toxic Heavy Metals" in the *Supplemental Information* section.)

Pyorrhea, Periodontal Disease

Pyorrhea is an inflammation of the gums and sometimes the outer covering of the roots of the teeth, with tender bleeding gums, advancing until the teeth become loosened from the supporting gums and the tooth dies. The jawbone develops osteoporosis from the erosion of the tooth socket by the infection and inflammation. It is essential to recognize this problem early if one is to prevent further damage and loss of teeth.

Stress affects the immune system, making it less able to fight against the type of bacteria that cause pyorrhea, making the persons more prone to gum infection. Pyorrhea is a marker for hardening of the arteries. Researchers at the University of North Carolina's School of Dentistry found that people with pyorrhea are more likely than others to have hardening of the arteries and heart attacks. Other research has indicated that poor dental hygiene is also a factor in general disease (*Lancet* 352 [1998]: 121).

Examine the teeth and gums for tenderness or redness. Should any develop at the tooth margin, this could be the onset of pyorrhea. Very carefully control this problem as it could result in tooth loss; it is the commonest cause of tooth loss in America after the age of 25.

Treatment

With the onset of redness or tenderness, do not use a commercial toothpaste. Instead, moisten a toothbrush, dip it in powdered charcoal, and brush after each meal. Sleep with a bit of charcoal paste in the mouth, made by mixing a tablespoon of charcoal with a few drops of water to make a thick paste about the consistency of thick peanut butter. Use dental floss after eating along with thorough rinsing, even if brushing is not possible.

Since a refined food diet is a common cause of pyorrhea, the total elimination of all refined fats, sugars, and proteins can be helpful. Switch to a diet high in fresh, raw fruits and vegetables, whole grains, and some nuts and seeds. A diet high in fresh fruits and vegetables will often stop acute pyorrhea in a few days, even if nothing else is used. A purely vegetarian diet produces less plaque than nonvegetarian diets, and cleanings may be delayed for years without significant plaque buildup in some vegetarians. Avoid between-meal snacking of any kind. Studies show that the more times a person eats in one day, the greater the buildup of plaque and the likelihood of pyorrhea.

Use the same measures as used for osteoporosis to prevent bone loss. Chewing food is important because of the massaging effect on the gums and bones of the jaw. The chewing action makes the teeth rise and sink in their sockets, promoting circulation and preventing gum disease and osteoporosis of the jaw.

Use large quantities of water, 8 to 10 glasses per day, as dry mouth encourages bacterial growth. Dehydration reduces tissue resistance to infection.

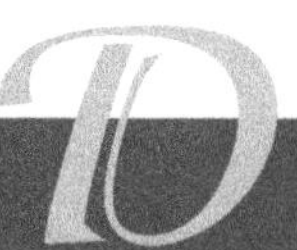

Do not smoke. Smoking doubles the risk of pyorrhea. Do not use oral contraceptives, coffee, tea, colas, chocolate, or dilantin as they increase the risk of gum disease.

Exercise is helpful to build the body's resistance against infection. Also take hot baths, garlic, chaparral, echinacea as in any acute infection. (See "Hydrotherapy" in the *Natural Remedies* section for information on hot baths.)

Use a soft, small toothbrush with rounded bristles and a flat brushing surface. Use short horizontal strokes and a jiggling motion, holding the brush at a 45 degree angle with the teeth at the gum line to allow the bristles to slip between the gums and the teeth. After brushing and rinsing, floss carefully, using unwaxed floss if possible. Use dental floss after each meal to prevent periodontal disease (pyorrhea). The use of dental floss and a soft bristle toothbrush allow longer periods between professional cleanings for most people.

Regular and thorough cleaning of teeth by a dental hygienist helps to remove plaque buildup, which otherwise promotes inflammation and leads to pyorrhea.

Hydrogen peroxide swished in the mouth for five minutes after brushing will often help. Continue this for several weeks.

For bleeding gums, rinse the mouth with salt water—one teaspoon of salt to one-half cup of hot water six times daily—being careful to avoid swallowing the salty water.

An astringent tea such as golden seal, comfrey root, witch hazel, nettle, or chamomile may be used hot as a mouthwash after each brushing. The astringent action encourages healing. Use golden seal powder with a moist toothbrush as a toothpaste three times a day. The golden seal helps to heal gum disease.

At night aloe vera should be swabbed onto the gums with a cotton-tipped swab.

Application of CoQ-10 on the gums improves adult pyorrhea. Following flossing and brushing, apply the CoQ-10 to the thoroughly rinsed gums at the junction between the tooth and the gum one to four times a day. Two or three layers of cotton gauze should be trimmed to the length of the area of pyorrhea and slightly moistened. A 50 or 60 milligram capsule should be opened and half the CoQ-10 sprinkled sparsely along the entire length of the gauze. A single layer of gauze should be placed over the CoQ-10 and then applied directly to the gum at the tooth line, avoiding spilling. Then the side of the jaw should hold the compress in place for an hour or two. Avoid talking, eating, or drinking during this time. Prepare similar applications for each area of the mouth involved, applying the single layer of gauze next to the gum, and the two or three layer gauze toward the jaw (*Molecular Aspects of Medicine* 15 [1994]: S241-8). You should also take CoQ-10 by mouth, about 300 milligrams a day, for healing periodontal disease.

Cinquefoil potentilla capsules or tea, along with 50 milligrams of vitamin B6, can often save a tooth loosened by pyorrhea.

Temporomandibular Joint Syndrome, TMJ

An estimated 20 million Americans, mostly women, have a wide array of distressing symptoms associated with TMJ—pain in the jaw muscles or in front of the ear, clicking or popping sounds in the joint, locking, difficulty chewing or talking, dizziness, headaches, neck pain, and even back aches. Approximately $32 billion is spent annually in this country seeking relief. About 40 percent of Americans have some form of temporomandibular disorder that includes TMJ. Only 5 to 10 percent require treatment by a dentist. At least 75 percent of patients treated still have pain, leaving us to believe dental treatment is ineffective, or only partly so.

The most common complaint is pain in one ear or in front of the ear, which may go to the temple or the side of the neck. The most common symptoms are frequent headaches, stiff and sore neck and shoulders, backache, jaw and tooth pain, popping of the jaw, ringing in the ears, and dizziness. Pain in the joint and dysfunction may be severe enough to interfere with chewing. It is a dull, constant ache worse in the morning, especially if the patient has tooth grinding (bruxism). Pain and limitation of movement with talking may be present. There may be tenderness in muscles and clicking and popping in the joint. In our experience the presence of food sensitivities is regularly found, and tooth grinding is also most often because of food sensitivities. An occasional case is quite disabling. The disorder may persist for a few years. The initiating factor appears to be the stretching of an abnormal pain focus which starts a self-sustaining pain-spasm-pain cycle.

Patients with the disease fall into two groups.

- Organic joint abnormalities (tumor, arthritis, chronic dislocation, muscle imbalance, or joint stiffness or fixation).
- Without organic joint disease but with facial pain, noise in the joint, and restricted movement. The second group is much more common.

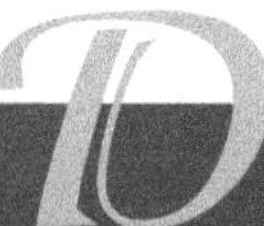

Treatment

For a period of one month use the jaw as little as possible. That means chew soft foods and blend any hard foods so that pressure on the temporomandibular joints will be avoided.

Avoid chewing ice, eating sticky foods, cracking nuts with the teeth, and chewing or biting pencils, pens, etc. Never chew gum, and do not grind granola or hard cereals with the teeth.

Do not sleep on your stomach or with your hands under your head as this may push the jaw to one side, straining the joints. When the head rests on the pillow if sleeping on the side, care should be used not to put pressure on the jaw. Lying for long periods of time on one side can strain the joints of the jaw.

Using a properly positioned scarf during sleep, either around the neck so high that it props the jaw shut or slung under the chin and tied on top of the head, may be helpful.

Chew slowly on both sides of your mouth. When chewing allow no motion that causes pain or popping of the jaw. If a side-to-side motion causes pain, do only up and down movements. If up and down movements cause pain, do only a sliding, grinding, or side-to-side movement. Sometimes jutting the jaw forward a bit can be helpful. In some people all food must be pureed or ground, then taken into the mouth in small bites and simply swished, to thoroughly mix with saliva, and not chewed.

Drink through a straw, keeping the jaws closed and relaxed.

Try to keep the lips together and teeth apart while awake. A specially constructed device called a bite plane may be needed.

Forego resting the telephone between your shoulder and neck as it puts a strain on the jaw.

Refrain from sitting with your chin in your hands.

Correct any slouching posture and keep the chin tucked in. While sitting, sit straight with feet on the floor. While traveling in the car, support the neck with a pillow.

Do not carry heavy bags, and never use a shoulder bag, as imbalance of the skeleton anywhere can cause an imbalance in the jaw.

Eat only two meals daily (breakfast and lunch) to allow for a long rest period for the jaw.

Use a heating pad as hot as can be tolerated, or a hot water bottle, 20 minutes two or three times a day.

Fever treatments, herbal treatments (feverfew, white willow bark, wild lettuce), and, for some patients, zinc and/or selenium supplements seem to be very helpful.

Some naturopaths believe TMJ and bruxism are symptoms of intestinal parasites. It is recommended to chew well five to six tablespoons of pumpkin seeds three times a day for four weeks. At the same time take a course of wormwood *(Artemisia annua)* to get rid of worms. Charcoal powder—two tablespoons in a glass of water twice a day—can help rid a person of parasites.

Of course, the most important matter is that of a carefully done "Elimination and Challenge Diet" evaluation, which can be found in the *Dietary Information* section. Foods that cause the pain must be carefully eliminated.

Toothaches

Drink a cup of black cohosh or catnip tea to help relieve pain. Comfrey root, echinacea, and golden seal tea may also be drunk for toothache, washing the mouth with each sip of the tea. Use two tablespoons of each herb to one quart of gently boiling water, simmer for 10 minutes before straining.

Wintergreen oil can be placed on a small cotton ball about the size of a pea and placed on the affected tooth and around the gum to help relieve pain.

Some recommend a supplement of calcium, magnesium, vitamin C, and vitamin E for five days to improve nerve impulses, nutrition, and circulation of the gums and teeth. The dosage should be 500 milligrams of calcium, 300 milligrams magnesium, 200 milligrams vitamin C, and 300 to 400 IU of vitamin E.

Put a drop of clove oil on the tooth and on the gum next to the tooth as a temporary measure of pain control.

Swish mouthfuls of warm salt water around the teeth, using one tablespoon of salt to a large glass of warm water, as warm as it can be tolerated. The salt has an astringent and slightly anesthetic action. Use care not to swallow the salt.

Rub an ice cube into the v shape in the middle of your palm on the same side as the aching tooth for a full minute or more. Some have received relief from the toothache with this very simple treatment.

Put an ice bag against the jaw next to the toothache.

Sleep with the aching jaw on a partly filled hot water bottle or an electric heating pad.

Toothpaste formula

The following toothpaste formula was developed by Andrew Thrash. You can make a larger amount by tripling the formula.

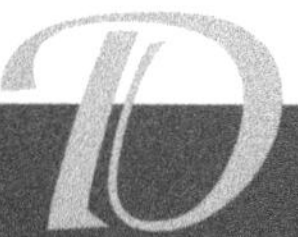

- ¼ cup baking soda
- ¼ cup charcoal powder
- 1½ tsp of hydrogen peroxide
- 4½ tsp of Bronner's peppermint soap

Depression

(See "Mental Health" in the *Conditions and Diseases* section.)

Dermatitis

(See "Skin Diseases" in the *Conditions and Diseases* section.)

Diabetes

(See also "Weight Control" in the *Conditions and Diseases* section.)

More than 150,000 Americans die each year from diabetes and its complications—blindness, kidney failure, nerve damage, and cardiovascular disease. Good monitoring of diabetes includes an annual hemoglobin A1c, a twice a year blood fats profile (cholesterol, HDL, LDL, and triglycerides), and twice a year eye exam, quarterly blood pressure exam, and daily foot exam by the patient.

Diabetes is two separate kinds of diseases, but both are linked to a genetic predisposition to get diabetes, but probably not through the same mechanism. Type I diabetes, which is also called juvenile diabetes, occurs because a virus (or sometimes a toxin or other substance that may injure the pancreas—see #9 below) has attacked the beta cells (insulin-producing) of the pancreas and caused inadequate quantities of insulin to be produced. In adult-onset diabetes, or Type II diabetes, insulin is usually in generous supply, even 10 times more than needed, but the tissues and cells of the diabetic person have become resistant to insulin so that insulin cannot bring sugar into the cells.

Predict Your Risk for Diabetes

Begin a good program early in the child's life when there is a family history of diabetes in siblings, parents, or grandparents. Even the early indications cause an acceleration of aging. There is much in lifestyle modification that can be helpful.

1. Birth weight greater than eight pounds.
2. Easy weight gain in childhood or youth—some 10- to 15-year-old children can gain one-half to one pound a day for weeks so that weight balloons.
3. Frequent infections—bladder, tonsils, appendix, skin.
4. Early menstrual periods in girls or beard growth in boys before 12 ½ years of age.
5. Carious teeth, especially if there are as many as one carious tooth per year of the child's life.
6. Lab tests beginning to show abnormalities:
   a. Blood sugar level above 85 milligrams per decilitre fasting.
   b. Insulin levels above 25 microunits per deciliter fasting.
   c. High total cholesterol, low HDL (less than about 40), high triglycerides (more than about 100).
   d. Uric acid above 5.
   e. Hemoglobin above 13.5 for females, 14.75 for males.
7. A variety of organic complications begin—varicose veins, hardening of the arteries, skeletal problems, bunions, hammer toes, backache, or sciatica, visual difficulties, digestive system symptoms, kidney and bladder problems, foot symptoms such as plantar fasciitis, chronic backache, neuropathy, or depression.
8. Measurement of waist to hip ratios can help to predict the likely development of diabetes in the future. For men, the waist to hip ratio should be no more than 1 to 1 and for women no more than 0.8 to 1. Measure your waist and divide the number in inches by the number of inches of your hip measurement. Example: Your waist measures 30 inches and your hips 33. By dividing 30 by 33 you get .9, a number indicating an increased risk for diabetes.
9. John Classen, MD, an immunologist at Classen Immunotherapies, published papers linking the immunization against hepatitis B and other diseases to the development of insulin dependent diabetes, an autoimmune disease. Dr. Classen's work revealed that immunization starting after two months of life was associated with an increased risk of autoimmunity. Data from a small study published by the US government appears to support his data and showed that when hepatitis B immunization was given starting after two months of life it was associated with an

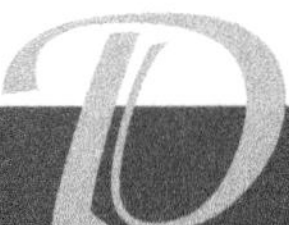

almost doubling of the risk of diabetes. Vaccine-induced autoimmunity is a major public health problem because of the number of vaccine doses given and the large percentage of people with undiagnosed inflammatory conditions. (BMJ, "Public should be told that vaccines may have long term adverse effects," 318 [January 16, 1999]: 193).

10. Gestational diabetes and adult-onset diabetes are probably a part of the same disease (*Diabetes* 20, no. 4 [1997]: 509). If a woman has had diabetes during pregnancy, she must carefully avoid becoming overweight in order to keep from getting adult-onset.
11. A high-fat diet, especially saturated fatty acids that come principally from animal products and margarine, increase one's risk of having glucose intolerance and subsequently developing adult-onset diabetes (*Diabetes Care* 18, no. 8 [1995]: 1104). Diabetics who eat one egg per day double their risk of having a heart attack or stroke according to a 14-year study done at Harvard University (*Journal of the American Medical Association* 281 [1999]: 1387).
12. Low magnesium levels in the serum have been reported in children with Type I diabetes. Low magnesium levels are present in at least 25 percent of all diabetics, and possibly in all people with frank diabetes, and in many who do not have diabetes but have a tendency toward diabetes by family history or by weight gain in early life (*Archives of Internal Medicine* 156 [1996]: 1143).
13. A birthday in the spring and summer is more likely to be associated with childhood diabetes (*Medical Tribune News Service,* June 11, 1996). The reason may have to do with the viral epidemics that more frequently hit in the fall. The mother gets a viral infection, which affects the unborn baby's pancreas, resulting later in Type I diabetes.
14. Insulin resistance is a good predictor of gain in body weight in the phase of childhood from age 5 to 15 (*Diabetes* 44, no. 1 [May 1995]: 7A). Any child or adult who can consistently gain from one-half to one pound a day or is steadily getting fatter year by year can be diagnosed by this fact alone as being resistant to insulin, regardless of the blood level of sugar. A profile to recognize those with insulin resistance includes central obesity (obesity in the trunk more than in the extremities), hypertension, and diabetes. These patients usually have an increase in triglyceride levels and a decrease in HDL cholesterol. With these findings, it is not necessary to do expensive tests for insulin in the plasma (*Lancet* 346 [1995]: 120). Insulin resistance syndrome is uncommon in non-diabetic populations.
15. Menstrual irregularity may be more strongly associated with Type II diabetes than had been previously thought (*Diabetes* 44, no. 1 [May 1995]: 181A). The reason for this may be in the area of fat/steroid/estrogen metabolism.
16. Oral contraceptives make blood sugar difficult to control. The diabetic should not smoke or use alcoholic beverages. These tend to damage blood vessels, and increase insulin requirements.

Prevention

A strain of Chinese hamsters genetically programmed to develop diabetes could be prevented from developing diabetes in adulthood by a low-fat diet. Parents should study their children's growth patterns and be certain they do not grow up too fast. They should supply plenty of fats from nuts, beans, whole grains, olives, avocado, and seeds, but not much (and preferably none) from margarine, mayonnaise, cooking fats, salad oils. This is highly desirable if they are growing rapidly, tend to be overweight, or have a diabetic family history (*Resident and Staff Physicians* 30, no. 4: 20).

In one study rats took one of several diets containing from 5 percent up to 22 percent fat from corn oil or beef tallow. The diets were given from three weeks before mating until after the birth of rat pups. In those on 22 percent fat, either from corn or beef fat, there was a deterioration of glucose tolerance and a reduction in survival and fertility of the young rats to only 50 percent of that in control rats fed a 5 percent fat diet. Human gestational diabetes may be well treated by a low-fat diet (*American Journal of Obstetrics and Gynecology* 161, no. 1 [1989]: 234).

Diabetes would be better named if it were called "accelerated aging." Another acceptable name would be "fat diabetes" rather than "sugar diabetes," since disordered fat metabolism is as serious a matter in the diabetic as disordered sugar metabolism. The cause of death in diabetics is regularly related to the problems of fat metabolism, and not directly to high blood sugar. However, the presence of even small amounts of extra insulin or sugar in the blood can cause blood vessel injury if it is long sustained. This injury leads to both hardening of the arteries as well as injury to nerves.

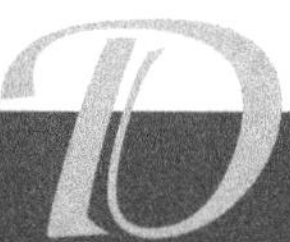

Diets high in animal fat rather than simply total mixed plant and animal fat appear to increase the risk for progression of a person already at risk for adult-onset diabetes (*Internal Medicine News* 24, no. 16 [August 15, 1991]: 44).

Calorie restriction was given to young rats at 70 to 85 percent of what other young rats ate if they took food anytime they wished. Those on only 70 percent of the amount of food given to the rats that could eat anytime, developed no diabetes compared to 67 percent who developed diabetes of the high calorie group. And of those on 85 percent of the feed-anytime group only 13 percent developed diabetes. The abdominal fat was two-and-a-half times as thick in the feed-anytime group as in the 70 percent calorie group. Insulin resistance developed in the feed-anytime group, but not in the 70 percent calorie group. These results demonstrate that calorie restriction is effective in preventing adult-onset diabetes in diabetes-prone rats, and certainly also in diabetes-prone humans (*Diabetes Research and Clinical Practice* 27 [1995]: 97).

Nicotinamide (vitamin B3) protects the beta cells of the pancreas from being destroyed by antibodies that develop apparently as a result of an infection by a virus such as mumps or encephalitis. Children who have developed antibodies can be tested and these antibodies discovered. Then these children can be given vitamin B3, which gives the child only a 7.1 percent chance of developing diabetes as compared to 20 and 21 percent as occurred in two control groups not given vitamin B3, a reduction of more than 50 percent (*Nutrition Reviews* 53, no. 5 [1995]: 137). Green leafy vegetables, especially collards, are high in vitamin B3.

Avoid giving infants and young children cow's milk. A no-cow's-milk program can protect against later development of diabetes. Up to 100 percent of newly diagnosed insulin-dependent patients have antibodies to a protein in cow's blood, which is also present in the milk (*Lancet* 347 [1996]: 1464). The more consumption of cow's milk, the greater the incidence of diabetes in a population. On the other hand, prolonged breastfeeding decreases the risk of later diabetes. But if cow's milk is introduced early along with breastfeeding, regardless of the duration of breastfeeding, diabetes still increases at a later time (*Diabetes Care* 17, no. 1 [January 1994]: 13–9).

Cow's milk proteins (particularly bovine serum albumin, BSA) stimulate the production of antibodies that destroy the insulin producing pancreatic cells. In 142 diabetic children, 100 percent of the children studied at the time the disease was diagnosed had antibodies to BSA. It is believed by some that cow's milk exposure is the major cause of Type I diabetes (*New England Journal of Medicine* 327 [1992]: 302–7; *Archive Diseases in Childhood* 57 [1982]: 369–72; *Diabetologia* 26 [1984]: 24–9).

Breastfeeding infants have a strong advantage over formula feeding to prevent Type I diabetes. Introduction at a young age to dairy products and high milk consumption increases the level of antibodies to cow's milk, indicating that these antibodies may be a factor in the production of juvenile diabetes. Additionally, dairy products are independently associated with an increased risk of Type I diabetes even in the absence of antibodies. Studies have been done by introducing cow's milk and the other dairy products early into the diet of children. The later milk is given, the lower the risk of early development of diabetes. Studies were done in London, Finland, the United States, Italy, and Canada, beginning with studies done back in the mid-80s in Minneapolis (*Diabetiologia* 29 [1986]: 784).

It seems quite clear that early exposure to cow's milk protein triggers Type I (insulin-dependent) diabetes and later on encourages Type II diabetes, one reason being because of the much greater likelihood that cow's milk and its products will lead to being overweight, which is the single most common cause of the development of adult-onset diabetes. The best food for an infant is breast milk, and the child should be breast fed until good teeth have developed and the child can chew solid food. Then the child should be weaned to table food, not to dairy milk. In many countries and in subsections of the population of the United States children have been successfully and healthfully reared from the cradle to adulthood and into advanced old age never having used any animal products.

The use of coffee during pregnancy increases the risk the unborn baby will get diabetes later in life. We recommend that pregnant women stay off coffee, tea, colas, and chocolate (*British Medical Journal* 300 [1990]: 641). These items are especially harmful for diabetics. Six hours after having been given coffee, diabetic rats had blood sugar levels twice their usual levels. Coffee can also depress blood sugar levels in rats not having diabetes. Children who consume coffee or tea regularly are at an increased risk of developing Type I diabetes (*European Journal of Clinical Nutrition* 48, no. 4 [1994]: 279).

The intake of nitrates and nitrites by children and their parents from food (such as foods at salad bars, meats, fish, and preserved animal products) as well as some drinking water, increased the risk of the development of Type I diabetes (*Diabetes Care* 15 [1992]: 1505; *Diabetic Medicine* 11, no. 7 [1994]: 656).

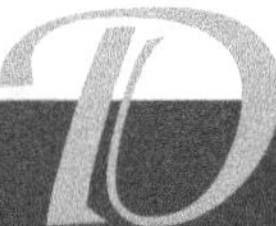

Diets low in fiber and high in starchy foods like sugary junk foods, white bread, soft drinks, etc., increase one's risk of getting diabetes according to a Harvard study of 65,000 nurses. The pancreas simply begins to refuse to respond to the frequent elevation of blood sugar such diets cause (*Self* 101 [April 1997]). Refined foods cause blood sugar to rise quickly because of the low fiber content of the food. Women are particularly at risk of developing diabetes from refined grains such as white rice, white flour, white pastas, etc. The incidence of diabetes in women can be reduced if they simply maintain a diet using whole grains rather than refined grains (*Journal of the American Medical Association* 277 [1997]: 472).

Phytosterols inhibit excessive inflammatory activity of immune cells and can reduce C-reactive protein. Good sources of phytosterols include legumes, whole grains, tree nuts such as almonds, Brussels sprouts, and olives.

The use of tobacco, alcoholic beverages, and many medications can increase the likelihood of diabetes.

Persons with diabetes who do not attend religious services are more likely to have elevated levels of CRP (C-reactive protein) than diabetics who attend services regularly (*Diabetes Care* 25, no. 7 [July 2002]: 1172). C-reactive protein elevation increases one's risks of coronary heart disease and strokes.Develop a program of guided Bible study and daily prayer. Learn to control the thoughts and to dwell on heavenly themes.

Treatment

The diabetic is well advised to avoid the oral antidiabetic agents, as these have toxic side effects. Several studies have shown that the use of these products is associated with an acceleration of the rate of sclerosis of the small and medium sized blood vessels, which is bad news. Being overweight increases the risk of getting diabetes, as 80 percent of overweight adults will get significant degrees of diabetes. There is an hereditary tendency for this type of diabetes. It will not usually be expressed, however, unless the person becomes overweight. If a child is born weighing more than eight pounds, the greater the weight the greater the likelihood that both the parents and the child will develop diabetes at some point.

There are several objectives in handling the "adult onset" type of diabetes, Type II. One of the most important management principles is that of weight reduction. This should be done by eliminating (not just cutting down, but positively cutting out) free fats and free sugars from the diet, getting plenty of exercise, using regularity in all things, and aiming toward a plant-based diet, which is the most favorable diet for reversing diabetes.

Exercise

Physical exercise is quite an effective preventive treatment and remedy for diabetes. Some of the same results obtained from exercise can also be obtained from partial immersion in a hot tub. Five men and three women ranging in age from 43 to 68 years sat in a hot tub at an athletic facility with water up to their shoulders. The hot tub was used for 30 minutes a day, six days a week for three weeks. The patients' diet, exercise, and treatments were all the same as they had been and were stable for eight weeks before the study and during the time of the study. The temperature of the bath water ranged from 100°F (37.8°F) to 105.8°F (41°C), and the patients' oral temperature rose an average of 1.6°F (0.8°C) during each session. After 10 days one patient reduced his dose of insulin by 18 percent. In order to prevent hypoglycemic reactions, the weight of the patients decreased by a mean of five pounds and their mean fasting plasma glucose levels decreased from 182, plus or minus 37 milliliters per deciliter, to 159, plus or minus 42. Their mean glycosylated hemoglobin levels decreased from 11.3 to 10.3 percent. When the water temperature was greater than 103°F (40 °C), the patients reported feeling hot. They became slightly dizzy on getting out of the tub if they hurried to stand. This kind of treatment would be especially helpful for diabetics who are not able to exercise (*American Journal of Physiology* 266: E 248-E 253).

Only a few people get adequate exercise. One of the most important aspects of exercise is that it is enjoyable, affordable, and accessible. It does not matter what type of physical activity is performed—sports, household or yard work, gardening, occupational tasks—all are beneficial in increasing energy expenditure. Regular exercise as a lifestyle behavior must be emphasized for the diabetic. Young individuals must adopt this good habit before the onset of irreversible damage when lifestyle changes may be more acceptable (*Diabetologia* 40 [1997]: 125). Physical fitness in one's thirties will reduce one's probability of getting diabetes in the fifties.

Diet

The optimum diet for diabetics is a totally vegetarian diet, very high in complex carbohydrate calories (70 to 80 percent of daily intake), very low in fat calories (only 10 to 20 percent), and very high in dietary fiber (10 to 40 grams) (*Let's Live*, November 1985, 8–11). The beneficial effect of a

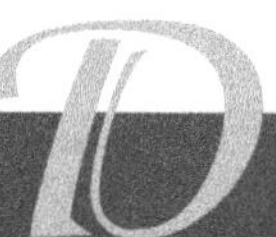

high-fiber diet may be in part because fiber increases insulin sensitivity in cells (*Metabolism* 32, no. 11 [November 1983]). A group of diabetics studied at Georgetown University who were given a plant-based diet with only 10 percent fat lost 46 percent more weight and had a 59 percent greaneter reduction in blood sugar than a group of diabetics who ate a meat-based and dairy-based diet, which contained 30 percent fat (*Self,* December 1996, 69).

Type II diabetes was effectively reversed in laboratory mice given a very low-fat diet (*Geriatrics Society* 46 [1998]: 143).

Many studies have shown repeatedly that whole grains are a must for diabetics and that white or polished grains are very detrimental to proper control (*British Medical Journal* 298 [1989]: 1616). Whole grain breads and cereals, as compared to white bread and refined grain cereals, give much superior control over blood sugar (*British Medical Journal* 297 [1988]: 958). This type of diet also lowers onc's risks for cancer, strokes, and other complications of diabetes.

Lemons and lemon juice will probably help most diabetics to lower blood sugar—*New England Journal of Medicine*, January 19, 1984, 310:171. Several studies indicate that beans of all kinds help diabetics to control blood sugar and to delay complications. A small serving of one quarter to one-half cup should be taken daily.

Laboratory mice given a gluten-free diet from birth developed a significantly lower incidence of diabetes than mice given the traditional laboratory diet. The grain highest in gluten is wheat, followed by rye and barley. Rice, corn, and millet are grains that do not contain gluten. Alternatives to grains include seeds not from the grass family as are all grains. (See "Grain Substitutes" in the *Dietary Information* section.)

Populations such as Korea and Japan who have a traditional diet almost free from gluten, as well as high in soy products, have reduced diabetes rates (*Diabetes, Research and Reviews* 15 [1999]: 223).

Barley has been long alleged to be useful in the treatment of diabetes. A study showed that diabetic animals had more normal blood glucose concentrations, water consumption, and weight maintenance on barley than on wheat (*Annals of Nutrition and Metabolism* 35 [1991]: 61). Various species of barley contain different amounts of chromium, some very high and some only moderate amounts. Barley is also rich in fiber, varying from 15 to 31 percent compared with less than 10 percent for whole wheat flour (*Journal of the American Dietetic Association* 94 [1994]: 1259).

The mineral magnesium is important in improving diabetes complications. Foods high in magnesium should be emphasized in the diet. (See "Food Sources High in Certain Nutrients" in the *Dietary Information* section.)

A diet consisting of 9 percent f, 70 percent complex carbohydrates, and 21 percent protein was fed to a group of 20 diabetics. During the test period the average dosage of insulin was halved from 26 units to an average of 11 units. In nine patients receiving from 15 to 20 units of insulin per day, and in two receiving 32 units, insulin was no longer needed (*American Journal of Clinical Nutrition,* November 1979, 2312–21). The protein content of this diet is probably higher than ideal for diabetics, as a high protein diet is hard on the kidneys, an organ already susceptible to damage in a diabetic. Complex carbohydrates (not refined variety) should comprise closer to 80 percent of the diet.

Free fats (margarine, mayonnaise, fried foods, cooking fats, and salad oils) interfere with the action of insulin and are actually more important as a cause of lack of control of diabetes than sugars that have always been recognized to cause the diabetic to lose control. Diets must be fashioned that will be highly palatable yet contain little or no free fats.

A study done in Norway on 2,000 men over a 22-year period found that those men consistently carrying a fasting blood glucose level greater than 85 milligrams were 40 percent more likely than average to get cancer and Type II diabetes. They also noted that men with high normal blood glucose levels also tended to have a clustering of several other unfavorable cardiovascular risks such as elevated blood pressure, increased blood lipid levels, and complications that attend these conditions (*Diabetes Care* 22 [1999]: 45–9). Measures should be taken to keep the fasting blood sugar levels below 85, including fasting, weight control, and avoiding overeating and stress.

Injury to organs from excessive blood sugar contributes to the development of insulin resistance in the person who has a genetic likelihood of developing diabetes. The higher the blood sugar, the greater the likelihood to progress to the development of insulin resistance. If glucose is controlled there is improvement in the insulin resistance. The glycosylated hemoglobins can be used to get an idea of blood sugar levels at times when not being tested. It tells the average blood sugar level over about the last one to three months (*Postgraduate Medicine* 101, no. 2 [1997]: 87).

Diabetes inhibits the formation of collateral coronary vessels, increasing the diabetic's likelihood of having a heart attack (*Circulation* 99 [1999]: 2224). If the fasting level of blood sugar routinely runs above 100, there is a four-fold increased risk for heart attacks.

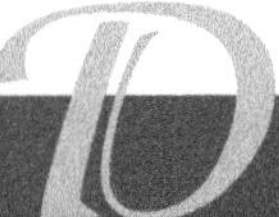

An extract of alfalfa gave beneficial results in the treatment of diabetes (*Diabetic Medicine* 11, no. 2 [1994]: S20). Whole leaf alfalfa tablets are available for those not having fresh alfalfa available.

In one study the use of canned fruits and fruit juices, when not prepared with sugar, showed a similar effect on the blood sugars as whole, fresh fruits, provided the amounts of carbohydrate were the same in all forms (*International Journal of Food Sciences and Nutrition* 43 [1993]: 205). Canned fruits may be judiciously used by the diabetic.

Onions are capable of lowering blood sugar as effectively as some prescription diabetic drugs. They should be eaten in the quantity of approximately half an onion cooked and half an onion raw with a meal.

Smoking may cause the usual factors used in bringing blood sugar down to fail to bring results. It is important to encourage diabetics not to smoke (*Diabetes* 44 [May 1995]: 99A).

The biotin levels of diabetics are generally significantly lower than that of healthy control subjects, and they tend to go down as blood sugar levels go up. Restoring the biotin levels encourages better control of the blood sugar (*Journal of Clinical Biochemistry and Nutrition* 14 [1993]: 211). Most of the biotin the body needs is actually produced in the intestines. (See "Food Sources High in Certain Nutrients" in the *Dietary Information* section).

Since omega-3 and omega-6 polyunsaturated fatty acids have been associated with better insulin sensitivity in laboratory animals, it seems reasonable that introducing walnuts and flax seed into the diet could do the same thing (*Journal of Nutrition* 126 [1996]: 1549). These foods are highest in these essential fatty acids.

It is possible to improve insulin sensitivity by cutting down on calories, losing weight, exercising, being regular in all one's habits, and taking certain herbs and supplements. Improving insulin sensitivity will reduce blood sugar.

For some diabetics suffering from numbness, tingling, and pain of diabetic neuropathy, they found relief by wearing magnetic shoe pads, which can be obtained through health food stores (*Bottom Line Health*, September 1998, 9).

Fasting for one to five days may be very useful in overweight, adult-onset diabetes. If on insulin, it must be omitted during the fast. Immediately after the is terminated, the insulin requirement will be markedly decreased or even gone. At times, with careful attention to diet and exercise, blood sugar will return to near normal levels without the use of insulin. It should be noted that the Type I, juvenile diabetic, should never fast. Acidosis can develop from fasting, which might be dangerous.

There are no safe, "responsible" snack foods for diabetics. There are no "vacations" from the diet. The more consistent you are, the longer you will live free from complications. Whole foods such as white potatoes with skin, lentils, kidney beans, peanuts, nuts, carrots, fruits and vegetables, and whole grains are handled much better by the diabetic than juices, purees, and milled foods.

Olives are a very important addition to the diet of diabetics and may be used in place of free fats. A spread can be prepared from green ripe olives that can substitute for margarine or mayonnaise. A spread from avocado can be prepared in a similar manner with a little salt if desired.

Herbal Remedies

Bilberry and blueberry leaves are useful in controlling blood sugar because of anthocyanosides which increase circulation and prevent complications. The following remedy was given to me by Esther Curry of Columbus, Georgia, who got it from an "old woman." It will prove useful only to those who have access to huckleberry bushes or other wild blueberry roots. Take one and one-half quarts of cut up huckleberry roots and add one gallon of water in a kettle. Simmer for one hour. Drain and save the liquid. Put the roots again in the kettle and add another one gallon of water. This time, gently simmer for 15 minutes. Remove from the stove and let it cool in the pot. Save the first gallon for use after the second gallon is gone. Drink three-fifths of a cup four times a day of the second batch, which is more diluted. Then begin using the first gallon drained off, in the same dosage. Watch for low blood sugar. If you feel weak or faint, you may need to take some unsweetened fruit juice to bring your blood sugar back up. Be sure to take 8 to 10 glasses of water daily, and even more in hot weather.

Fenugreek seeds contain trigonelline which has the property of reducing blood sugar. The seeds of fenugreek (Trigonella foenum-graecum) have been used traditionally because of antidiabetic properties. Recently, these properties were investigated in diabetic animals and found indeed to be effective. No effect was found on glucagon secretion by the pancreas, but there was an immediate and relatively strong increase in plasma insulin levels accompanied by a decrease in blood sugar. The extracted compound is nonsulfonylurea but directly stimulates insulin secretion (*Diabetologia* 36 [August 1993]: A119). In another study, fenugreek seed powder was fed to 60 adult-onset diabetics who showed a significant improvement in glycosylated hemoglobin after eight

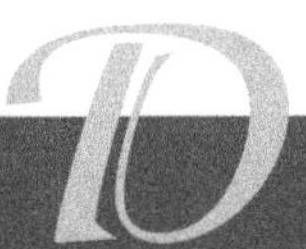

weeks of the fenugreek seed feeding (*Nutrition Research* 16, no. 8 [1996]: 1331). Glycosylated hemoglobin and similar tests are good ways to keep up with general levels of blood sugar.

Gymnema sylvestre has been used for hundreds of years in Indian herbal remedies to balance sugar levels and reduce the appetite for sweets. It is believed that *Gymnema* can actually regenerate and repair pancreatic beta cells that are responsible for producing insulin. Also bilberry (*Vaccinium myrtillus*) has been found helpful for blood sugar and to protect nerves, veins, and eyes from degeneration in diabetics. *Gymnema sylvestre* extract helps to promote the production of insulin, and some believe to promote the number of insulin-producing cells in the pancreas. All parts of the plant can be used.

Goat's rue contains galegine, a nutrient that reduces blood sugar.

Coleus forskohlii assists in normalizing the release of somatostatin and glucagon, other hormones from the pancreas.

Ginkgo biloba increases blood circulation to internal organs by a beneficial effect on blood vessels and helps to prevent complications of diabetes.

Purchase clean, untreated broomcorn seed. Boil one-forth cup of seed in five cups of pure water and simmer. Let stand overnight and then strain. Take one-half cup on rising and one-half cup on retiring. This formula immediately reduces blood sugar levels. You should probably not take insulin while taking this formula as the blood sugar may drop too low. One could do an Internet search for possible sources. The principal nutrient is sparteine, which also has uses in heart rhythm disturbances and uterine bleeding.

Cinnamon increases the ability of insulin to handle blood sugar up to nine-fold, according to research done at Human Nutrition Research Center of the United States Department of Agriculture. Take one-forth teaspoon one to three times daily (*Vogue* [1993]: 56). Chromium may be the most active agent in cinnamon.

Ginseng has the ability to reduce blood sugar because of some other factor than ginsenosides, which are without hypoglycemic action. The whole crude root or extract from the whole crude root should be used (*American Journal of Natural Medicine* 3, no. 6 [1996]: 28).

Agrimony eupatoria has certain factors that reduce blood sugar, enhance sugar metabolism in the body, and stimulate insulin secretion (*Diabetic Medicine* 13, no. 4 [1996]: S22). The longer the herb is taken the more beneficial it becomes. Take one-half cup of tea three times daily, made from one teaspoon of the herb to one cup of boiling water, steeped for 30 minutes.

Momordica charantia (bitter melon) and *Vaccinium myrtillus* (bilberry) can both help normalize blood sugar levels (*Planta Medica* 42: 205–12; *Journal of Ethnopharmacology* 30: 295–305; *Indian Journal of Physiology and Pharmacology* 33: 97–100).

Dried fig leaves boiled in water for 30 minutes showed a factor capable of reducing blood sugar (*Phytotherapy Research* 10 [1996]: 82). The factors in fig leaf tea enhances the uptake of glucose by cells by increasing the number of insulin receptors, thereby reducing blood glucose levels (*Diabetes* 39 [1998]: 19).

Turmeric, bay leaves, and cloves can all act to enhance insulin production. Chromium may be the active ingredient in these foods, as in cinnamon.

For insulin resistance use the following dietary supplements and herbs:

- Dandelion, sage, bay, cedar berries, and oregano teas
- Magnesium salts; magnesium sulfate, magnesium aspartate, magnesium citrate, etc.
- Vanadyl sulphate
- Chromium, 200 micrograms before each meal

Use one teaspoon of cascara sagrada in a quart of chia tea daily. If the cascara is too laxative, cut it in half. Not only is this remedy good for the pancreas and diabetes, but also for gallbladder and liver problems, diabetic cataracts, and glaucoma.

For visual problems associated with diabetes, the above remedy is quite useful, along with a cup of chopped or pureed nopal (prickly pear) every day. If nopal is not available, three spears of pureed celery may be substituted.

For diabetic cataracts, and glaucoma, wash the eyes once daily in eyebright tea. Drink one cup of eyebright tea daily.

Among many herbs and foods considered good for diabetes the following should be used: aloe, apple, asparagus, blackberry, black cohosh, coriander, dandelion, garlic, golden seal, marshmallow, meadowsweet, raspberry, sage, and white willow.

Nutrient Supplements

Vitamin E in large doses (900 IU daily for four days) can help the diabetic gain control of blood sugar levels. Then the vitamin E levels should be maintained with daily use of whole grains, nuts, beans, etc (*Let's Live,* December 1993, 12). If vitamin E continues to be taken, it should be only

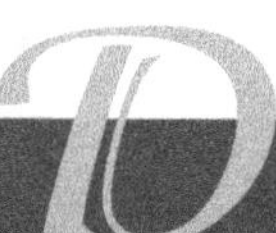

around 200 to 400 IU daily. It is believed by some researchers that too much vitamin E might cause internal bleeding in the bowel or brain.

The daily dietary requirement for vanadium is very small, probably 10 micrograms per day. Most diets supply between 15 to 30 micrograms of vanadium per day. Good dietary sources of vanadium include vegetables, whole grains, and cereals. Meats, fish, butter, and cheese are poor sources of vanadium. This mineral is also in the air and water of most, if not all, regions of the United States (*The Journal of Alternative and Complimentary Medicine* 5 [1999]: 273).

Since vitamin C administration has beneficial effects upon blood sugar control, it would be wise for a diabetic to eat large quantities of raw fruits and vegetables that are high in vitamin C (*Journal of American College of Nutrition* 14, no. 4 [1995]: 387). (See "Food Sources High in Certain Nutrients" in the *Dietary Information* section.)

In a group of 3,575 subjects, it was found that as the intake of zinc went up, there was a lower incidence of diabetes, glucose intolerance, coronary artery disease, hypertension, and high blood cholesterol levels (*Journal of the American College of Nutrition* 17, no. 6 [1998]: 564). (See "Food Sources High in Certain Nutrients" in the *Dietary Information* section.)

Complications of Diabetes

Magnesium is the fourth most abundant mineral in the body. It affects the transport of potassium and calcium. It affects healing of cells, nerve transmission, energy metabolism, bone strength, etc. Magnesium deficiency is not uncommon, and its intake has steadily decreased over the years. Magnesium deficiency is a regular condition in those prone to have diabetes, and their relatives, even if they do not have a high risk of diabetes. Fiber-rich cereal products have been shown to decrease diabetes risk. The high magnesium content of these foods may be the greatest reason for this phenomenon. There is no room in the menu for refined grains for those who have diabetes or are at high risk of developing diabetes.

Elevated insulin levels cause an increase in magnesium excretion through the kidneys. The insulin can be either naturally produced or injected. Magnesium supplementation helps in the regulation of diabetes, prevention of hypertension, and the complications of diabetes. Magnesium supplementation apps to help reduce the risk of atherosclerosis, obesity, and Type II diabetes associated with the over secretion of insulin in the metabolic syndrome X (*Diabetic Medicine* 12 [1995]: 664–9). Further, their lifespan was significantly increased.

The proper action of insulin requires magnesium in order to control blood sugar. Conversely, magnesium cannot do its proper function without insulin. Individuals who eat foods lower in magnesium have one-third greater likelihood to develop diabetes than those who consume sufficient quantities (*Journal of the American Medical Association* 277 [1997]: 472). Similar results have been found in studies on high blood pressure and strokes. Even migraines may be associated with inadequate intake of magnesium. (See "Food Sources High in Certain Nutrients" in the *Dietary Information* section.)

For at least 50 years it has been known that the control of diabetes was better if the person ate less foods high in calories. Now a study in laboratory animals reveals that a low calorie diet will actually prevent diabetes. Sixty-seven percent of diabetes-prone rats developed diabetes on an unlimited food supply, but none of the rats given a diet that was only 70 percent of the food they would have taken if they had had an unlimited supply developed diabetes (*Diabetes Research and Clinical Practice* 27, no. 2 [1995]: 97–106).

A person with diabetes is approximately eight times more likely to develop arterial disease in the extremities than non-diabetics. Since smoking, hypertension, and an HDL cholesterol below 35 spell very serious problems for the arteries, we need an easy way to make an assessment of the arteries in smokers. One easy way is by the comparison of the ankle with the arm blood pressures. The systolic blood pressure above the ankle as measured by a Doppler blood pressure instrument and compared with the systolic blood pressure in the arm is 95 percent sensitive and is almost 100 percent specific for arterial disease such as . The ankle systolic blood pressure is divided by the arm systolic pressure. A result less than 0.90 is diagnostic. The normal reading should be between 0.95 to 1.20. Between eight and 10 million people in the United States have arterial disease in the extremities, a condition posing serious health risks. Only about half have symptoms such as lameness on walking a short distance (*Internal Medicine News*, September 1, 1999, 18).

For many years we have known that foods that have been overly browned contain toxic substances. Research indicates that Advanced Glycolated End products (AGEs) from excessively browned foods of all kinds, whether it is roasted chicken, or overly browned toast, produce AGEs, which are dumped quickly into the bloodstream and contribute to the serious complications of diabetes. These risks are particularly high if the diabetic has kidney damage, making it difficult for the body to dispose of the AGEs rapidly. If AGEs build up in the blood, they hasten the onset of the dreaded complications of diabetes (*Your Health,* August 20,1996, 80).

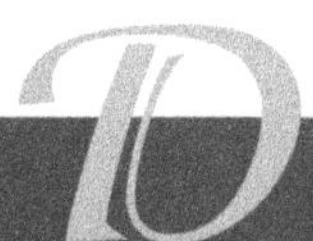

The browning reaction (Maillard) of foods has been under study for several decades. It is a very complex reaction that results in both desirable and undesirable food attributes and some nice flavors. On the undesirable side the Maillard process produces a union of glucose and protein that makes a stiff molecule, causing accelerated aging. The Maillard reaction is not always detrimental and can improve the properties of some food proteins. It is for this reason that the Maillard reaction or browning of breads and long cooking of grains boiled for use as cereals improve the digestibility and healthfulness of the grains. The Maillard reaction occurs in the body, also, being continuously formed but removed by macrophages in the healthy, normal person. Diabetics operate this removal process much less briskly than normal people. When these products are not removed, they may contribute to the complications of diabetes (*Food Technology* 48 [July 1994]).

Protein restriction in diabetics slows down the rate at which kidney damage occurs from diabetes. Even a slight reduction has been found to be beneficial. It has been observed that plant protein protects the kidneys. Soybeans especially contain a protein that specifically protects and heals the kidneys. As an animal-based diet is replaced by a vegetarian diet, the diabetic will benefit in many ways, not just with the kidneys (*Nephrology, Dialysis, and Transplantation* 14 [1999]: 1445).

Magnesium helps slow or prevent the progression of complications of diabetes (*Trace Elements and Electrolytes* 15, no. 4 [1998]: 163). Diabetic neuropathy is particularly related to low levels of magnesium in the tissues. High levels of magnesium in the diet improve nerve conduction.

Type II diabetes is associated with an increase in free radicals that results in damage to fats, proteins, and DNA. When overweight people lose weight, there is a corresponding drop in free radicals.

Fourteen volunteers drank two cans of a cola drink in the laboratory before blood was drawn for tests at one hour and two hours. The free radical generation increased significantly at one hour and more than doubled at two hours. The level of vitamin E also fell about 4 percent by the second hour.

General blood vessel diseases increase by six times when diabetes is out of control. Coronary heart disease, strokes, hypertension, glaucoma, and premature births in pregnant diabetics are all increased. Gangrene of an extremity is increased 25 times in diabetics. Blindness in the United States is caused by diabetes in 25 percent of cases. It is the number one cause of blindness apart from macular degeneration. Cataracts develop earlier. Life expectancy is decreased by one-third and in pregnancy a woman can expect larger babies with more complications and a longer gestational period. Control diabetes carefully when there are complications, as it is impossible to control the complications if diabetes is not brought under perfect control.

Since diabetes is a metabolic acceleration of the rate of aging, it is understandable that cancer, heart disease, hypertension, and strokes are more likely to occur in diabetics. These diseases are also more likely to develop because diabetes reduces the effectiveness of the immune system, making it less capable of warding off viruses.

Insulin-dependent diabetics should not apply heat to the feet at a higher temperature than about 102°F. The application should always be monitored carefully. Heating pads are dangerous for persons with poor arterial blood supply to the lower extremities as the amount of heat delivered to the skin cannot be accurately measured. A warm footbath can be tested by a thermometer, insuring a safe level. If there is any doubt, use a large fomentation to the groin to reflexively dilate the blood vessels in the feet.

Problems with the feet and legs in the diabetic are directly related to reduction in blood flow to these extremities. Intermittent claudication (lameness that comes and goes during exercising) is because of reduced blood flow in the arteries to the legs. Exercise is an important way to encourage circulation to the lower extremities. Extreme care should be taken to avoid infections in cuts and abrasions of the feet. Protective footwear must always be worn, even inside the home.

It has been discovered that in persons with foot and leg ulcers and gangrene the blood is quite thick and has a slow-flow condition somewhat like honey on a cold morning. It is not known whether the ulcers come first and cause the thick blood or whether the thick blood comes first and causes the ulcers. We favor the latter position. We believe that too many red blood cells and plasma containing too many nutrients and wastes promote the development of intermittent claudication (*Blood Viscosity in Heart Disease and Cancer*, eds. L. Dintenfass and G. V. F. Sean [Pergamon Press: 1981]). If a diabetic is not taking medications and can properly answer the questionnaire of the Red Cross, it is beneficial to donate blood as often as allowed.

Diabetic Neuropathy (Nerve Damage)

This condition is characterized by unpleasant or painful symptoms caused by degenerative changes to the nerves. This complication is one of the most dreaded because it has been considered to be incurable, but with the introduction of a low-fat, plant-based diet, alternative medicine practitioners

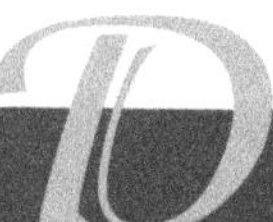

have recognized diabetic neuropathy as a curable disorder. The sharp, burning pains characteristic of polyneuropathy, when treated with exercise, diet, and regularity in lifestyle, will often begin to subside in one month (*Journal of Nutritional Medicine* 4 [1994]: 431). In some individuals, taking vitamin B12 can help clear lost vibratory sensation and diabetic neuropathy.

Diabetic neuropathy is improved by taking myoinositol, a nutrient found especially in beans, cantaloupe, citrus fruits—especially grapefruit—and many other vegetarian foods. (See "Food Sources High in Certain Nutrients" in the *Dietary Information* section.) On the other hand, myoinositol is quite low in meat, milk, eggs, and cheese. The myoinositol content of foods is one of the reasons the plant-based diet is superior to a diet that contains animal products (*Nutrition Research* 16, no. 4 [1996]: 603).

A form of carnitine called acetyl *L-Carnitine* is helpful in diabetic neuropathy. It can be obtained on-line or at health food store. It is also sold in Europe over the counter.

Soy protein is also specifically nutritious for the kidneys and can slow the progress of diabetic nephropathy. The best form is whole, unprocessed soybeans. Only one-fourth cup of cooked soybeans a day is required to yield sufficient protein for the healing benefit.

Diabetic Nephropathy (Failing Kidneys)

A low sodium diet coupled with a low protein diet can be very effective in slowing down the development of diabetic nephropathy, the gradual loss of kidney substance. All diabetics should be counseled to use both a low protein and a low salt diet. Diabetic rats showing enlargement of the kidneys and protein in the urine (signs of beginning kidney failure) were given 5 percent guar gum in their diet. Glycosylated hemoglobin was significantly reduced in the treated group as compared to those not given guar gum. Kidney weights were significantly reduced, indicating the kidneys had an improvement in renal function, and protein in the urine was decreased, although with the passage of time the protein in the urine and the kidney function again deteriorated. Guar gum slows the progress of nephropathy. Lowering cholesterol can retard diabetic nephropathy (*Diabetologia* 38 [1995]: 604).

Diabetic Retinopathy (Failing Vision)

Persons with Type II diabetes usually develop poor blood circulation in the retina, which results in long-term damage. The failing vision of diabetics can be improved by eating at least one pint of blueberries per week, according to a diabetic in California with failing vision. We suggest about one-half cup per day.

Case Reports

We received the following letter from a man in California: "I am a 57-year-old, married, white male minister, weight 295 lbs., height 5 feet 10 inches. I have never smoked. Before reading your book I exercised daily. Frustrated with stubborn obesity, I welcomed your book *Diabetes and the Hypoglycemic Syndrome*, which was recommended to me by my chiropractic doctor. Until I read your book, I ingested some sweets, meat, poultry, fish, and dairy products in 'moderation'—which is to say three or four times per week—along with lots of fruit, whole grains, and vegetables. But after careful study of your book, I adopted your recommended strict plant-based diet to complement my other habits of avoiding all alcohol, caffeine, coffee, tea, and chocolate.

"But what seemed a slight dietary change to lots of water, two-meals-a-day, strict plant-based diet, has had amazing and profoundly excellent results in quick order.

"Within five days, persistent swelling in my lower legs and feet began to subside. A troublesome, three-month old sore on my lower left shin, about four centimeters in diameter, which often filled with bloody liquid as in a blister, began to heal rapidly and is now gone, replaced with healthy skin merely two weeks after beginning the lifestyle change. I am losing excess fat steadily while continuing my one hour daily exercise. My blood pressure is consistently in the 136/80 to 128/76 range. I have no swelling (now) of my lower extremities. Dry, flaky athlete's foot and rough patches of foot skin, especially at the heels, is clearing and becoming soft and smooth. My endurance and flexibility seem to improve daily. Even osteoarthritis of both knees, because of old knee injuries and subsequent surgeries, has abated.

"Every time I grow hungry (which is most evenings) I look at my unswollen feet and ankles, thank God for your work, and renew my resolve to stick to this the rest of my life. Then I have a cup of herbal tea with stevia."

A 55-year-old woman came to Uchee Pines complaining of feeling as if she were in a fire or in an ant bed. She had not smiled for over a year and constantly felt miserable. She had deteriorated from a dignified and prim school teacher to a whining and simpering person who had no thoughts except for how bad she felt. Her fasting blood sugar was only 125, which is sometimes typical of those with diabetic neuropathy,

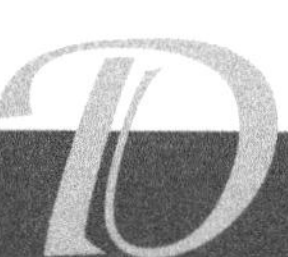

the neuropathy being the first sign of their disease. Her cholesterol was 305 and triglycerides 230. Her primary doctor in her hometown had not diagnosed her with diabetes or noticed the high blood fats.

We gave her lots of whole grains, cantaloupe, and citrus fruits, which are all high in myoinositol. Her diet was plant-based and her exercise was to tolerance. We gave her neutral baths for the stinging sensations, lots of water to drink by mouth, treated her pain with massage, heat, cold, and range of motion movements. Occasionally we would give her an enema as a pain control measure. Within eight weeks she was walking eight miles daily and was smiling for the first time in over a year. Within another month she was totally well and was able to go home feeling well enough to keep house again.

One man reports that a few weeks after beginning drinking a juice he made, his diabetic neuropathy, which he had had for over a year, cleared almost miraculously. He had experienced weakness and lack of feeling in his legs. While driving his car and stopping at a traffic light, his right leg was used to apply the brake. After a short while of waiting for the light to change, he would have to place his hand on his knee in order to keep the foot on the brake. If the light were especially long, he had to place the car in park.

Several days after beginning juicing, he noticed while parked at a traffic light that he had no difficulty whatsoever in holding his foot on the brake the entire time before the light changed. The juice consisted of collard greens, kale, and mustard greens, about equal parts of each as available. He also put about a cup of the white and green watermelon rind through the juicer with the greens. In addition, he ate about a handful of raw parsley each day. He could only take one to two ounces of the green juice because of the very strong taste. He attributes his healing of the neuropathy to the use of these juices and parsley. Myoinositol is high in all these foods, a substance present in nerve cells, but lost from the cells in diabetes.

A 63-year-old lawyer with diabetes came to Uchee Pines Institute having a fasting blood sugar level of 310. He suffered persistently from angina and took 28 units of insulin daily. Because he also had gout, we did not give him a period of fasting as usual, but merely gave him a plant-based diet, sufficiently low in calories, which resulted in 20 pounds weight loss in six months. Within five weeks his blood sugar was down to 115 fasting, and he was taking no insulin.

His angina totally disappeared while on this diet, which included no free fats. He also engaged in a program of walking with the instruction to keep the extremities warm and avoid cold blasts of air on the chest. Four years later his gout has totally disappeared, his angina has never returned, and his blood sugar levels never exceed 100 fasting.

Diaper Rash

Ordinarily an infection is not involved, and the rash is simply the result of irritation of the skin by a wet diaper, aggravated by the ammonia from the urine. The ammonia is formed by bacteria working on urea, a waste product in urine.

The finest treatment is a slightly warm vinegar water sitz bath for five minutes every hour until better, and then every several hours as needed. Put one-half cup of vinegar in the bathtub with water. If the vinegar burns the baby, use as little as one tablespoon of vinegar, gradually increasing as the rash heals.

At night, petroleum jelly or a zinc ointment may be applied generously to the diaper area to minimize the night time contact of wet diapers with the skin.

Sunning and drying the diaper area are excellent for diaper rash.

Diarrhea

The condition of loose bowel movements with or without painful cramping may occur because of some toxic, irritating, or infected food, such as unripe fruit, highly spiced foods, alcoholic drinks, or spoiled foods.

The treatment of choice is a heaping tablespoonful of powdered charcoal stirred into a full glass of water and taken after every loose bowel movement or with every feeling of discomfort in the abdomen. You cannot overdose on charcoal when taken with a lot of water. Be generous in the dosage.

Diarrhea can be treated with several foods and herbs: apple, bayberry, blackberry root, carob, catnip, dill, fennel, garlic, golden seal, meadowsweet, mullein, psyllium, raspberry, turmeric, and uva-ursi.

A spoonful of arrowroot starch in a small amount of water will often cure diarrhea.

Garlic, about one-half to one teaspoonful of dried garlic powder, may be sprinkled on food to good advantage.

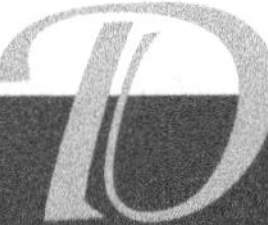

Ripe green bananas, the large cooking bananas, are usually tolerated well and may assist in the control of diarrhea.

Carob paste may be eaten, or a carob milkshake, or carob-nut milk-fruit smoothie may be prepared, using one tablespoon of carob blended with a few nuts, water, canned or frozen fruit, or fruit juice to make a nice smoothie.

For soreness or rash on the bottom, apply coconut oil.

Since dehydration may follow diarrhea, it is especially important that large quantities of water be taken during the course of the diarrhea. The water will also serve to dilute the influence of toxins or infectious germs.

Since much potassium can be lost in diarrhea, it is well to take a broth made of potato peels called "potassium broth" (see "Potassium Broth" in the *Dietary Information* section), and to drink fruit juices high in potassium—tomato, citrus—and to eat bananas and other high potassium foods.

If the diarrhea becomes chronic, an investigation should be made to determine the cause. Food sensitivity is often the culprit. Follow the "Elimination and Challenge Diet" in the *Dietary Information* section to determine those foods to which the person is sensitive. Sometimes an intestinal parasite is the cause. (See "Parasites" in the *Conditions and Diseases* section.)

Dietary Deficiency

(See "Nutrient Deficiency" in the *Conditions and Diseases* section.)

Digestion

Poor digestion may be helped by digestive enzymes such as papain and bromelain from papaya and pineapple respectively. For those needing assistance in digesting their food, the following herbs may be helpful: anise, catnip, dandelion, dill, fennel, golden seal, hops, mint, oregano, rosemary, sage, savory, slippery elm, thyme, turmeric, or yarrow. Some of these may be chewed, but some may need to be made into teas.

Transit time is the time required for food to be processed by the digestive tract, from the time food is eaten until the residue appears in the stool. You can check your transit time by swallowing two or three tablespoons of moistened sesame seed. Record the time of swallowing and count backward to get the number of hours when you see the last of the sesame seed in your bowel movement. Normal transit time should be less than 30 hours, but the average American has a transit time of more than 89 hours. Mustard seed and turmeric can significantly shorten the transit time in healthy volunteers (*American Journal of Gastroenterology* 90 [1995]: 668).

Diphtheria

Following is a story that was related to us by a family who immigrated to America. "During an outbreak of diphtheria in Europe a family lost several children to diphtheria, and then the husband came down with a fever. During this plague an old woman came to the mother with a jar of kerosene and said, 'Take a clean white linen and wrap it around your finger. Touch the tip of your finger into this pure kerosene. Remove any excess to prevent any from entering the airway. Gently swab out your husband's throat. Then have him swallow a drink made of water or tomato juice and two cloves of garlic blended together until smooth. This should cause him to vomit and bring up some mucus, getting rid of the deadly film on his throat that would cause the throat to close off and suffocate the life.'

"The wife and mother followed the instructions and within a few minutes her husband wretched and vomited the deadly mucus membrane on his throat. His fever broke, and her husband gradually recovered."

We leave this story in this book although we have had no experience with the use of kerosene and sore throat. Use care that the patient does not inhale liquid kerosene. It could cause pneumonia.

We have not treated a case of diphtheria during all the time we have been using natural remedies, but should we get a case we would use any form of hydrotherapy which would be applicable: fever baths, hot foot baths, fomentations to the throat and chest, cold mitten frictions, hot mitten friction, etc. We would practice scrupulous cleanliness, regularity, and faithfully follow the natural laws of health.

We would treat with the various herbs that might be beneficial such as golden seal, echinacea, myrrh, and propolis especially, but also with grapefruit seed extract and aloe vera. We would emphasize garlic in several forms to maximum dosage (raw, steamed, the powder on food, the aged extract both as pills and as liquid), etc. We would give the treatments around the clock. Massage to the full body should not be neglected. Massage will boost the immune system. Gargles with the antimicrobial herbs, charcoal powder, or warm herbal irrigations should be done.

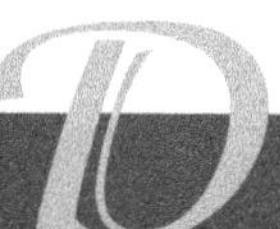

Diverticulosis/ Diverticulitis

Diverticula are small pockets caused by a ballooning out of the lining between muscle bundles of the wall of the colon because of increased abdominal pressure.

They usually occur in groups or patches so that in one place in the colon perhaps three to five diverticula might occur and in another, perhaps five to six. This condition is called diverticulosis. It commonly develops in middle-aged and elderly people. It may exist without infection or inflammation. In the person with diverticulosis, the objective is to keep them free from inflammation. The symptoms are pain, gas, cramping, constipation, and, if the inflammation is severe, there may be fever and diarrhea. Bleeding may occur.

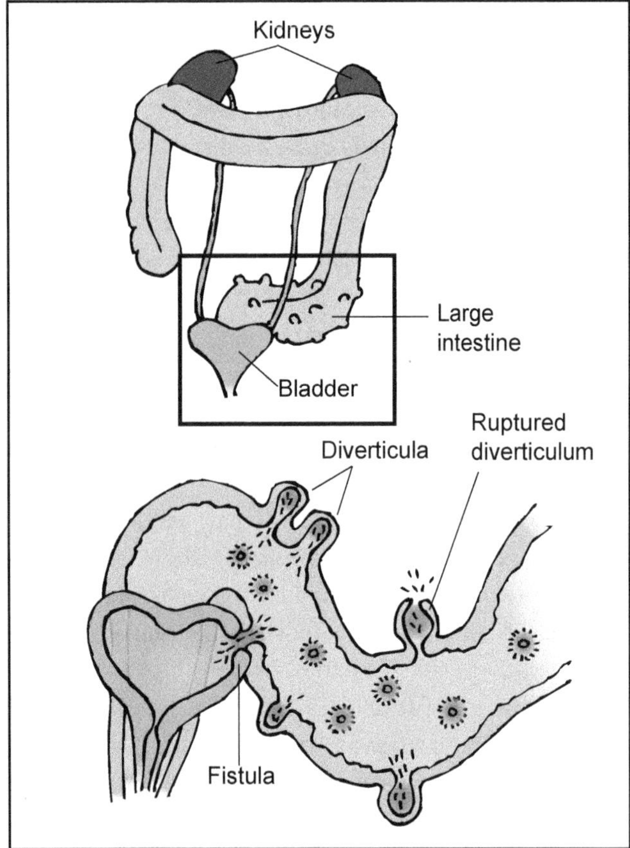

The inflammation of diverticulitis is usually brought on by constipated fecal matter or small seeds impacting them. When inflamed they cause pain, most frequently in the left lower abdomen, but it can be in any part of the bowel, often with diarrhea and fever. The pockets can in rare instances abscess and rupture, resulting in peritonitis. Prevention, by avoiding constipation, is definitely the best route. A high fiber diet rarely allows diverticula to develop.

To treat diverticulosis use a diet high in fiber such as would be obtained from a purely vegetarian diet. Apples, pears, peaches, bananas, oranges, grapes, raisins, all dried fruits, carrots, broccoli, limas, turnips, and whole grains are all very helpful in diverticulosis and the inflamed condition of diverticulitis.

Many persons with diverticulosis or diverticulitis are sensitive to certain foods. These generally tend to be nuts, corn, popcorn, raw celery, tomatoes, cucumbers, grapes, figs, strawberries, raspberries, and breads with poppy, caraway, and sesame seeds (*Patient Care,* January 30, 1979, 167). Chocolate should also be avoided.

Fiber-less foods such as all animal products—meat, milk, eggs, and cheese—refined grains and white sugar, as well as other concentrated sweeteners, encourage diverticulitis. Of course, the cause of increased intra-abdominal pressure should be removed. Get plenty of exercise and drink water copiously, 8 to 10 glasses daily. The use of stomach irritants such as vinegar, spices, sugar, baking powder and soda, alcoholic beverages, and fermented foods must be avoided.

If occurs, fomentations to the abdomen should be used. If there is marked inflammation and abscess formation, heat may cause more congestion and increased pain. In this case, an ice pack should be used. Never take laxatives, as they may cause rupture of the abscessed diverticulum and result in peritonitis. Very gentle and careful small enemas may be tried using one-half cup of golden seal tea as a retention enema. The tea must be at body temperature. Use golden seal, one cup of tea or two capsules every four hours around the clock until the fever is gone. Take this along with garlic. Use raw or steamed garlic, two cloves four to eight times a day; or Kyolic liquid, one to two teaspoons four to eight times daily, depending on how sick the patient is.

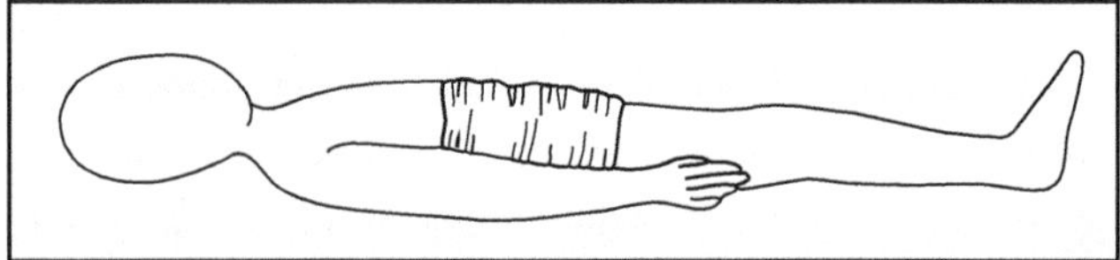

Persons who take a diet high in fiber from fruits, vegetables, whole grains, and nuts rarely if ever have diverticulosis. Prolonged transit time, tight belts, overweight, pregnancy, constipation, and increased pressure within the colon are factors that lead to diverticulosis. You may check your own transit time by taking two tablespoons of sesame seed stirred in a little water and swallowed whole. This will be a marker for you to tell how long the seed took through the entire intestinal tract. The ideal time is less than 30 hours. The average American takes more than 90 hours.

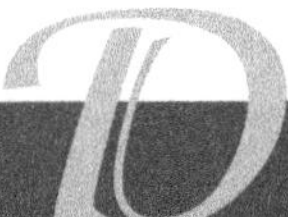

A totally vegetarian diet, avoiding all animal products, has been found, in all countries where it has been used, to prevent diverticula in almost all people. Use a diet high in fiber, which would include fruits, vegetables, whole grains, nuts, and seeds. Since meat and all other animal products are totally devoid of fiber, they are an active cause of diverticula.

Avoid milk and all dairy products. This is the primary treatment of diverticular disease. Often diverticulitis can be cured with no other measure than a milk-free diet.

Avoid all stomach irritants—spices (ginger, cinnamon, nutmeg, cloves, black and red pepper), vinegar and all products made with vinegar, brown drinks (coffee, tea, colas, and chocolate), sugar and all refined sweeteners, baking powder and baking soda. Avoid overeating or eating too frequently or off schedule.

Take large quantities of water to make the fecal material softer and encourage evacuation.

A hot water bottle or electric heating pad laid over the abdomen can relieve pain, as can hot compresses. A self-administered gentle massage over the painful area has been helpful for many.

Dizziness, Ménière's Disease, Vertigo

(See "Ménière's Disease" in the *Conditions and Diseases* section.)

Dizziness produces a sensation of swimming in the head and, like a cough, it may be the sign of something wrong elsewhere. It may follow recovery from all kinds of diseases, poisoning by drugs or other chemicals, sensitivities to foods, or accompany acute illnesses such as a cold or the flu. It is a symptom in high blood pressure, menopause syndrome, headaches, eye strain, brain injury, punctured eardrum, malformations of the inner ear, syphilis, alcoholism, and many other diseases and conditions.

Low sodium in the blood can cause a significant loss of surefootedness and falls with fractures. It should not be overlooked when a person falls that the cause of the fall may have been low sodium in the blood which causes unsteadiness, attention deficits, and potential falls (*The American Journal of Medicine* 119, no. 7A [July 2006]: S83).

Unsteadiness on the feet is especially seen in older people who are taking Benzodiazepine or drugs in which it is used (Valium, Xanax, Librium, and many others). These people have a serious risk of falling because of unsteadiness, which greatly increases the risk of bone fractures (*Journal of the American Medical Association* 262, no. 23: 3303).

Many elderly patients experience episodes of vertigo. One milliliter of vitamin B12 given every 12 to 14 days can cause vertigo to disappear soon after the first injection in many elderly persons. A vial of the B12 can be obtained from a pharmacy along with 27-gauge needles and 1 or 3 cc syringes (*Cortlandt Forum*, August 1994, 65).

Occasional dizziness is no cause for alarm. It is a common complaint and rarely has a serious or organic cause. Recurring dizziness could be because of high blood pressure, low or high blood sugar, an inner ear problem, a heart disorder, a food reaction, or, rarely, brain or nerve trouble. Simple dizziness may be helped by the following suggestions:

- Correct all known causes, and if the dizziness disappears, there is no need for further investigation.
- Avoid eating between meals, drinking much fluid with meals, heavy evening meals, or eating too many varieties at one meal. These practices promote the formation of toxic aldehydes, esters, amines, and alcohols in the intestinal tract that can cause dizziness. Since certain foods cause many people to get dizzy, a list of foods causing food sensitivities should be eliminated for 10 days to see if the dizziness disappears. (See "Elimination and Challenge Diet" in the *Dietary Information* section.)
- Avoid all stimulants such as caffeine, spicy foods, and rich or concentrated foods. These all cause unsteadiness on the feet.
- Keep well hydrated to avoid variations in the concentration of fluid in the inner ear. Such variations can set up currents in the fluid, which result in dizziness.
- Avoid tobacco smoke and other fumes.
- Avoid looking up or down from contrasting heights. The difference may be visually disturbing and result in dizziness.
- Avoid hot or crowded rooms. The combination of hot, stale air and crowds is often a cause of dizziness.
- Avoid unnatural body positions. Standing from the bending position, or any abrupt change of head position can cause dizziness. Change positions slowly. Take a quick, deep inhalation upon changing your position to minimize the discomfort of sudden changes.
- Keep ears and shoulders warm. Blood that has been chilled can be reflected from the ears or shoulders to the structures of the head, causing fluid currents in the inner ear with resultant dizziness. This is especially true if only one side is chilled.

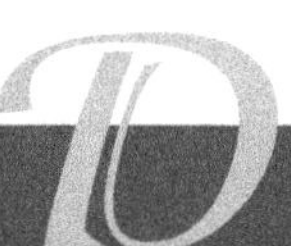

- The use of ginger root is very good for vertigo. Make a tea of it and drink it four times a day, or as needed for dizziness or vertigo.
- Tyrosine can elevate the mood of elderly people, relieve dizziness, normalize blood pressure, and improve the appetite (*Pharmacology, Biochemistry, and Behavior* 47, no. 4 [1994]: 935–41).

Repositioning Treatment

There is a form of dizziness called vertigo that occurs at irregular intervals when the patient assumes certain positions or makes certain types of movements. If it occurs often enough it can become nearly impossible for its victims to function. One of the causes is displacement of the calcified bodies (otoconia, otolith canalith) inside the semicircular canals. With a change in position the displaced concretions move inside the canals and cause dizziness. The condition can be caused by a head injury, which displaces the otoconia. In elderly people a degeneration of the inner ear can be the cause. Various positions can be used to help reposition the otoconia.

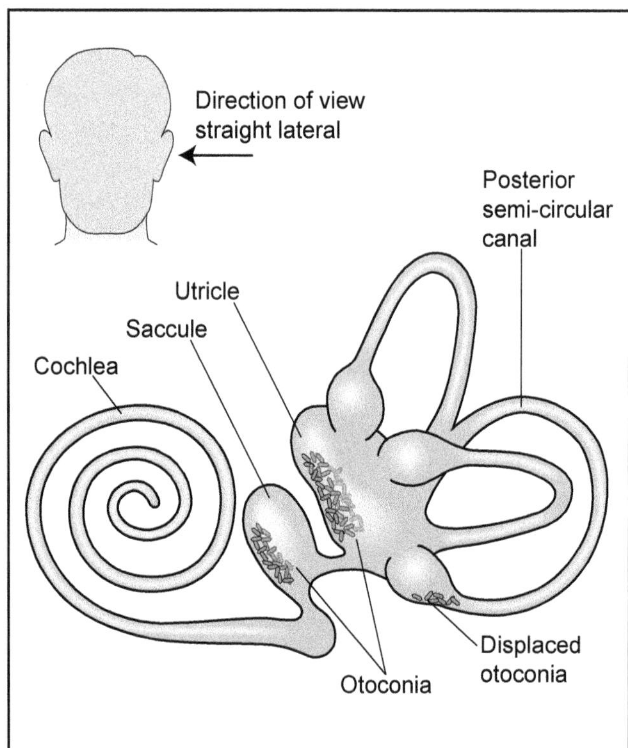

Some types of vertigo can be helped by the canalith (otolith) repositioning maneuver, followed by maintaining the upright position for 48 hours. Patients treated in this way had complete resolution, or greatly decreased intensity, of the vertigo, although some patients needed a repeat of the positioning maneuver. The use of a vibrator, which was originally used in this procedure, was not found to be essential.

The repositioning maneuvers have four steps. First the patient sits on a table. Second the patient moves to the vertigo provoking position, such as the right ear down (if this is the position that brings on the vertigo) and holds that position for two minutes. The third step is to turn smoothly and continuously so that the opposite ear (in this case the left) is pointing down toward the floor, with the nose at a 45-degree angle to the floor. Hold that position for two minutes.

The fourth position is that the patient is brought smoothly with a continuous movement to the upright sitting position. Then the patient is instructed not to lie down or make sudden head movements for 48 hours. A recliner chair can be prepared for the patient to rest, tilted not more than 45 degrees to the horizontal position. With pillows and cushions the head is maintained in the upright position. A foam neck cushion is also helpful in maintaining the proper position.

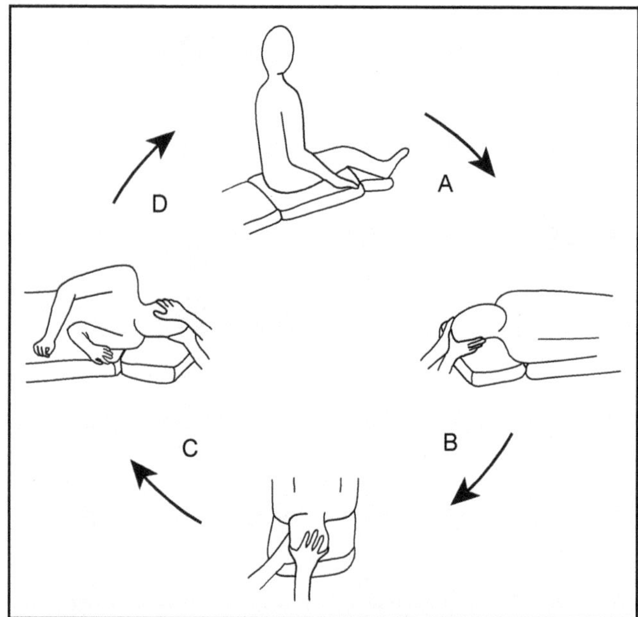

About 80 percent of patients with vertigo have a satisfactory response. If symptoms recur, the patient repeats the maneuvers. A word of caution: If the patient is not put in the correct position during these maneuvers, the otoliths can slide into the superior semicircular canal (before treatment the otoliths were in the posterior semicircular canal), rather than in the utricle, their natural position. In the superior semicircular canal vertigo may continue, but be related to different positioning of the head than at the beginning. Watch for hearing loss, as it may sometimes be associated with vertigo.

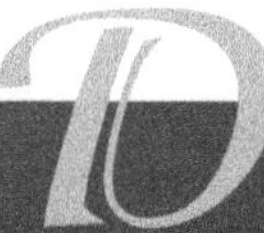

Drugs

Adverse reactions to both prescription and over-the-counter medicines kill approximately 106,000 Americans and seriously injure an additional 2.1 million Americans every year. These reactions do not include prescribing errors, patient or caregiver mistakes, or drug abuse and represent the fourth leading cause of deaths in the United States, behind heart disease, cancer, and strokes. This also does not include those deaths from the use of experimental drugs in testing or those from self-administered proprietary drugs or illicit drugs. Serious injury was defined as being hospitalized or having to extend a hospital stay or suffering permanent disability. Adverse drug reactions rank between fourth and sixth among leading causes of death, depending on whether they used their most conservative or most liberal estimates. More than two-thirds of the cases involved reactions occurring outside the hospital settings (*Journal of the American Medical Association* 279, no. 15 [April 15, 1998]: 1200).

Antibiotics

Many strains of bacteria we thought we had about eliminated, and indeed for a while were subdued after sulfonamides and antibiotics were introduced in the 1930s, have come back with a vengeance. There is also the emergence of new strains of "super bugs." In theory antibiotics are a good thing, and in life-threatening situations they may still be useful in the standard medical system. But through misuse and overuse of antibiotics, some germs have developed defense mechanisms that allow them to produce stronger cell walls and other features to both cause disease and resist antibiotics. It is believed that the overuse of antibiotics has not only caused many old diseases to reappear but may also lie behind a host of baffling new ones (*What Doctors Don't Tell You* 8, no. 1 [1997]: 1).

Aspirin

Reye's syndrome is a potentially fatal disease. Although the exact cause is unknown, many believe it is caused by taking aspirin to treat viral diseases during childhood. As the quantity of aspirin goes up every day, so does the risk of a child getting Reyes' syndrome. Even at low doses of aspirin intake there is some risk of this complication (*Modern Medicine* 57, no. 2 [1989]: 115).

Drugs and Unnecessary Surgery

Reducing the amount of time you stay in the hospital may very well prevent you from getting overloaded with drugs or catching a hospital infection. Also, you may experience improved recovery possibilities of being in the familiar and pleasant surroundings of home.

A study done by Harvard Medical School researchers revealed that of 2.7 million patients hospitalized in New York one year, 3.7 percent of the people suffered injury from medical intervention. Over 70 percent of these injuries produced a disability that persisted for at least six months, and 9 percent suffered a disability lasting more than six months. More than 14 percent died, at least in part, as a direct result of the injury (*Public Citizen Health Research Group* 6, no. 4 [April 1990]: 4, 5).

Lariam

An antimalaria drug named Lariam has been associated with aggression, depression, paranoia, hallucinations, and suicidal thinking. Lariam is also called mefloquine. This drug is suspected to have played a role in the murder of three wives of soldiers stationed at Fort Bragg who had just returned from Afghanistan and were taking the medication.

Steroids

After taking corticosteroid medication, most people have a sense of immediate well-being, but many people experience a sense of uneasiness, unhappiness, and insomnia not long after that. In some, the emotional problem progresses to deep depression, and the person may become suicidal (*British Medical Association* 316 [1998]: 244).

Dry Eye Syndrome

(See "Collagen Diseases" in the *Conditions and Diseases* section.)

Dry Mouth Syndrome

If a person is taking four or more drugs daily there are good chances they will get a dry mouth from the medications.

Toothpaste or mouthwash can cause dry mouth. Certain substances in toothpaste such as sodium lauryl sulfate or peroxide can initiate or perpetuate dry mouth syndrome. Even too frequent rinsing of the mouth with water can also cause dry mouth as it rinses away the mucinous material from the saliva.

A lubricating jelly is a good remedy for dry mouth syndrome. Lubricate the dry mouth two to three times or more a

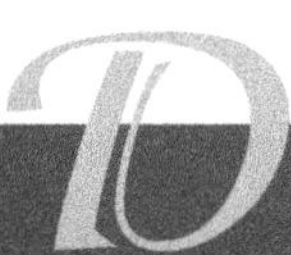

day with the jelly or a similar product, which can be obtained from a pharmacy.

Fifteen milligrams of zinc taken daily may help to increase saliva and tears.

Read the material for dry eyes. All items applying to dry eye syndrome will also apply to dry mouth syndrome. (See "Collagen Diseases" in the *Conditions and Diseases* section.)

In severe cases, a good bit of extra water may be required with meals to chew the food sufficiently for swallowing.

Dupuytren's Contracture

Baron Guillaume Dupuytren, a French surgeon, described the surgical treatment for Dupuytren's contracture in 1832, and reported it in *Lancet* in 1834. This is a disease of the connective tissue in the palms and fingers that results in drawing the fingers toward the palms. It features a painless onset, is self-progressive, and declares itself by typical visible trademarks often beginning with stiffness of a finger with a dimple in the palm near the crease closest to the finger. Knuckle pads may appear on the hairy side of the finger.

The commonest first sign is a fleshy nodule in the palm, usually located at the base of the ring or small finger in the crease where the finger joins the hand. The nodule may be painful or itch, and it may reach one-half inch in diameter. Puckering of the skin of the palm over the involved tendon follows it. The cause of it is not understood well, but some things have been learned in recent years.

Causes

Inheritance is the most important factor; whites, especially those of Celtic origin, have the highest incidence, and it runs in families. It is uncommon in pigmented races, and males are at least twice as often affected as females, in some reports as high as seven to one. The peak incidence is between the fifth and the seventh decades of life. The younger the patient, the more rapidly it progresses.

High blood fats (cholesterol and triglycerides) have been associated with Dupuytren's disease (*Journal of Bone and Joint Surgery* 74B [November 1992]: 923–27). The ideal levels in the blood are 100 plus the person's age for cholesterol, and the same as the age for triglycerides.

Several associated diseases have been observed, including epilepsy, diabetes, alcohol abuse, heart disease, and pulmonary disease. Note that each of these diseases is usually treated with powerful drugs, which may unite the side effects of the drugs with the metabolic disturbance of the disease to cause abnormal growth of the connective tissue in the palms and fingers.

One study showed alcoholics have a higher rate of this disease than others—28 percent as compared to 8 percent (*Journal of Hand Surgery* 17 [1992]: 71–4).

Several studies have indicated an association between some kind of immune disorder and Dupuytren's contracture in susceptible persons (*Journal of Hand Surgery* 16 [1991]: 267–71).

Type II diabetes (adult onset) with absent or reduced insulin receptors on cells of the palmar connective tissue, with a disturbance of the smallest blood vessels and nerves, (micro angiopathy and neuropathy), as well as cigarette smoking, and other factors such as barbiturate use, promote the development of connective tissue disorders (*Diabetes Research and Clinical Practice* 11 [1991]: 121–5; *Archives of Internal Medicine* 149 [1989]: 911–4; *Journal of Hand Surgery* 11 [1986]: 463, 464).

Being overweight, or other metabolic factors may be involved in causing Dupuytren's. Some believe Dupuytren's to be an autoimmune disease or excessive free radical production (*The Journal of Bone and Joint Surgery* 48B, no. 2 [1966]: 312).

It was once thought occupational trauma and Peyronie's disease, a male genital tract disease, were factors, but many in this field now believe these are not factors. Yet, the right hand is more often affected, the ring finger (fourth) being most often involved, followed by the small, middle, and index fingers. We believe trauma is a factor in producing the disease, and also any problem with the nerves.

Physical forces seem to be indicated by some research in causing Dupuytren's contracture, particularly electrical fields. Electrical fields have had bad press in many areas of abnormal tissue growth, including cancer (*Annales De Surgery Chirugie De La Main Ee Du Membre Superieur* 11, no. 5 [1992]: 355–61). It seems wise not to live within 200 feet of a transformer station or high tension electric lines.

Treatment

The treatment has been said to be only surgical, and there are controversies over the type of procedure that should be used, whether it is extensive excision or limited excision of the connective tissue in the palm and fingers, as well as exactly what time in the progress of the disease it is best to operate, whether it should be early or late. There is controversy over whether the wound should be left open or closed after the surgery.

In all methods of treatment currently used in standard medicine, we find a disappointingly high rate of recurrence after what appears to be successful operations. We believe alternative methods should be applied as soon as the first symptom appears. Every attempt should be made to arrest the progress of the disease before it becomes disabling. However, if natural remedies fail to halt the disease, we believe delaying surgery as long as possible to be the more desirable course. Then, as soon as the wound healing is well underway (three to five days after surgery), the natural remedies should be started again and continued for four months to reduce the likelihood of recurrence.

Several natural remedies have been tried and found to be unable to completely stop the disease, but may be of some help to delay or reduce the severity of the disease. The objective of treatment is avoiding surgery.

Most surgeons seem to feel that delaying surgical correction of the condition is reasonable since there is marked individual variation in the rate and severity of the progress of the contracture. Some people have such slow progress they actually outlive the need for an operation. It has been said that successful non-surgical treatment is possible only at the very beginning of the disease. While it may be that only at the start you could hope to cure the disease, there may be some remedies that would stop or slow its progress (*Seminars in Arthritis and Rheumatism* 3, no. 2 [1973]: 155). Therefore, at whatever stage you are, we recommend the following home remedies be applied very carefully:

- The most favorable diet is a totally plant-based diet—no meat, milk, eggs, or cheese. Damage from xanthine oxidase, which is found in homogenized milk, was discovered in the palmar connective tissue of patients with Dupuytren's contracture. Xanthine oxidase has also been found in the joints of both normal and rheumatoid joints, suggesting these joints may be the target of damage by free radicals promoted by this enzyme (*British Medical Journal* 296 [1988]: 292, 293).
- Use *no* free fats—margarine, mayonnaise, fried foods, cooking fats, salad oils, or nut butters. Free fats cause tissue proliferation in certain diseases (cancer, keloids and other skin lesions), and could be a factor in Dupuytren's contracture. Free radicals are compounds with unpaired electrons, making them chemically unstable and active. Since they are not harnessed in any way, they can shoot around and cause damage. They are developed from fats and play a part in inflammation, autoimmune diseases, and possibly help cause Dupuytren's contracture (*Journal of Bone and Joint Surgery* 70-B [November 1988]: 689).
- While free fats and oils of all kinds should be removed from the diet, nuts, seeds, avocados, and olives may be used as desired. All free sugars should also be removed from the diet such as sugar, honey, syrup, molasses, etc. Fruits may be eaten freely, however.
- Be regular in your schedule—especially with mealtimes, bedtimes, etc. Do not overeat.
- Do physical exercise to tolerance, at least six days a week. This should be done with religious consistency. Finger and wrist exercises have helped in trials also using heat and massage (*Journal of American Geriatrics Society* 16 [1968]: 531). Get a sponge ball from a toy department and try to make your thumb meet each finger, one by one, through the sponge ball using a pinching motion. Begin with five repetitions with each finger and build up to 20. Then squeeze the ball as firmly as possible. While squeezing the ball tightly, slowly bend the wrist up and down as if waving goodbye.
- Soak hands and wrists in hot water four times a day for 20 minutes each time, for two months. After the hands become warm, the fingers should be manipulated and stretched by firm massage and pulling or pushing. The use of ultrasound with the heat has proved beneficial in many cases (*Heat Therapy and Ultrasonics* 208 [1972]: 125). Some cases have been effectively treated and corrected with ultrasound. Severely contracted hands will sometimes improve considerably (*Physiotherapy* 66 [1980]: 55).
- A long period of fasting, three to five days, at the beginning of the treatment may be helpful. This should be followed by a diet sufficient to keep the fasting blood sugar level between 70 and 85, the blood pressure under 120/80, and the blood cholesterol and triglycerides in the ideal range.
- If hypertension is also present, the patient should be given a very strict routine of blood pressure control. (See "Blood Pressure" in the *Conditions and Diseases* section.)
- A few studies have indicated that 2,000 IU per day of vitamin E has been found helpful, although in a few studies it has not been found helpful. It might be worth a trial of three months using high doses of vitamin E, from 200 to 2,000 IU per day unless the use of so much vitamin E might be contraindicated in your case.

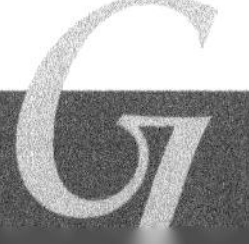

Case Reports

A 66-year-old man with Dupuytren's had surgery to correct the contracture. During surgery his arm was accidentally put in a position that cut off the blood supply. Although the surgery healed well, the arm was weak and painful after the surgery and was immobilized for a few days. Immobilization seemed to increase the symptoms and pain developed in the fingers and along the forearm. Severe weakness developed in several fingers, which after many months had returned to perhaps only 30 percent of original strength. The pain developed into causalgia, a condition in which there is a lot of continuous pain.

The problems resulted from failure of the anesthetist to properly position and move the arm frequently enough to prevent irreversible muscle and nerve damage. From this case one can readily appreciate the fact that any surgical procedure can be hazardous. It is no light matter to be put to sleep. Nevertheless, surgery can be most helpful to restore function in a severely contracted finger.

Virginia Neumann, a 70-year-old woman from Cobb County, Georgia, began working as a deputy sheriff at about age 45. Part of her duties included pulling open and closing heavy steel doors in the jail multiple times daily. She began to develop Dupuytren's contracture. For years it got gradually worse until she began to think perhaps some self-treatment should be attempted. She began to press her left thumb into the mound of tissue that had developed beneath the middle finger of the right hand, and she massaged it with some pressure, enough to be almost painful. Then she would open and stretch the finger and hand as far as possible, then close the hand and repeat. This action was repeated throughout the day at intervals until the finger returned to its normal state. Probably a few weeks or months were spent in this treatment; but the patient does not remember the length of time.

She states, "I just realized one day the mound had shrunk to a very small place." The duration of treatment will depend on how far advanced the condition is. She believed that soaking the hand in very warm water or in a paraffin bath prior to treatment seemed to help. The stretching of the hand should be continued indefinitely to keep it flexible.

Dyslexia

This condition is characterized by being unable to read with understanding. There are varying degrees of the condition from very mild disability to severe. The difficulty apparently has its origin in the brain. Individuals who have dyslexia in childhood are more likely to develop depression later in life (*Internal Medicine News* 29, no. 10 [1996]: 38).

Dr. David Horrobin, a British researcher and editor of the medical journal *Hypotheses*, reports that dyslexia, dyspraxia (poor coordination), and attention deficit disorder are often associated with low levels of essential fatty acids (*Let's Live*, September 1997, 45). Supplementation with essential fatty acids can dramatically improve both the behavior and the intelligence of children. Research was reported in *Medical Hypotheses*.

Both omega-6 fatty acids and omega-3 fatty acids are required for proper development of all tissues, but they are especially important for the brain and nervous system. Omega-6 fatty acids are essential for the normal growth of infant brains and omega-3 fatty acids are needed for the brain's normal functioning. Both of these groups of fatty acids must be converted from the form they are found in vegetable oils and dark green vegetables to other tongue-twister fatty acids that have been abbreviated GLA, DGLA, EPA, and DHA. Breast milk is the primary source of essential fatty acids for infants. One study revealed that eight-year-olds who had been breast-fed as babies scored higher on intelligence tests than did formula-fed children. They also developed sharper eyes and minds when they consumed generous quantities of essential fatty acids.

Dysmenorrhea, Painful Menstruation

(See "Women's Conditions and Diseases" in the *Conditions and Diseases* section.)

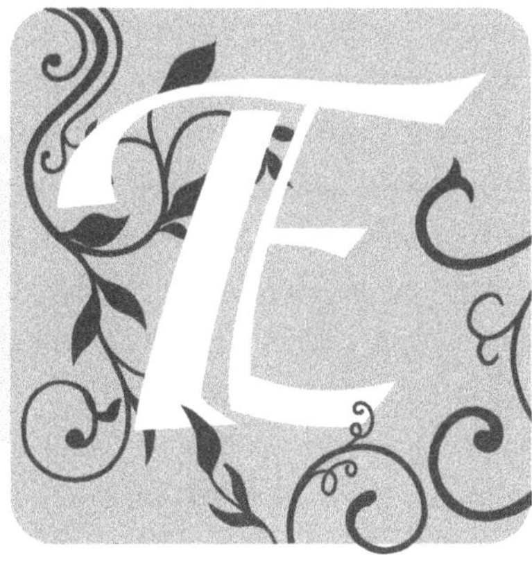

Earache, Otitis Media, Mastoiditis

Children with earaches may have a low grade fever, diarrhea, and a loss of appetite. Infants may tug occasionally at the ear that is bothering them, and they are usually irritable and cry often.

Even without treatment the course of otitis media is generally toward healing, but much can be done to make the patient more comfortable and encourage the body's healing mechanisms.

Avoid sugar and sweets since they cut down on the body's ability to combat infections. Also avoid refined foods.

Children with repeated earaches should be tested for food allergies. The most highly suspect food is cow's milk and all foods prepared with any kind of dairy product, including breads, cakes, crackers, ice cream, etc. Dr. Frank Oski authored a book titled *Don't Drink Your Milk* that, among other findings, indicated that earaches was associated with milk. This has been our experience also, not only with strep throat but with earaches as well. We believe that either an allergy to cow's milk itself, or some infectious agent in the milk promotes earaches.

Avoid common allergenic foods such as dairy products, citrus fruits, chocolate, eggs, and any of the brown drinks related to coffee or colas. The diet during the attack should eliminate not only the common foods known to be allergens, but should contain no free sugars or free fats (margarine, mayonnaise, fried foods, cooking fats, salad oils and nut butters), as both decrease the activity of the white blood cells. The diet should consist of simple fruits and vegetables, with whole grain breads.

Babies should be breast-fed rather than bottle-fed. If breastfeeding is impossible, soy-milk based formula should be used. Breastfeeding will eliminate much, if not all, earaches in very small infants.

Children with recurrent ear infections should guard against forceful blowing of the nose during upper respiratory infections, as blowing may force infected secretions into the middle ear.

Drink plenty of water to mobilize secretions in all of the structures of the upper respiratory tract, including the eustachian tube which connects the middle ear to the outside air in the back of the throat.

Do not use antihistamines, decongestants, or cough syrups as they have a vasoconstricting and drying effect on the middle ear and promote fluid behind the eardrum or "glue ears," one of the most common causes for insertion of tubes in the ears.

Recent studies have shown that putting tubes in children's ears for fluid behind the eardrum may be ill advised. Those who get the tubes are more likely to experience some degree of hearing loss in the years following the procedure. Even in those children in whom the tubes were removed one year after insertion, hearing loss continued according to an article published by A. Scheck titled "Tympanotomy Tubes May Cause Hearing Loss" for as long as twelve years and is probably permanent (*Family Practice News*, March 15, 1993, 3, 24).

Fluid in the middle ears of children almost always disappears within three to six months without any kind of treatment. Antibiotics should not be used as they are of no value

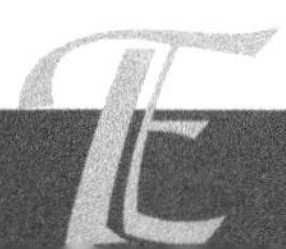

and can cause many side effects. The fluid is almost never infected with germs, and will soon subside. The standard American treatment for an earache is Amoxicillin. A study published in *Medical Tribune* on Thursday, January 16, 1992, showed that the antibiotic is no more effective than placebo in the treatment of earache and fluid in the middle ear, and increases the risk of recurrences up to six fold! Antibiotics used for earache can cause serious side effects.

Smoking, either by the patient or persons around the patient, can promote recurring earaches. It must be forbidden in the area around a child.

The ears may be treated quite effectively by a throat gargle. Use plain hot water and continue the gargle for at least 10 minutes. A gargle with plain hot water or salt water (one teaspoon per glass of water) can open up the eustachian tube. Repeat the gargle every hour.

Warm glycerine or olive oil may be instilled into the ear for pain relief.

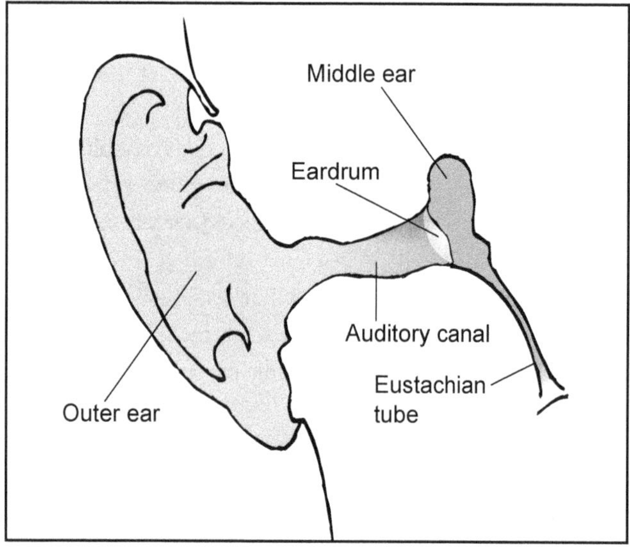

Local heat may be applied to the ear. Deliver heat to the ear from a table or desk lamp, or by sitting in a closed car parked in such a way that the sun can shine on the painful ear for half an hour or more. Other methods to deliver heat are fomentations, a partly filled hot water bottle wrapped in a towel, a heating pad (use with care in infants), or hot salt or sand bag (oven heated). A small child may be placed on the affected side with the ear placed over the heat source.

An ice bag may be used to reduce swelling and pressure and thus decrease pain. Some patients prefer this to heat.

Alternating hot and cold compresses (three minutes for the hot, 30 seconds for the cold), applied to the face and sinuses will assist in decongestion of the head.

Hot foot baths will draw blood from the head, providing relief from pain and congestion. Put the feet in a tub of hot water, as hot as the patient can endure. Keep it hot for 20 to 30 minutes by adding more hot water as tolerated. Keep the head cool with a cloth wrung from ice water. At the conclusion of the hot foot bath remove the feet from the foot tub and pour over them the ice water used to keep the head cool. Dress the patient warmly (particularly the feet) to prevent the slightest chilling of the skin of the extremities.

Fever treatments may be given daily. Hot baths using as hot a temperature as can be tolerated for three minutes for a child three years of age or under, and one additional minute for each year of the child's age. Finish off the bath with a cold water pour and a friction rub with a dry towel. Put the child to bed as quickly as possible after standing out of the hot water. Children will often sleep after this treatment.

A hot mitten friction to the entire body is often helpful.

Steam inhalations in the form of a hot bath or shower may be helpful.

A charcoal poultice may be applied to the ear. This would be particularly helpful if the ear were draining. A charcoal poultice secured over the ear with an ace bandage around the head should be used every night until the earache heals. Use the same treatment for mastoiditis, a rare infection of the bone behind the ear, as it is a part of the same disease process.

Charcoal tablets held in the mouth may help earaches.

An earache can be treated by dropping ice water in the ear, from an ice cube over the ear and letting the ice water drip off into the ear canal until the canal is filled with the cold water. Then turn on the side to drain the water. Pain relief will often be dramatic, and the patient may go to sleep and wake up free from the earache. But occasionally the treatment must be repeated two or more times, draining out the water and dripping it in again. The next day after such a treatment, the ear canal should be filled with ordinary rubbing alcohol, and then drained in the same way. The little finger should be used with a tissue to dry as much of the alcohol as can be reached with the finger. Do not insert anything in the ear smaller than the little finger.

Elevate the head of the bed about four inches with bricks or similar material to promote better drainage of the middle ear through the eustachian tube. Elevation causes the eustachian tube to have a more perpendicular position.

Sometimes a foreign body such as a hair or other irritant can cause pain in the ear or in the back upper wall of the mouth. Such a foreign body can also trigger a cough reflex or dizziness that can become chronic. Irrigation of the ear can remove the foreign body and stop the pain or cough or dizziness (*Cleveland Clinic Journal of Medicine* 56 [1989]: 273).

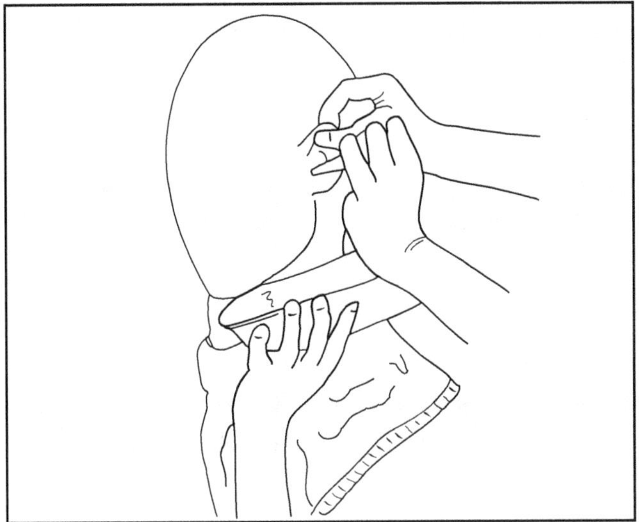

We no longer recommend drying the ears, after swimming or showering, with a hair dryer. Even with the hair dryer on low, hearing can be damaged by frequent use of a blow dryer. Use sponge ear plugs when the dryer is on. The use of ear plugs while showering or swimming can help prevent moisture in the ear canals, which can lead to infection. Prevent bacteria and fungi from causing chronic otitis externa or swimmer's ear by pouring rubbing alcohol into the ear to fill the ear, then tilting the head to empty the ear. Dry the ear as far as you can reach with a tissue and the little finger.

Use antimicrobial herbs. See the *Herbal Remedies* section for a list of such herbs.

Earwax

To dissolve earwax put one-half teaspoon of baking soda in two ounces of warm water. Drop enough of the water into the ear to fill it up. Repeat this process twice a day for one to two weeks. Irrigation may not be necessary to remove wax if this procedure is used. Ear irrigation, however, is not difficult. (See "Irrigation Fluids" in the *Natural Remedies* section.)

Eczema, Infantile Eczema, Acrodermatitis Enteropathica

(See "Skin Diseases" in the *Conditions and Diseases* section.)

Edema, Swollen Legs

Sitting in a tub of neutral water for 30-60 minutes will bring visible results quickly for swollen legs. Walking in water about three feet deep is excellent to remove fluid in the legs. The shallow end of a swimming pool is a good place to accomplish this.

Emergencies

(See the *Home Emergencies* section.)

Emphysema

This disease is the condition that results from over-dilation of air sacs and the tiniest bronchi of the lungs, making them first into small cysts which break open into adjacent small cysts to make ever enlarging cysts. These cysts may be as small as the naked eye can see or as large as a football. The condition can result from anything that causes chronic coughing or wheezing, such as asthma, chronic bronchitis, smoking, or air pollutants. Smoking is by far the main culprit. Once the disease begins it is permanent, because of the destruction of the walls of the air sacs. However, much can be done to bring relief of symptoms.

There is also the kind of emphysema caused by breathing certain types of particles of silica or dust. Some people develop emphysema because they have had asthma since early in life, which causes breaking of the tiny partitions between air sacs in the lungs with subsequent emphysema. Another kind of emphysema comes from a continual cough and other childhood illnesses in which there is coughing.

The objectives in treating emphysema are to reduce bronchitis and bronchial spasms, to improve breathing, and to avoid infection and progression of the disease.

Treatment

The first objective must be to remove all lung irritants—smoke, fumes, pollens, animal dander, house dust, etc.

A fat-free diet promotes easier breathing. This means avoiding all free fats, including margarine, mayonnaise, fried foods, cooking fats, salad oils, dairy butter, cream, peanut butter, and other nut butters made by high speed grinding. The most favorable diet for someone with emphysema is the totally vegetarian diet. Do not overeat.

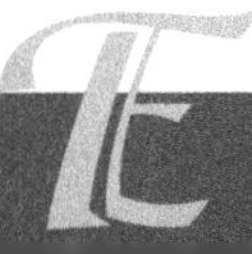

Secretions must be kept moist and moving by drinking plenty of water, using a vaporizer in the bedroom, or taking nebulized water inhalations using a small hand nebulizer available in department stores and pharmacies.

Long, slow, deep breathing relieves shortness of breath better than rapid shallow breathing.

Exercise to tolerance every day to keep the breathing muscles strong and the air passages cleared.

Living at a high altitude (above 5000 feet) can be detrimental to emphysema patients. For people with emphysema there is a premium on following the basic laws of health—good nutrition, exercise, water, sunshine, self-control and discipline, fresh air, rest, and trust in divine power—because the disease can only be controlled, not reversed.

An exercise called "controlled coughing" will be very beneficial. The exercise is done by inhaling slowly and deeply and exhaling through tightly pursed lips while coughing in a burst of short, fairly gentle, almost silent huffs. This can help to remove secretions.

Be very careful to breathe only fresh air. The air should be as clean as possible and not heavily charged with moisture. A steamy bathroom can cause a poor exchange of gases in the lung. Learn to breath from the diaphragm, having no tight bands from clothing or other constricting bands (even underwear or panty hoses can cause a problem). In cold weather a scarf or mask can be worn over the nose and mouth when outdoors.

The extremities must be kept warm at all times to avoid congestion of the chest.

Every effort should be made to prevent infection. That would include promoting proper drainage. Three to five inch blocks can be placed under the foot of the bed which will help prevent the accumulation of mucus in the lower parts of the lungs during the night. Do not lie in the same position more than two or three hours to promote drainage from all portions of the lungs.

These patients should avoid persons who have any type of respiratory tract infection, and should keep the immunity always at the highest possible level.

Generally speaking, the thinner the patient is and the smaller amount of flesh which must be supplied with oxygen and nutrients, the better the patient will fare. Being overweight is definitely a handicap for the emphysema patient.

Endometriosis

(See "Woman's Conditions and Disease" in the *Conditions and Diseases* section.)

Encephalomyelitis

(See "Fatigue, Chronic Fatigue Syndrome" in the *Conditions and Diseases* section.)

Enuresis

(See "Bed-Wetting" in the *Conditions and Diseases* section.)

Epilepsy

(See "Convulsions" in the *Conditions and Diseases* section.)

Erythema Multiforme

This is an acute inflammatory disorder of the skin and moist tissues such as the oral cavity, vagina, etc. Typically erythema multiforme appears as a rash on the palms of the hand, then spreads to the soles and other areas of the arms and legs, and then spreads to the face and rest of the body. In the majority of cases it is self-limiting and relatively benign, but it can be potentially quite severe.

In the severe form it is known as Stevens-Johnson syndrome. The lesions are symmetrical from one side of the body to the other, raised, fluid-filled red spots. It is sometimes painful or burning. The lesions often look as if they are targets with clear centers and concentric red rings. They usually clear within two to three weeks. Fever, headache, sore throat, diarrhea, and a tendency to recur in the spring and fall characterize the disease. It can be caused by a viral infection such as herpes simplex or by medications such as sulfonamides, penicillins, salicylates, barbiturates, etc. If the disease is a reaction to a drug, it may not occur until 7 to 14 days after beginning using it.

Treatment includes stopping any medications. Use an anti-inflammatory program of light exercise, anti-inflammatory herbs, and appropriate hydrotherapy. Bed rest for a short

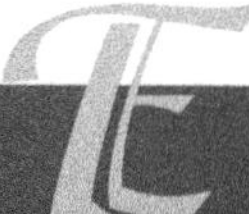

time is recommended if fever is present. The diet should be totally plant-based with an emphasis on fruits and vegetables and their juices. Also the use of wet dressings and soaks for soothing the skin, as well as lukewarm baths three times a day for half an hour may be soothing.

Esophageal Reflux

Heartburn is the most prominent symptom of esophageal reflux. It is caused by a weakened sphincter muscle at the lower end of the esophagus. Poor posture can intensify the problem.

Many things can be done to help someone with reflux. Never lie down after eating; elevate the head of your bed six inches; avoid coffee, tea, colas, chocolate, alcohol, and smoking; and do not bend over after meals, especially to pick up heavy loads. Many drugs are known to cause reflux, including the following: all anticholinergics, calcium channel blockers, alcohol nitrates, progesterone, theophylline, and tricyclic antidepressants.

For esophageal reflux, we have found people receive good benefit by sitting and standing in very good posture and by yawning. If you are aware that you are having reflux, if you can induce a good yawn, sometimes that will help to relieve the sensation. If you take pills of any kind, the best time to swallow them is when you have in your mouth already thoroughly chewed food ready to swallow. Introduce the pill, and swallow it all together.

Essential Tremor

(See "Parkinson's Disease" in the *Conditions and Diseases* section.)

Eyes

Blindness

To prevent blindness you should do the following:

- Purchase sunglasses that block out UV rays up to 510 nanometers and all infrared light.
- Eat a good quantity of antioxidant foods every day. (See "Food Sources of Certain Nutrients" in the *Dietary Information* section.)
- Know what your cholesterol level is and keep it well below 180. A cholesterol level of no more than about 100 plus your age is probably ideal.
- Walk at least two miles every day to keep circulation to the eyes optimal.
- Eat a diet low or devoid of free fats—margarine, mayonnaise, fried food, cooking fats, and salad oils. Limit nut butters such as peanut butter to one teaspoon daily until eyes are healthy again.
- Do not smoke, and avoid secondhand smoke.
- Check regularly for signs of glaucoma if you are over the age of 50. Regular eye examinations always include an examination for glaucoma.

Eye Floaters

The vitreous is an actual structure of the eye, not merely a fluid as was initially believed when the eye parts were named. The vitreous can get diseases of its own, even flakes of it can "turn lose" from the remainder of the vitreous, or the entire vitreous can separate from its attachments to the retina and actually turn or tilt. In either case the portions that have turned lose are visible as floaters because of variations in the density of the various layers. This can make worm-like or dot-like floaters. In the case of the entire vitreous turning lose, the "tail" of the vitreous often turns in such a way that it can be seen. The tail has greater density than other parts and may even have tiny fragments of the retina still clinging to it, which can create round or spider-appearing floaters.

Case Report

A woman in her late fifties, who was a proofreader for a large newspaper and spent several hours reading for her job, became profoundly dehydrated on a business trip to Florida. Apparently the effects of the sun, her acute dehydration, and water deprivation for almost two days caused sudden development of symptoms like lightning flashes in her left lateral visual field with certain eye movements. After a few weeks she began to notice the flashes of light disappeared but she now saw floaters that, while they generally maintained the same position in the visual field of the left eye, would float after movement of the eye, slightly downward and centrally.

Although she enjoyed her job, she became severely handicapped and took a short leave of absence. Examination of her eye by an ophthalmologist revealed no basic pathology except in the vitreous where the barely visible floaters were identified. I will now outline how we handled her case and how others can treat for eye floaters.

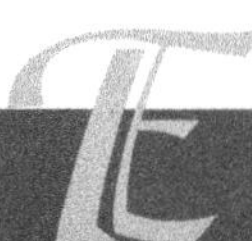

- She was instructed to ignore the floaters. I pointed out that many with congenital accidents or developmental problems were in much worse condition than she, and yet were successful along academic lines, doing much reading and studying. Thousands of people with permanent floaters learn to ignore them every year, many of them much older than she. The younger the person the more able to adjust to floaters. The key is to fasten the mind on the material being read rather than on the floaters. It is mandatory to learn to do that. Determine that the floaters will be ignored.
- You should spend 10 minutes each hour reading a passage in a book such as *Ministry of Healing*. Set a timer for 10 minutes and at the end of 10 minutes you should have read a reasonable length passage for your level of education. Then you must write a summary of what you have read without referring back to the text. If your floaters are disabling, this reading exercise, practicing ignoring the floaters and focusing on the text, should be engaged in for one year—10 minutes three times a day.
- You should do a series of eye exercises in which the eyes are turned to the farthest extent of their capability, up then down, left then right, and in each of the two diagonals. The exercise should be done 10 times per day.
- You should drink 10 eight-ounce glasses of water every day as a minimum, even if you are not thirsty.
- You should use no dairy products, lactose or galactose (milk sugars) in anything you eat. Dairy products are known to have a deleterious influence on the eyes, as are aspirin and other drugs.
- You should take a six- to eight-ounce glass of fresh carrot juice on a daily basis. The beta-carotene in carrot juice will be strengthening to the eyes.
- Make certain you are not low in taurine. This amino acid can be found in beans, nuts, seeds, and food yeast (take no more than one teaspoonful per day). This product is also called nutritional yeast, or seasoning yeast, and is used in cheese substitutes by vegans who avoid all dairy products.
- Bilberry and ginkgo tea are both excellent for the eyes. Of ginkgo tea you should take one caplet three times daily, or one cup of the tea four times daily, using one rounded teaspoon of the tea leaves per cup. You can make it all at once by bringing five cups of water to a boil and adding the four teaspoons of the tea leaves, covering it, and setting it aside (do not boil) to steep for 30 minutes. If the bilberry comes as leaves it can be prepared along with the ginkgo in the same water, but if it comes as a root bark or chopped plant, it must be boiled gently for 20 minutes prior to the addition of the ginkgo leaves.

Foreign Body

To remove something from the eye, take a flax seed and put it in the eye. The speck will stick to the flax seed which can then be easily removed with the corner of a facial tissue. (See also "Eye Care" in the *Home Emergencies* section.)

Macular Degeneration

The macula is the small central point of light-sensing retina in the back of the eye responsible for reading and detail vision. Symptoms of macular degeneration include blurring, darkness, or other visual deficiencies, although peripheral vision is not affected.

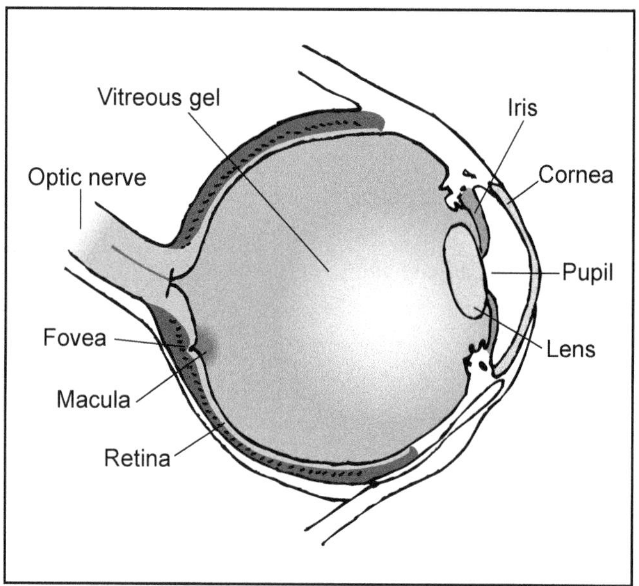

Macular degeneration is caused by a general aging of the eye, but some researchers believe that highly active chemicals called free radicals contribute to the onset of the disease. These free radicals are formed by environmental factors such as a diet generous in meat, dairy products, salt, refined sweets, or refined fats and exposure to toxins or sunlight striking the retina. Antioxidants in the diet turn off the free radicals and prevent damage to the retina. Those who are at high risk for macular degeneration are smokers, diabetics, the elderly, and those with high levels of cholesterol.

The commonest cause of blindness after the age of 50 today is macular degeneration. It affects almost 13 million Americans. The incidence of age-related macular degeneration (AMD) rises sharply after the age of 60. It is more common in women. Smoking makes a woman three times more likely to develop AMD than women who have never smoked. AMD tends to run in families, and certain genes have been linked to the disorder—fair skinned, blue-eyed people are more susceptible, but no race or ethnic group is immune.

Hardening of the arteries compromises blood flow to the retina and increases the likelihood of AMD. Low intake of fruits and vegetables increases the risk of AMD.

AMD is caused by small deposits of waste products called drusen, and a high level of fat in the blood increases the production of drusen. Prolonged exposure to direct sunlight while gardening, fishing, or attending a sporting event, and so forth, can damage the eyes. UV filtering sunglasses and a hat with a big visor or broad brim should be worn during sun exposure.

Another form of sun exposure is more serious and can progress rapidly to blindness. In this form new and fragile blood vessels begin to grow in the tissue beneath the macula. If these fragile vessels rupture, leaking blood or plasma into the macula, a reduction can occur in vision.

A simple test you can give yourself in your own home is the Amsler Grid test. The Amsler Grid is simply lines that cross, making many equal-sized boxes. The test is done by looking at the very center of the grid and detecting if the center of the grid fades out with a spot or vacant space which moves as you move your eyes. Your doctor or a public library can give you an Amsler Grid, which looks much like a blank calendar. One eye is checked at a time, so the eye not being checked is blocked by a card. If the center of the grid pattern looks broken, distorted, wavy, or any of it appears to be missing, you should visit your doctor right away (See Figure 4 on page 146).

Another symptom may be that you require more light in order to read clearly. Another symptom is requiring longer to adjust to dim light after having come from the outside in bright sunlight.

The sooner one stops smoking, the lower the risk of macular degeneration. Over the years, people who have once smoked gradually lessen their risk of getting macular degeneration. In 20 years the risk is still about 40 percent greater than in people who have never smoked, therefore, the sooner one stops smoking, the better.

Aspirin or any drug with a similarity to aspirin such as Aleve, Motrin, Nuprin, etc., encourages bleeding from capillaries and tends to initiate or make macular degeneration worse. Researchers examining 109 patients afflicted with macular degeneration found that all patients had been taking frequent dosages of aspirin. It is of concern that the present counsel to take an aspirin a day to keep from having a heart attack may cause increases of unnecessary blindness in the 50-plus age group in the coming years. In one study of three adult males, given large doses of nicotinic acid to treat high blood cholesterol, there was a loss of central vision. The nicotinic acid can cause retention of fluid and swelling in the retina, which could lead to a loss of vision. After the vitamin was discontinued some improvement of vision occurred.

Lowering blood cholesterol also reduces the risks of blindness from this disease. Large doses of vitamin E, such as over 200 IU per day, may increase the risk of macular hemorrhage, the same as aspirin. Diabetes should be kept in perfect control to reduce the risks of blindness in diabetics.

Researchers have found that four servings of spinach weekly can to some degree reverse macular degeneration (*Alternatives*, April 1999, 172). For macular degeneration, one-half cup of spinach, prunes, or blueberries four times a week will reduce the likelihood of coming down with this disease by one-third.

Certain antioxidants such as lutein, zeaxanthin, and lycopene are helpful to prevent macular degeneration. These carotenoids are found in dark green leafy vegetables and red and yellow colored fruits and vegetables. Such fruits as peaches, persimmons, kiwis, apricots, etc., and such vegetables as tomatoes, watermelon, beets, etc., contain generous quantities of these carotenoids, which have a protective value for the eye. People whose intake of leafy greens was high had 43 percent lower expectation of developing age-related macular degeneration than people whose leafy greens intake was very low (*Journal of the American Medical Association* 272 [1994]: 1413).

Dr. Lloyd Rosenvold found some improvement in his central vision in the four months he used pycnogenol (bioflavonoids found in pine tree bark and grape seeds). Bioflavonoids are available as well in true extracts from lemon peel.

It has also been found that the greater the use of raw foods with a high vitamin C content and other antioxidants such as beta-carotene, vitamin E, selenium, etc., the lower the incidence of macular degeneration (SER Abstracts, *American Journal of Epidemiology* 138, no. 8 [October 15, 1993]: 659). Vitamin C is found in practically all raw fruits and vegetables, highest sources being citrus, kiwi, green peppers, strawberries, raw cabbage, green leafy vegetables, tomatoes, and white potatoes. Vitamin E is found in nuts, seeds, whole grains, and vegetables.

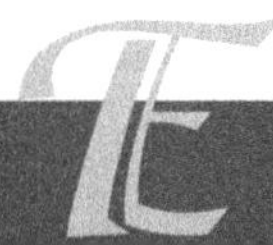

Figure 4: Amsler Grid

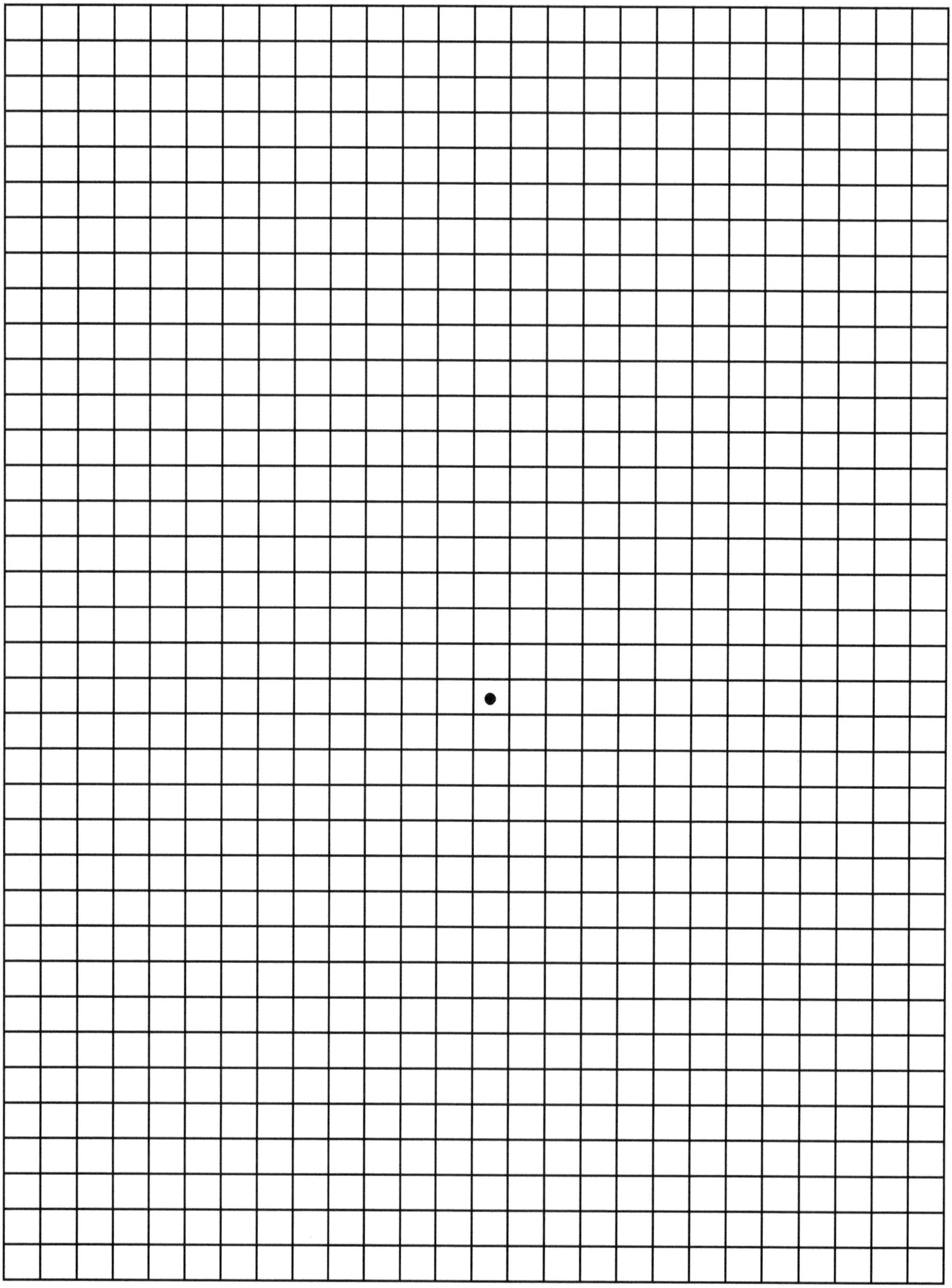

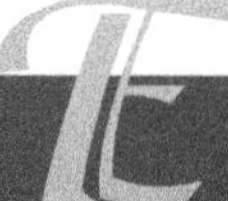

Five ounces of grape juice taken twice a day can greatly reduce the likelihood of developing macular degeneration, as well as heart attack and stroke (*Journal of the American Geriatric Society* 46:1, 98).

A diet rich in saturated fat and cholesterol can increase the likelihood developing macular degeneration by 80 percent. Healthful eating appears also to lower the risk of cataracts. A number of very good health benefits result from leaving out all animal products from the diet (*St. Petersburg Times*, October 11, 1995, 5A).

Macular degeneration can be treated with hawthorn, ginkgo, and bilberry tea. Take four cups daily. Make the tea fresh every morning by gently simmering the freshly ground hawthorn berries for 20 minutes in one quart of water, then adding one heaping tablespoon of both ginkgo and bilberry tea leaves, setting it off the heat immediately, and steeping for 30 minutes. In addition get plenty of outdoor exercise.

Evidence points to the fact that zinc (with a trace of copper added) can retard and possibly even reverse certain eye ailments, including macular degeneration. Taurine is an antioxidant, and it has been shown to greatly help some cases of nerve disorders such as epilepsy and macular degeneration. Copper supplementation may be able to help. A daily supplement of zinc may also help, but should not be used in quantities greater than 20 to 30 milligrams per day (*Journal of the American Medical Association* 276 [1996]: 1141, 1147, 1178; *Ophthalmology* 103 [1996]: 878). Small doses of selenium may also be helpful. One Brazil nut may contain 50 to 60 micrograms of selenium, depending on its size. The daily requirement is only about 70 micrograms. Two Brazil nuts will generously provide.

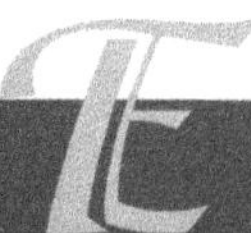

Fainting

To prevent impending fainting raise both arms over your head. Yawn and stretch and contract your abdominal muscles. Persons with heart or circulatory problems should perform these maneuvers before getting to their feet if they have been sitting for quite a long time, such as in an airplane flight (*Lancet* 350 [1997]: 744). If you know the cause of fainting, such as dehydration, you should correct that promptly.

Fasting

(See "Fasting" in the *Dietary Information* section.)

Fatigue, Chronic Fatigue Syndrome

A more and more common complaint heard in physicians' offices today is that of fatigue. Since the beginning of the 1960s, fatigue has become a very common condition. During the early 1980s, fatigue became associated with a syndrome named chronic fatigue syndrome. We will discuss that condition separately after discussing general fatigue. Fortunately there are a number of simple causes for ordinary fatigue; if we eliminate these, the fatigue will usually disappear.

Other treatable conditions causing debilitating fatigue include the following:

1. Narcolepsy (See "Sleep" in the *Conditions and Diseases* section.)
2. Reactive hypoglycemia, especially at night, with or without laboratory evidence of decreased glucose tolerance
3. Hypervitaminosis E from supplementation
4. Excessive ingestion of aspartame (NutraSweet)
5. Hypothyroidism (if the iodine level is low and the TSH is higher than normal limits)
6. Excessive toxic metals (ingestion of mercury in contaminated dolomite or bone meal, hair dyes containing lead, dental amalgam)
7. Vitamin B12 deficiency with or without anemia in those past age 50 and in patients with prior gastrectomy or the resection of the terminal ilium or cecum
8. Hepatitis with or without jaundice
9. *Myasthenia gravis* in the earlier stages

Fatigue

There are certain conditions of the body associated with fatigue that must be diagnosed by chemical tests. If the thyroid is either overactive or under active, a sense of fatigue may result. The same thing can be said of blood sugar if it is up or down. The ideal blood sugar range in the fasting state is 70 to 85. Any deviation from the ideal may mean a trend toward an error in metabolism. A special program should be followed. (See "Diabetes" in the *Conditions and Diseases* section.)

The *Townsend Newsletter for Doctors* editorial of July 1992 indicated that toxic substances not properly dealt with by the liver could be the cause of many vague symptoms in humans that cause chronic ill health and fatigue. Improved detoxification can be achieved through a high fiber diet and herbs, fasting, taking milk thistle, or eating one-half bunch of cilantro with each meal.

If the hemoglobin or blood iron are either too high or too low, the person can sense fatigue. Almost everyone is aware that a low hemoglobin is associated with fatigue, but it is the rare person who understands that rich, heavy blood can also cause fatigue. Pushing around the heavy blood taxes the heart and arteries, uses up energy, and results in fatigue. Often the true source of fatigue in cases of high hemoglobin is not even understood in the physician's office. In order to bring the hemoglobin down, one should exercise more, eat more fruits and vegetables prepared simply or eaten raw, avoid all rich or concentrated foods, avoid overeating, drink plenty of water, and avoid stress. Very high levels of hemoglobin (over 14 for women and 16 for men) may represent a serious disease of the blood-forming organs and should be investigated.

A class of stressful stimuli can be listed as fatigue producers. These include working around a lot of noise, being in a stressful or anxious state, having periods of lack of sleep or rest, and depression. All of these are stress factors for the body and can bring on a state of chronic fatigue. Often one of the first indications of depression is fatigue. On the contrary, depression is not only a cause of fatigue, but fatigue can bring on depression. Often a person would be able to cope with all life's stresses were it not for the fact that there are certain factors in the life that are bringing on "excessive and cumulative fatigue," causing the person to have inadequate strength left over to resist depression or cope with situations.

Physiological Causes

One of the most important treatments for fatigue is restoring proper hydration. This must be done by approaching the problem in several ways. The first thing to be aimed at is the proper quantity of water taken during the day. For some people this may be as little as six glasses, but for most people the quantity is probably eight, and for men and women after age 50, as many as 10 or 12 glasses, and more if there is sweating. A standard glass is eight ounces. Next, the person must not take such concentrated foods that the blood becomes dehydrated through a chemical process. Everyone is aware that such things as salt and sugar make one thirsty. Any kind of very concentrated nutrient tends to concentrate the blood and cause dehydration. The best diet is one high in fruits and vegetables. The pattern of drinking is also very important. Do not take all the water for a day at one time, as the large quantity of water has a diuretic effect, causing the kidneys to put out more water than is taken in. Chronic dehydration is often caused by diuretics such as coffee, tea, colas, and chocolate. Further, if large amounts of water are taken at one time, it can cause pressure in the eyes to increase.

Poorly conditioned muscles have greater difficulty maintaining the skeletal frame in good posture without fatigue. Add to that the fact that poor circulation decreases the ability of the body to eliminate toxic products and to receive nourishment and oxygen and one has a physiologic cause for severe fatigue. Our indoor living customs promote fatigue. Exercise in the great out of doors is curative in many cases, and helpful in all.

A very common cause of fatigue is overeating and eating too great a variety of food. The meals should consist of two or three foods prepared in a simple yet tasty way without a lot of mixing of food groups to make a complex mixture. Eat enough only to satisfy hunger. You can never eat enough to satisfy a perverted appetite without overeating. Metabolizing food of itself requires much energy from your quick energy storage, and overeating may drain off more energy than it supplies for quick energy, while storing the excess calories as fat. Overweight and overwork are often related, and both of course cause fatigue. If one eats only enough to satisfy the essential needs of the body, the overall effect will be a sense of well-being and energy. Eating more will sap the strength and give a sense of fatigue. It would seem that a snack, or between meal feeding would be the very thing to help cure fatigue, but the reverse is often the case. Never should one overeat, use between meal snacks or have heavy suppers. While a heavy and late supper may enable one to sleep the sleep of the drugged, it does not cause refreshment, and the next morning the person awakens in a partial stupor.

The use of stimulatory beverages (coffee, tea, colas, and chocolate), or highly concentrated foods, is a common cause of fatigue, as are most medicines, including those bought over-the-counter. Most drugs can cause fatigue. Blood pressure medications, sleeping pills, diuretics, and alcohol are famous fatigue producers. Insecticides and radioactivity, fluorides, lead, mercury, cadmium, and copper all cause fatigue. Cigarette smoking robs the system of energy.

Inadequate fresh air causes fatigue. Be certain there is a current of fresh air in the bedroom at night, summer and winter, good weather and bad. The toxic substances blown off in the breath are fatigue producing and when taken back into the lungs, double energy must be put forth to get rid of them again, leaving less energy behind.

A diet high in sugar causes fatigue as does too much protein, particularly that of animal origin. Vitamin and mineral supplements can imbalance the body's economy and induce fatigue after a period of stimulating metabolism and temporarily providing more energy. An imbalanced diet that fails to provide adequate quantities of nutrients from easy to process foods such as fruits, vegetables, whole grains, and a few nuts can cause fatigue. Refined foods, artificial colorings, many additives, and high dietary fat levels encourage fatigue.

Regularity in all things is essential, and failure to be regular wastes energy and puts a strain on the body. If one has an irregular schedule, the body does not have the ability to control the expenditure of energy, and the loss of energy with resultant fatigue is a usual companion of an irregular schedule. One should schedule all major events of the day and stick to the schedule, especially eating time and bedtime.

A large number of physical factors in the environment can cause fatigue. White shiny colors are more fatiguing than subdued colors. Glare causes fatigue, making those who must look into it more tired than those in more protected environments. A cluttered and disordered work area not only reduces efficiency but leads to fatigue and sometimes dissatisfaction with life. Loud noises in the immediate vicinity cause fatigue.

Television watching, both because it promotes inactivity and because it produces an excess of stress hormones, is fatigue producing. Dr. Wilhelm Raab reported many years ago on the increase in catecholamine levels in urine of persons watching any kind of commercial television except simple pictures of nature. Television is designed to make the viewer react. That uses emotional and chemical energy and can lead to fatigue. Also, TV robs one of sleep, which makes it a true thief.

One of the most common, yet less readily diagnosed causes of fatigue is allergies. Most people who try it find that their fatigue greatly diminishes if they use a diet that contains no foods to which they are sensitive. To discover these sensitivities, you must follow the "Elimination and Challenge Diet" in the *Dietary Information* section. You may be surprised how much better you sleep and feel rested.

Persons with even a mild case of celiac disease (a sensitivity to gluten in wheat, rye, and barley) may have fatigue as their only symptom. For these persons, eliminating gluten will bring slow improvement, perhaps not recognized for one to six weeks.

Check iron, B12, and sodium levels to be certain they are adequate but not too high. Iodine deficiency can also cause fatigue. Large amounts of soy products daily can inhibit the thyroid. Vegetarians need to be careful about that point. Seaweed products are good sources of iodine, as is sea salt. Up to 80 percent of those who eat a plant-based diet can become iodine deficient, compared to 9 percent of people on a mixed diet.

Psychological causes

Depression, boredom, stress, anxiety, excitement, and over-stimulation can all cause fatigue. The varieties of psychological conditions in people that increase the likelihood of fatigue include the following: people who are compulsive; people who are bored; people who work or live with someone who is unpleasant or overbearing; people whose work is largely mental rather than physical; people who are under a great deal of stress or nervous tension; people who are depressed; people who are always either in a hurry or are sluggish and indolent; and people who do not observe Sabbath.

Chronic Fatigue Syndrome, Post Viral Syndrome, Epstein-Barr Virus, Myalgic Encephalomyelitis (ME)

Chronic fatigue syndrome (CFS) appears to be a modern society disease that is growing in importance as more and more people come down with disabling fatigue of a nature never experienced before. We can say that "to know chronic fatigue syndrome is to know medicine" because of the wide nature of the symptoms and the number of conditions that must be excluded before the diagnosis can be nailed down. It is one of the most challenging disorders we have ever encountered in medicine. It is felt that it could be toxic or pharmacologic in origin because of our "chemical society" or that it might be an autoimmune disorder, a post-infection state, or a post-traumatic condition as in PTSD (post-traumatic stress disorder).

One-third of cases of chronic fatigue syndrome seem to be because of a retro-viral cause, virus X. It causes immune suppression and can activate latent viruses that have been sleeping in the body for years. There is no medical cure for this virus, but there are some very hopeful physiologic remedies that put the disease in remission if not cure it.

Others believe CFS may even be genetic, involving the chromosomes. Some have suggested that it might be developmental, representing some normal development that went astray, possibly some missing enzymes. We should bear in mind that developmental, genetic, and immune system problems are commonly caused by some kind of chemical or pharmacologic trauma, possibly striking even before birth. Some have suggested childhood immunizations as the cause of this disease.

Spontaneous recovery occurs in 20 percent or more of persons. It appears that there must be genetic predisposition in order to develop CFS. It can be documented in the

Laboratory Values often Helpful in Diagnosing CFS

Test Name		Reference Range
CMV ELISA	2.41H	<0.80 = Negative 0.81 - 0.99 = Equivocal >1.00 = Positive
Cytomegalovirus IGM, ELISA		<0.80 = Negative 0.81 - 0.99 = Equivocal 1.00 = Positive
Herpes I and II		
Herpes Virus I, IGG	3.02H	<0.99 = Negative >1.00 = Positive
Herpes Virus II, IGG	2.12H	<0.99 = Negative >1.00 = Positive
Rubella		Immune
Rubazyme Index		2.395
Index of 1.000 or greater indicates presence of Rubella IGG Antibody Index less than 1.000 indicates absence of Rubella IGG Antibody CLIA # 41-1021		
Immunoglobulins AGM		
IGG	1160	639-1349 MG/DL
IGA	1727	70-312 MG/DL
IGM	312	56-352 MG/DL
Epstein Barr Virus-Panel		
IGM ANTI-VCA	<1:10	<1:10
IGG ANTI-VCA	1:640	<1:10
ANTI-EBNA	1:8	<1:2
EBV-EA	1:20	<1:10

laboratory that these persons have a decreased immunosurveillance. Because of this a variety of viruses may invade the body as well as spirochetes (such as the Borrelia which causes Lyme disease), Candida, chlamydia, Mycoplasma, protozoans, and certain bacteria. There is abnormal antigen processing and diminished function of natural killer cells. There has been a report of increased risk of cancer in persons with CFS, although other investigators seem not to reach that conclusion such as Dr. Seymour Grufferman from the Pittsburgh Cancer Institute.

Dr. Allen D. Aken of California has presented evidence that many cases of chronic fatigue syndrome may be related to the rubella (German measles) vaccine. We suggest extreme caution in the use of any vaccines.

Symptoms

While fatigue is by far the most common symptom, and this complaint must always be present for this diagnosis to hold, there are 30 to 50 other symptoms recognized as being associated with this condition.

Some people with CFS can pinpoint the onset of their symptoms to the exact day, sometimes almost to the hour. The symptoms often begin as a flu-like illness. Clusters of people in the same work place or school with CFS have been reported (*Journal of the American Medical Association*, May 1, 1987, 2303–7). The person with chronic fatigue syndrome usually exhibits increased chemical sensitivities.

In order to make the diagnosis, the following symptoms must be present:

1. Persistent or recurring fatigue that limits daily activity to less than half its previous level and lasts for at least six months in a person who was previously well.
2. All other causes of fatigue must be eliminated.
3. Six of the following 11 features must also be present:
   a. Mild fever
   b. Sore throat
   c. Painful lymph nodes in the neck or armpit
   d. Generalized weakness of the muscles
   e. Muscle pains or discomfort
   f. Disabling fatigue lasting more than 24 hours after exercise that could previously be easily tolerated
   g. Headaches
   h. Joint pains that come and go
   i. Visual complaints or other symptoms involving the central nervous system
   j. Sleep disturbance
   k. Onset of the condition at a definite time, generally over a matter of hours to days
   l. Excessively emotional or dramatic, schizoid, depressed, suicidal, avoidance, narcissistic, or aggressive behavior; sleep disturbances, changes in the function of IQ (such as processing information, orientation in time and geography, memory control areas, etc.), insomnia, nausea, and vomiting

The current theory is that Epstein-Barr Virus or some other virus of a similar type infects the body and produces illness such as mononucleosis, hepatitis, flu, shingles, or fever blisters. The symptoms disappear as usual, but the viruses stay around in what is called a "latent" state, a condition in which there are no symptoms, but the viruses are still inside the cells for years or decades. They remain quiet unless activated by a triggering event. The triggering event is followed by another round of symptoms.

The triggering agent may be yet another virus, and this other virus is the "real culprit." A prime suspect is the human B-lymphotropic virus (HBLV not related to HTLV which causes AIDS). It does not appear to be easily transmitted from one person to another. The cornerstone of CFS treatment in standard medicine is Acyclovir, an antiviral drug with many toxic side effects, and it is felt, that relapse will almost always occur after Acyclovir is stopped. Many patients do not respond to this kind of treatment even from the beginning. Alpha interferon has had limited use but is not helpful in CFS.

While the condition tends to get worse and get better, there is no evidence at present that the disease causes the general constitution of the person to deteriorate. This disease is associated with high levels of certain antibodies in the blood.

Treatment

The reason why some patients respond to certain treatments and others do not is an enigma. When the diagnosis is made treatment is begun until one is found that works for that particular patient. Treatment is a trial and error experience.

Since no drug therapy has had lasting benefit in scientific studies, save your money and turn your attention in another direction. Observe all the suggestions given above in the general discussion of fatigue.

Many have benefited temporarily from a short cold bath, but more have benefited from a series of fever baths. See instructions for this bath in the "Hydrotherapy" entry in the *Natural Remedies* section. Take a series of 15 fever treatments, five treatments a week for three weeks. Skip one week. If you feel well, you may discontinue future fever baths. If you still feel tired or if fatigue at first abolished returns, take another series of 15 treatments. Again, skip a week and repeat a third time if required to cure the fatigue. We have had a few cases that required even more than three series.

Learn to budget your time to minimize fatigue and take advantage of days or periods during the day in which you have more energy.

Take a short nap before lunch every day, but never after lunch as doing so may interfere with sleeping at night. Do mild exercise after each meal.

Be regular in all your habits: have meals on time, go to bed and arise on time, schedule everything on time as much as possible, and systematize all of life.

Full body massage one to three times weekly may be helpful, as may regular bathing in cool water (slightly lower than skin temperature) to help fight off viruses and stimulate the circulation. A cold mitten friction stimulates the immune response and may be done every morning upon arising.

Certain herbal remedies have proven helpful. Keep up treatments for six months or more except where noted.

- Whole garlic – Fresh or dried garlic may be taken up to the equivalent of three cloves per day.
- Kyolic – Two tablets three times a day. Kyolic has been shown to have an antiviral effect.
- Echinacea – Two capsules three times a day.

- Golden seal tea – One cup twice daily for 30 days.
- Evening Primrose oil – Six capsules per day.
- Flaxseed oil – Two tablespoons per day.
- Ground flax seed – Up to four tablespoons per day.
- Shizandra – See package instructions for dosage.
- Essiac tea – One cup four times daily.
- Lauric acid – One tablespoon of dry, shredded coconut with each meal.
- Ashwaganda – One capsule daily.
- Super charged silver – One teaspoon every three hours for two weeks, then drop down to one teaspoon three or four times a day.

Diet

Unproven but possibly helpful remedies include:

- Vitamin C – Inhibits suppressor T-cells, breaks antibody disulfide bonds.
- Germanium – 450 milligrams a day seems to increase natural killer cell activity.
- Vitamin B12 – Some with psychiatric symptoms have been helped, and there is a transient energy boost.

It is now suspected by some researchers that chronic fatigue syndrome may sometimes represent a shortage of the mineral magnesium (*Lancet* 9337 [1991]: 757–69). Magnesium has been shown to be effective in the treatment of chronic fatigue syndrome, as well as non-specific fatigue and heart disease. Magnesium appears to be used up when one exercises. Athletes show a decline of the magnesium in red blood cells after running in a race. Perhaps this explains why people who are endurance athletes do best on a vegetarian diet that is naturally high in magnesium (*International Journal of Sports Medicine* 11 [1990]: 234–7).

Beta-carotene therapy in CFS has been demonstrated to increase natural killer cells. Since natural killer cell activity is usually reduced in CFS, patients suffering from this disorder can be helped by eating foods and drinking juice high in beta-carotene. This would include deep yellow foods or very dark green foods.

Many people with CFS will find a marked benefit by strict adherence to the following diet:

- Avoid yeast, free fats (margarine, mayonnaise, all nut butters, fried foods, cooking fats, and salad oils), mushrooms (except the therapeutic ones), wheat, rye, oranges, apples, pineapple, tomatoes, peppers, unpeeled white potatoes, eggplant, oats, bread, plums.
- Eat rice, corn, peeled white potatoes, bananas, avocados, pears, nuts of all kinds, seeds of all kinds, especially sunflower and pumpkin seeds, and certain dried fruits (raisins, prunes, apricots, and figs).
- Most people will fare well on a simple vegan diet with no visible fats added (other than the oil supplements noted above). The plant-based vegetarian diet is the most favorable for recovery.

Case Reports

A 46-year-old professional woman had felt well and energetic until she got what seemed to be the flu one January. She got over the acute illness but continued to deal with sleeplessness, overwhelming fatigue, depression, and hopelessness. Her symptoms continued unabated despite various simple measures. Finally we tested her for chronic fatigue syndrome and found a typical pattern of antibodies. Her treatments began the last Sunday night in April. Monday morning she felt better than she had since January. One series of treatments was effective for her. But another patient we had whose symptoms had gone on for two years required the third series. About halfway into the second week of that last series she began to feel like her old self. The first two series gave only partial relief. Another patient required several five hour fever baths before getting well.

A 32-year-old man previously in excellent health, strong, ambitious, and always positive began to feel as if he had the flu a day after his second son was born. In a few days he recovered without any difficulty, only to get sick again in less than a week. Again he seemed to recover a bit, but was again sick within less than a week. After his sore throat and sore muscles cleared, he was left each time with a sense of fatigue that he felt was the recuperation period from the flu. After recovering the next time, he did not have a cessation of fatigue for the next six years.

While some days were better than others, most of the time he felt disabling fatigue. There were times that the fatigue would be so disabling that getting out of bed was entirely out of the question for three or four days at a time. Yet his family had to be supported, and some suggested that the condition was "all in his head," that the arrival of a second child imbalanced his mind and made him unable to face life. He denied that assessment but was willing to see a psychiatrist on the urging of several friends. The psychiatrist made a diagnosis of depression and offered him an antidepressant.

For over six months he refused the medicine, but finally decided that he must try to get relief somehow, and accepted the antidepressant. The medicine caused his condition to get much worse, and he became unable to function. When he stopped the medication, he was able once more to go to work several days each week as he had before, but often felt such overwhelming fatigue that he simply could not lift his hands.

Almost immediately after starting the treatment program suggested in this book, he became functional. While he could not describe his condition as totally recovered and in as good health as before his son was born, he recognized a clearing of his mind so that he was as sharp as he had been before, and he never again spent a whole day in bed. For seven months, his condition steadily progressed day by day and his sense of well-being improved until he felt almost as good as before the onset of chronic fatigue syndrome.

Fever Blisters, Cold Sores, Herpes I

Fever blisters most commonly occurs on the lip just at the border between the hairy part and the non-hairy part, but it may occur anywhere around the mouth or nose and occasionally on the face, chest, lower trunk, or genital area.

While the virus lives in the tissues in some way, there are certain triggering agencies that cause the blisters. Exposure to sun or getting a sunburn is one of the common triggering agents. Allergies to food will trigger fever blisters for some people, especially chocolate and dairy milk, but other foods are also common triggers.

Failure to get regular exercise outdoors will weaken the body and make it more susceptible to blisters. Excessive stress has induced fever blisters in many susceptible people. A cold or any kind of upper respiratory tract infection will cause fever blisters.

Treatment

An extract of witch hazel (Hamamelis virginiana) using a diluted alcohol base was found to have an antiviral effect in treating fever blister (*Quarterly Review of Natural Medicine* [Fall 1996]: 179).

With the first hint of tingling, burning, or itching in the area where one recognizes a fever blister might occur, begin rubbing with an ice cube within 20 minutes of feeling the first symptom. Keep the ice moving on lip for 45 to 60 minutes and the fever blister will almost always not develop.

If the lesion develops, alternately apply hot and cold compresses to the lesion for 20 to 30 minutes two or three times daily until the fever blister disappears. Use three minutes for the hot compress and 30 seconds for the cold.

Powdered golden seal may be applied directly to the fever blister by making a paste with some of the powder and a drop or so of water, spreading it over the lesion.

A tincture of cayenne may be made by putting a teaspoon of red pepper into a small jar having a screw-top lid. Pour about two ounces of rubbing alcohol onto the red pepper and swirl. The alcohol can be applied immediately with a cotton tip applicator, but it does not develop its full strength until after three weeks of mixing with the red pepper. Pour the alcohol mixture into a dark bottle after three weeks. The alcohol extract can be applied once an hour to a fever blister to promote healing. This tincture may be diluted 10 times with alcohol and is good for many other skin lesions such as acne rosacea, shingles, and herpes genitalis. Do not use undiluted—use 1 part of the tincture to 10 parts of alcohol.

Apply a single drop of balsam sap to the blister. The sap protects the blister and greatly increases the rate at which it heals.

Echinacea, chaparral, and osha will sometimes break the cycle of repeated herpes outbreaks. Osha is an antiviral and antifungal herb.

The following drink can be boiled for 20 minutes and set aside to cool before being ingested slowly over one week, more during the first part of the week:

- 3 quarts water
- 2 whole heads of garlic (10 to 20 cloves)
- 2 grapefruit, chopped (peel off the superficial yellow part with a sharp knife, leaving the white)

Fevers

Fever is a symptom of disease. It is not an enemy, but a friend. Temperature regulation is an important duty of the body. To provide this service, the body is equipped with a variety of mechanisms that effectively work to control body temperature in a very low tolerance of variation—around 98.6°F—the usual midday oral temperature. A degree or so up or down is about all the variation we will see in resting conditions. Chills and fevers in children do not usually represent a serious illness and can be allowed to run their course with no treatment. However, there are measures to make the patient feel better and get over the fever quicker.

About 75 percent of the time a respiratory tract infection produces the fever—sinuses, ears, mastoids, pharynx, tonsils, eyes, or nose. Other causes of fever in children are intestinal infections, urinary tract infections, or lung infections.

Other things that cause fever in children and adults include inflammation or overactivity of the thyroid, vigorous physical activity, hot baths, or being too warmly clothed. Most drugs may cause "drug fever." If one is on drugs of any kind and develops unexplained fever, the first thing to do is to stop the drug for a few days in consultation with one's physician.

Other causes of fevers may be bacteria; some viruses; Rickettsiae; protozoa; fungi; cancer, especially lymphomas such as Hodgkin's disease; tissue death from chemicals used or accidental traumatic injuries; myocardial infarction; or pulmonary embolism. Other causes may be foreign proteins in the blood as from milk leakage into the blood during breastfeeding, venomous bites, intestinal malabsorption, dehydration, excessive sweating, or heat treatments, prolonged heavy exercise, labor of childbirth, work in hot environments, various drugs and chemicals, pyrogens, toxins, hyperthyroidism, stress, fear, or excitement. Even recently eating a meal can cause a mild fever.

Serious Versus Non-serious Fevers

Most fevers, especially in small children, represent only a mild, self-limited illness. To distinguish between serious and non-serious fevers, there are several signs that can be very helpful. Have other children in the family or those with whom the child spends time been ill? Does anyone have diarrhea, a sore throat, a rash, vomiting, a tummy ache, a runny nose, or the flu? Has the child been traveling, especially to places where serious diseases such as Rocky Mountain Spotted Fever are likely to be?

Now, check the patient's temperature. With temperatures below 102.5°F, the risk of anything serious is quite low, and even above that, the likelihood is only around two percent. Check for a rash, a lump, a scar, or a skin lesion. Observe the child's appearance and the response to people and food or fluid. If a child takes a bottle eagerly, we can be pretty certain the child is not dreadfully sick. If the child can put up a vigorous struggle, the child is not very sick.

There are certain signs that may indicate a more serious condition in children. They are as follows:

- The child is a newborn or less than two months old and the rectal temperature is 101 or above.
- The fever has gone unabated for three days and is associated with vomiting, difficulty breathing, and the person looks seriously ill.
- There are strange features, twitching, abnormal movements.
- Heat elevation is likely if the circumstances include high humidity and heat, and still, closed-in air.
- A sore throat that lasts more than a week.

Keep the child nearby for observation for several hours or be in close contact to observe any changes. A culture of the upper respiratory tract is usually a waste of time and money because the results are too frequently the same in both sick and well children. They both have H-influenza, pneumococci, and certain streptococci as normal residents in the nose and throat.

Mechanisms to Regulate Temperature

A dry skin surface promotes heat conservation, but it can be made wet by millions of tiny sweat glands, which cool the body.

Temperature is regulated by the shunting of blood from the outside of the body to the interior of the body by the mere stimulus of a bit of chilling on the surface, thereby conserving heat.

The "natural" body posture helps regulate heat, especially folding the arms, drawing up the legs, hunching over the shoulders to conserve heat. When the temperature of the body falls, one tends to draw the body into a small ball and take shallower respirations to minimize heat loss. With overheating, the opposite posture and breathing pattern will be seen.

Relaxation of muscles or contraction of muscles can substantially alter body temperature. If all the muscles that can raise goose bumps on the skin surface are contracted at one time, the temperature can rise as much as one and a half degrees in half an hour. Shivering for half an hour will cause similar elevations in body temperature. On the other hand, relaxation that occurs during massage can lower body temperature by a similar mechanism in the opposite direction over a similar period of time.

Dehydration can cause the temperature to rise, while rehydration will help to regulate temperature. The drinking of large quantities of water is essential if the body is to do its best work with a fever. Offer water as frequently as possible, and make the meals light, as heavy foods, salted or fatty foods, sugary or concentrated nutrients, can all increase the requirement for water beyond that which the appetite for water can supply.

A small infant's crying spell may cause the temperature to rise by two or three degrees.

Public speakers notice that they often become dehydrated after speaking, thus resulting in their temperature rising. The pulse increases about 10 beats per minute for each degree elevation in temperature.

Treatments

Ice water and ice applications were once used in emergency rooms to reduce fevers in children. Any cold application prolonged over 15 to 20 minutes can cause marked internal congestion. The forcible reduction of temperature in fevers by ice water applications is usually not wise. The body begins to work against you, and the immune system is weakened.

Do not apply ice to the head, but you can apply cool water or cold compresses. Also, apply hot fomentations to the bowels, stomach, and liver. This will quell the fever much sooner even than cold. The reaction after the cold applications raises the fever, in the place of killing it (Ellen G. White, *Manuscript Releases,* no. 1481, Letter 112a).

Even if the fever is up to 104°F, a brief exposure to a warm water bath or mild fomentations will often treat the underlying infection, bring the blood to the surface, relax the muscles, increase the depth of respiration, and reduce the fever. The bath water temperature should be slightly lower than the mouth temperature by about one degree when the fever is over 103°F.

By warming the skin, a number of activities in the body are cranked up that assist in fighting disease. White blood cells become more rapid in their movement and much hungrier. Interferons and other blood proteins are made in larger quantities in a fever. Interleukin I and Interleukin II are also made more rapidly during a fever. Because heart rate is increased and circulation quickened, the immune process is enhanced.

Because skin blood vessels are opened up, white blood cells come to the periphery of the body, giving them access to other white blood cells stationed permanently in the skin, with which they communicate to intensify the defense efforts against a disease process. The chemical substances already mentioned that cause foreign elements and bacteria to be more easily destroyed by white blood cells are released more readily during a fever, both artificial as well as natural. The fixed macrophages in the skin help to purify the blood as the blood is brought more to the surface, making germs easier to destroy. Wastes are removed more quickly from the blood by the increased body temperature.

In vigorous adults and children with mild fevers, a hot half bath is a useful treatment. The patient should enter the tub with water at 104°F, raised after half a minute or so to 108°F to 111°F, and held there one minute for each year in age for children, and 10 to 15 minutes for adults. Keep the face generously sponged with cold water and an ice cap to the head. Note that some people get a headache if cold is applied to the head. These persons should have cold only to the face. Keep a thermometer in the mouth and discontinue the treatment if the mouth temperature exceeds 104.6°F, or if the pulse exceeds 150. Finish the treatment with a cold shower for 10 to 20 seconds followed by a brisk rubdown with a coarse towel. Some prefer a cold mitten friction to finish. Remember that successful treatments bring large quantities of blood to the surface, a condition that can cause momentary faintness. Be prepared to support the patient until the sensation passes, or if it is a self-treatment, bend over, tighten the abdominal muscles, and run to the bed.

For fevers of 103°F and over, the water temperature and the length of time spent in the bath should be less—the higher the fever the shorter the time. The objectives of treatment are the reversal of the heat conservation gear into the heat dissipation gear, and the stimulation of the immune system. As soon as one sees the skin getting red, indicating that blood has come to the skin surface, as soon as any degree of sweating is observed, or the person becomes comfortably relaxed in the bath, and begins to breathe deeply, one can assume that the objectives are accomplished and the bath may be terminated. For high fevers in infants under six months, over 104.5°F, as brief a bath as 30 seconds at 100°F to 102°F (this bath temperature will be less than body temperature) followed by a five second cold water pour and a brisk frictioning of the skin with a dry towel, may be successful in bringing down a fever. If the treatment is long enough, and of proper temperature, a child invariably, and most adults usually, will sleep after the treatment and will awaken with a fever reduced or entirely gone. For children use one minute in the water for each year of their age.

Short treatments can be repeated in infants and children under three as often as every two hours, but only once daily for baths lasting more than 10 minutes, since prolonged sweating can result in excessive mineral loss.

Herbs for Fever

Bayberry, black haw, catnip, chaparral, echinacea, feverfew, garlic, golden seal, meadowsweet, parsley, white willow, and licorice are all helpful.

Ginger has anti-inflammatory and antiemetic actions. It also has properties that make its use identical to the use of cayenne. Its anti-inflammatory activity makes it useful for arthritis, migraines, collagen diseases, etc. The anti-inflammatory activity may be because of inhibition of the enzyme cyclo-oxygenase. Ginger can reduce a fever, in most instances almost as well as aspirin. Take one teaspoon of powdered kitchen ginger in a teacup of hot water or blend one-half to two thirds of an inch of fresh ginger root in a cup of hot water.

Using Water to Reduce Fevers

If the fever is *106°F or above*, follow these procedures:

1. A tepid or neutral bath at around 98°F.
2. Cold compress to head and neck.
3. Ice bag or cold compress to the heart in a feeble patient.
4. Cool (95°F) rectal irrigation or enema—3 to 4 ounces for a child.
5. Fresh, cool (60°F to 68°F) air in the sickroom.
6. Cool water (40°F to 55°F or tap temperature) taken by mouth to promote sweating.

If the fever is *104°F to 105°F*, use one of the following procedures instead of #1 above; then proceed with #2 to #6 above:

1. Short warm bath almost the same as normal skin temperature, or repeated warm water friction-sponging with a coarse washcloth to bring blood to the surface.
2. Very warm fomentations to the abdomen or spine for five to seven minutes.
3. Cold mitten friction or hot mitten friction.

If the fever is mild, *99°F to 104°F*, give a hot treatment by one of the following methods:

1. Hot half bath, prolonged to the point of elevating the oral temperature to 102°F to 104°F. Finish the bath with a pail pour of cold water or a cool shower, followed by a dry friction rub or cold mitten friction.
2. Hot foot bath with blanket pack to elevate temperature. Finish off as above.
3. Hot fomentations to chest and spine with cold mitten friction at the end.
4. Hot water or hot ginger tea to promote sweating.
5. Measures #2 and #3 listed above under treatment of a fever to 106°F.

Fibrocystic Breast Disease

(See "Breast Conditions" in the *Conditions and Diseases* section.)

Fibroids

(See "Women's Conditions and Diseases" in the *Conditions and Diseases* section.)

Fibromyalgia

This disorder affects between 1 and 5 percent of the population, making it one of the most common rheumatological disorders. Irritable bowel syndrome occurs in 34 to 50 percent of patients with fibromyalgia. This brings up the question as to whether this disorder might be casued by "leaky bowel syndrome" (*Internal Medicine World Report,* March 1–14, 1991, 10).

Sixty percent of those with 11 or more tender points (the standard definition for fibromyalgia) did not have chronic widespread pain. The number of tender points rose with age and were significantly higher in women. Aches, pains, stiffness all over, combined with numbing fatigue are all made worse by the disturbed sleep and depression that many persons with fibromyalgia suffer. It is thought to affect three to six million Americans, most of them women (*American Journal of Epidemiology* 138, no. 8 [October 15, 1993]: 641).

Spinal fluid levels of homocysteine are increased and B12 levels are decreased in fibromyalgia (*Scand J. Rheumatol* 1997; 26(4): 301–7). A nutrient imbalance or a malabsorption of nutrients may be a feature of this disorder. Perhaps poor chewing is also a factor that then causes "leaky gut" problems. A viral infection that strikes primarily the respiratory and autonomic nervous systems may be involved in the development of fibromyalgia. Many patients give a history of upper respiratory infection followed or associated with neurologic symptoms prior to the onset of full-blown fibromyalgia.

Diagnosis

The American College of Rheumatology has agreed on certain guidelines for diagnosing fibromyalgia by tender points (*Arthritis & Rheumatology* 33, no. 2 [1990]: 160–72). If a patient has widespread pain and no other obvious cause, as well as tenderness in at least 11 to 18 of the fibromyalgia sites (see diagram), the diagnosis is probably fibromyalgia. The locations are specific and symmetrical. When the sites are palpated the patient flinches, withdraws, shudders, yelps, or even cries in pain.

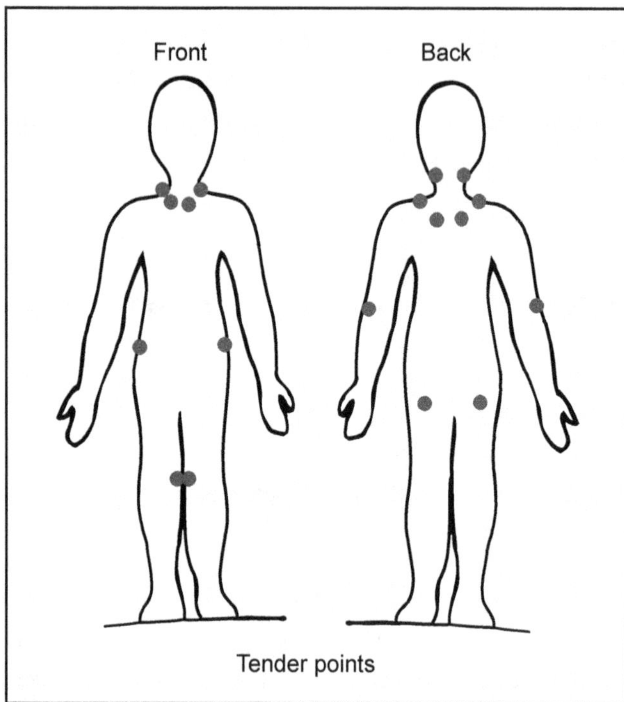

Tender points

The most outstanding symptoms:

Muscular pain	100 percent
Badly disturbed sleep	nearly 100 percent
Symptoms worse in colder, humid weather	nearly 100 percent
History of injury within the year before the symptoms started	nearly 100 percent
Depression	0 to 100 percent

Also many suffer from irritable bowel syndrome (which could be the herald of a food sensitivity), severe migraines or non-migraine headaches, Raynaud's phenomenon (30 to 50 percent), anxiety, dry eyes or mouth, osteoarthritis, rheumatoid arthritis, and substance abuse.

Treatment

Treat like chronic fatigue syndrome. (See "Fatigue, Chronic Fatigue Syndrome" in the *Conditions and Diseases* section.)

Physical fitness is an absolute must. This is not optional; it is part of the cure. Begin a program at once. Low impact aerobics, walking, bouncing on a rebounder or trampoline, and any other kind of exercise equipment placed on a porch, patio, or under the shade of a tree, can all be very helpful. Of course purposeful labor in the yard or garden is probably the very best exercise for most people.

Use all the treatments suggested for depression. (See "Mental Health" in the *Conditions and Diseases* section.)

Use the treatment for sleep to treat sleep disturbances. (See "Sleep" in the *Conditions and Diseases* section.)

A dear friend of the author says her fibromyalgia is made better by sunlight, rest, regularity, and carefully regulating her food sensitivities and made worse by poor posture, stress, and winter weather.

A woman who had suffered with fibromyalgia and been almost disabled for nearly 10 years told me that leaving off dairy products from her diet helped her more than anything else had up to that time. She discovered two other things that helped her have less pain and less fatigue and disability. The first, getting a good night of sleep; this could make night and day difference in the way she felt. The second was using a very heavy vibrator (the kind held in both hands and used on big athletes) in the areas of her greatest pain. This would often stop the pain long enough for her to get a good night of sleep if the vibration was done just at bedtime.

The most favorable diet is a strictly plant-based diet. A gluten free diet may also be helpful for fibromyalgia. The gluten grains are wheat, barley, rye, and possibly oats.

Nutrient supplements found helpful are malic acid, inositol, other antioxidants, hydrochloric acid, digestive enzymes, essential fatty acids, anti-inflammatory supplements, and choline. The immune regulators such as vitamin E, vitamin C, vitamin B12, and vitamin B1 may also be given a trial of several weeks to see if a benefit is derived.

A carefully performed "Elimination and Challenge Diet," found in the *Dietary Information* section, should be done. Those foods discovered to cause increase in *any* symptom should be banished from the diet for one year before testing even a small amount again. Then give yourself a challenge with the food to see if your body can now tolerate it. If you again get an increase in any symptom, eliminate that food again for another year.

Autoimmune diseases often respond to antifungal treatments. Eliminate sugar and its relatives, animal products, yeast, refined carbohydrates, peanuts and peanut butter, mushrooms, and moldy foods.

Some physicians consider fibromyalgia to be one expression of low thyroid function. Indeed, there are features that are common to both: increased risk of vitiligo, water retention, low body temperature, weight gain, cold sensitivity, dry skin, muscle weakness, arthritis, high blood pressure, slow heart rate, and constipation. These patients may be started on thyroid hormone, the smallest dose, and then increased by that amount every two weeks until the milligrams are equal to approximately one-tenth of a milligram for their weight in pounds.

Many sleep in rooms poorly supplied with fresh air during the night. Any illness or disability from which one suffers can be made worse by poor oxygenation of tissues and by rebreathing the wastes just excreted through the lungs. It has been discovered that low oxygen content of the blood and muscles may be a factor in the production of fibromyalgia syndrome. In an overnight sleep study of patients with fibromyalgia and healthy patients, the fibromyalgia patients had an oxygen saturation of 86.8 as compared to 90.7 in controls. It may be that part of the cause of pain in fibromyalgia is low oxygen saturation in arterial blood (*American Journal of Medicine* 101 [1996]: 54–60). To correct this problem, a positive pressure breathing machine can be purchased for nighttime use.

A Dr. Kim from New Jersey locates each tender point and injects bee venom over the point. After a few weeks of daily stings,the patient becomes completely asymptomatic. He says they can be taken off all their pain killers, tranquilizers, mood elevators, or other pharmaceuticals. There are some who say there is nothing more effective than bee venom. We have had no experience with it , but it may be worth a try.

Herbal remedies are numerous. All herbs described under pain control, sleep, or depression can be used for fibromyalgia. Herbs for other symptoms one suffers should also be tried. Some may help one person that would not help another. It is best not to mix more than six to eight herbs at one time. In addition to other herbs, you should try pycnogenol, cat's claw, echinacea, black cohosh, comfrey, white willow bark, feverfew, devil's claw, yarrow, yucca, and marshmallow. Comfrey can be used in compresses. Garlic, tea tree oil, and grapefruit seed extract may be helpful to some. The hormone herbs such as licorice root, black cohosh, and red raspberry leaf can help regulate the endocrine system, which can be under par in this disorder.

First Aid

(See the *Emergencies and Hazards in the Home* section.)

Fistula

(See "Fissures and Fistulae" in the *Women's Conditions and Diseases* section.)

Foot Odor

Often the only remedy needed is a daily light spraying of the foot with plain vinegar, white or brown. Vinegar discourages the growth of fungi and bacteria and improves the health of the skin of the feet.

A foot spray made from witch hazel and cyprus essential oil can be used twice a day. In most cases it will completely solve the problem of foot odor.

Frostbite

The toes, fingers, ears, and tip of the nose are usually the first parts of the body to be affected. They turn pale, the blood and moisture in the tissues freeze, and the circulation stops. Frostbite is deceptive since there is no feeling of pain. Treatment should begin at once with warming the affected area by immersing it in tepid water or bundling it up in woolen clothing. Warming too fast produces pain and can accelerate tissue breakdown. Do not rub the frostbitten area as the friction can break down the cell structure of the cold tissue. If the skin is warmed immediately, the color will usually return. If the frostbite is severe or long standing, however, the area will remain white. In time the blood will seep back into the tissues and the affected area will appear purplish or black. In these severe cases the tissues may be damaged beyond repair and gangrene may develop. This may necessitate amputation of a toe, finger, or entire limb. Long-term consequences possible from frostbite are persistent pain; numbness and tingling; arthritis; dry, cracked, discolored skin; increased susceptibility to future frostbite; and excessive sweating.

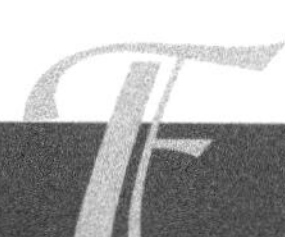

As soon as rewarming has been accomplished, apply aloe vera juice from plant leaves or commercial products every hour. Cover with clean dry dressings. Aloe vera counteracts an injurious agent called thromboxane released from the damaged cells. It is the counteracting of thromboxane that reverses loss of tissue oxygen in burns, and it is just as helpful for frostbite.

To prevent frostbite, do not wear tight fitting shoes, socks, and gloves as they restrict circulation. When the temperature is below 8°F, persons who must work out of doors should not remain out longer than two hours at a time without a warming period. Persons with diabetes or heart disease are particularly susceptible.

Fungus Nails

(See "Skin Diseases" in the Conditions and Diseases section.)

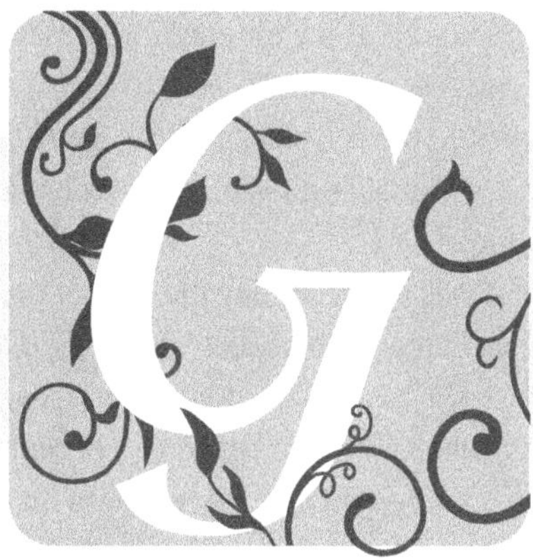

Gallbladder Disease and Gallstones

The typical patient with gallstones was once described by the three F's: fat, female, and forty. In the early days of my medical training, a fourth F was included: fair, since gallstones were seldom seen except in Caucasians in the mid-twentieth century. Now, however, blacks eat the same unhealthful diet and lead the same sedentary lives that whites do, and the incidence of gallstones is virtually the same in both races. Furthermore, each generation is producing gallstones younger and younger because of the richness and refinement of the diet. Decreased exercise is also instrumental in the formation of saturated bile. It is not uncommon for a young person in their teens to get gallstones.

Symptoms from gallbladder disease include indigestion, pain or discomfort—especially after rich or fatty meals—gas, bloating, belching, regurgitation of food, and finally obstructive symptoms including pain in the right upper abdominal quadrant. With an acute attack of biliary colic, one may have fever, chills, and jaundice along with nausea, vomiting, and cramping. The pain comes in waves, and is often intense and accompanied by severe nausea with active vomiting.

The crucial factor in the development of most gallstones is the presence of over nutrition. Refined carbohydrates are a prominent culprit. In countries taking their food in a natural state, people do not produce gallstones. When fiber is removed from food and it is rendered less bulky, less chewy, sweeter, and more fattening, it is prone to cause saturation of the bile. When fiber in the diet is low, cholesterol in the bile goes up. Fiber tends to bind bile salts. It decreases intestinal transit time of food wastes, and interrupts the enterohepatic circulation of bile as it makes its circuit from the intestine to the blood, then to the liver, then to the gallbladder, and back to the intestine where the cholesterol gets bound to the fiber.

When the bile becomes saturated, it may crystallize certain of the solid materials dissolved in bile, forming a tiny nidus on which other crystals develop to form gallstones. Those who do not drink water, or who drink dehydrating beverages such as soft drinks and coffee, tend to get more gallbladder disease.

Refined fats are as instrumental in the production of gallstones as are refined carbohydrates. The more free fat in a meal the more bile is released, and the more concentrated it is with cholesterol and bile salts. Free fats are margarine, mayonnaise, fried foods, cooking fats, salad oils, and any food to which these are added. Extremely fast weight loss can dump large amounts of cholesterol into the bile. Cholesterol then crystallizes into gallstones, which then may cause an acute gallbladder attack.

Treatment and Prevention

Drugs used in treating gallstones may cause unwanted side effects. Such drugs can cause elevation of low density lipoprotein (LDL) cholesterol, the kind of cholesterol associated with increased coronary heart disease risk. Therefore, it is very desirable to follow simple remedies for this disease.

The first and easiest treatment should be directed toward making certain the person drinks plenty of water. Concentrated bile is more likely to form gallstones. It has been found that drinking about one pint of plain water causes the gallbladder to empty within about 20 minutes. An empty gallbladder does not form stones, and when fresh bile runs

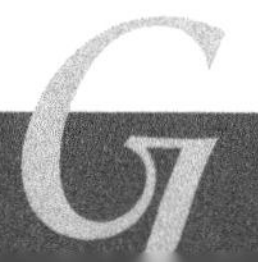

into the gallbladder, it is not as concentrated as after remaining a while in the gallbladder.

The first dietary measure should be to remove free fats from the diet and decrease the number of rich and spicy foods served. One may eat freely of fruits and vegetables prepared in a simple way without sugar or fat or spices. The diet should certainly be totally vegetarian, as all kinds of animal products have been shown to increase the risk of gallbladder disease.

A food allergy can irritate the gallbladder. Foods that have been associated with gallbladder irritation in order of their occurrence include the following: eggs, pork, onions, fowl, milk, coffee, oranges, corn, beans, nuts, apples, tomatoes, peas, cabbage, spices, peanuts, fish, and rye. An "Elimination and Challenge Diet," found in the *Dietary Information* section, should be done to find those foods that cause symptoms. Those foods should be cut out of the diet for one year before testing again. If you are still sensitive, continue another year.

In order to treat gallstones, one should immediately begin to reduce one's weight and maintain normal weight. One can calculate normal weight by allowing 100 pounds for the first five feet, and five pounds for each inch of height thereafter for women, and six to seven and a half pounds for men depending on how muscular they are. Since losing weight can increase slightly the ratio of cholesterol to lecithin in the bile, persons losing weight must drink quite a lot of water to keep the bile thin to prevent stones made of cholesterol in the first few days of beginning a weight-loss program. One should especially avoid alternately gaining and losing weight as this seriously increases the risk of forming stones. (See also "Weight Control" in the *Supplemental Information* section.)

One should reduce or eliminate salt since salt is dehydrating to many body fluids, including the bile. If one is already overweight, sugar, oil, and margarine should be permanently omitted, as you have proven them to cause overweight.

Vitamin C has been reported to reduce the incidence of gallstones. To insure plenty of vitamin C, something raw should be eaten at each meal. Remember that for the average person taking vitamins by pill is upsetting to the body's nutrient economy and should probably be avoided, especially if one is at risk for gallstones. A diet that does not contain adequate raw foods to give a high intake of vitamin C is associated with gallstone formation in guinea pigs.

Use care with gas-forming foods such as radishes, Brussels sprouts, cucumbers, dried beans, prunes, sauerkraut, and so forth. Bloating increases gallbladder irritation. (See "Gas, Flatulence" in the Condiitions and Disease.)

Use no fresh-from-the-oven yeast-raised breads, as they increase the likelihood of forming gas. You may eat freshly baked quick breads as cornbread and tortillas.

The beneficial effects of dietary fiber are so pronounced that a high fiber diet makes gallstone formation unlikely. Eat plenty of raw foods.

The more meals eaten per day the greater the likelihood of getting stones in the gallbladder (*New England Journal of Medicine* 288 [1973]: 24–7). Two meals per day, with nothing between meals—food, or beverages except water and unsweetened herb tea—and nothing but these fluids taken after 3:00 p.m. represents the ideal diet pattern for gallbladder disease.

Coffee, tobacco, and candy should be avoided.

Any kind of surgical procedure can also increase the likelihood of getting gallstones.

Stay away from drugs that are reported to reduce gallstones as they have serious unwanted side effects. These drugs include Estrogen-containing medications, Gemfibrozil, Fenofibrate, and Octreotide.

Oral contraceptives, clofibrate, and heavy supplementation with B vitamins, have been reported to increase the likelihood of developing gallstones.

Physical exercise tends to prevent gallstones. One should bear in mind that a number of other diseases are also associated with gallstones—cancer of the colon, hiatus hernia, angina pectoris, and coronary heart disease, most of which are benefited or prevented by exercise and a proper diet.

There are many herbal remedies for gallbladder disease, one of which is fringe tree. Use the tea or pills. Mint oil is also very good to settle the gallbladder, as is mint, sage, or catnip tea.

Some have recommended a liver and gallbladder flush to get rid of gallstones. The procedure can be tried and is sometimes successful, but most of the time it is not, at least in our experience. We have felt that there is a faint possibility that taking so much oil might cause a stone to enter the bile ducts and not be able to get through; however, many people have tried the gallbladder flush and we have not heard of an impacted stone occurring. Perhaps it is not likely to occur.

Liver and gallbladder flush

Cleanse #1

To encourage the gallbladder to empty itself of stones, the following routine has been suggested:

- Day One – Fast, except for water and taking one pint of carrot juice three times a day at mealtimes.

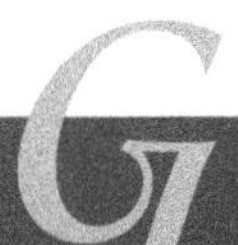

- Day Two – Take one pint of apple juice three times a day at mealtimes. One quart of hot water to which is added 3 tablespoons of charcoal powder can be used for an enema. If constipation results from either the juice fast or the charcoal enema, Cascara sagrada can be taken to relieve the constipation.
- Day Three – One cup of olive oil should be taken on the following schedule. Early in the morning, about 7:00 or 7:30 take two ounces of olive oil with two tablespoons of freshly squeezed lemon juice and one tablespoon of pineapple juice mixed. Lie on the right side. Every fifteen minutes repeat the dose until the cup of olive oil has been consumed. Then lie on the right side and try to sleep, using a hot water bottle over the abdomen.

Cleanse #2

- Take a five-day juice fast as from Sunday morning through Thursday night. Drink as much apple juice, grape juice, pineapple juice, or other fruit juice at mealtimes as the appetite indicates you should. Sip it slowly to allow saliva to mix. Take no solid food.
- On Thursday evening at about 5:30 or 6:00 take some grapefruit juice or other citrus juice, or the entire fruit may be eaten, as desired. At bedtime, drink either one-half cup of olive oil followed by a small glass of grapefruit juice, or one-half cup of warmed, unrefined olive oil blended with one-half cup of lemon juice. Go to bed immediately and lie on the right side for half an hour.
- On Friday morning take two teaspoons of Epsom salts dissolved in two ounces of hot water. The dark green irregular-shaped ball-like objects passed may or may not be stones. Your own examination should tell you readily. With a tongue blade or strong plastic spoon or knife, press on the rounded objects. If they are hard as a rock, they are probably stones. If they can be compressed with the firmest pressure you can give, they are not stones but are portions of fecal matter comprised of dead bodies of germs, shed portions of gastrointestinal lining, coagulated bile, etc.

Treatment for Acute Gallbladder Attack

Start with a 15-minute continuous fomentation over the gallbladder area followed by rubbing with ice, repeated three times. Treatment should be suspended for an hour and can then be repeated as often as necessary.

Be certain the patient stays well hydrated, even if that means giving retention enemas.

Use a rich paste of charcoal in water, spread it on a paper towel, fold, and apply to the area of pain. When the poultice is in place, cover it with kitchen plastic and hold it in place by using a binder. Charcoal by mouth, one tablespoon in a glass of water, can help relieve nausea and assuage pain.

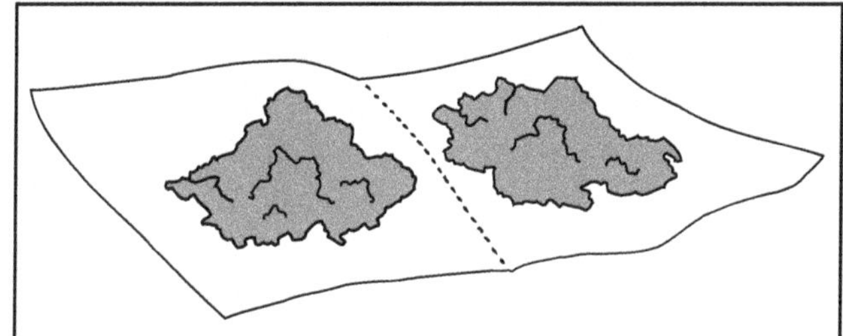

The use of catnip tea can quiet the gastrointestinal tract and the gallbladder. Use mint tea or sage tea in place of, or in addition to, catnip. Celandine, turmeric, Java tea, and milk thistle are other herbs that are very helpful for gallstones.

An ice rub over the area of pain can give great relief. Swelling and inflammation around the bile duct may produce a large portion of the pain, and both heat with cold, or either one alone, can help to reduce swelling and promote drainage. They both increase the concentration of white blood cells that move into the area to help eliminate products of inflammation.

An enema is sometimes helpful to relieve gallbladder pain.

A fingertip massage over the abdomen, or a firm back rub or foot rub can sometimes bring relief.

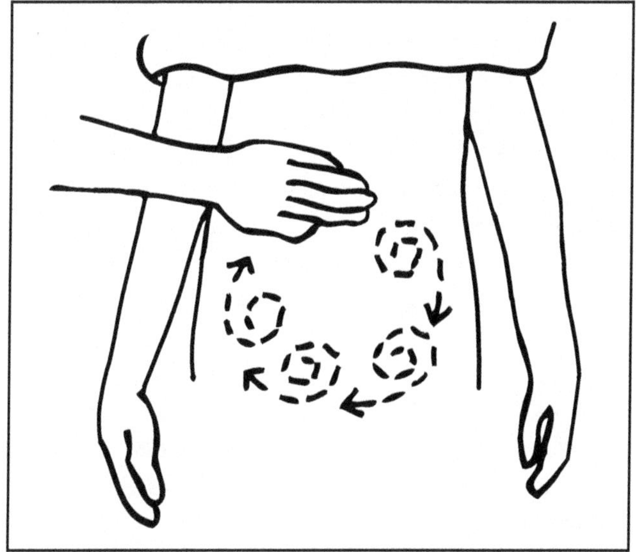

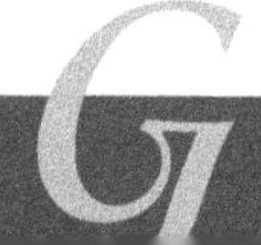

The question always arises as to whether a person with "silent gallstones," those not causing any symptoms, should have them surgically removed. In most cases it is better to leave the silent gallstones in place. While it is said that there is an increased incidence of cancer of the gallbladder in those who have gallstones, it is quite rare and certainly no more common than the incidence of death from the gallbladder surgery, which is also rare. Cancer of the gallbladder is unusual and more often not associated with stones. It has been found that removing the gallbladder doubles the risk of cancer of the colon. Further, intolerance to foods tends to be worse after the loss of the gallbladder. A group of surgeons were asked if they would recommend surgery to their patients who had silent gallstones. Eighty percent responded that they would. However, when asked if they themselves would have surgery to remove silent gallstones, only 20 percent responded that they would. Our advice is usually similar for our patients to what we choose for ourselves.

Case Report

The following is a case report on a patient who had a gallbladder full of stones with regular bouts of gallbladder colic about once a month. She had been recommended to have a cholecystectomy when she wrote to us to ask if there were any alternatives to surgery. I recommended a totally plant-based diet with no free fats, two meals a day, and plenty of exercise. Since she was quite heavy, I recommended that she swim and do leg and arm exercises in the pool beginning with 10 to 15 minutes five days a week. While that was not much, it was definitely more than she had done before.

Recognizing that a sedentary lifestyle contributes to gallbladder disease, she began to be more active. She had only done housework before, but now began to do aerobic exercises as well. She started a steady weight loss program, averaging about a pound and a half each week. Several months went by without a single attack. Then she had two severe attacks of gallbladder colic, each occurring 8 to 12 hours after eating a vegetarian gluten patty in a casserole, which had spices in it. She remembered my stating that she might be sensitive to concentrated gluten. Avoiding all gluten products has kept her free from another gallbladder attack.

Ganglion Cysts

(See "Skeletal Problems" in the *Conditions and Diseases* section.)

Gas, Flatulence

Dr. Michael D. Levitt of Minneapolis is considered one of the world's leading experts on flatulence. He considers flatulence to be entirely normal, but cites several reasons for an increased production of intestinal gas such as hard to digest complex carbohydrates that escape digestion and pass into the colon where the intestinal flora ferment the residual food into gas. Milk is also likely to cause gas because of the persistence of lactose that passes the digestive process of most adults. Food allergies may also be a cause.

Some foods are more prone to form gas than others. These include all foods containing dairy products, dry beans, corn, apples, raisins, bananas, prune juice, apple juice, grape juice, onions, celery, carrots, apricots, pretzels, bagels, wheat, wheat germ, Brussels sprouts, pastries, potatoes, eggplant, citrus fruits, bread, broccoli, cauliflower, kohlrabi, radishes, cucumbers, cabbage, artificial sweeteners (such as sorbitol), and inadequately cooked grains. The reason some foods produce gas more easily is that they have more residue left after digestion and the food residues are then made into gas by gas-forming germs that inhabit the colon.

The major gases of the intestinal tract are oxygen, hydrogen, carbon dioxide, and methane, which are odorless. Those components of intestinal gas that have a bad odor, comprising much less than one percent, include ammonia, hydrogen sulfide, volatile amino acids, short-chain fatty acids, and highly disagreeable amines such as indole and skatole. Fats and proteins have the unpleasant smelling residues whereas carbohydrates tend to have the odorless components of intestinal gas. Acids are often produced when intestinal gas is formed. It is these acids that cause much irritation and discomfort in the colon, which we associate with gas.

Following are some additional causes of gas in the colon:

- Overtaxing the digestive system:
  - Eating too fast or too slowly. A desirable meal length might be 30 to 50 minutes.
  - Inadequate chewing, or chewing with the mouth open. Chunks escape that cannot be completely digested. Chewing with the mouth open encourages swallowing of air. Saliva needs to be well mixed with the food to insure proper digestion.
  - Eating too much. The digestive tract is unable to handle the excess food.
  - Meals too close together or off schedule.
- Drinking with meals or too much liquid foods, milks, soups, and juices.

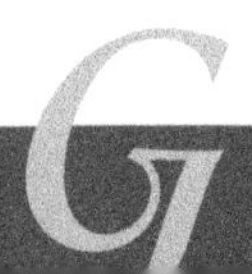

- Tension, noise, or distraction at mealtime.
- Improper cooking. All grains and some legumes require several hours of cooking time.
- Wrong combinations—fruits and vegetables; milk, fats, eggs, and sugar in any combination.
- Inadequate water between meals. This causes thick saliva that more readily traps air than watery saliva.
- Eating foods that disagree with one another. Milk sensitivity is a frequent cause of gas. An intolerance to lactose, the chief carbohydrate of dairy products, is the most common food sensitivity in America.
- Reclining after meals or failure to get mild to moderate exercise after eating.
- A number of things that worsen gas include the following:
  - Laxatives
  - Tight fitting clothes
  - Sedentary job with lack of exercise
  - Sucking air in with hot beverages
  - Carbonated drinks, beer, or champagne
  - Drinking from fountains
  - Chewing gum
  - Smoking
  - High-fat diet
  - Swallowing air when one is under stress
  - An airline flight

Treatment

Grains prepared by boiling should be cooked more than two and one-half hours, except for rolled oats, which can be prepared in 60 to 90 minutes.

To encourage beans to be less gas forming, rinse the beans, soak them overnight, and then freeze them in the soaking water. Thaw and pour off the first soaking water, rinse thoroughly and cover again with water, which will be frozen a second time. The first water may contain some of the oligosaccharides, raffinose, and stachyose, which are soluble fibers responsible for gas formation. The freezing will break up the fiber somewhat so that it is more water soluble and digestible. If this is followed by long cooking, many can eat beans who cannot without this treatment. In tests done on beans, it was found that pressure cooking, sprouting, soaking beans for eighteen hours, and dehulling beans all had a favorable influence on the digestibility of beans (*Plant Foods for Human Nutrition* 46 [July 1994]: 71–6). We have found that cooking beans for 8 to 10 hours overnight in a slow cooker has a very salutary effect on beans to prevent the formation of intestinal gas. But no method of preparation will prevent gas if too many beans are eaten and your digestive system is overtaxed.

Activated charcoal is the number one treatment for gas. Start with a one-fourth teaspoon taken twice daily, and increase it to as much as one teaspoon taken four times daily. Simethicone, the most commonly used pharmaceutical agent for gas, is only a fraction as effective as charcoal.

A commercial product containing alpha-D-galactosidase, an enzyme produced from Aspergillus, a type of mold, is quite effective against the gas produced not only by beans but by any foods containing high amounts of indigestible fiber. It is a very potent enzyme that will break down fiber so that it can be digested. It is available in health food stores and many supermarkets. Directions are on the package. For those with the candida-related complex, use with caution, as it is a mold product. We have noted few ill effects so far, but one person reported that her heart seemed to be affected by its use.

Enzyme production by the intestinal tract can be boosted by the eating of fresh, raw fruits and vegetables and seeds and nuts. Chew them well.

Garlic is capable of relieving gas in the majority of individuals. The enzymes of garlic help in the digestion of beans.

You can take certain herbs that are rich in aromatic oils—fennel, anise, and ginger—to reduce flatulence.

Dandelion root and artichoke leaf both stimulate the secretion of digestive juices to make digestion of gas-producing foods more complete. Because of their bitterness they taste better when mixed with other greens, as in a green salad.

Caraway or dill tea is excellent for gas, as are spearmint and thyme tea, particularly in children.

Mix two ounces chamomile, two ounces fennel, one ounce peppermint leaves, and one ounce anise seed. Use one teaspoon of the herb mixture per cup of boiling water. Steep for 15 to 20 minutes. Use one cup per day as needed.

Mix two ounces sarsaparilla, two ounces fennel, one ounce dandelion root, half an ounce licorice root powder, one-eighth ounce artichoke leaf, and one-eighth ounce ginger. Use one teaspoon of the mixture per cup of boiling water. Steep for 15 to 20 minutes.

Kneel over a low table such as a coffee table and maintain that position for a few minutes. This posture promotes bowel movement and gas expulsion.

A rocking motion of the abdomen may help. While lying flat in bed, push the heel of the right hand into the right side at the waist, alternate with pushing the heel of the left hand into the left side to set up a rocking motion for about five minutes. This will often move gas out.

A heating pad may bring prompt relief for many people.

Do not postpone bowel movements, as gas is formed progressively when residue remains in the colon.

A glass of water every 10 minutes for one hour will relieve gas pains for most people.

Gastritis

A stomach upset or inflammation of the stomach is called gastritis. It may be acute or chronic and caused by food poisoning, spoiled food, overeating, the use of alcohol, not drinking sufficient water (enough to keep the urine very pale), aspirin, vinegar, or spices such as ginger, cinnamon, nutmeg, cloves, and black and red pepper. It may be treated in the same way as intestinal flu. Treat acute gastritis with charcoal, mint tea, a glass of water or tea every 10 minutes for an hour, and an ice bag over the stomach.

Chronic severe gastritis as from alcoholism leads to atrophy of the stomach, with progressively decreased acid and pepsin. This causes a deficient digestion, malabsorption of vitamin B12 (pernicious anemia), and increased risk of stomach cancer.

Persons with persistent stomach problems should be checked for helicobacter, a common cause of chronic complaint with the stomach. Helicobacter can be treated with golden seal, echinacea, myrrh, grapefruit seed extract, and garlic for one month. Simmer one quart of water and add one slightly rounded tablespoon of golden seal powder, myrrh, and one heaping tablespoon of echinacea. Gently simmer for 20 minutes, strain, and drink throughout the day each day for 30 days. To each cup of tea, add 8 to 10 drops of grapefruit seed extract.

Additionally, eat 12 to 20 cloves of garlic steamed for 8 to 10 minutes at each meal. For simple gastric acid overproduction, drink a mixture of charcoal powder, one tablespoonful, in a large glass of water four times daily.

Gastroesophageal Reflux Disease, GERD

Gastroesophageal reflux disease (GERD) causes significant disability in an estimated 20 percent of the population of the United States who suffer symptoms at least once a week. GERD can lead to prolonged esophagitis, which may cause a scarring of the lower end of the esophagus, even to the point of reducing the ability to swallow. It may also encourage esophageal cancer. Several factors are known to increase the likelihood of developing GERD are obesity, lack of physical exercise, the use of aspirin and non-steroidal anti-inflammatory drugs (NSAID), antidepressants, and tranquilizers (*Annals of Epidemiology* 9 [1999]: 424). Treat the same way as hiatus hernia (see "Hiatus Hernia " in the *Conditions and Diseases* condition).

Geographic Tongue

This condition is not serious or life threatening, but it can be quite annoying. Tender areas develop on the tongue caused by denuding of the papillae of the tongue, the structures giving the tongue a slightly rough or velvety appearance. The lesions move around from day to day, as they begin healing in one place, but do not complete healing before another area begins. It is of unknown origin.

Of 25 patients with geographic tongue causing symptoms, serum zinc was low or marginal in 85 percent (21 people). Four cases (33 percent) had a complete resolution of the geographic tongue with three months of zinc sulphate. The researchers used 200 milligrams three times a day. We believe a smaller dose of 50 milligrams may be adequate and just as effective. A total of 10 of the 25 stopped having symptoms of pain or tenderness in the tongue in three months (*Journal of Trace Element Experimental Medicine* 3 [1990]: 203-8). We feel uncomfortable advising such a large dose of zinc for a long period of time as several other minerals may become unbalanced. Certainly if one decides to take the larger dose, it should not be taken for longer than three months. Its association with Alzheimer's disease has not been clarified yet, and even the chance that zinc supplementation for long periods (the research indicates some years) could cause Alzheimer's disease is reason enough to urge restraint.

Germs on Food

Germs on fruits and vegetables such as *Salmonella*, *E. coli*, *Listeria*, and *Pseudomonas* often come from the colon of some person, being transferred by the fingers. Washing fruits and vegetables in water with a detergent dissolved in it, and then rinsing well, or dipping into a non-toxic mix of vinegar and hydrogen peroxide, half and half, will remove these germs and many toxic substances. The mix can be used for repeated washings. About twenty drops of grapefruit seed extract in a kitchen sink of water can be used to soak vegetables

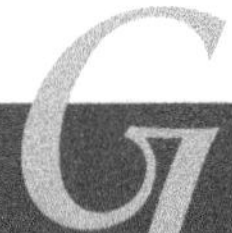

for 10 to 20 minutes. Then rub the skins of the fruits as much as possible as they are being rinsed. The rubbing will remove particles of dust and dirt.

Glaucoma

Increased pressure within the eyeball is called glaucoma. Normal pressure is about 15 to 20 millimeters, but in glaucoma the pressure may go up to 40 millimeters. It is estimated that one million Americans may have some degree of glaucoma. It is the commonest cause of blindness over the age of 65. It tends to run in families. The buildup of pressure is caused by inability of the fluid that is constantly produced in the eye to drain through the tiny tubules which normally drain away this fluid. Symptoms include redness of the eye, decreased vision, colored haloes seen around artificial lights, sometimes headache or pain in the eye, enlargement of the pupil, and nausea and vomiting. People over 40 should have an eye exam for glaucoma once every year.

There are certain drugs that make glaucoma worse, including corticosteroids, even cortisone creams rubbed on the skin for eczema; nasal decongestants; many cough medicines; drugs that inhibit stomach acid secretion; antiasthmatics; antidepressants; some blood pressure-lowering and sedative drugs; appetite suppressants; and caffeine. Since so many drugs worsen glaucoma, it is a good policy not to use medicine except as a lifesaver, and only when there is no natural remedy available. Antihistamines taken for asthma or other allergies can induce glaucoma (*American Family Physician* 51, no. 1 [1995]: 191). Cataracts and glaucoma have both been found to be increased in incidence by the use of corticosteroid ointments (*Lancet* 345 [1995]: 330).

Treatment

Obey all known health laws, those dealing with fresh air, sunshine, rest, proper diet, exercise, abundance of water, moderation in all things, and trust in divine power.

Glaucoma should be treated naturally in the very same way that high blood pressure is treated. Use the method for treating high blood pressure given in this book, and follow it to the letter, even if you do not have hypertension.

Become a total vegetarian. Breakfast should be essentially fruits and whole grains with a few nuts and seeds, and lunch should be vegetables and whole grains with a few nuts and seeds. If a third meal is required, that can be of fruits and whole grains with no nuts or seeds. These basic four food items (fruits; vegetables; whole grains; and seeds) can be prepared in thousands of delightful ways. This type of diet reduces both systemic hypertension and the pressure within the eyes.

Use a fat-free, sugar-free, and salt-free diet. Remove all added sodium and high salt foods from the diet—monosodium glutamate, salt, non-fat dry skim milk, soy sauce, any product containing a sodium compound, including many medicines (even the official name of penicillin is "penicillin-sodium"). Remove all sources of free fats (butter, mayonnaise, margarine, fried foods, cooking fats, salad oils, peanut butter, etc.). Reduce to the barest minimum all concentrated foods such as sugar and its relatives, refined foods of all kinds, high protein foods, and any other concentrated nutrient. Even concentrated vitamins and minerals may be a big problem. The sweet fruits may be taken in abundance, as can creamy fruits such as avocado and bananas, which can be mashed and used as a spread for bread.

Remove all spices from the diet—ginger, cinnamon, nutmeg, cloves, black and red pepper, etc. All of these hot spices contain such substances as capsaicin, myristicin, eugenol, etc. These are aromatic oils that injure the delicate structures of the sensory organs (balance, vision, hearing, smell, etc.). Some people are damaged by one, and others by another. Still others may appear to come off problem free, or nearly so. Do not use any fermented foods of any kind, whether it be fermented soy, or products such as kim chee. These contain toxic amines known to damage delicate tissues. Fermented garlic extracts, such as Kyolic, should not be used with this diet.

A four-day water fast can bring the pressure down as much as five units. One woman brought her pressure from 30 down to 26 during a four-day fast. One should then take four to six days to break the fast, using only a plant-based diet thereafter, as it is the most favorable diet in glaucoma.

If diabetes is present, it should be corrected through diet and exercise, as it increases the severity of glaucoma.

Glaucoma is often related to a food sensitivity, and every attempt should be made to discover the foods to which the person is sensitive. The blood pressure may respond to the diet, giving one an index to the foods involved. (See "Elimination and Challenge Diet" in the *Dietary Information* section.)

Do not overeat as that raises the pressure in many organs. Do not drink more than one glass (eight ounces) of water or other fluid at one time as pressure in the eyes is raised by quickly drinking a large amount of water, especially more than two glasses at one time.

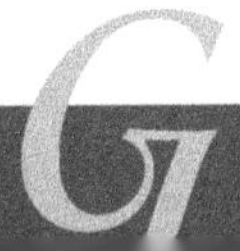

Lose weight. Being overweight increases the incidence and severity of all diseases.

Avoid coffee, tea, colas, and chocolate, even if they have been decaffeinated. There are toxic alkaloids other than caffeine present in these things.

Nicotine is an optic nerve toxin and should be avoided. Damage to optic nerves is much worse if the tobacco user also has glaucoma.

Do not use drugs, alcohol, and medications known to make high blood pressure worse. Cortisone type drugs, even for skin disorders, motion sickness drugs, and drugs for angina can make glaucoma worse. Many drugs also cause damage to the optic nerve and encourage deterioration. These include ibuprofen, aspirin, tranquilizers, antidepressants, antidiabetic drugs, antibiotics, and steroids.

A helpful treatment is the application of hot compresses to the eyes for nine minutes, then exchange with one minute of cold compresses. Repeat the process six times, making the hot application as hot as can be tolerated and the cold water compress as cold as you can get it. Continue the treatment for a month or two until improvement is obvious.

Take a hot foot bath (if not diabetic) every morning and every evening, and again at noon if possible. This decongests the head. This is best done simultaneously with the hot compresses to the eyes.

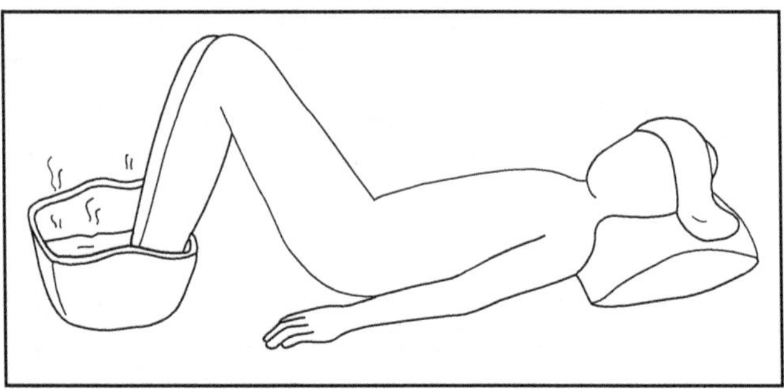

At night one should put a very light pressure bandage on the eyes, about the equivalent of pressure from a folded wet washcloth laid on one eye when one is lying down, if the washcloth were folded so that all the weight of the wet washcloth rested on the eyeball. That much pressure can be held in place by a knit cap pulled down over the eyes and secured by a scarf tied around the head. The small amount of pressure is to encourage the eyeball to drain excessive quantities of fluid from the eyeball structures. Do not overdo the pressure.

One should perform a series of eye exercises and facial and neck exercises to soothe the eyeball. The primary exercise is to turn the eyes to the full extent of their ability in all four quadrants and four diagonals while keeping the nose pointed straight in front. That means to look as far to the left as possible, then as far to the right; then as far to the top, and as far to the bottom. Then split each of those by looking up to the upper left and lower right, upper right and lower left. This series should be repeated once every 10 minutes as often as it can be remembered.

In addition, there are some facial exercises that will be of help. Tighten the eyelids by doing what is called the "silent scream," which consists of contracting all the muscles of the face, forehead, chin, eyes, and even neck muscles while keeping the mouth as wide open as possible as if mimicking a scream. It is somewhat of an exaggerated yawn and can be treated as a yawn when done in public. Again, if one can do it once every 10 minutes, one may get a benefit from it.

Intense exercise for at least 15 minutes daily will drop the intraocular pressure by as much as five millimeters of mercury. Even mild exercise can be expected to drop the pressure in the eyes by at least one millimeter of mercury (*Japanese Journal of Ophthalmology* 38 [1994]: 191). The reduction in pressure continues for at least two hours following the exercise.

Avoid emotional upsets. Stress increases blood pressure and is just as likely to increase eye pressure.

Avoid heavy straining either in having a bowel movement or in lifting or pushing.

Avoid slant-boards or other upside down positions or lying face down unless you lie on a wedge elevator.

Hypothyroidism has been associated with glaucoma and increased pressure within the eyes. Treat the person with glaucoma for two weeks with the thyroid routine in this book, and retest the eye pressure.

Coleus forskohlii seems promising to reduce the pressure within the eyes. Several studies have indicated help from this common herb (*Japanese Journal of Ophthalmology* 30 [1986]: 238).

Large doses of vitamin C are claimed to cure "open angle glaucoma." The patient should take as much as possible without getting diarrhea in three daily doses. A group of 30 patients each showed a reduction in their eye pressure on the vitamin C supplements. Dr. Hershell Boyd commented that he had never seen a case of glaucoma in any patient who routinely took fairly large quantities of vitamin C (*Journal of Orthomolecular Medicine* 10, no. ¾ [1995]: 165–8).

Gluten Sensitivity

(See also "Celiac Disease" in the *Conditions and Diseases* section.)

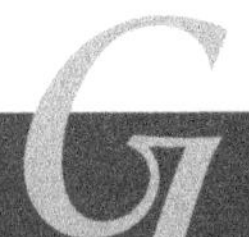

Gluten is composed of gliadin compounds. Some 18 different gliadin-associated medical conditions have been identified. They include dermatitis herpetiformis, rosacea, celiac disease, autism, and pervasive developmental disorders, some forms of epilepsy, brain atrophy, intellectual deterioration, some forms of chronic schizophrenia, chronic neurologic disorders of unknown cause (ataxias and peripheral neuropathies), dental enamel defects, low bone mineral density, recurring aphthous ulcers (mouth ulcers or canker sores), small bowel lymphomas, arthritis and other joint symptoms, loss of fertility and menstrual periods, as well as miscarriages in women and infertility in men.

Gluten sensitivity can cause or worsen certain autoimmune diseases, thyroid diseases, some forms of insulin-dependent diabetes (2 to 4 percent of insulin dependant diabetics), and iron-deficiency anemia in infants and children, abnormally elevated liver enzymes (alkaline phosphatase, etc.), and abnormal intestinal permeability (*Lancet* 349 [1997]: 1755).

Goiter

(See "Thyroid Disease" in the *Conditions and Diseases* section.)

Gonorrhea

Gonorrhea is a sexually transmitted disease. Symptoms include a discharge from the urethra and burning and frequency of urination, with or without fever.

Treatment

Since gonorrhea is becoming resistant to more and more drugs, hydrotherapy treatments for this disease take on added importance. Adminster a 30-minute fever treatment five days a week for three weeks, bringing the mouth temperature up to 104°F each time. Culture the secretions for gonorrhea from the vagina or penis before beginning the treatments and again after two weeks. If the secretions continue to contain the gonococcus, continue the treatment for one or two more weeks and get a final culture. About 10 percent of patients will be cured after one session, about 30 percent after two sessions, and an additional 40 percent after four sessions. Some cases may require the additional weeks of treatment, but eventually more cases can be cured by this method (over 95 percent) than by giving antibiotics. Re-culture male patients three weeks after discontinuing the treatments, and re-culture female patients on the first post menstrual day after three consecutive periods. If there is no evidence of the gonococcus, the patient is dismissed as cured. If gonococci are found on culture, continue treatments two more weeks.

Prevention should be rather obvious, but in this age of sexual promiscuity, we would like to urge abstinence from any sexual contacts outside of marriage. "Safe sex" means the use of condoms to much of the world; however, the high failure rate of condoms—in several studies up to 20 percent—should give everyone pause to reflect on just what "safe sex" means. To us, "safe sex" means no sex outside of marriage. *This* is the norm; not promiscuity, as is generally accepted as normal.

Gout

Gout is a form of arthritis because of accumulation of uric acid as a result of abnormal purine metabolism. Purines are found in certain foods as follows:

- High levels – Liver, kidneys, brains, heart, sweetbreads, mussels, anchovies, sardines, meat extract, consommé, gravies, fish roes, herring.
- Moderate levels – Fish, except as noted above, other seafoods, all meat, all fowl, yeast, lentils, whole-grain cereals, beans, peas, asparagus, cauliflower, mushrooms, spinach, oatmeal.
- Negligible levels – Vegetables, fruit, refined cereals, cereal products.

More men than women suffer from gout in the ratio of six to one. The typical joint involved with gout is the great toe. The disease is by no means limited to that joint but can involve any soft tissue of the body, any internal organ, and any one or multiple joints with the sudden onset of severe pain, which increases over the first 12 hours with exquisite tenderness of the joints involved. One attack usually lasts 10 to 14 days. Between attacks the patient feels quite well, and attacks may recur months or years later, with individual attacks getting closer and closer. Any metabolic condition that reduces the excretion of uric acid in the urine or makes the system more acidic can trigger a gout attack. Starvation, because it increases the amount of uric acid produced from tissues, can precipitate a gout attack. Minor injury, alcohol, overeating, etc., can cause an attack of gout.

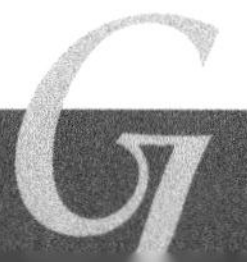

Certain triggering agents for acute attacks include foods to which the patient is allergic, notably milk, tomatoes, eggs, and all animal products. These articles should all be avoided. Fasting may, in some persons, trigger an attack.

Colchicine, the common antigout medication, is toxic and should be avoided, as the disease can easily be controlled by natural means in most cases. Side effects of the medication include hair loss, anemia, reduced immunity, liver damage, cramping, nausea and vomiting, etc.

Diagnosis is made by a blood test in which the uric acid is checked. Since patients with gout also tend to be prone to diabetes and heart disease, cholesterol and blood sugar levels and triglycerides and SGOT levels should also be obtained. Hypertension is also common in these patients. The most disabling of the features of gout is kidney failure. Uric acid damages the kidneys, leading to kidney failure. Tests for kidney function (creatinine, GFR and BUN) should also be obtained.

Treatment

The most important single thing to treating gout is weight control. It should begin slowly but proceed with perfect control. Too rapid loss of weight may precipitate attacks of gout in susceptible individuals.

Fluids should be taken at a high level. It is recommended that 10 to 14 glasses of water be taken every day to encourage elimination of uric acid and to protect the kidneys from the irritation of the uric acid.

Use a diet high in unrefined carbohydrates and low in protein and fat. There must be absolutely no free fat in the diet, only that which nature has placed there. Free sugars such as honey, molasses, sugar, syrups, etc., are also difficult foods for the gout patient to handle. However, sweet fruits, vegetables, and melons may be taken freely.

Cut out all high purine foods and eat sparingly of vegetarian foods having a moderately high purine level. Emphasis should be given to fruits and vegetables, which may be freely eaten.

Take cherries of any kind and drink the juice of canned cherries (canned in water pack, not syrup). The quantity is anything up to half a pound (about one heaping cupful) of fresh or canned cherries daily. The severity of the attack and the availability of the cherries may determine how many can be taken. One tablespoon of unsweetened cherry concentrate daily brings good relief in some patients. The active nutrient in cherries reducing uric acid is ellagic acid. It is also present in grapes and many other fruits.

Charcoal lowers serum uric acid levels. Take one to four tablespoons two to four times daily, depending on the need of the person. As the symptoms reduce, the level of charcoal can be reduced.

Charcoal compress applications to the joints, fomentations or hot baths, a daily paraffin bath, and compresses of comfrey root or leaves can bring relief. In addition, mud packs and hot baths have been of substantial help in the treatment of gout. (See "Hydrotherapy" in the *Natural Remedies* section.)

Avoid those drugs that are known to increase uric acid: thiazides, ethacrynic acid, penicillin, thiamin, vitamin B12, insulin, folic acid, sulfa drugs, ergotamine tartrate, mercurial diuretics, and many other drugs.

Grief

Any major loss will probably be characterized by the following stages: 1) Numbness; 2) Rejection; 3) "Why me?"; 4)Depression; 5) Acceptance; and 6) Reinvestment of time and interests.

A number of physical and emotional symptoms may accompany grieving: sadness, yearning for return of the lost person, a sense of emptiness, depression, guilt, anger, anxiety, social withdrawal, loneliness, forgetfulness, weight change, nightmares, dreams of the lost object or deceased person, and visualizations or other illusions of them.

Prolonged grief (in excess of about three months) may indicate an abnormal relationship with the deceased such as dependent, ambivalent, complicated, or troubled. Prolonged grief may follow suicides or a missing person. It may also be caused by the lack of social supporters or being perceived by someone as not handling the situation, sickness, or funeral well. If the loved one died in a socially unacceptable way such as being executed, prolonged grief may occur. Abnormal grief may also include slow movements or functional impairment such as inability to think well, sleeplessness, eating disorders with weight loss or gain, etc. Normal acute grief should not last longer than about two months after the loss. While life will never be the same, life can again be good if properly invested.

Resolution of grief is recognized by easing of or freedom from intense emotion referable to what has been or may be lost in the near future and a move toward new activities and new relationships. The time and affections must be reinvested for a proper resolution of grief.

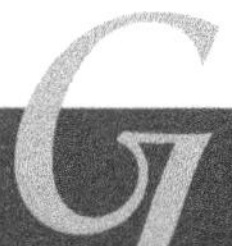

Stages of Grief

Do not make the mistake of failing to tell the terminally ill person that he or she will die. It is rarely new information, and the patient may be relieved that discussion has begun. If the family persistently refuses to talk about the impending death, the dying person may think that it is simply too horrible to bring up, a thought that intensifies the total grief process the dying person goes through and cuts him/her off from free and open communication with those closest to him/her.

Any person learning about a life-changing diagnosis, or a fatal condition needs to be handled delicately.

The following stages of grief may be experienced by the terminally-ill patient and/or loved ones who experience a death in the family:

1. Realization – Gently explain the medical status, but do so in an emphatic way. Some of your words may echo in the mind for days or weeks; choose them with gentleness and care.
2. Anger – Accept the patient's anger undefensively. Provide updated health status reports even if doing so causes venting of more anger. Chances are good the patient may have passed to the next stage.
3. Bargaining – Facilitate discussion. Be a good listener. Try to inspire hope that there is much or at least something that can be done to ease the situation, even if there is no cure. In the bargaining stage, the patient may wish to survive just long enough to complete a duty or experience a significant life event, and then the idea of death may be less onerous.
4. Depression – With depression comes sadness, anxiety, insomnia, poor appetite, and withdrawal from family and others. Be supportive and do not suggest medications to dull the mind, or a psychiatric referral, but use natural measures to control strong emotions—massage, neutral baths, walks, or other exercise, charitable deeds, etc.
5. Peace – In the fifth stage of grief, the patient has peacefulness, calmness, improved sleep, improved appetite, and concern for family and others.

Physicians and other caretakers may have a pronounced grief reaction when a patient dies. The grief reaction should be anticipated. The physician should attend wakes and funerals of their patients where this is appropriate or needed. These activities are useful to ease acceptance of death.

"Every draught of bitterness will be mingled with the love of Jesus, and in place of complaining of the bitterness, you will realize that Jesus' love and grace are so mingled with sorrow that it has been turned into subdued, holy, sanctified joy" (*Selected Messages,* book 2, 274). Do not indulge in prolonged grieving. "Grief, anxiety, discontent, remorse, guilt, distrust, all tend to break down the life forces, and to invite decay and death" (*Ministry of Healing,* 241). Therefore, you must pray for courage and strength to bear all trials.

"If we would think and talk less of our trials, and more of the mercy and goodness of God, we would find ourselves raised above much of our gloom and perplexity. Try singing a cheerful song. You may say, How can I sing, with this dark prospect before me, with this burden of sorrow and bereavement upon my soul? But have earthly sorrows deprived us of the all powerful Friend we have in Jesus?" (*Selected Messages,* book 2, 268).

The assurance of God's approval will promote physical health. It fortifies the soul against doubt, perplexity, and excessive grief that so often saps the vital forces and induces nervous diseases of a most debilitating and distressing character.

How to Live a Worry Free Life

Peace is the objective of many people rather than happiness or excitement. There are certain things that can be helpful to you in learning to live a worry free life.

First, you should remember who you are. You are a son or daughter of God if you have given your heart to the Lord. If you have not surrendered to Him, let this be the first order of business. Your eternal welfare is more important than your temporal welfare, as the eternal life is more important than the earthly life.

Live one day at a time. Worriers tend to make poor decisions. The happiest people are those who love the world around them. Do not feel that you must live your entire life in one day. While it is well to look at the future so you can plan the present, you must not worry about the future as it is in the hands of God.

Seek first the kingdom of God. This is a Bible injunction, and it makes good sense more than any other single option you have. You should covenant with God to spend one hour per day with Him in Bible study, prayer, and meditation on His Word.

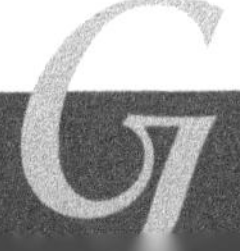

Guillain-Barre

This syndrome results from inflammation and destruction of the sheath that covers nerves. It results in progressive muscle weakness, and also in tingling or numbness. The symptoms usually spread upward from the legs to the arms and then the face. Generally it is said that the cause is unknown, but it was epidemic after the swine flu shots of the latter part of the twentieth century. It also occurs after many viral infections, after surgery, or such illnesses as AIDS. Most people recover gradually over several months. Physical therapy can help to regain strength and flexibility of muscles during the recovery process. Fomentations to muscles or extremities can also be very helpful.

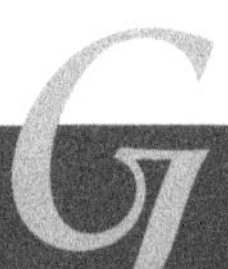

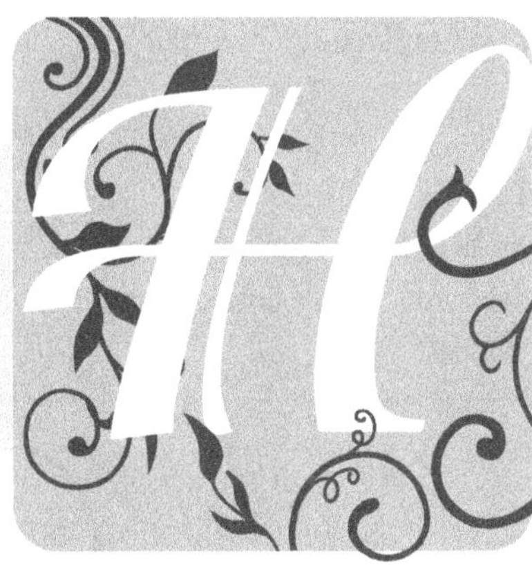

Hair Loss, Baldness, Alopecia

(See "Skin Diseases" in the *Conditions and Diseases* section.)

Hay Fever, Allergies, Sinusitis

(See "Allergies" in the *Conditions and Diseases* section.)

Head Injuries

Consumers Union Medical Consultants say that the head does not require X-rays, CT scans, or MRIs after most automobile accidents or with headaches unless the headaches are:

- accompanied by weakness of one or both limbs, loss of balance, or changes in vision or speech;
- accompanied by nausea, vomiting, fever, or disorientation;
- lasting longer than 24 hours;
- severe or frequent, even if they don't last long;
- worse on bending over, straining during bowel movements, coughing, or doing any other straining activity; and
- getting worse over the course of days or weeks.

Headaches

Headaches are invariably caused by some factor that can be discovered, and every attempt should be made to discover the cause of recurring headaches so as to eliminate it. Unless other symptoms are present, headaches are usually not serious. Skull X-rays and EEG's should not be done unless there are specific signs other than headache that indicate the need, such as loss of consciousness, confusion, disorientation or weakness, or numbness or paralysis in some part of the body. If a headache has been recurring for years, you can be certain it is not because of a brain cancer.

General, Tension, and Allergy Headaches

Tension headaches can continue for weeks or months with only brief periods of relief. The headache may begin any time of the day in contrast to other headaches that may come on mainly at night or upon awakening. It can often be described as a tight band, but it is rarely throbbing and never associated with fever. Exercise and gentle stretches greatly help to relieve tension.

Headaches because of poor health habits can be prevented by following the natural laws of health. Use general measures for the treatment of headaches.

Allergy-related headaches can be treated in the same way as those because of poor health habits. In addition it is important to discuss what food one is allergic to. (See the "Elimination and Challenge Diet" in the *Dietary Information* section.) Often inflamed sinuses are associated with a sinus headache. You can spot this kind of headache in that it usually begins during or after a bad cold and there is a postnasal

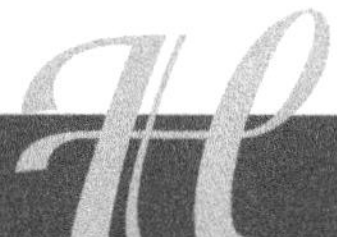

drip. It is often localized to one specific area of the face or head and comes on very quickly. It can be aggravated by coughing, sneezing, or sudden movements of the head, and it is usually worse in the morning before the sinus mucus has drained. It is intensified by alcohol, sudden temperature changes, winter, and going out into the cold.

Prevention

Avoid all exposure to toxins, tobacco, licit and illicit drugs, coffee (even if decaffeinated), tea, colas, chocolate, and any sweet drinks. Also avoid alcohol, odors, fumes, air pollution, rotting leaves or compost, or molds from shrubs or vines growing near the house.

Caffeine withdrawal is notorious for causing headaches. The headache often comes on one to three hours after taking the food, drink, or medication containing caffeine, but may sometimes not appear until one to three days later.

Morning headaches are often the result of stale air during the night. Keep fresh air in the bedroom.

Check during sleep time for an uncomfortable bed or pillow, or chilling of the head, neck and shoulders.

Keep the extremities warm at all times.

Keep a strictly regular schedule.

Never eat even so much as a peanut between meals.

Avoid eating too much protein, which can give you a "protein hangover."

Dispense with the third meal. Meals should be at least five hours apart.

Use a limited quantity and variety of food at meals. Do not mix fruits and vegetables at the same meal. Milk-sugar-egg combinations tend to cause intestinal fermentation, leading to headaches.

All dairy products tend to be associated with headaches, especially cheese. If you have difficulty accepting your recurring headaches are food related, as a test, for six weeks avoid all foods of animal origin—meat, milk, eggs, and cheese—then systematically remove other groups of the most suspect foods.

Check the intestinal transit time. Keep the time under 30 hours by using whole grains, extra bran, raw fruits and vegetables, exercise, plenty of water, and a regular schedule.

Practice deep breathing; learn to maintain good posture; and exercise from one to five hours daily out of doors.

Drink plenty of water, enough to keep the urine quite pale.

Prevent constipation, a common cause of headaches. (See "Constipation" in the *Conditions and Diseases* section.)

Doses of more than 25,000 IU (five times the RDA) of vitamin A can lead to liver damage, hair loss, blurred vision, and headaches.

Treatment

At the very beginning of a headache, soak both the feet and hands in hot water, with a cold compress to the head, for 20 minutes or more.

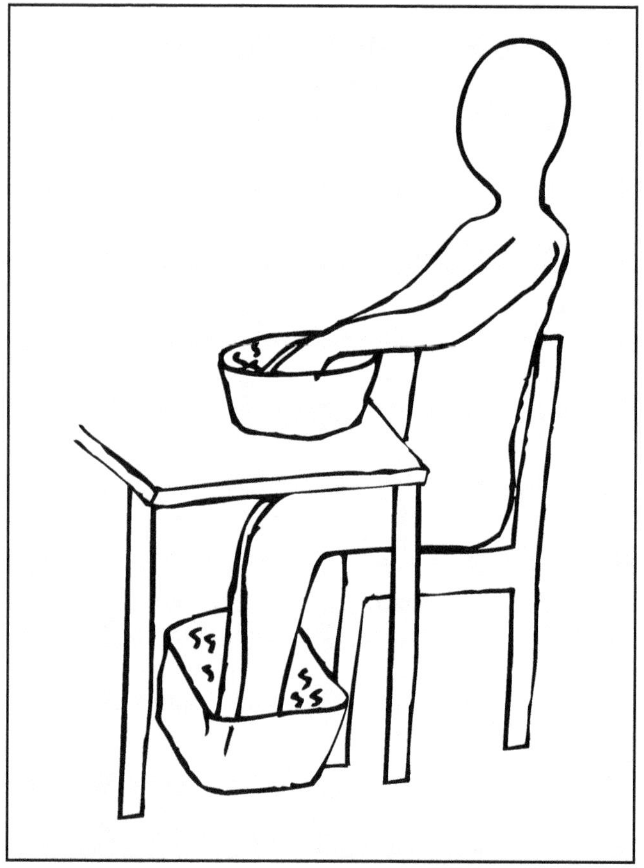

Some get relief from a neutral bath for 30 to 45 minutes.

Drink a cup of red clover tea or catnip tea at the onset of a headache. Try also black haw, feverfew, meadowsweet, white willow bark, and wild lettuce. Usually the teas are more beneficial when taken on a regular basis, not just at the time of pain.

Induce vomiting with the finger if undigested food is fermenting in the stomach, or take two to three heaping tablespoons of powdered charcoal. Eating too many varieties of foods at one meal is a common cause of headache. The many nutrients from the various foods, even though naturally produced, still are chemicals that make a war inside the system. For people with headaches it is wise to take two dishes at a meal of very simple foods such as baked potatoes and string beans along with bread and spread and a raw dish of some

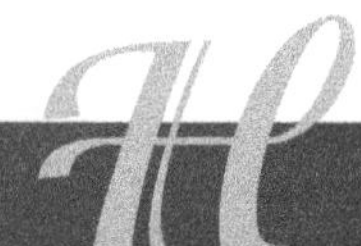

kind for salad such as sliced tomatoes, lettuce wedges, simple coleslaw, or fruit, etc.

Give enemas until clear, using hot water or charcoal water.

Take a brisk walk with the extremities well protected from dampness or chilling. Keep your head up, shoulders back, breathing deeply to relieve congestion.

A tension headache is best treated with a steam pack on the shoulders and back of the neck for 20 minutes, followed by massage of the neck and shoulders and finger stroking over the forehead and back through the hair to relax the scalp. A simultaneous hot foot bath will assist with the decongesting effect.

Maintain a sustained traction for 1 to 10 minutes on the head. Position the patient on a bed with the head so that you can seat yourself to hook the fingertips around the base of the skull and the angles and under-surfaces of the jaw and give gentle traction. The patient can direct the most favorable position for your fingertips and the amount of traction you give. While the patient is lying on his/her back, simply lay one hand on the forehead and place the other hand at the base of the skull at the neck. An occasional headache patient finds this so relaxing as to induce sleep.

Moving the head in such a way as to mobilize the vertebrae in the neck has a good effect on headaches in most cases. It is always worth a try to do an exercise for neck muscles and a complete range of motion in all possible head movements (*Journal of Orthopedics and Sports Physical Therapists* 21, no. 4 [April 1995]: 184).

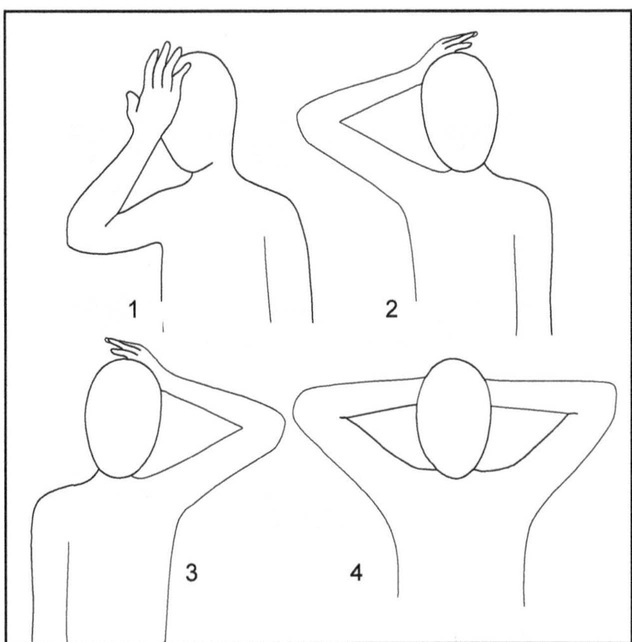

Muscle spasm in the neck sometimes because of injury can be relieved by strengthening the overly stressed muscles. This will relieve headaches. A good exercise for the neck muscles requires the patient to press the head into the heel of the hand with as much force as possible, holding it for 10 seconds; first the forehead, then over the right ear, then the left and finally pressing backward into the clasped hands.

Peppermint oil is an effective pain-killer without the side effects of aspirin and similar drugs. Just dab a little on the forehead, temples, and nape of the neck.

Migraines

Migraine headaches are usually one sided and may change sides from time to time, occurring anywhere in the head, face, or neck. They may be preceded by visual disturbances—blurring, spots before the eyes, etc. Nausea and vomiting are common as the attacks come on.

Migraine patients may have a deficiency of omega-3 fatty acids and an increase in platelet serotonin release (a brain neurotransmitter contributing to migraines). Omega-3 fatty acids may help to moderate migraine headaches and rheumatoid arthritis symptoms.

Prevention

Migraine headaches appear most often in a tense meticulous and obsessional person who tends to have allergies. Treat the person with prayer, study, and counsel to receive insights to correct these personality traits. A well ordered, temperate life is essential.

Attacks are triggered by numerous factors other than allergies such as overeating, gastrointestinal upsets, emotional stress and resentment, hypothyroidism, fatigue, bright or flickering lights, bright sunlight, a cold wind on the face or forehead, high altitudes, chilling, constipation, salty foods, the menstrual period, too little sleep, smoking, chocolate, mushrooms, seafood, fried foods, caffeinated beverages, food additives, antibiotics, odors and inhalants, and foods containing cheese, Chianti wines, chicken liver, pickled herring, monosodium glutamate, cured meats, pressed meat and pork products, as well as other factors.

The most important feature of preventing migraines is discovering those foods to which one is sensitive and removing them from the diet. (See the "Elimination and Challenge Diet" in the *Dietary Information* section.)

Remember that drugs can cause migraines as well as foods, especially birth control pills and caffeine.

Avoid tyramine, a metabolic product from tyrosine, an amino acid. Tyramine is found in various cheeses, wines,

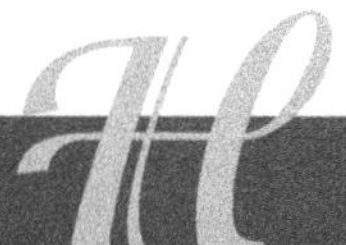

avocados, raspberries, plums, oranges, and bananas. Except for cheeses and wines, the others contain very small amounts.

An excellent herbal preventive for migraines is feverfew, a member of the chrysanthemum family. Drink a cup three times a day. If the herb is not available, use two capsules three times a day. Since the powdered herb in the capsules is not well absorbed, it may be necessary after a week to increase to three or even four capsules, three times a day if migraines continue. This herb may do little or nothing for the acute headache, but double blind studies in England show it to be a very capable preventive. It also has anti-inflammatory effects.

Migraine headaches can be caused by medication actually given *for* migraines. Persons who take pain medication on a regular basis can have what is called the rebound effect that happens after the medication for the acute headache begins to wear off. Medications that cause vasoconstriction such as Midrin, eventually cause blood vessels to swell more when the drug wears off, requiring higher doses to get the same effect. Caffeine-containing medications such as Excedrin can also have a rebound effect.

Many foods are involved in triggering migraines. Sometimes a food will trigger a migraine within a few hours, but the next time it is eaten a headache does not develop. The person then thinks the food is not involved whereas it is one of the culprits. It takes most people about two months to learn how to get the maximum benefit from a migraine-preventive diet.

Diet, exercise, and adequate sleep go far toward keeping women who get migraines at the time of their menstrual period from having headaches (*Medical Tribune* 40, no. 6 [1999]: 25).

A group of migraine sufferers showed a 50 percent reduction in frequency of headaches after they began engaging in vigorous exercise 30 minutes per day, three days a week (*The Physician and Sports Medicine* 9, no. 8 [1981]: 24, 25).

Treatment

Alternate hot and cold to the head using the following procedure: hot water bottle or hot fomentation to the base of the head and cervical spine, ice water compress to the face and temples, ears, and forehead. After three minutes switch the hot for cold compresses, and the cold for hot compresses. Give three complete sets of hot and cold. Always use with a moderately hot foot bath, 103°F to 106°F.

Some headaches may continue unabated, or recur. If so, try the following variation of the above treatment. Simultaneous hot and cold to the head: ice bag to the base of the skull, a second ice bag to the forehead, and ice bags or ice compresses over both carotids in the neck; a simultaneous application of hot compresses on the face, covering the ears and forehead. Maintain the treatment from five to 45 minutes or more, determined by the reaction of the patient. If the headache abates quickly, discontinue the treatment, but continue even for several hours if it persists. Always use with a moderately hot foot bath, 103°F to 106°F, unless the patient has insulin-dependant diabetes. This person should not have a hot foot bath at temperatures over 102°F.

Rest in a darkened room with an ice cap to the head.

Re-breathe into a paper bag for 10 to 20 minutes off and on as many times as you can.

Get in a very hot shower, head and all, and rotate around and around until you are red all over (about 12 to 15 minutes), then turn off the hot water and turn on the cold, continuing to rotate until you are shivering. Then dry off and rest in bed for 45 minutes.

Apply light pressure on the neck over the carotid arteries, applying the pressure for a few seconds only one side at a time.

At the first sign of a migraine—dizziness, blurred vision, black or colored spots in the visual field, nausea, etc., try the following procedure:

- Seat the person in a chair with the head hanging between the knees.
- Apply a gentle flow of ice water to the base of the skull, allowing it to flow forward through the hair roots over the scalp for 45 seconds. Catch the run-off water in a pan placed between the feet. Briefly dry the hair and scalp by blotting with a towel, taking no more than 10 seconds.

Allow the person to sit up promptly after the water pouring procedure, elevating the feet on a stool. Direct a stream of cold water under pressure if possible, to the soles of the feet for one and a half minutes. If water under pressure is not available, use one quart of ice water poured over the feet for 90 seconds. You will need a time keeper.

- After the cold water pour, apply pressure to the temples with the heels of the hands, exerting as much pressure as can be generated between the palms, for two to five minutes. Gradually reduce the pressure—do not suddenly let go—using about one minute to accomplish the full release.
- Repeat every two hours until the headache is gone.

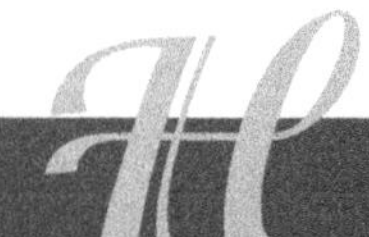

- In treating migraines it is sometimes necessary to go through your entire arsenal of treatments. Sit for a while at the head of the patient and simply lay one hand on the forehead and place the other hand at the base of the skull at the neck. Even this simple touch can often bring some relief. Then start all treatments over again. Sometimes a second application is more effective than the first time, sometimes less.

A frequently neglected treatment for migraines is an enema. (See "Hydrotherapy" in the *Natural Remedies* section.)

Persons who suffer from recurring migraine headaches may find good results, both preventing the headaches, as well as treating one that has occurred, by taking 200 milligrams of magnesium daily (*Headache* 31 [1991]: 298). Magnesium sulfate is probably best.

One sufferer from migraines says that if she catches her migraine very early, she can take five to six ginger root capsules and two valerian capsules and that will stop her migraine.

Use an extract of cayenne pepper applied inside the nose on the same side as the headache. (See cluster headaches below for method.) The migraine will almost always stop within five minutes of the application. The treatment is not as painful as one might think.

Wrap a tight bandage around the head in such a way as to compress the swollen blood vessels at the temples and forehead. A headband made of elastic material can be of great help in migraine patients. The elastic headband can be sewed, securing it with velcro and inserting rubber disks for additional local pressure over the areas of maximum pain. The rubber disks should be firm, about one centimeter in thickness and three centimeters in diameter. These can be slipped under the elastic band, one or more disks layered at one spot once the pain reaches above 5 on a scale of 0 to 10. The amount of pressure exerted by the band should be determined by the patient. Thirty minutes of the band in place and 30 minutes with the band off can be effective in some patients. Repeat if needed. In one study 60 out of 69 headaches were relieved by the use of the band.

Other Forms of Headaches

Bleeding Into the Brain

A sudden blinding generalized headache that continues despite any kind of treatment, especially if it is in an older person and associated with a stiff neck, raises the possibility of internal bleeding. A physician should be consulted immediately.

Cluster Headache

It occurs mostly in men and is often situated behind one eye. Cluster headaches come on suddenly, become very intense, and disappear usually in about half an hour. It does not fluctuate in severity once established, but may be worse in the morning, aggravated by exertion, straining, coughing, sneezing, lifting, or triggered by alcohol. They may occur several times a day for weeks and then stop for several months, only to start again. Successive recurrences may be characterized by worsening.

A water extract of cayenne pepper applied inside the nostril on the same side of the cluster headache, can stop a cluster headache attack and can be curative after about 5 to 10 days of applications four to six times daily. The application can be from a squirt or spray bottle or may be done with a cotton tip applicator.

Fever Headaches

Treat the fever, and the headache will disappear. (See "Fevers" in the *Conditions and Diseases* section.)

Glaucoma Headaches

Successful treatment of the glaucoma will cure the headaches. (See "Glaucoma" in the *Conditions and Diseases* section.)

Head Injuries

Even a small injury in elderly persons can cause internal bleeding. Any unusual headache that persists may require a physician to make the diagnosis.

High Blood Pressure Headaches

(See "Blood Clotting, Anticoagulation, Intravascular Clotting" in the *Conditions and Diseases* section.)

Ice Cream Headaches

Drinking or eating icy cold beverages or food can give some people a headache. These persons must either avoid ice cold food or drinks, or must take only tiny bites and hold it in the mouth until warm before swallowing.

Medication Headaches

Drugs such as nitroglycerine and related drugs (Isordil or Isosorbide Dinitrate), antibiotics, hormones, heart medications, and almost any kind of medications can be

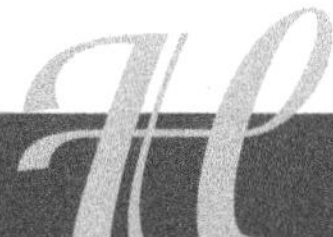

associated with headaches. Also, black cohosh can cause headaches if taken in large quantities.

Temporal Arteritis

This kind of headache is serious and often exhibits impaired vision and pain in the temple on chewing. It is associated with aches and pains all over the body, sometimes fever and weight loss. It is localized to one side of the head and has a tender spot near the ear opening.

Temporal arteritis is very difficult to treat and requires attention to detail. The first item on your treatment schedule is to institute all known laws of health. That includes getting plenty of fresh air in your bedroom at night, using the most favorable diet possible—a plant-based diet with no free fats of any kind (margarine, butter, mayonnaise, fried foods, cooking fats, salad oils, and all nut butters)—avoiding excessive salt, all spices, free sugars, including honey, and any food you know will hurt you. Strict control of the diet is mandatory as is determining if there are any food allergies.

Fomentations over the painful area and fever treatments may be helpful. (See "Hydrotherapy" in the *Natural Remedies* section.)

Treat the patient in much the same way we suggest for lupus. Some believe this disorder to be a form of an autoimmune disease.

Painting the tender spot four to six times daily with the cayenne extract described above for cluster headaches may bring some relief. After relief comes, the applications can be reduced to twice a day.

Exercise should be taken in the amount that is correct for you. It should be described as vigorous, but not violent. Water should be taken in sufficient quantity to cause your urine to be quite pale. Use purified, distilled, well, or spring water.

Be out in the sun either early in the morning or late in the day for at least 15 minutes on every sunny day. You may be fully clothed while sunning on cold days.

Get adequate rest at night, going to bed at least two hours before midnight, and preferably three. A short nap, even five minutes, but up to half an hour, before lunch every day rather than after lunch, is very helpful to boost the functioning of the immune system.

Temporomandibular Joint Syndrome, TMJ Syndrome Headaches

(See "Dental Care" in the *Conditions and Diseases* section.)

Trigeminal neuralgia—Tic douloureux

This kind of headache develops mainly in middle age and older persons and is an inflammation of the fifth cranial nerve, a major nerve in the face. Shooting pains that last only a few seconds are caused by a trigger activity such as brushing the teeth, chewing, touching a sensitive spot on the face, talking, and yawning. Hot compresses and fever treatments may be helpful, as will determining any food allergies. The cayenne extract should be rubbed over the area, both inside the mouth as well as on the side of the face four to six times daily for 10 days. See instructions under cluster headaches above.

There are persons practicing the healing arts usually as chiropractors or naturopaths who use apitherapy (bee stings for treatments) and declare it to be curative for tic douloureux. I would certainly give it a try if I had this distressing condition.

Hearing Loss

Nearly all drugs currently used for arthritis cause ringing in the ears and some degree of hearing loss. After stopping the drugs, it quickly goes away. Other drugs, however, including some antibiotics, can cause complete inner ear destruction with total and permanent deafness.

Dr. Norman Childer describes hearing problems that people get who have aches and pains when they ingest mint, either mint candy or mint tea. Usually the problems go away in a few days after stopping the mint.

A build-up of ear wax can cause loss of hearing, a feeling of fullness in the ears, earache, or rattling or ringing in the ear. To remove the wax, follow these steps:

- Soften the wax by applying a few drops of mineral oil with an eye dropper twice a day for several days.
- Fill a three-ounce rubber bulb syringe with water at body temperature. With the head upright pull the top of the ear up and back. Then gently squirt the water into the ear canal, directing the stream at one wall or other, not straight into the ear, unless the syringe is kept a quarter inch outside the ear to avoid putting pressure on the internal structure of the ear.

  The process must be repeated several times until the wax appears in the drainage water, which can take 10 to 30 minutes or more. Sometimes, if you are fortunate, it is dislodged in the first few squirts. Catch the run off water in a bowl held just under the ear with

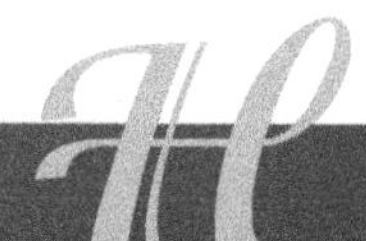

a large towel placed under that to protect the person from spills.

Dry the outer ear with a towel and the inner ear with an eye dropper full of rubbing alcohol. Then tip the head to drain the alcohol. Have the patient dry the ear with a thin towel or tissue over the little finger, not with a cotton-tipped applicator as it might be inserted too far and push wax deep within the ear canal or next to the eardrum.

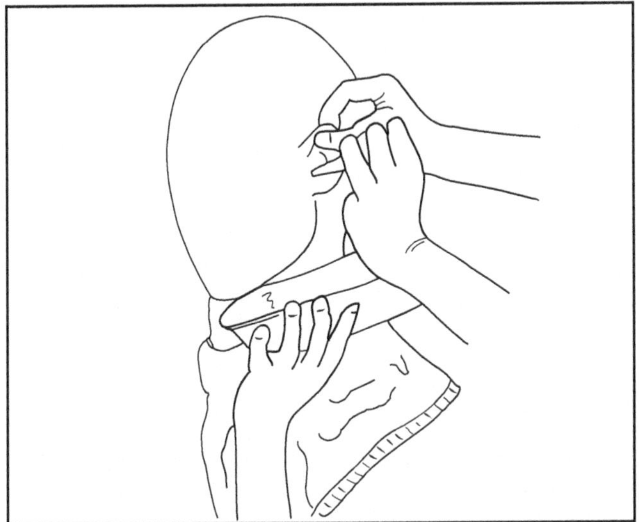

Babies are often born hearing impaired because of loud noises from machinery or other noisy sources experienced during the prenatal time. Sounds of greater than 85 decibels intensity reaching the fetus through the mother's abdomen may not only damage the ears but can cause growth retardation and prematurity. Machinery noise is most often to blame. The average city bus emits about 80 decibels, just below the safe upper limit, whereas a moving subway train is about 100 decibels, which is well above it. The mother's voice is the sound most often reaching the fetus, and when she is speaking loudly, its intensity in the uterus is just under 85 decibels because of the better transmission through the mother's tissues.

Just after birth, during the first few days, babies may be injured by noise of only 45 decibels intensity. We can warn expectant mothers not to work in noisy factories and certainly not to try to shout above the noise of machinery.

The noise of jack hammers, chain saws, and blenders can cause a reduction in hearing if it lasts long enough. There is a special muscle that reflexively tightens the eardrum to prevent the drum's vibrations from being big enough to injure the inner ear. Alcohol and sedatives interfere with this reflex muscle tightening, and increase the likelihood of getting injury to the inner ear from continued loud noises—another reason for avoiding alcohol or sedatives. The longer the loud noise continues, the more likely it is to cause injury.

Protective earmuffs or ear plugs should be used when operating guns, hair driers, lawn mowers, vacuums, leaf blowers, blenders, and other kitchen machines, and when any loud noise is near you. Noise so loud that it interferes with our hearing other people's conversation, that causes a ringing in the ears, or even temporarily causes hearing loss can be hazardous. Exposure over a lifetime to loud noises causes loss of hearing in older people. This damage is permanent, and the hearing loss it causes develops progressively over a period of many decades.

The following sounds and their related decibels show you when damage to your hearing may occur:

1. The softest sound a healthy young adult can hear is 0 decibels (dB).
2. A whisper or background room noise is 30 dB.
3. Rainfall, a breeze, or a refrigerator is about 50 dB.
4. Normal conversation or an air conditioner is about 60 dB.
5. City traffic or a crowded restaurant is about 70 dB. Noise at 70 dB with constant exposure may begin to damage your hearing.
6. An alarm clock, heavy traffic, or vacuum cleaner is 80 dB.
7. A motorcycle, lawn mower, or heavy truck is 90 dB.
8. A jet plane taking off is 120 dB, about the same as a close up blender at top speed.
9. A cheering crowd at an athletic event can reach 125 dB.
10. A live rock concert is 130 dB.
11. A gunshot or firecracker is 140 dB. At that level, exposure without earplugs may be damaging.

Heart

Congestive Heart Failure

This is the condition that results from the inability of the heart to beat forcefully to completely empty all blood from the heart with each heartbeat. Causes include previous heart attacks, high blood pressure, atrial fibrillation, rheumatic heart disease, myocarditis, and other causes.

Persons with congestive heart failure (CHF) benefit from exercise. Being prescribed rest as we once did for CHF has a depressing effect on most patients, but an exercise

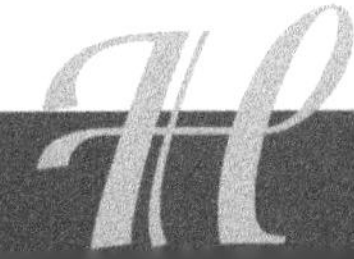

program maintained for 12 weeks in one study showed no adverse effects. Patients reported greater physical stamina, better respiratory function, and improvements in quality of life (*European Heart Journal* 20 [1999]: 851). Arterial blood flow is improved in congestive heart failure by exercise, possibly by increasing the release of nitric oxide by blood vessels. Nitric oxide relaxes arterioles, thus increasing blood flow and reducing blood pressure. Walking more than four hours a week significantly reduces the risk of heart disease or death from heart disease in the elderly (*Journal of American Geriatrics Society* 44 [1996]: 113–20).

Digoxin used for congestive heart failure *may* improve the quality of life *but* does not increase the length of the life (*New England Journal of Medicine* 336 [1997]: 525). With carefully selected exercise and herbs, and a determination to stick with it, much can be done with these simple measures to improve the quality of life as much or more than with pharmaceuticals. You will be very fortunate if you have a physician who will work with you on such a program and check on your progress.

Follow a diet absolutely free from salt and dairy products until the condition is under control. These foods cause the retention of fluid.

CoQ10, available from health food stores, has been shown since 1976 to be of value in congestive heart failure. Even 30 milligrams daily will help mild congestive heart failure in most; 200 to 400 milligrams per day can be used for more severe heart failure (*Clinical Investigation* 71 [1993]; S134-6).

Persons with congestive heart failure were given exercise tolerance tests on days 7, 28, and 56 of a study comparing hawthorn berry with Captopril for eight weeks. Nine hundred milligrams of hawthorn extract or 37.5 milligrams of Captopril were administered daily. Both groups showed a 50 percent decrease in shortness of breath and fatigue after exercise. No adverse effects were reported using hawthorn, and, of course, none would be expected since hawthorne is a close relative of apples. Considering the potentially serious side effects of Captopril as well as other pharmaceuticals, we strongly recommend the herbs. Some of these serious side effects include very low white blood cell count, serious or even life-threatening allergic reactions, kidney damage, extremely low blood pressure, and others.

A very good diuretic is made of burdock, and a mixture of equal quantities of dandelion leaf, corn silk, and buchu. Take a tablespoon of burdock and a quart of water and simmer gently for one-half hour. Pour into a container with one tablespoon of a mixture of dandelion, cornsilk, and buchu. Let it steep for half an hour, strain and drink daily in about four doses. Make it up fresh every day. If more diuretic activity is needed, increase the herb mixture from one tablespoon to three tablespoons, but do not increase the burdock.

Hawthorne berry, one tablespoon simmered gently in a quart of water for 20 minutes, set off the heat, to which is added one tablespoon of yarrow and one dandelion leaf and steeped, covered for 30 minutes, can be taken daily in four doses. This mixture is quite good for CHF or atrial fibrillation.

Heart Attacks

Approximately 1.2 million people a year in the United States have an acute heart attack and about 50 percent die. Of these deaths, between 50 and 65 percent occur before the patient reaches a hospital. About 25 percent of the deaths occur within 10 minutes of the onset of symptoms. Those patients who are at high risk include middle-aged men with high blood pressure, diabetes, high blood cholesterol or triglycerides, a family history of heart attacks, a history of heavy cigarette smoking, and/or preexisting angina.

The usual cause of myocardial infarction is a blocked coronary artery. This condition is usually associated with an elevated homocysteine level, cholesterol level, and triglyceride level in the blood, and a history of heart attacks in the family.

Definition and Symptoms

The death of a portion of the heart muscle usually causes acute pain in the chest and is associated with fever and multiple other signs and symptoms such as nausea, low blood pressure, vomiting, sweating, shortness of breath, and bluish lips and fingernails. The pain is generally severe and prolonged and described as intolerable, crushing, clutching, and viselike with a sense of impending doom or agony.

The pain may continue for hours. It may be confined to the chest, or it may be referred to the upper abdomen, down the left arm or right arm, up into the left jaw or head, or to the back of the left chest. When the pain is referred to the right upper abdominal quadrant and back, it may be confused with acute gallbladder pain. When confined to the upper abdomen, especially if it comes on suddenly and is associated with dilation of the stomach, an acute surgical abdomen may be suspected. There may be abdominal signs such as muscle rigidity and guarding, fever and elevated white blood cell count, which can often confuse the diagnosis. The patient may believe he has "acute indigestion." Some patients feel as if they must belch but can't. Later, the left hand may become

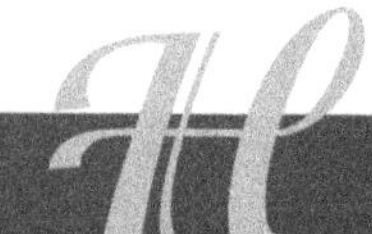

swollen, glossy, stiff, and painful on motion and be labeled, "shoulder-hand syndrome."

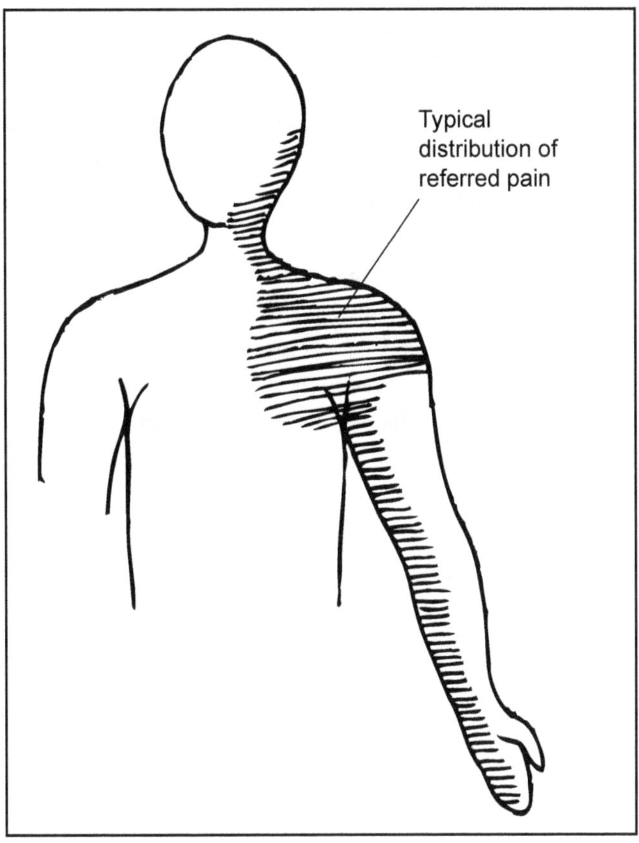

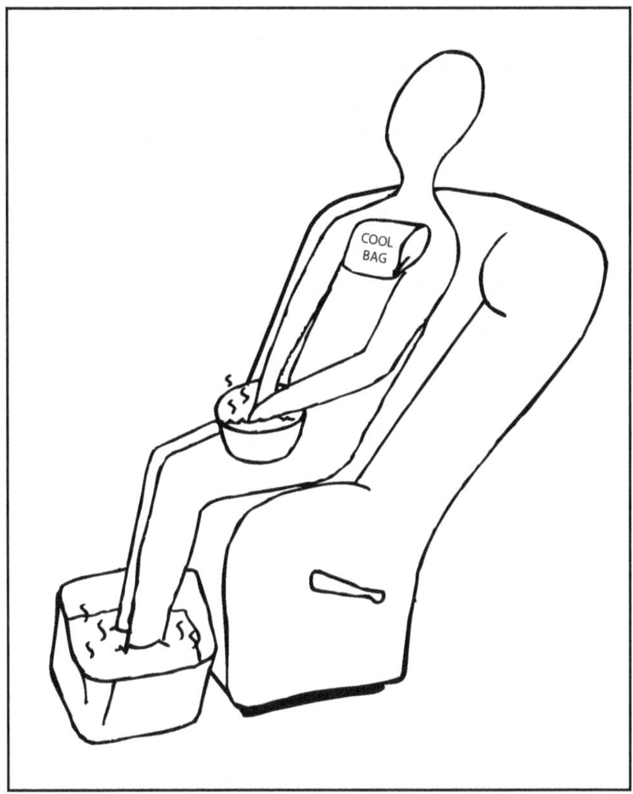

First Aid for the Acute Attack

1. Sit in a seat with a back, preferably leaning slightly backward in a semi-reclining or semi-sitting position. Do not lie down.
2. Sip a glass of water at room or tap temperature, never ice water. Empty the entire glass within five minutes.
3. Put an ice bag over the heart and keep all four extremities warm to decongest the heart.
4. Put the hands in very warm water, a large bowl on each side. Set the feet in a tub of warm water. Gradually add hot water to the tubs to make both the hands and feet hot unless the patient has insulin dependant diabetes, in which case treat only the hands. The ice bag over the heart and the heat to the extremities redistributes the circulation, decongesting the heart and lowering elevated blood pressure. Interestingly, if the heart is not congested, and the blood pressure is not elevated, the treatment will have minimal effect. Therefore, one need not fear any harm from this treatment.
5. Get fresh air.
6. If available, sniff peppermint oil.
7. Take a large amount of garlic—three cloves or a triple dose of extract—right away. The capsules or tablets may be taken with cool (not cold) water. Drink a large glassful.
8. Massage extremities and back. Full body massage causes hemodilution and a fall in blood viscosity, which improves the ease of blood flow and reduces the workload on the heart. Heart attacks are frequently associated with a high hemoglobin or high blood concentration (*Physiotherapy* 73 [January 1987]: 43–5).
9. Take a quarter to one-half teaspoon of cayenne mixed with a little water and swallow. Even if only held in the mouth, it could save your life by dilating coronary arteries and strengthening the heartbeat. Arnica tincture taken by mouth is also said to be lifesaving in a heart attack.
10. Don't take any food or beverages by mouth except for water or herb teas. Hawthorn berry should be given as soon as it can be prepared. Put one tablespoon of the freshly ground berries in one cup of gently simmering water for 25 minutes. Repeat the dose every two hours until pain subsides. Avoid coffee, alcohol, and tobacco.

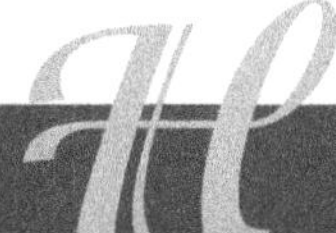

11. Give one teaspoon of magnesium sulfate (Epsom salts) in a glass of cool water. Magnesium has been found to reduce the incidence of death and the frequency of arrhythmia when given within 24 to 48 hours after a suspected heart attack. Give one tablespoonful immediately to anyone experiencing chest pain for more than 20 minutes.
12. Make a potassium broth by boiling the peelings of two potatoes in two to four cups of water until the potato peelings are well cooked. Pour off the water and drink it, unsalted.
13. Get complete rest in bed for five days apart from using the restroom and eating meals while sitting comfortably in the bedroom.
14. Do not strain when having a bowel movement. Use a small cold enema if necessary, administered as one-half cup of cold water to initiate a reflex to defecate.

Heart Disease

Heavy proteins in the diet increase the likelihood of developing high blood cholesterol and hardening of the arteries. Several proteins were studied for their ability to cause these disorders in the blood and arteries. In order of their ability to produce these disorders, soy protein was at the bottom of the list, next up was wheat gluten, then pork, beef, lactalbumin (from milk), skim milk, and whole eggs, which was the worst. The release of insulin is controlled to a large degree by the type of protein one eats. With plant protein the quantity of insulin the pancreas must produce goes down, but with animal protein insulin goes up. A high level of insulin in the blood is a predictor for cardiovascular disease independent of all other factors. Subsequent studies indicate even a protective factor for proteins from beans, vegetables, greens, and fruit.

Both bananas and potatoes are known to make cholesterol go down as these foods are high in potassium. Top potassium sources include broccoli, tomatoes, and orange juice. Breakfast brings many advantages. One is that it keeps the blood cholesterol level lower than without it. Eating breakfast is the best possible method of keeping a proper control of the appetite. (See "Food Sources of Certain Nutrients" in the *Dietary Information* section.)

A 10 to 15 pound weight gain after age 18 should be taken seriously as it indicates that diet and exercise alterations are required if one wishes to avoid heart disease later in life. Women are especially at risk, having a 25 percent greater than normal risk of heart disease compared to those who maintain the same weight. If one gains as much as 25 pounds after the age of 18, there is a 65 percent increased risk, 200 percent for those gaining up to 44 pounds, and 300 percent for those gaining more than 44 pounds (*Journal of the American Medical Association* 273 [1995]: 481).

Women who ate five ounces of nuts a week were only 65 percent as likely to suffer from coronary artery disease, including fatal heart attacks, as those who rarely ate nuts (*Clinical Pearls News*, March 1999). Coronary heart disease is 50 percent decreased in men eating one ounce (two tablespoons) of walnuts per day compared to men eating no walnuts. Blood platelets are less sticky. Triglycerides, cholesterol, and blood pressure are lowered, apparently because of a high content of omega-3 fatty acids.

A study done by researchers from Harvard and the University of Minnesota on 34,486 post-menopausal woman over seven years revealed that those who regularly consumed diets highest in vitamin E were 62 percent less likely to die of heart disease than those whose diets were not rich in vitamin E (*New England Journal of Medicine,* May 2, 1996). Beans, nuts, seeds, green leafy vegetables, and whole grains are high in vitamin E.

Get six to nine hours of sleep each night. Take time to rest when needed during the day, including short naps.

Healthy appearing older women who were found to have an ankle/arm index of 0.9 or less are at high risk of death during the next four years. Persons in this group died not only from heart disease, but also other cardiovascular diseases, cancer, and several other causes. The method for testing is that of comparing the systolic blood pressure in the arm with that in the leg (the brachial, at the elbow, and the posterior tibial, behind the knee or on the foot). Those women with a positive test should be aggressively treated with lifestyle change (*Journal of the American Medical Association* 270 [1993]: 465).

Usually a casual blood pressure reading taken after five minutes of lying down is considered an appropriate measure of blood pressure. But it has been shown that blood pressure taken during six minutes of moderately vigorous exercise was a better predictor of the development of a heart attack with either sickness or death resulting. Among 520 men with a casual blood pressure at around 140, about half increased their systolic blood pressure to 200 during the six minutes of exercise. These men had about twice the risk (18.8 versus 9.5 percent) as the 1,294 men with a casual blood pressure less than 140 and an exercise blood pressure less than 200. More than half (58 percent) of those suffering a heart attack died compared with 33 percent for all other groups having heart attacks, including those with a casual blood pressure of 140

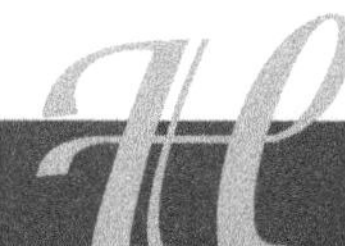

and an exercise blood pressure less than 200 (*Hypertension* 27, no. 1 [1996]: 324).

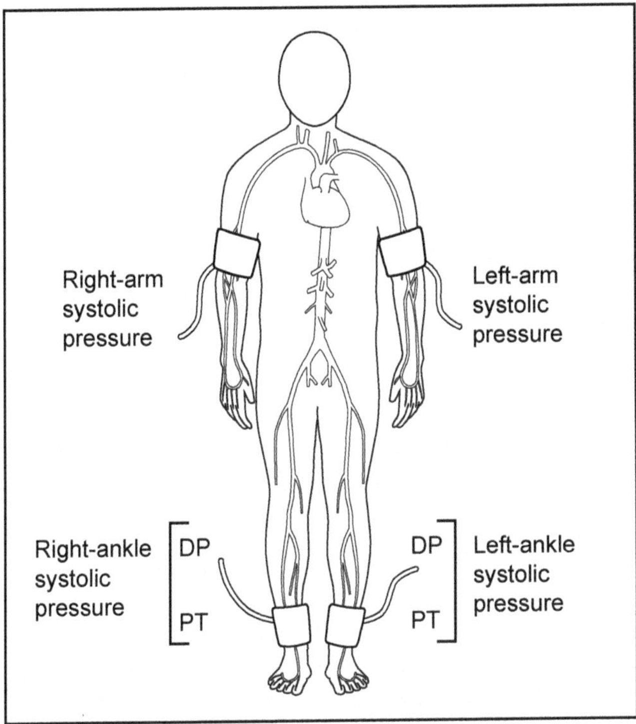

Moderate activity through gardening can reduce the risk of heart attacks about as well as jogging or aerobic exercise. Brisk walking for at least an hour a week lowers the cardiovascular risk by 73 percent, whereas gardening reduced the risk by 66 percent according to a 1998 study by the University of Washington Cardiovascular Health Research Unit in Seattle.

The size of red blood cell clusters or clumps fluctuates, depending on the flow speed and friction qualities of the blood and blood vessels. The lower the rate of flow, the larger the aggregates formed. This accounts in part for the desirability of remaining active following meals. Heart and cancer patients usually show higher degrees of aggregation than well persons. The more clumps or aggregates, the greater the viscosity. An increase in blood viscosity usually comes before the appearance of symptoms. Cigarette smoking increases blood viscosity as does chronic anxiety, dehydration, etc (*Blood Viscosity in Heart Disease and Cancer*, eds. L. Dintenfass and G.V.F. Seaman [Pergamon Press, 1981]).

There is a direct association between high body iron levels and the risk of coronary heart disease. Periodic blood donations to the Red Cross can be very helpful in this situation (*Clinical Cardiology* 19 [December 1996]: 925–9). Several studies have shown that men having a higher blood level of iron as measured in ferritin have an increased risk of suffering a heart attack. It has also been observed that after menopause women's blood iron goes up and their incidence of heart attacks also increases proportionate to the increase in iron. Male blood donors have an 88 percent reduced risk of suffering a heart attack compared to a group of non-blood donors of the same age. During a nine-year period, 2,862 men age 42 to 60 showed this marked difference. Only one man in every 153 who donated blood in the 24 months preceding their first evaluation suffered a heart attack compared to one in eight who did not donate blood (*American Journal of Epidemiology* 148 [1998]: 445).

Remember that stressful emotions are wearing on the body and mind. Therefore, move constantly toward becoming gentle, appreciative, loving, and lovable.

People with gum infections have three times the heart attack risk of people with healthy gums (*Psychology and Health Update* 9, no. 1 [January-February 1999]: 2). Pyorrhea (peridontitis) is a marker for hardening of the arteries. Researchers at the University of North Carolina's School of Dentistry found that people with periodontitis are more likely than others to have hardening of the arteries and heart attacks. This is not the first research that indicates poor dental hygiene as a factor in general disease. If you have gum or tooth disease, it may be to your advantage to get an electric toothbrush that gives a more thorough brushing at the gum line than can be done by an ordinary toothbrush (*Lancet* 352 [1998]: 121).

Minimize the environmental toxins to which you are exposed such as automobile exhaust fumes, chlorinated water, industrial emissions, and cigarette smoke.

By taking one tablespoon of powdered charcoal in water four times a day for three to six months, serum triglycerides will fall an average of 36 percent and serum cholesterol by an average of 67 percent.

Zinc may be a factor in heart attacks, especially if there is a deficiency of copper, which acts to balance zinc. Copper prevents cardiovascular disease, whereas zinc may promote it. Excessive intake of zinc by humans—100 to 150 milligrams per day—was implicated as a cause of heart rhythm disturbance, high blood cholesterol, and heart disease. While zinc stabilizes cell membranes, has an anti-inflammatory effect, promotes wound healing, and improves immune functioning, too much can harm the heart. If zinc is taken as a supplement, copper is also needed in supplement (*Indian Journal of Medical Research* 94 [1991]: 316–9).

Dr. Castele of Framingham Heart Study states that measurement of total HDL cholesterol should be made in every age group, including newborn infants. The cord blood from an infant would identify one of every 20 babies who should

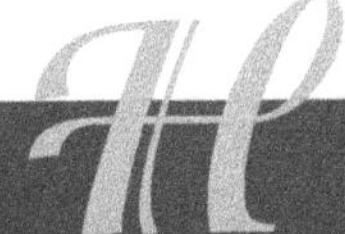

be put on a soy formula if they are not breast fed. Average HDL cholesterol for men is 45 milligrams and for women 55 milligrams, possibly accounting for lower rates of coronary heart disease in women than men.

Apolipoprotein B-100 (Apo-B), which is made in the liver, is a better predictor of atherosclerosis than cholesterol or LDL levels. Apo-B is the key to LDL-cholesterol receptors pulling in LDL from blood as it is the part that connects with the receptor. Some people have only one (not the usual two) genes for LDL receptors on cells, and some have no genes for this—only one in a million Americans. They are handicapped in dealing with cholesterol.

Alpha-lipoprotein A is 10 times more toxic to the heart and arteries than LDL. This substance can be measured in some laboratories.

In the physical examination, checking a patient's waist-hip ratios should be as routine as checking the weight. The American Heart Association recommends a waist-to-hip ratio for women of no more than 0.80 and for a man no more than 1.00. A ratio much under these figures is quite a lot better. To calculate waist-to-hip ratio, stand relaxed without pulling in the abdomen and measure the waist at the level of the navel. Then measure the hips over the buttocks where the hips are the largest. Finally, divide the waist measurement by the hip measurement.

Cholesterol, Atherosclerosis, and Stress

In addition to the total fat contained in it, animal muscle tissue of all kinds—beef, pork, lamb, poultry, fish, shellfish, etc., and especially organ tissue (liver, brain, kidney, etc.) and eggs (chicken eggs, fish roe, etc,)—introduce preformed cholesterol. While some cholesterol is needed by the body, it can produce all it requires.

Stress hormones and sex hormones both use cholesterol as a part of their molecules, and those who are under emotional tension will find this to be a cause of elevated blood cholesterol. The body can handle (although not so easily) the amount of cholesterol present in about three ounces of animal protein (meat, fish, etc.) daily. That would be a small piece of food approximately 1 x 1 x 3 inches. Any more than that gets stored in the blood and tissues. The excess stored cholesterol forms plaques inside the blood vessels, and in time, these plaques begin to ulcerate and give off fragments that travel in the blood to organs such as the lungs or brain. This condition is known as atherosclerosis. In some countries atherosclerosis is almost unknown and cholesterol levels run 60 to 90, whereas in the Western world, which has a diet high in animal products, cholesterol levels run 200 to 250 or more. The ideal for an American should probably run no more than around 100 plus the age. The heart attack rate is four times higher if the cholesterol is more than 260, than if it is below 200. A mere 10 percent reduction in cholesterol reduces by about 25 percent the likelihood of a heart attack.

To understand how free fats cause problems for the body, we need to observe what happens after we eat free fats. It enters the blood as microscopic fat balls. These can stick onto red blood cells, causing them to clump together in formation resembling stacks of coins. These have lost much of their efficiency in picking up and transporting oxygen and carbon dioxide.

This process of depriving the body cells of oxygen is one of the causes of atherosclerotic plaques. The artery walls become much more easily penetrated by fats and cholesterol when the blood that bathes them is deficient in oxygen, thus encouraging the plaques to form. The plaques cause a gradual deterioration in hearing, vision, joint function, digestion, and finally, brain function, leading to senility. With a change to a proper diet and lifestyle, the plaques will begin to shrink and gradually disappear so that near normal circulation will be restored.

A low level of thyroid function can cause the cholesterol to rise. Both low thyroid levels and extremely high cholesterol levels can cause slow mental processing. The stresses of life can raise blood cholesterol.

Lack of sunshine can raise the cholesterol. Low Vitamin D levels are also a sign that cholesterol is not being used up from the skin or blood.

A number of general factors can lead to high blood cholesterol. They include smoking, poor posture, low vital capacity, lack of exercise, irregular schedule, underactive thyroid, deficiency of fiber and vitamins C, E, and B12, elevated blood pressure, tension, noise, unstructured lifestyle, too much work, being overweight.

Cholesterol Reduction

The diet in technologically advanced countries has an average fat content of 30 to 50 percent of the calories consumed. It is also very high in refined carbohydrates. An especially damaging food combination is refined fats and refined sugars. Investigators have found that in poorer countries where the people eat 20 percent or less of total calories in free fats, where the diet consists mainly of unrefined carbohydrates such as whole grains, fruits, and vegetables, degenerative diseases are almost never found.

The use of diets high in soluble fibers (oat bran and beans) will lower cholesterol significantly. Insoluble fiber

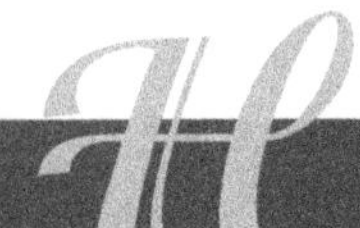

(wheat bran) is not so effective. Extra water, at least two eight-ounce glasses a day, should also be taken with the soluble dietary fiber, as that will increase the effectiveness of the fiber. If gas or flatulence is a problem from the extra fiber, the use of digestive enzymes such as papaya, bromelain, etc. can be very helpful (*American Family Physician* 51 [1995]: 419). These enzymes may also independently reduce cholesterol.

Blood Cholesterol Elevated by Protein

Heavy proteins in the diet increase the likelihood of developing high blood cholesterol and hardening of the arteries. Several proteins were studied for their ability to cause these disorders in the blood and arteries. In order of their ability to produce these disorders, purified soy protein was at the bottom of the list, next up from the bottom came wheat gluten, then pork, beef, lactalbumin (from milk), skim milk, and whole eggs (being the worst).

The high cholesterol level caused by saturated fats can also be caused by trans fats. These fats are formed when manufacturers process oils in any way, such as to hydrogenate vegetable oils. The product can be labeled without cholesterol, but still stimulate the liver to produce cholesterol in excess. Check your commercial foods such as cookies, crackers, canned soups, frozen or dry foods, and even cereals for hydrogenated fats. Fast foods such as French fries, onion rings, fried chicken, doughnuts, and so forth, along with vegetable shortening and margarine, also contain trans fats. Human breast milk is often a very rich source of trans fats because of the mother's diet (*New England Journal of Medicine* 341 [1999]: 1396).

Almost 120,000 doctors, dentists, and nurses completed a questionnaire every 24 months over a period lasting 8 to 14 years. Harvard University conducted the study and found that for diabetics in the study eating an egg a day doubled the risk for coronary heart disease and stroke. We recommend for those who are genetically high in cholesterol that all animal products be removed from the diet. Even animal protein has a deleterious effect on blood cholesterol (*Journal of the American Medical Association* 281 [1999]: 1387).

Iron has been found in trace amounts in atherosclerotic plaques. It may be that the high iron content of certain animal products or supplemental iron accounts for some portion of hardening of the arteries. Many metals are becoming linked with disease such as the link suspected between aluminum and zinc and Alzheimer's disease, and the link between iron and Parkinson's disease. High iron levels have also been linked to bowel cancer and fatal coronary heart disease according to Dr. Michael Selley of Australian National University's Curtin School of Medical Research in Canberra (December 1992). It is not advisable to take supplements containing iron unless your hemoglobin is under 10 grams or your serum iron is under 20.

One meat meal per month keeps the liver turned up to produce an increased quantity of cholesterol. To reduce cholesterol a person must be off all animal products. The release of insulin is controlled to a large degree by the type of protein one eats. With plant protein the release of insulin goes down, but with animal protein the release of insulin goes up. Of course, this reflects the release of glucose as it is on the same control system of insulin. The level of insulin in the blood, just as the cholesterol level, is a predictor for cardiovascular disease, hypertension, diabetes, and cancer, independent of all other factors.

Diet to Lower Cholesterol

If you are even 10 pounds overweight, you have a greater likelihood of developing high cholesterol. Don't keep any extra weight, as it can nullify an otherwise excellent program in some people. Calculate 100 pounds for your first five feet, and for women five pounds per inch thereafter, six to seven pounds per inch for men, depending on how muscular he is. Example: If you are a woman who is 5'5", you could weigh as much as 125 pounds, plus or minus about 10 pounds.

People who eat breakfast have lower blood cholesterol than persons who do not eat breakfast. It was found that children who consistently skipped breakfast had significantly higher blood cholesterol levels. The national average for cholesterol in students ages nine to 19 is 165! Students who eat breakfast as a routine have cholesterol levels from 140 to 150. Even this level is higher than ideal. Those who regularly skip breakfast average about 172. The study by Dr. Ken Resnicow was reported in *USA Today* on March 18, 1991.

Basic Daily Needs on a Therapeutic Diet

- Fruit: Two or more servings of any kind of fruit, including olives and avocados. (Note that the whole fruit has 6 to 10 times as much fiber as the juice. Fiber attaches to cholesterol and takes it out of the body.)
- Vegetables: Two or more servings of any type of vegetables, greens, or herbs, but especially green or yellow vegetables.
- Legumes: One serving of beans, peas, garbanzos, or lentils.
- Cereal: Two servings of whole grains, varied from time to time.

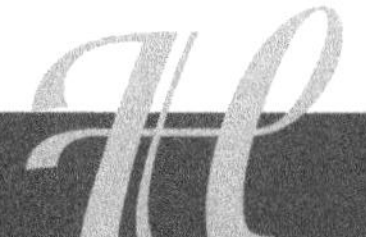

- Tubers: Use as needed in place of vegetables or grains or to increase the total number of calories if needed. Yams, potatoes, beets, carrots, radishes, etc. fall into this category.
- Nuts and Seeds: One ounce daily of any, roughly two tablespoons. Good options include walnuts, almonds, some peanuts and cashews, pecans, and all seeds.
- Foods to Avoid: Sugar, syrup, honey, molasses, oil, margarine, shortening, peanut butter, other nut butters, all animal products, including all animal protein, alcohol and caffeinated beverages, and strong spices and excessive salt.

Garlic and Onions

Even as far back as 1962, and especially more recently, garlic has been shown to inhibit the synthesis of excess lipids in the liver and to increase the utilization of serum insulin, benefiting both heart disease and diabetes (*Medical Science Research* 20 [1962]: 729–31). In a study on the effects of garlic to lower cholesterol and triglycerides, 20 healthy volunteers were fed garlic oil (0.25/mg/kg per day in two divided doses for six months).The treatment significantly lowered average cholesterol and triglyceride levels while raising levels of high-density lipoprotein cholesterol (HDL, the good cholesterol).

Sixty-two patients with coronary artery disease and elevated cholesterol levels were assigned to two subgroups. One group was fed garlic for 10 months, and the second group served as the untreated controls. Garlic decreased cholesterol, triglyceride, and low-density lipoprotein cholesterol, while increasing HDL. The anticoagulant properties, cholesterol-lowering properties, blood pressure-reducing properties, and most others are not lost when cooking garlic, although they may be reduced.

A study conducted by Tulane University revealed that total cholesterol levels in those taking garlic tablets dropped by 6 percent and LDL cholesterol was reduced by 11 percent. Researchers at the University of Kansas discovered that garlic tablets reduced the susceptibility of LDL oxidation by 34 percent compared to the placebo group.

One way to raise HDL cholesterol is with the juice of one white or yellow onion a day. The HDL cholesterol should rise by 30 percent in three to four months. Onions are also remedial in stimulating a weak heart, but the benefit is in the bite. Mild onions lack the HDL-elevating effect.

Soybeans

Soybeans contain isoflavones that have a very marked influence on reducing high blood cholesterol, yet it does not reduce HDL (*Health Letter on Current Research on Nutrition and Preventive Medicine* 9, no. 1 [1999]: 9). One serving daily of one-half cup of soybeans reduces LDL cholesterol an average of 10 percent in about four months.

Nuts and Flaxseed

Walnuts have a more favorable ratio of total to saturated fatty acids than any other food. A couple of tablespoons of walnuts taken daily can be an important factor in controlling cholesterol. The total cholesterol to HDL ratio, considered by many to be the most accurate measure of heart attack risk, dropped from 4.0 to 3.7 for 31,000 Seventh-day Adventists eating nuts at least five times a week. They had half the risk of fatal heart attacks of those who had nuts less than once a week. Even in as short a time as two months the difference can be seen. Volunteers took a diet containing 20 percent of calories from walnuts, as compared to a diet entirely nut free: the no-nuts volunteers had a 6 percent reduction in cholesterol, and an additional 12 percent when they switched to the walnut diet for two months. Walnuts contain omega-3 fatty acids that have a cholesterol lowering effect ("Walnuts Lower Lipids," *New England Journal of Medicine,* July 1993). Flaxseed has a similar fat content to walnuts, can often be purchased at a fraction of the cost of walnuts, and are just as effective.

Herbs

Cholesterol can be helped by a number of herbs: ginger root, hawthorn berry, myrrh, psyllium, and turmeric. A tea made from one teaspoon of powdered myrrh steeped for 10 minutes in boiling water is reported to bring cholesterol down. Use two cups per day. Another tea can be made from one tablespoon of powdered hawthorn berries, with or without one tablespoon of powdered turmeric, and/or one tablespoon of powdered ginger root boiled gently in one quart of water for 20 minutes. Strain and drink the entire quantity in one day. Milk thistle can be helpful to bring cholesterol down. Take the standard dosage. Psyllium seed, one to three teaspoons stirred into a glass of water two or three times daily, has a cholesterol lowering effect and also helps prevent cancer of the colon. The cost of these treatments is one-tenth that of cholesterol lowering drugs, is just as effective, or more so, and does not come with the serious side effects that can be seen with the drugs (*FDA Bulletin,* #92 to 1182).

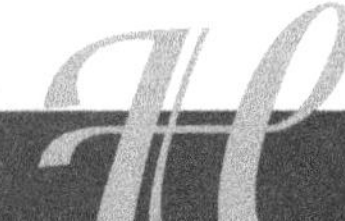

The following herbs are good for the heart: alfalfa, apple, buchu, garlic, hawthorn berry, motherwort, myrrh, tarragon. Geranium, rosemary, and grape seed extract are good anticlotting herbs.

Certain Fruits

Prunes help reduce cholesterol. Eating 12 prunes a day helped reduce blood cholesterol levels in 41 men with elevated levels of LDL. Three ounces of prunes contain 239 calories, seven grams of fiber, and 745 milligrams of potassium—more than a banana. Prunes are high in iron and are a good source of beta-carotene. Prune paste can replace high-fat shortening in a variety of baked goods. Prune paste is made of pitted prunes, vanilla and water. You can make your own by blending one cup of pitted prunes with six tablespoons of water and two teaspoons of vanilla. It can be kept in the refrigerator for several days. When substituted for shortening in baked goods, prune paste reduces the fat in the recipe by at least 75 percent.

Resveratrol, a nutrient found in purple grapes and purple grape juice, has been found to lower cholesterol in rats. It is present also in raisins. Resveratrol is also an anticoagulant to prevent blood clots in deep veins. A five-ounce glass of grape juice is sufficient, once or twice daily.

Women who ate enough avocados to comprise around 30 percent of the calories in the diet had a significant drop, 10 percent, in both total and LDL cholesterol with no change in HDL.

Citrus fruits and juices given to rabbits caused a reduction in LDL cholesterol. When orange juice or grapefruit juice was mixed with their drinking water, their LDL cholesterol was reduced by 43 percent and 32 percent respectively (*Nutrition Research* 20 [2000]: 121). Try eating a grapefruit twice a day that has been peeled, de-seeded, and blended in a blender. Continue this practice for as long as the cholesterol is elevated. Reports show that pectin in grapefruit can reduce cholesterol by 7 to 20 percent, which is better than the drugs (*Science News,* July 25, 1987, 63). Cholesterol-lowering drugs work by poisoning the liver's ability to make cholesterol. It is this feature that causes liver cancer or hepatitis which have been reported because of Mevacor or Pravachol; further, about 15 percent is the expected drop in cholesterol, which is a very modest number. It is not worth taking the risk with these drugs (*Modern Medicine* 60, no. 6: 70, 92).

An Ancient Grain

Use amaranth, the ancient Aztec seed that was lost for many centuries but has recently been re-found. It contains a form of vitamin E and is able to substantially reduce cholesterol. It can be used as a breakfast cereal or to make vegetarian roasts. The flour can be used in waffles. It is not actually in the family of grains, but grows on a bushy plant with broad leaves.

Nutrient Supplements

Chromium picolinate, 400 milligrams daily, has been shown to be quite effective in the treatment of high cholesterol and triglycerides. It also decreases high insulin levels in insulin resistant persons too (*Health Letter on Current Research on Nutrition and Preventive Medicine* 9, no. 1 [January 1999]: 16).

Inositol in a 500 milligram supplement is good to bring cholesterol down. It is best taken with choline. It is also helpful as a stress neutralizer and to bring blood pressure down.

A supplement of 60 milligrams of vitamin C can help to prevent oxidation of LDL, thus making it so that arteries do not get atherosclerosis as fast. Vitamin C also limits the production of fibrinogen, a principal precursor of a blood clot, and a cause of poor ability of arteries to dilate as age increases. Vitamin C thereby reduces the likelihood of strokes and heart attacks (*British Medical Journal* 310 [1995]: 1548–63).

Drugs and Cholesterol

Certain prescription drugs such as Dilantin can cause an increase in serum cholesterol, which increases risks of coronary heart disease (*British Medical Journal* 4 [1975]: 85). Serum cholesterol levels were found to be 6 to 48 percent higher during the first three months of treatment with Dilantin and remained high through the treatment period. The mechanism for this increase is probably through damage to the liver.

Charcoal

Activated charcoal has been found to lower the concentration of total lipids, cholesterol, and triglycerides in the blood serum, liver, heart, and brain. A study reported by the British journal *Lancet* found that patients with high blood cholesterol levels were able to reduce total cholesterol by 25 percent. About the best hoped for with drugs is around 15 percent. Not only that, but while LDL was lowered as much as 41 percent, HDL was increased. The patients took the equivalent of roughly one quarter ounce (approximately one heaping tablespoon) of activated charcoal three or four times daily for six to eight months. It should be taken upon rising, mid-morning, midafternoon, and bedtime. Another study conducted by the National Institute of Public Health in

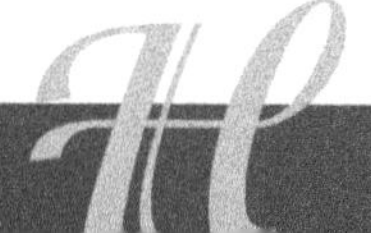

Finland suggested that activated charcoal was as effective in reducing high cholesterol levels as the drug Lovastatin.

Charcoal should not be taken near mealtime as food interferes with its best action. It will take up any kind of pharmaceutical type of medication as being poisonous. Since it will absorb most poisons and inactivate them, it is necessary to take charcoal at least two hours from the time medication is taken, and even longer is desirable. For example: If you take blood pressure or epilepsy medication in the morning, take the charcoal in the evening. Charcoal therapy is certainly less expensive, while possessing none of the dangerous side effects of anticholesterol drugs. Our own experience has been that charcoal is a valuable part of a total cholesterol reducing program, but long-term lifestyle changes must be maintained to permanently reduce high cholesterol.

A group of 60 patients ranging in ages from 60 to 74 were divided into two groups. Forty were given activated charcoal for their high cholesterol, and 20 patients were treated with a placebo. The course of treatment lasted for four weeks. There was a 20 percent reduction in total cholesterol, 27 percent reduction in triglycerides, 20 percent reduction of apolipoprotein A, and Apo B dropped by 32 percent in the patients taking the charcoal. There were positive changes in the circulation, and in the clinical status of patients in 60 percent of cases, and exercise tolerance improved in 12 percent of the patients. At the same time the control patients did not present any noticeable changes (*Klin-Med (Mosk)* 69, no. 6 [June 1991]: 51–3).

Melatonin

The pineal gland and its melatonin secretion are associated with the control of levels of cholesterol. It may be that very high and difficult cholesterol levels which are not brought down by ordinary means might respond to a trial of sun baths four or five days a week for 20 minutes each time, along with an early bedtime in a dark room, or if all else fails, melatonin administration (*International Journal of Neuroscience* 76 [1994]: 81).

Exercise

Probably the single most widely beneficial thing, having great effectiveness in bringing cholesterol down, is exercise. Begin your program today. Start with what you can easily do, and build up both the length of time and the intensity of the exercise as your level of physical conditioning improves. Exercise neutralizes tension. Face squarely those things that trouble you, and deal with each one dispassionately, patiently, and kindly.

Vital capacity is the amount of air blown out after a full breath. The more air we can take in, the more oxygen in the blood, and the less likely we are to damage our blood vessels to start the process of atherosclerosis. Smoking and a sedentary lifestyle both decrease the vital capacity, whereas exercise increases vital capacity.

Triglycerides and HDL

The ideal for triglycerides is below 140, and probably below 100 is safer. Many people can achieve an enviable triglyceride level around the same as their age. The heart attack rate is two times higher if the triglyceride level is above 250 as compared to below 170. Ninety percent of overweight people have increased triglycerides. Other causes of increased triglycerides are alcohol, sugar, the type of fats in dairy products and refined carbohydrates such as white bread, white flour products, white pastries, and white starch. Even large quantities of fruit juices or very sweet or dried fruits (dates, raisins, and figs) may increase triglycerides.

There are a few things one can do to increase HDL cholesterol levels. Fast a day or two each week. Increase the amount of vegetables and whole grains in the diet. Eliminate nitrites (from salad bars and aging foods), free sugars, free fats, junk foods. Use salt sparingly. Increase physical activity.

Homocysteine

The amino acid homocysteine has a strong relationship to human health and disease. This amino acid can influence both directly and indirectly all methyl and sulfur metabolism occurring in the body. This substance is critical for the production of essential compounds, including carnitine, taurine, glycocyamine sulphate, coenzyme Q-10, and melatonin. If levels of vitamins B12, B6, and folic acid are deficient, the complete transformation into these substances is low, and homocysteine begins to build up until its level is above ideal range. Elevation of homocysteine has been linked to a long list of diseases: alcoholism, Alzheimer's disease, coronary artery disease, deep vein thrombosis, depression, diabetic nephropathy, diabetic retinopathy, intermittent claudication, low birth weight, multiple sclerosis, myocardial infarction, diabetes, neural tube defects, osteoporosis, Parkinson's disease, peripheral vascular disease, placental abruption, premature birth, renal failure, retinal vascular occlusion, rheumatoid arthritis, schizophrenia, spontaneous abortion, and stroke.

The only treatment that has been shown to be effective is nutritional intervention—supplementation with folic acid, B12, B6, betaine, and N-acetylcysteine. Findings of either

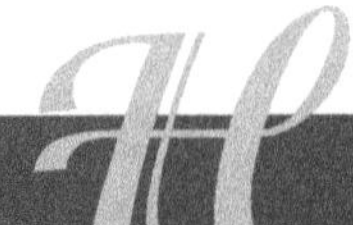

increased creatinine or uric acid levels on a routine blood chemistry panel justifies further testing for elevated homocysteine. The daily treatment includes 650 micrograms of folic acid, 400 micrograms of vitamin B12, and 10 milligrams of vitamin B6. With this treatment, in one group of 100 men with high homocysteine levels, the levels were reduced 50 percent in six weeks (*Alternative Medicine Review* 2, no. 4 [1997]: 233). The nutritional intervention mentioned helps to optimize the metabolism so that a number of essential nutrients, enzymes, and the hormone epinephrine can be produced in normal quantities. Levels of homocysteine go up with age.

In a case control study 185 patients with recurrent venous thrombosis and 220 controls had serum homocysteine levels measured. The thrombosis patients had over three times the likelihood of having an elevated serum homocysteine level!

There is an association between coffee drinking and the elevation of total homocysteine in plasma. It may be that the daily use of coffee has its adverse effect on heart disease through the homocysteine elevation. Cigarette smoking and alcohol ingestion both make the level go up. While normal levels are considered to be between 4 and 10, as the level goes up even in the "normal" range, so does the risk for coronary artery disease. Homocysteine increases the likelihood of production of hydrogen peroxide, which acts as an oxidant in the body, changing cell membranes of blood vessels so that the damaged blood vessels can take up cholesterol; then hardening of the arteries occurs.

Mitral Valve Prolapse

What is now agreed to be the most common valvular disorder of the heart was not even recognized until around the early 1970s. The advent of echocardiography, which for the first time allowed the cardiologist to see what was going on inside the heart in real time, allowed the diagnosis of mitral valve prolapse. It involves a thinning of the valve with ballooning upward into the left atrium (upper chamber of the heart), on contraction of the left ventricle. Apparently the disorder is congenital, and it is said to involve between 25 and 30 percent of all women in the United States, most being diagnosed in the 25 to 35 age group. It is a strange disorder, generally quite benign, but fraught with much mystique.

Bondelais, writing in the October 1989 issue of the *American Heart Journal*, proposed that it be divided into two groups: the first he called the anatomic group, and the second, the Mitral Valve Prolapse (MVP) Syndrome group. The anatomic group is older, with an average age of 67 years—85 percent were over 50 years of age when symptoms developed. This group had much more severe symptoms with more severe valvular involvement. Eighty-five percent had had at least mild degrees of congestive heart failure, and 58 percent had atrial fibrillation, the erratic "quivering" arrhythmia of the upper heart chambers. Eighty-eight percent of these patients required valve surgery. Fortunately, this group is much less common than the other, even rare.

The Mitral Valve Prolapse Syndrome is said to be characterized by a symptom complex of palpitations, chest pains, easy fatigue, exercise intolerance, shortness of breath, easy fainting, anxiety, and predisposition to panic attacks. The average age was 30 years. The symptoms, which can cause extreme anxiety in some, can be disabling, even though the disorder is generally quite benign. There is evidence of increased activity of the sympathetic nervous system with increased levels of stress hormones (catecholamines) in the blood and urine.

The causes of the symptoms are poorly understood. The chest pain may be due to stretching of the chordae tendineae, the "heart strings," which anchor the mitral valve to the interior wall of the heart. It is usually described as a dull aching beneath the breast bone and under the left breast, with much anxiety. It can last for hours and is not aggravated by exercise, in contradistinction to angina, which comes on after exercise and emotional upsets and usually lasts only a short time after resting.

Treatment of the symptomatic group involves a great deal of support and reassurance. Patients may become "cardiac cripples" if not handled properly. It is common for cardiologists to give strong medication, such as the so-called "beta blockers," examples being propranolol or atenolol and antiarrhythmic drugs to these patients. While the beta blockers slow the heart and often give a measure of relief, they should not be used in most cases. In fact, it is well to avoid the pharmacological treatment of the MVP syndrome. Besides frequent reassurance, graduated exercise out of doors is an excellent method of physiological dissipation of the excess catecholamines. The resting pulse is slowed naturally with exercise, chest pains melt away, and anxiety and fatigue are relieved.

If anything is needed for the palpatations, some simple herbs such as hawthorn berry tea are very helpful. Since most of these patients have a total body deficiency of magnesium, for unknown reasons (perhaps because of poor absorption), supplementation with Epsom salts (magnesium sulfate, one teaspoonful in a glass of water twice daily) or magnesium chloride or magnesium oxide tablets, two tablets three times a day, are also quite helpful. These seldom need to be

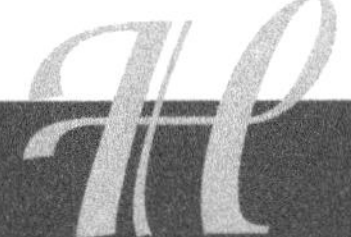

continued very long if the patient embarks on a serious exercise program.

Do not use prophylactic antibiotics before dental manipulation for these patients, as they are prone to develop the candida related complex (chronic yeast syndrome). In fact, one study of candida patients showed over 60 percent with MVP.

Rhythm Disturbances or Arrhythmias of the Heart

Atrial Fibrillation

This irregularity of heartbeat is common among the elderly. It should be treated vigorously when it first starts to try to get it to convert to a normal rhythm again. If it persists for six months, it becomes chronic and much more difficult to convert.

Work on getting the digestion perfect—meals on time, no spices, eliminate refined foods of all kinds (fats, carbohydrates, proteins, salt, etc.)—until the condition is either converted to a normal rhythm or the condition has become manageable—pulse under 100, and preferably in the 70s, minimal swelling of the feet. Be certain not to overeat.

Use digestive enzymes. Homeopathic physicians believe that digestive disturbances are often at the basis of the rhythm disturbances of the heart.

Administer alternating hot foot baths, three minutes hot, 30 seconds cold for four exchanges. The first week of treatment do three treatments a day; then do one treatment a day for a month.

Use herbs to restore normal rhythm—slippery elm, golden seal, licorice, hawthorn berry, barberry, Oregon grape.

Kyolic and garlic help to prevent clotting inside the atrium, one of the most serious complications of atrial fibrillation.

Take magnesium, as most people with basic heart disease are magnesium deficient. First take one-half teaspoon of Epsom salts (magnesium sulfate) morning and night. If you tolerate that quantity without getting diarrhea, increase the dosage to one teaspoonful at least one of those doses and preferably both of them.

Take ginkgo as arrhythmias may be due to reduced oxygen in the heart. Ginkgo also helps prevent strokes from blood clots.

The heavy use of coffee or tea—nine or more cups daily—has been associated with nearly twice the incidence of premature beats of the heart as compared to those who consume two or fewer cups daily (*Journal of Chronic Disease* 33 [1980]: 67–72). It appears likely that atrial fibrillation may have its initiation in the heavy use of coffee at some time in the person's life.

A naturopath from Oregon told us that lycopus (also called gypsy wort and bugle weed) are the best botanicals we have for atrial fibrillation in conjunction with cayenne and CoQ10.

CoQ10 is excellent to minimize symptoms of heart consciousness from the irregular rhythm. Start with 400 milligrams per day for one month, then 200 to 300 milligrams per day, in two or three doses for two weeks. Then switch to a maintenance dose of 100 milligrams per day.

Take *Lactobacillus* powder, one-half teaspoon, twice a day between meals.

If the herbs and magnesium sulfate alone do not help one's heart within one week, we suggest one take any three of the following diuretic herbs as well: corn silk, burdock, buchu, watermelon seed, and chamomile. Try the first routine for at least a month before adding the others.

Of course exercise to tolerance on a daily basis can slow the heart rate, even in atrial fibrillation.

Paroxysmal Auricular Tachycardia

Paroxysmal Auricular Tachycardia (PAT) is a benign, non-threatening condition that causes a good bit of anxiety and discomfort. If prolonged, it may result in fatigue, but it is not serious. Individual attacks may be merely a short run of very fast heart beats, or may last for 10 seconds to 10 hours or more. The heart is usually normal, although PAT may coexist with organic heart disease, such as coronary heart disease. In these cases, the rapid rate may cause significant problems. Our recommendations have two objectives: (1) to prevent attacks and (2) to treat the acute attack and convert to a normal rhythm.

Lobelia has been reported to slow palpitations of the heart.

We have had several patients who have been able to calm down a PAT attack by taking magnesium salts. We generally use magnesium sulfate (Epsom salts), one-half teaspoon in the morning and one-half teaspoon in the evening, increased to one teaspoon twice daily if tolerated. Dr. Coleen Izdale from Texas had complete relief from troublesome PVC's and cardiac arrhythmia after about three weeks of taking Epsom salts. We believe it possible to keep many people off medication if they were simply knowledgeable about magnesium supplements. (See "Food Sources of Certain Nutrients" in the *Dietary Information* section.) If you get diarrhea from Epsom

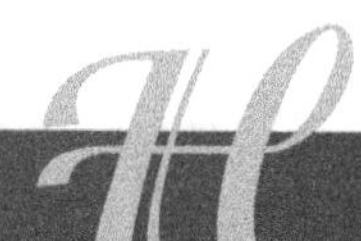

salts, take magnesium oxide, which is available in health food stores, two tablets three times a day.

Hawthorn berries contain procyanidines, which help stabilize the heart rhythm (*Aizneim Forsch* 55, no. 5: 490). When the arrhythmia is caused by a lack of oxygen to the heart, ginkgo biloba may be of help. The active ingredient in ginkgo is ginkgolide. It has been shown to be as effective as anti-arrhythmic drugs such as Lopressor and Cardizem (*Euro J Pharm* 89, no. 164: 293–302).

Heartburn

Probably everyone has suffered from heartburn at one time or another. It comes about from reflux of acid stomach contents into the lower end of the esophagus, which is not equipped to handle acid. The result is a burning pain, usually starting beneath the lower end of the breast bone and often causing spasms of the esophagus. The pain can progress up to the root of the neck. At times it may resemble angina pain. Some differences are that it is not provoked by exercise, often lasts for a long time, does not radiate to the jaws or arms, and is not associated with sweating and weakness. Yet some cases are so difficult to differentiate that a physician may be required.

The cause of heartburn is an irritation of the stomach and esophagus because of alcohol, eating too much, foods that don't agree, eating between meals, lying down after meals, bending over, especially to lift something heavy, taking pills or tablets without water, and eating foods that cause the upper portion of the stomach to dilate so that stomach contents can run back into the esophagus. (See "Food Sources of Certain Nutrients" in the *Dietary Information* section.) A diaphragmatic (hiatus) hernia is a common cause. (See "Hiatus Hernia" in the *Conditions and Diseases* section.)

Many drugs cause paralysis of the sphincter muscle that usually prevents back-flow of stomach contents. One inhaled puff of cigarette smoke will paralyze the sphincter for 20 minutes or more, so all smokers are subject to heartburn.

One of the commonest times for heartburn to occur is after a person has been lying down for some time. Reclining after meals is particularly likely to lead to heartburn.

One of the important things a person with heartburn can do is to lie on the left side. Lying on the right side makes heartburn worse because the esophagus is more straight in relation to the stomach on the right side than on the left.

Avoid eating while driving, working, or playing. Do not bend over shortly after eating, especially to pick up something heavy.

Eat slowly, take small bites, and chew thoroughly.

Finish all eating at least three to four hours before going to bed. Never eat just before lying down.

Never eat between meals, as this practice encourages slow peristalsis of the stomach and regurgitation of stomach contents into the esophagus.

Don't overeat, and avoid fatty foods, red wine, coffee, tea, colas, fried foods, spicy foods, and chocolate. Never use alcohol.

Watch your weight. Being overweight increases intra-abdominal pressure.

Avoid constipation, tight waist bands, and any other condition that increases abdominal pressure. Avoid tight-fitting clothes.

Do not smoke, or even breathe secondhand smoke, as tobacco relaxes the muscle sphincter at the top of the stomach.

Elevate the head of the bed six inches with blocks under the feet of the bedposts.

Check all your medications, as many are capable of causing heartburn. Check Physicians' Desk Reference Web site for your medications.

Avoid the use of antacids and the potent stomach acid blocking medications. They have many potential complications, and besides that, they result in rebound high acid a few hours after the last dose.

Heat Stroke

(See "Heat Stroke" in the *Home Emergencies* section.)

Heel Spurs

(See "Skeletal Problems" in the *Conditions and Diseases* section.)

Hematocrit

(See "Lab Tests" in the *Supplemental Information* section.)

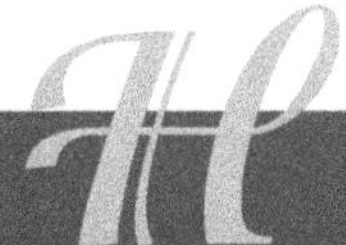

Hemochromatosis

Hemochromatosis is a disease that interferes with the body's ability to absorb and store iron and results in too much iron being absorbed from the gastrointestinal tract and stored in various tissues of the body, including the skin. A bronze discoloration of the skin occurs when the iron storage is heavy. Because excess iron is both an irritant and an oxidant, tissues are damaged where the iron is stored. Thus, the pancreas can be damaged and diabetes result; the liver damaged and cirrhosis result; the blood damaged and a stroke result, etc.

The only way we have treated hemochromatosis is with repeated blood draws, removing about 500 cc or two cups of blood with each blood draw, until the hemoglobin is well below 15 grams in men and well below 13 grams in women. Then we labor diligently to keep it always below those levels.

In addition to that, we use a very carefully planned physical conditioning program with special emphasis on a proper diet. The most favorable diet for hemochromatosis is a totally vegetarian diet using no animal protein of any kind. That means the person should restrict breakfast to fruit and whole grains, and lunch to vegetables and whole grains. Either meal may contain bread, spread, nuts, and seeds. These meals should be very simple, the menu containing only about three dishes plus bread and spread. Salt should be used very sparingly. Stomach irritants promote a greater absorption of iron. These include vinegar, hot spices, such as black and red pepper, ginger, cinnamon, nutmeg, cloves, and allspice and all fermented foods, such as sauerkraut, cheese, kim chee, etc. No mineral or vitamin preparations should be taken, and drugs should be avoided as much as possible as they irritate the intestinal tract and promote excess absorption of iron.

Water should be used in large quantities to thin out the blood as much as possible. We have not had much success in treating poisonings from iron pills (often seen in children) with charcoal, as charcoal does not adsorb nutrients well, even in over abundance. While this is one of its benefits as it enables the long-term use of charcoal, but it is a drawback in treating poisonings with vitamins, minerals, proteins, or heavy metals.

Hydrotherapy, consisting of three hot baths per week (after the hemoglobin gets below 15 grams), may assist in keeping the iron levels low. While the hemoglobin is above 15 grams, give cold mitten friction treatments to prevent pressure from building up in the head.

Daily exercise should be followed by a cool shower with a brisk rubdown, as some bits of iron can be lost through the skin if the skin is kept healthy.

Hemorrhage

Very hot or very cold water can be used to stop hemorrhaging as blood vessels will close up tightly when touched by heat. Hot water is usually more effective than cold if applied properly.

To stop bleeding with hot or cold applications, the temperature of the water must be either very hot (115°F to 123°F), or very cold (32°F to 40°F). After three to six minutes of application, either of the hot or cold, the blood vessels will cease to react to the extreme temperature by contraction and will begin to dilate. That tends to encourage hemorrhaging; therefore, the applications *must be kept short.* Usually within a minute the bleeding checks, certainly by three minutes. An even hotter temperature may be used and is more efficient in stopping hemorrhaging, but must be carefully regulated. At 125°F to 127°F, usually 10 to 15 seconds only are required, and no greater than 30 second exposure is allowed. Longer could cause burns.

Direct applications of extreme heat to stop bleeding are generally more useful than extreme cold in nosebleeds, menorrhagia (excessive menstrual bleeding), postpartum hemorrhaging, a blood ooze from raw surfaces, and bladder hemorrhaging. Hot water packs at 115°F to 120°F placed on the spinal column for two to three minutes *only*, extending from the lower thoracic to the sacral region have arrested postpartum hemorrhaging. The old doctors used to stop bleeding after childbirth by irrigating the vagina with water at 118°F to 120°F for one to two minutes. (That is why the husband put the water on to boil.)

"Hot lap packs" have been used successfully in surgery for generations in the treatment of bleeding from large surface areas, C-sections, and mechanical injuries.

When applying extreme heat to the skin, one must use caution to not burn the skin. The following chart provides information about the length of exposure that will may result in a burn.

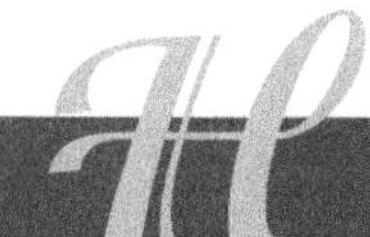

Water Temp	Length of Direct Exposure	Degree of Skin Burn Possible
158°F (70°C)	1 second	Full thickness of skin
149°F (65°C)	2 seconds	Full thickness of skin
140°F (60°C)	3 to 5 seconds	Full thickness of skin
135°F (57°C)	10 seconds	Full thickness of skin
133°F (56°C)	15 seconds	Full thickness of skin
127°F (53°C)	60 seconds	Full thickness of skin
124°F (51°C)	3 minutes	Full thickness of skin

General Bleeding

Almost all bleeding from the outside of the body can be stopped by placing gauze or a clean handkerchief or washcloth directly against the wound and applying pressure. A bleeding tooth socket can be controlled by filling the socket with cotton or gauze and applying gentle pressure by biting on the cotton.

A powerful constriction of the blood vessels in the extremities occurs with cold application to the soles of the feet, abdomen, or legs. This treatment may be used in acute blood loss to cause the blood from the extremities to move to the more vital organs. It is well for those having a major hemorrhage to be kept slightly cool.

Intracranial Hemorrhage

An ice cap and ice cold compresses to the head and neck are most appropriate, also the hot foot bath. Restlessness and agitation can be combatted by cool facial sponging, cool water or ice collar, warm steam packs to the spine or chest, and fomentations to the low abdomen and upper thighs. Massage of the extremities, moist abdominal bandage, and hot immersion arm baths are all helpful. The patient must be kept very quiet, and in a room with subdued light. Visitors are strictly forbidden.

Lung Hemorrhage

The patient should be kept quiet in bed without visitors. The assistant should keep hot water bags to the feet, the lungs, and the stomach.

Place a very cold compress over the front of the chest and very hot fomentations (115°F to 118°F) between the shoulder blades, taking care to cover both the lower cervical and upper thoracic region. Do not extend the fomentations below the lower edge of the shoulder blades. Continue the fomentations and cold compress for no longer than three minutes. Remove the compresses and gently dry the skin. Keep the patient quiet in the upright or slightly reclining position; move the patient as little as possible, and combat sweating and a sensation of overheating by sponging the face with cool water or using a gentle breeze from a fan. Do not permit the slightest degree of chilling as that sends blood to the internal organs, including the lungs. A more reclining position can be assumed as the hemorrhage subsides, recognized by the cessation of coughing bloody foam.

Treatment includes all the following:

- Staying in bed with the head of the bed elevated several inches to several feet.
- Not getting overheated, and not overexerting your lungs.
- Slowly walking around once the coughing stops.
- Taking a sedative herb such as catnip, valerian root, chamomile, etc.

Use bugleweed tea, made by pouring one pint of boiling water over one ounce of bugleweed. Cover and steep for 30 minutes. Take eight ounces with each new episode of coughing of blood, up to 10 glassfuls per day. If bugleweed is not readily available, licorice root powder may be used until the bugleweed can be obtained. Put two level tablespoons of the powder in one and one-half quarts of water, gently simmer for 10 minutes. Drink eight ounces with each coughing bout, not to exceed sixcups per day.

Menstrual Bleeding

Since some women respond to one treatment and some to another, it is well to have a number of treatments available for use in gynecologic conditions.

The daily diet should be a plant-based vegetarian diet, including several servings of the following foods: corn, apples, carrots, peanuts, sweet potatoes, tomatoes, and white potatoes. These foods are high in plant sterols that have a hormonal influence in the body. Take one tablespoon each of shredded coconut (unsweetened) and wheat germ. Avoid all dairy products, which tend to have excessive estrogens.

Fasting is also helpful for persistent uterine bleeding, but if anemia or weight loss are a problem, fasting may not be a good choice. For anemia use a diet high in dark leafy greens and whole grains.

A hot vaginal douche at about 115°F to 122°F for one to three minutes only may temporarily stop menstrual bleeding. The high temperature is critical. Cooler temperatures may actually promote bleeding.

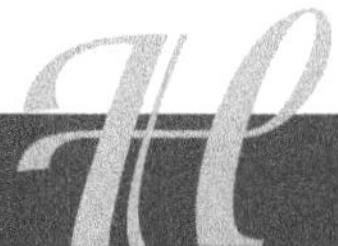

A hot foot bath for two minutes at 118°F to 120°F is often helpful along with a cold application to the low abdomen and inner thighs.

A very powerful vaginal treatment is a cold tap water irrigation for six minutes. The water temperature should be 40°F to 55°F, or ice should be used to cool the water.

Another good treatment is that of putting the patient in a shallow sitz bath at 50°F to 70°F for five to six minutes, the feet being placed in very hot water at the same time. Put a small tub containing the hot water into the bathtub containing cold water.

A valuable method is a fever treatment using an appropriate bath to briefly elevate the mouth temperature to 104°F before reducing it to 101°F and holding it at that level for 30 minutes.

Golden seal can be used both for bleeding as well as for prevention of infection in the uterus or vagina.

Herbs that are helpful include alfalfa, red raspberry, black cohosh, false unicorn, squaw vine, and garlic. Except for the black cohosh, which can cause cramping and headache in some people if more than three teaspoons of the herb are used daily, all the other teas may be used in any quantity up to 10 or more cups a day, sufficient to slow down the bleeding. Bring one quart of water to a boil, add three teaspoons of black cohosh and simmer 20 minutes. Set off the heat and add one-fourth to one-half cup of red raspberry and alfalfa. Cover and steep for 30 minutes. Strain and drink one cup four times a day.

Do not use black cohosh as in the above formula if you continue to bleed after three weeks of the use of black cohosh. Change to two tablespoons of chaste tree, three of red raspberry, and one of false unicorn, two each of witch hazel bark, milk thistle, beth root, and periwinkle leaf. Simmer the non-leaf herbs gently in one quart of water for 20 to 25 minutes. Then remove from the fire and add the periwinkle and red raspberry leaves for 30 minutes of steeping. Dilute to five to eight cups, and take this herb preparation throughout the day.

Take evening primrose oil, four capsules three times a day for two to three months, or until improvement is noted. Gradually cut back to two capsules three times a day.

For prolonged menstrual bleeding (several months or several years), set one and a half quarts of water in a gentle simmer and add two and a half tablespoons of chaste tree berries, two tablespoons of milk thistle seed, one tablespoon of false unicorn, and one tablespoon of witch hazel bark. Simmer gently 25 minutes, remove, and add four tablespoons of red raspberry leaf. Cover and steep for 20 minutes, strain. This is one day's supply. If this causes nausea, add one teaspoon of ready prepared soy milk powder per cup, and it should make it so that it doesn't cause nausea.

Another formula for use in uterine bleeding is as follows: beth root, two tablespoons; witch hazel, two tablespoons; periwinkle leaf, two tablespoons; and one quart of water. Simmer the first two ingredients 20 minutes. Take off the stove and add the last ingredient. Steep for 30 minutes. Drink one cup of the tea four times a day.

Certain other herbal remedies are often very helpful—catnip, chamomile, shepherd's purse, and peppermint.

Avoid free oils in cooking, baking, frying, and in salad dressings.

Nosebleeds

The blood vessels in the nose are very superficial, only covered over by a thin layer of mucous membrane. There are many causes of nosebleeds including trauma (a bump on the nose or putting some object such as fingers or a dry tissue into the nasal cavity), high blood pressure, physical exertion, stress, drug reactions, high altitudes, and unknown reasons. Nosebleeds may be in the front of the nose or high up in the back of the nose. In the latter case they are almost never related to trauma but to some of the other causes.

Ninety percent are because of picking the nose or faulty methods of cleaning the nose. Forceful rubbing or twisting the nose may also cause bleeding.

Although nosebleeds may be quite disturbing, they are rarely serious and do not represent a life-threatening condition. There are few disorders for which nosebleeds are a primary symptom.

Avoid blowing the nose or attempting to clear the blood out of the nose. Pinch the nose together lightly for 10 to 15 minutes, apply pressure on the upper lip and ice to the nape of the neck or under the upper lip.

Have the person lie on his or her back on one or two large pillows to lower pressure in the head. Bleeding usually stops in a few minutes. Sometimes the application of very hot or very cold packs will bring about the same result. Cold applications for one to two minutes may be put on the upper spine at the base of the skull for stopping nosebleeds. (See discussion above on the use of very hot compresses or irrigations to stop bleeding.)

Soak some cotton in strong witch hazel tea, twist the cotton into a cone, insert it into the nose, and apply gentle pressure for 15 minutes.

A coin under the upper lip, or a cold compress to the back of the neck, can often stop it in a few minutes.

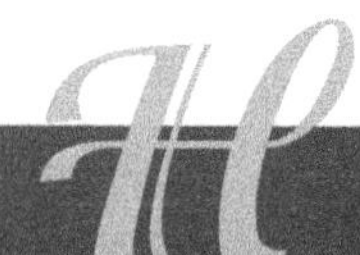

Also try placing the hands in ice water, or the feet in cold water for about one to three minutes *only*. A longer time than three minutes can cause blood vessels to dilate and bleeding to worsen.

Irrigate the nose with hot water or saline at between 118°F to 122°F. Use a bulb syringe, electric dental irrigator, or an enema type setup to irrigate the nostril from which the blood is coming. Continue the hot irrigation for 10 to 20 seconds, or until bleeding stops, but no longer than one minute.

If the hot application is unpleasant or cannot be tolerated or does not stop the bleeding, use a very cold irrigation, water or saline at 32°F to 36°F. Again, irrigate for about 10 to 20 seconds.

A physician from Saginaw, Michigan, tells of a treatment for nosebleeds using a swab full of Monsel's solution (ferrous subsulfate) for nosebleeds. Take a small piece of cotton, just enough to completely fill the nasal passage after having been wet in the solution, and insert into the nose. Put a small amount of pressure on the nose by gently pinching the sides of the nose together. After about five minutes slowly release the pressure. In some instances the removal of the cotton swab starts up the bleeding again; therefore, do not remove the swab until all danger of nosebleed has passed. Repeat the procedure if necessary.

To stop a nosebleed in the back of the nose is more difficult than in the front of the nose. These nosebleeds are likely to be more severe and could be unresponsive to pressure on the front of the nose. The person should sit in a chair and apply ice to the nose and cheeks while, at the same time, receiving a relaxing foot rub which will reduce the pressure and relax tensions which might continue to hold blood vessels open. If bleeding continues one may need to consult an otolaryngologist.

For Recurring Nosebleeds

Caution the person against forceful blowing of the nose or cleaning the nose with a dry tissue. Improper cleaning of the nose often causes an ulcer in susceptible persons. The nose can be cleaned with a moistened finger or with a moistened paper towel or handkerchief to prevent trauma to the surface lining.

Avoid putting objects, including dry fingers, inside the nostrils.

Keep the nasal mucous membrane properly hydrated by using a humidifier and by drinking adequate quantities of water. For persons over age 50, 10 or more glasses are needed.

People with high blood pressure should lower their blood pressure. (See "Blood Clotting, Anticoagulation, Intravascular Clotting" in the *Conditions and Diseases* section)

Those who take aspirin should eliminate the aspirin and use some other remedy for the purpose aspirin was taken.

Postpartum Hemorrhage

Keep the mother in bed with her knees tightly together for the first hour after delivering the placenta. Massage the top of the uterus about as firmly and vigorously as you would rub an apple to polish it; the uterus will be felt about halfway from the umbilicus to the top of the public bone. With massage it should contract and become very hard and will not bleed.

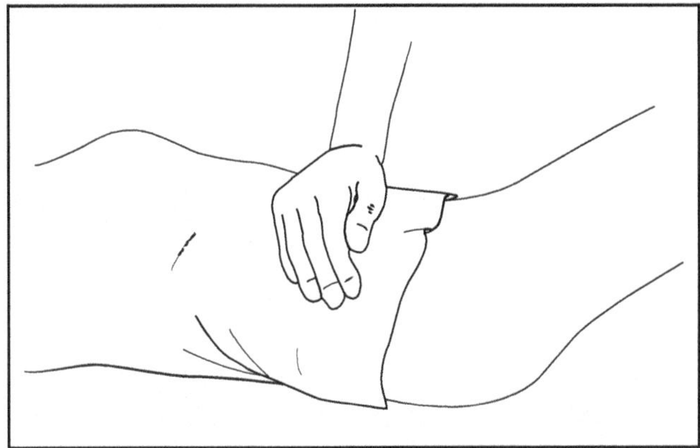

Watch carefully for excess blood, which will be recognized as bright red blood in a constant stream, not a gush of very dark blood and then no more blood. Then you may use shepherd's purse, motherwort, bayberry, and a pinch of cayenne. Make this into a tincture to be used in case of such an emergency.

If a mother begins to hemorrhage, work fast but deliberately as a lot of blood can be lost in half an hour. Symptoms of substantial blood loss are a loud ringing in the ears, lightheadedness, fast pulse (above 100) and eventually a fall in blood pressure. Extremes of temperature have the effect of stopping bleeding from small blood vessels. A very hot low abdominal and upper thigh compress (prepared from water at about 120°F), or a hot water douche at 118°F to 120°F, or both, may be used. The temperature is critical, not too cool or it will not be effective, and not too hot or it will burn, and not for more than three minutes, or bleeding will be encouraged instead of stopped.

Another method is to apply the compresses to the thighs and spine (from the waist to end of the spine), and a simultaneous ice bag placed over the lower abdomen. The hot compresses must be refreshed every 30 seconds for three minutes maximum—one minute is usually sufficient.

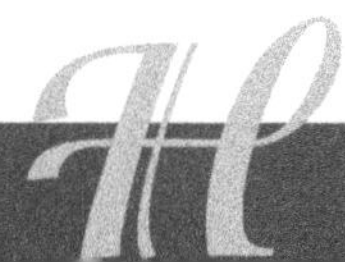

Often the hemorrhaging can be stopped, even while the hot and cold applications are being prepared, by simply putting pressure on the uterus. First, rub the top of the uterus.

If this simple maneuver to encourage contraction of the uterus does not stop the bleeding, the second pressure application is made by placing one hand on the abdomen on top and cupping it behind the uterus, and pressing the uterus with the other hand in front of the uterus, which is between the two hands, squeezing with quite firm but not intense pressure.

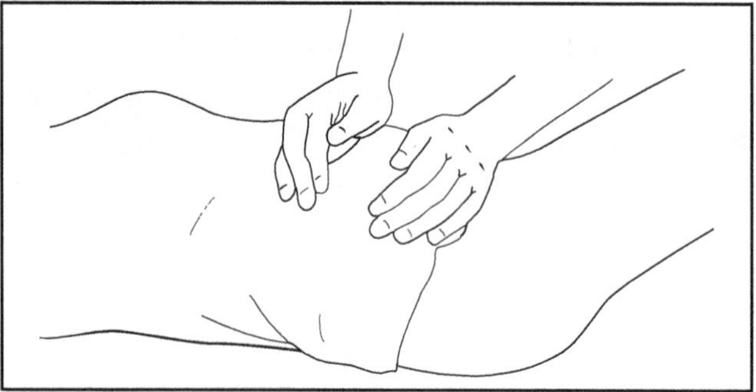

If this does not stop the bleeding the third maneuver is to insert your fist into the vagina and use it as a piston to press against the cervix while the other hand pushes down on the top of the uterus. Insertion of the fist may cause pain for a short while.

The fourth pressure maneuver is done with a sheet folded lengthwise to about two and a half feet wide and slipped under the hips, with one end hanging off the bed on one side, and the other end hanging off on the other side. Two people pick up the ends, exchange them over the top of the patient, and pull as firmly as possible, squeezing the hips. If the bleeding is from the cervix or from high in the vagina, the pressure can be helpful.

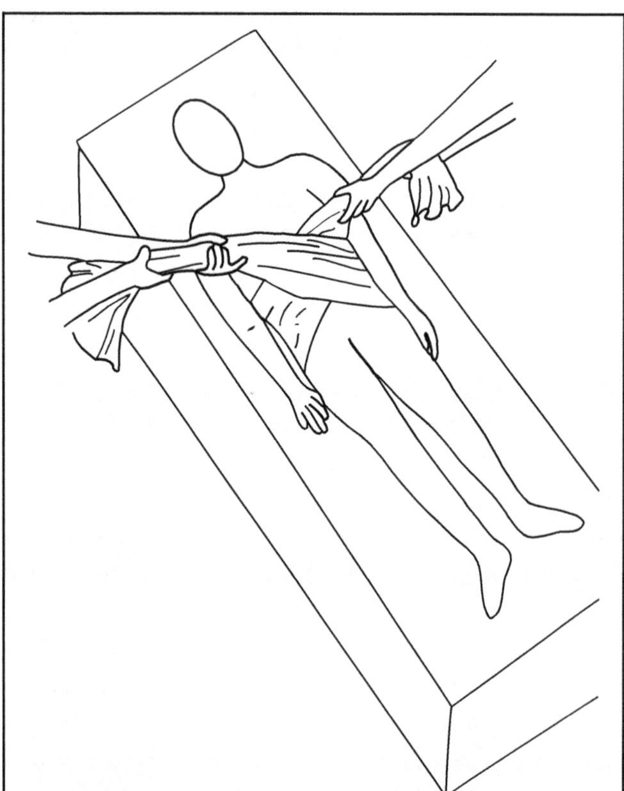

If the cervix is open, use blue and black cohosh. Place five drops of a tincture of each under the tongue. Hold the tincture under the tongue for 5 to 10 minutes without swallowing. Can repeat up to four times. It will lower the blood pressure. A blood pressure reading should be taken every two minutes for four readings. Then every 30 minutes or as needed.

If the cervix is closed use cramp bark root tea, red raspberry tea, and wild yam tincture. Make the tea as follows: Put one quart of water on to boil and add two tablespoons of cramp bark. Boil 25 minutes. Pour onto three tablespoons of red raspberry leaves; steep for 30 minutes. When cool, strain and then put 10 to 15 drops of the yam tincture in the tea. Use one cup at a time throughout the day.

Stomach Hemorrhage

If you vomit blood, there is a great chance that you have one of the following conditions. (1) peptic ulcer, (2) gastritis or an erosion of the esophagus or stomach, or (3) cirrhosis of the liver with esophageal varices. These three disorders will cause about 95 percent of all vomiting of blood from the stomach. Bear in mind also that blood which is vomited may have been blood that was swallowed during a heavy nosebleed, a tooth extraction, or an injury to the tongue or mouth. If it is foamy and frothy, it may have come from the lungs. If the blood is dark red or black and looks somewhat like coffee grounds, the bleeding is from quite some time before, perhaps even hours or days, and has stayed in the stomach long enough for the digestive juices to alter the appearance of the blood. If you feel thirsty or lightheaded, are sweating, or have ringing in the ears, the internal bleeding is substantial. The lightheadedness and ringing in the ears means your blood pressure has dropped. Vomiting blood should always be immediately evaluated by someone who has enough knowledge about stomach hemorrhage to make a proper decision as to treatment, as continued vomiting of blood is life threatening.

While awaiting emergency care, small lumps of ice may be swallowed, large ice compresses may be placed over the stomach for two to three minutes. Of course, the person should not ingest any food. A retention enema of eight ounces of lukewarm water can be made if the pulse rises, but blood replacement must be made if the patient vomits significant quantities of red blood. Vomiting as much as a cup or two of blood unmixed with food represents a dire emergency. A pulse above 100 or a drop in blood pressure may indicate a significant loss of blood and the need for immediate blood transfusion.

Hemorrhoids and Fissures

Hemorrhoids are caused by dilation of blood vessels at the end of the rectum, and fissures are caused by a division or crack between folds of the skin around the anus, usually at the depth of a fold in the purse string area of the anus. An anal fissure causes quite a lot of pain. So can hemorrhoids if they become thrombosed or ulcerated and inflamed. Bleeding from the rectum, often assumed to be from hemorrhoids, may be coming from many other sources. It is essential that the cause of the bleeding be identified. Cancer, polyps, inflammatory bowel disease, and occasionally diverticula can cause rectal bleeding.

Treatment

Use a high fiber diet. A dandelion salad eaten every day for six weeks, or fresh cooked dandelion root every day for six weeks, has been reported by one patient to completely cure her hemorrhoids, which had been a problem for several years since the birth of her last child. Psyllium seed may also be used. Take one dose of any method you choose, three times a day, until the hemorrhoids are gone.

Dr. Ludmilla Kolobanova from the Ukraine told me of a woman who had hemorrhoids following pregnancy that were very painful. For two months she had bled every day at the time of bowel movements. She got relief in two weeks from taking one tablespoon of strong, freshly squeezed onion juice three times a day. The total treatment period is four weeks, but often relief will come much sooner. The onion juice should be taken immediately before meals. As soon as the onion juice is swallowed, the person should drink a small amount of water, about two swallows. Dr. Kolobanova's patient obtained relief in about two weeks but continued the treatment for four weeks; she had no trouble during the next thirteen years.

Avoid gas forming foods as they promote painful hemorrhoids. A forceful expelling of intestinal gas can cause trauma of the anus and formation of a fissure or injury to a hemorrhoid.

Drink lots of water to avoid dry hard stools.

Avoid foods that are spicy and highly seasoned.

Daily out of doors exercise is very helpful for hemorrhoids.

Several times an hour, squeeze the muscles of the perineum and buttocks as if forcefully holding back the urine flow, and hold for 5 to 10 seconds. This procedure will empty the hemorrhoidal veins and bring in fresh blood for healing.

Avoid standing or sitting for prolonged periods unrelieved by walking, as this allows congestion of the hemorrhoidal veins.

Cleanse the tissues after a bowel movement by light rubbing or blotting with dampened toilet paper or a paper towel. Pouring warm water over the area and patting dry can also be used for cleansing.

An ice pack or a very warm compress can relieve pain. If the hemorrhoid becomes hard and has increasing pain, it means that the hemorrhoid has become thrombosed. It will gradually heal over several days. Vaseline or lecithin can be applied for soothing as can a golden seal, ice, or witch hazel compress. An astringent tea such as golden seal or witch hazel may be applied as hot or cold compresses. They not only sooth but heal.

The hot sitz bath is the treatment of choice for hemorrhoids. It brings pain relief and induces healing. It can be used for 10 to 20 minutes three to five times a day.

Boiled onions and raw garlic have been used as well as aloe. Three boiled onions should be eaten daily. The aloe is prepared by cutting a stalk and freezing it. Using a sharp knife, remove the tough green rind and the spikes. Cut a piece of the frozen blade into the shape of a lozenge or suppository and place it against the affected area, or insert it into the anal canal for internal hemorrhoids. Cover the area with a soft cloth or a panty liner. It is best done just before retiring because the plant "melts" and can get somewhat messy if up and walking.

If you are not sensitive to raw garlic, a garlic clove can be peeled, scraped to expose a moist surface, and inserted at bedtime as a suppository. To test if you are sensitive to raw garlic, peel and scrape the outside of a clove and put it in your mouth between your jaw and your teeth for two hours. If your mouth gets raw or tender, do not use it.

Avoid aspirin and local anesthetic agents as they tend to irritate.

Blackberry root, mullein, witch hazel, horse chestnut, and golden seal are good herbs for hemorrhoids.

An ointment may be made by putting one pint of petroleum jelly or a mixture of one-half cup of olive oil plus enough paraffin to make up one pint in the top of a double

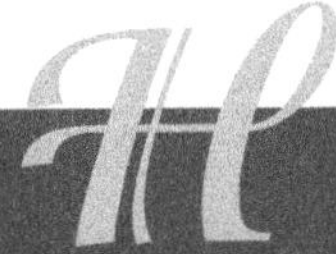

boiler. Add two ounces of one or more herbs such as plantain, calendula, yarrow, golden seal, or arnica. Thoroughly stir the mixture and boil in the double boiler for about two to three hours. The herbs may become crisp. Strain the mixture through a gauze lined kitchen strainer, squeezing as much of the oily material as possible into the container. Pour while it is still warm into clean storage jars. Plantain ointment is used to heal hemorrhoids, calendula or yarrow for skin rashes and fungus, golden seal for skin infections, and arnica ointment for muscle aches and pains. Obviously, more than one of the herbs may be needed. Use two ounces of each one you need.

Another salve for inflamed hemorrhoids may be made by putting two cups of coconut oil, one-half cup of dried yarrow leaves and flowers, two cups of dried plantain leaves, and one tablespoon of powdered golden seal root in a casserole dish. Mix the herbs and oil thoroughly. Put the mixture in an oven at the lowest possible setting for six to eight hours. While it is still warm strain it through a kitchen strainer lined with gauze or cheesecloth. Pour the oil into a wide mouth jar and store in a cool location. Apply a thin smear six times daily to hemorrhoids and after each use of the bathroom for either bladder or bowels.

An alternative preparation can be made by grating one-half cup of beeswax into one cup of olive oil. Add two heaping tablespoons of dried plantain and dried yarrow and one tablespoon of powdered golden seal root. Put the oil and herbs in a covered baking dish in a 200 degree oven for three hours. Strain while it is still warm and pour the oil into a glass jar and refrigerate. Note that it may be more convenient to add the beeswax after the oil and herbs have been removed from the oven and strained, but while still hot. Use for hemorrhoids as instructed above.

Elder flower oil is made by putting fresh or dry elder flowers in a jar and covering with olive oil. Tightly seal the jar and set it in a sunny location for two to three weeks. Strain and pour the oil into clean, airtight dark bottles. Store in a cool, dark place. Apply to hemorrhoids as instructed above, or to other skin lesions or rashes. Other flower oils may be made in a similar way.

Hepatitis

Hepatitis viral types are A, B, and C with less common varieties being D, E, and G, as well as other viral causes of hepatitis—herpes simplex virus, cytomegalovirus, and Epstein-Barr virus.

Hepatitis A

Hepatitis is an inflammation of the liver and gives signs and symptoms of jaundice, fatigue, lack of appetite, headache, backache, joint pains and stiffness, vomiting, diarrhea, constipation, muscle aches, and fever. Hepatitis A, the most common type, is spread by fecal contamination of water or food sources. Raw shellfish have been responsible for many outbreaks. It is usually benign and self-limiting, but it can cause several weeks of illness. It does not usually evolve into a chronic hepatitis infection, and only rarely is a death reported because of this type of hepatitis. About 15 percent of cases experience prolonged or relapsing hepatitis.

Should you contract hepatitis A, use every care to avoid spreading the disease, washing the toilet seat after each use or using a separate bathroom, washing your hands with soap and warm water after every bathroom use, and bathing very frequently. Avoid preparation of food or being in the food preparation area. Use disposable dishes and launder personal clothing and linens separately. It is not necessary to isolate yourself after the jaundice has been gone for two to three weeks.

Hepatitis B and C

Hepatitis B, which is shed in saliva, semen, and vaginal secretions, can be transmitted through sexual contact, and also through infected blood or blood products. Hepatitis B can live on dry surfaces for at least seven days, and is one of the most common causes of communicable disease, and the ninth cause of death worldwide. About 5 to 10 percent of adults and around 75 to 90 percent of children under the age of five who are infected with hepatitis B do not clear the virus from their bloodstreams within six months and are considered chronically infected.

Hepatitis C is primarily blood-borne but can also be transmitted sexually or through an infected mother to her newborn. Hepatitis C is responsible for roughly 90 percent of all cases of hepatitis contracted through blood transfusions. About one-third of patients who become infected with hepatitis C do not become chronically infected. But of those chronically infected, 70 percent will develop serious liver damage, and 20 to 30 percent of these will develop liver cancer or liver failure that requires a liver transplant. Monogamous sexual practices, a lifestyle promoting healthfulness, and a strong immune system are substantial preventive factors.

Not everybody who gets hepatitis C, not even all of those who get some scarring in the liver, have a lot of difficulty with hepatitis C. Unfortunately we have no way to predict

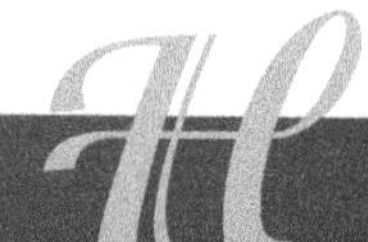

at the outset who may be more likely to have severe liver damage and who will experience no damage at all. There are several things that will serve very well for treating hepatitis C. We recommend milk thistle, two doses three times a day, taken with maximum doses of echinacea and golden seal, two herbs that can be obtained from a good herb shop. You should also be taking one teaspoon per day of high-potency lecithin having at least 50 percent phosphatidyl choline.

Some patients with the infection will develop B-cell, non-Hodgkin's lymphomas. When the lymphoma is diagnosed, if the spleen is removed and the patient given chemotherapy, a five-year survival rate of 80 percent may be obtained. The key seems to be the reduction in the hepatitis C virus. With simple remedies, which direct the treatments toward eliminating the hepatitis C infection, patients may put the lymphoma in long-term remission (*New England Journal of Medicine* 347 [2002]: 89).

Treatment for Hepatitis C

Treatment should include the use of large quantities of water (eight or more glasses), vegetable broths, diluted vegetable juices, and herbal teas. Solid foods should be restricted to brown rice, steamed vegetables, and legumes.

Free fats should be avoided such as margarine, mayonnaise, fried foods, and all refined oils as these fats can cause cellular damage and could contribute to blockage of bile flow.

Food containing added iron and iron supplements can combine with hepatitis C virus to form potent free-radicals that seriously damage liver cells. Be certain to avoid vitamin or mineral supplements containing iron, and if the blood iron is high, a therapeutic blood draw should be obtained through a blood bank.

Foods having high sulphur content such as garlic, legumes, and onions should be taken in generous quantities. So should foods containing water soluble fibers such as pears, oats, apples, and legumes. Other good foods having a therapeutic benefit in hepatitis include broccoli, Brussels sprouts, cabbage, artichokes, beets, and carrots.

Powdered charcoal, one tablespoon in water four times a day, may tie up the virus and transport it from the body.

Dandelion, turmeric, cinnamon, and licorice may also have a beneficial effect in the early treatment phase of hepatitis.

Selenium, N-acetyl cysteine (NAC), alpha-lipoic acid, licorice root, and milk thistle are very helpful.

A super charged silver solution has been helpful in some cases.

Treatment for All Types of Hepatitis

Do not overeat but maintain proper nourishment using a totally vegetarian diet, principally fruits and whole grains. Avoid free fats and oils, as in margarine and salad oils. Also avoid heavy protein foods even though vegetable in origin.

Drink water generously.

Avoid constipation and any other toxic condition.

Avoid any kind of toxic fumes, cleaning compounds and drugs, including birth control pills, aspirin, and corticosteroids (such as cortisone and prednisone as they encourage later relapses), all free fats, all free sugars, spices, vinegar, baking soda, baking powder, caffeinated beverages, alcohol and more than three dishes at a meal or anything or any practice that will put a burden on the liver.

It is quite proper even in the acute phase, to be active, but avoid becoming overly tired. Prolonged bed rest can lead to increased symptoms and weakness.

Hydrotherapy should be given in the acute phase in the form of hot baths and fomentations over the liver. The hot baths can be used to elevate the mouth temperature to around 102°F for 15 treatments. The fomentations over the liver should be kept hot for 15 minutes and followed by a cold compress for one minute and repeated three times each day for 45 minutes. In chronic active hepatitis, artificial fever treatments two or three days a week with fomentations over the liver on the off days can be beneficial. (See "Hydrotherapy" in the *Natural Remedies* section.)

Charcoal compresses and charcoal by mouth (one tablespoon three to four times daily) as well as oat or wheat bran by mouth (one tablespoon with each meal) can reduce the amount of bile salts and the degree of jaundice.

When jaundice produces itching, it can be relieved by giving guar gum (*European Journal of Clinical Investigation* 28, no. 5 [May 1998]: 359–63). It can also be treated the same as for pain, as itch and pain are carried over the same nerve pathways. (See "Pain Control" in the *Conditions and Diseases* section.)

Use silymarin, derived from milk thistle, to make tea. Drink one cup of tea or take two capsules three or four times a day. In chronic active cases, it should be continued indefinitely.

Artichoke capsules are liver protective. Use the same dose as for silymarin.

Japanese clinicians have used glycyrrhizin, an extract of licorice, for more than 20 years in hepatitis cases with good results. Since the extract is not currently available in

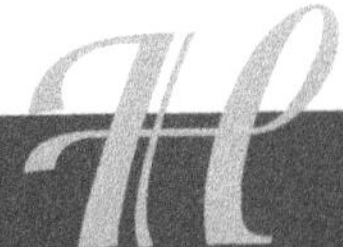

the United States, licorice tea may be used. A caution is that long-term use may cause salt and fluid retention and increase one's blood pressure. It should be used with caution in people with hypertension; and probably should be used only two weeks out of the month in individuals with normal blood pressure who start experiencing water retention or the rising of the patient's blood pressure.

Phyllanthus urinaria increased antibodies from 51 percent to 89 percent over a three-month period in one study. It is believed this herb can be of help in hepatitis (*Journal of Laboratory and Clinical Medicine* 126, no. 4 [1995]: 350).

Gently boil one and a half quarts of water to which has been added one-half cup of Echinacea purpurea root, three tablespoons of milk thistle seed, two heaping tablespoons of Oregon grape root, and two tablespoons of dandelion root. Remove from the stove after 25 minutes, strain. This is one day's dose. Give it in small divided doses throughout the day. If the patient tolerates it all right, the second day the dose should be doubled.

Astragalus root, licorice root, turmeric, and milk thistle are all good herbs to use in treating hepatitis, including hepatitis C (*Journal of Alternative and Complementary Medicine* 3 [1997]: 77). The dosage of turmeric is one-half teaspoon three times a day. We also advise that individuals with hepatitis C take ginkgo four times daily and flaxseed, two tablespoons freshly ground each morning on cereal or at lunch on salads or rice, etc.

Hernias

A hernia is a protrusion of a body part into a pouch of weakened wall of a cavity in which it is normally enclosed. It may occur through a weak spot in the abdominal wall, a weak point in the groin at the lowest point in the abdomen, at the navel, or in the area of the external sex organs. A hiatus hernia occurs if the stomach makes a small pouch at its upper end, which slides back into the chest through a weakening in the opening for the esophagus to go through the diaphragm to join the stomach.

Potential causes of a hernia include a muscular weakness present from birth, straining or lifting, childbirth, a surgical operation that did not heal properly, or a large tumor inside the abdomen.

Hiatus Hernia

This is a protrusion of the uppermost portion of the stomach up into the chest through the hiatus or opening in the diaphragm. Hiatus hernia is caused by increased intra-abdominal pressure just as are hemorrhoids and varicose leg veins. Major treatment is directed toward reducing the pressure by reducing gas, avoiding overeating, reducing weight, getting rid of tight bands around the waist, avoiding constipation or coughing, and avoiding heavy lifting, straining or bending immediately after meals. (See also "Hemorrhoids and Fissures," "Gas, Flatulence,"and "Constipation" in the *Conditions and Diseases* section.)

It is especially important to avoid all those foods known to relax the sphincter muscle, which guards the upper end of the stomach. Methylxanthines (found in coffee, tea, colas, and chocolate) are particularly troublesome. Alcohol, citrus juices, milk, spicy foods, tomato, tobacco, peppermint, and spearmint are all capable of relaxing the sphincter muscle.

Eat a wide variety of unrefined foods, avoiding all white flour products and sugar. Whole grain breads and cereals are very efficient in relieving straining when having a bowel movement. Fruits, vegetables, legumes, and nuts also contain good amounts of fiber.

Add one to three tablespoons of wheat bran to your diet each day; sprinkled on cereal, baked in bread, etc.

Eat only two meals a day, breakfast and lunch, no supper.

Drink 8 to 10 glasses of water daily.

Do not smoke or use tobacco in any form.

Get plenty of exercise. Especially helpful are walking and gardening. Do not lift heavy objects or work bending over. Do not lie down immediately after meals. These things encourage the opening up of the muscle that controls the junction between the esophagus and stomach, allowing stomach acids and food to run back into the esophagus, causing irritation.

Prop up the head of the bed four to eight inches on blocks.

Try three charcoal tablets chewed one and a half hours after meals to avoid gas.

Avoid aspirin and all its relatives.

Take one to two ounces of aloe vera juice or gel once or twice a day.

Drink one or two cups of slippery elm tea daily.

Inguinal and Femoral

These hernias occur through the lower abdominal wall and the same exercises in the treatments section benefit both conditions. No exercise should be employed until the hernia has been coaxed back into the abdomen and is entirely flat. Then lie flat on the floor (if over 45 so as not to increase pressure in the head and strain the blood vessels) or on a slant board with the head slightly lower than the feet (if under 45).

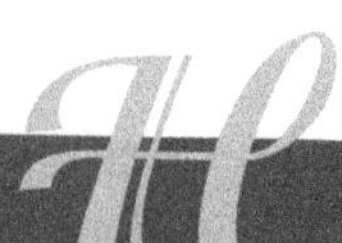

Don't expect miracles overnight as strengthening and repairing muscles is hard work and requires perseverance and concentrated, persistent effort. Slowly raise both legs about 14 inches. Now spread the legs apart. A variation of this exercise is to try to raise the legs while an assistant pushes them down.

The second exercise is also done while lying on the back or on the slant board. Hold the sides of the board for support. Now raise the knees over the head and do a cycling movement. Keep up the exercise for one minute, or until your tolerance is reached. Do not overdo. If you cannot do the exercise for one minute, continue trying until your abilities improve.

A chiropractor told me of a treatment he uses in women with small, recently (last year or so) developed hernias. He has the patient lie on a slant board or flat on the floor (if over 45), and then he gently massages the area to get the hernia to retract. Then he vigorously s the area where the hernia had been to try to stimulate ingrowth of new connective tissue, which will gradually form a scar under the hernia tract. If it is not painful, resulting in the development of slight tenderness the next day from the trauma, the scar tissue cannot grow in to strengthen the area. Repeat the treatment three times a week until the hernia quits bulging.

Treatment

Surgery is optional for hernia repair. You may try these simple remedies or simply live with the hernia.

A truss can be worn more or less permanently. If one is overweight, the weight should be brought to normal or slightly below normal. Fat gets into the ligament surrounding the fibrous tissue strands, weakening the ligament. Figure normal weight by allowing 100 pounds for your first five feet and five pounds per inch thereafter for women and six to seven pounds thereafter for men. Any increase in pressure inside the abdomen can make a hernia worse. The truss is a support that must be fashioned for the individual by someone who understands how to make such devices. Surgery can be used if the hernia gets too large or causes incapacitating pain.

An incarcerated hernia is one that is "stuck" and will not go back inside the abdomen when lying down. It may be treated by decreasing the tone of the voluntary muscles of the abdomen through the application of heat such as a mildly hot tub bath to reduce the tone of abdominal musculature so that the hernia may be released. A deep breathing exercise should be practiced during the bath to encourage decongestion of the hernia. After three or four minutes the abdominal wall should be nicely relaxed. Put firm sustained pressure on the hernia with the fingers while the patient forcibly sucks in his breath and reduces the pressure in the abdomen and chest. To apply the pressure, use a cold compress held firmly against the hernia. You may need to repeat the procedure several times. Small hernias are more likely to get caught than large ones, which can slip back and forth easily.

Those who have small hernias should carefully watch them, and if a portion of the abdominal contents gets caught in the opening, it should be replaced by lying flat on the back and putting pressure on the hernia to make the abdominal contents return into the abdomen. If it does not reduce, and if pain, bloating, and nausea occur, it is essential to seek medical attention as the bowel may eventually become gangrenous.

Herpes

Herpes viruses are a family of viruses; the most familiar ones cause fever blisters (Herpes simplex), genital herpes (Herpes genitalis), and chickenpox (Herpes zoster). The first two named are also known as Herpes I and Herpes II, respectively.

Herpes Simplex, Herpes I

The natural element lithium, as well as selenium, vitamin C, and lysine all inhibit the replication of the herpes virus and can discourage outbreaks of herpes blisters. Quercetin (from onions), rutin, and hesperidin are also helpful to reduce the outbreaks. See "Food Sources of Certain Nutrients" in the Dietary Information section for foods high in lithium, selenium, and vitamin C. (Also see "Cold Sores, Fever Blisters, Herpes I" in the *Conditions and Diseases* section.)

Genital Herpes, Herpes II

This disease is incurable and is referred to as the silent epidemic. The infection can often be silent and remain dormant for years before suddenly causing an acute outbreak of painful blisters. Approximately one in three to four women in the United States is infected, and the frequency increases with age. Almost everyone (89 percent) who has one outbreak of genital herpes lesions will develop at least one recurrence in the next year. About 35 percent have frequent recurrences (six or more in one year) with men having about 20 percent more recurrences than women (*Annals of Internal Medicine* 121 [1994]: 847). The typical genital herpes female patient suffers three or four flare-ups with painful blisters on the genitals each year, but more severely afflicted patients may have 12 to 16 recurrences a year.

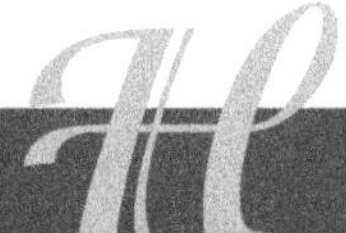

There are a wide range of symptoms, including vaginal discharge, genital tenderness, and vaginal bleeding. Men may suffer from blisters or ulcers on the genital area or adjacent skin. Both men and women may have painful urination, painful intercourse, fever, swollen glands in the groin, itching, loss of appetite, a sensation of loss of well-being, and localized abscesses if the lesions become secondarily infected. Complications of genital herpes include neuralgia, meningitis, urethral strictures, scarring and fusion of the labia, and lymphatic abscesses with long-term drainage. Herpes recurs more frequently during pregnancy, which increases the risk of premature delivery of the baby. Infected babies die about half of the time at childbirth. Birth defects include blindness and abnormalities of the central nervous system. An active herpes episode in the mother within a few days preceding delivery could be dangerous for the infant. At least 85 percent of these episodes are accompanied by easily detected lesions, and the baby should be delivered by cesarean section (*Science News*, December 24 and 31, 1983, 413).

A diet containing large amounts of arginine (another amino acid) appears to aggravate herpes. Foods to avoid include chocolate, nuts (especially peanuts, almonds, cashews, walnuts), seeds (sunflower and sesame), and coconut. Foods containing a moderate amount of arginine should be eaten with discretion. These include wheat, soy, lentils, oats, corn, rice, barley, tomatoes, and squash. Those suffering from an outbreak should avoid these foods until the blisters have disappeared.

Treatment for an outbreak includes compresses, sitz baths, hydrotherapy, soothing ointments, pain killers, and abstinence from sexual intercourse. The external use of calendula ointment, spirits of camphor, and aloe vera make the lesions heal faster.

For herpes II, when the blisters break out, take 1000 milligrams of lysine twice a day until the blisters have disappeared. Other remedies for the blisters are golden seal and echinacea, one teaspoon of tincture every hour until the blisters begin to recede. Of course, a totally plant-based diet with no margarine, mayonnaise, fried foods, and cooking fats or salad oils can be very helpful.

A naturopath who has treated herpes says that bee venom can be very successfully used. Build up from 1 sting per day to 10 stings. He has found that 10 stings per day will discourage the eruption of the blisters. The most favorable place for the stings is in or near the area where the blisters customarily erupt.

A high lysine and low arginine regimen has been shown by Dr. Christopher Kagan of San Francisco to inhibit recurrent outbreaks of blisters in about 85 percent of cases. After going on this routine, patients may have one additional outbreak, and then no more in the vast majority of cases, according to Dr. Kagan. Unfortunately, all foods high in lysine are also high in arginine. Therefore, the patient would be facing taking lysine supplements for about a year while reducing legumes (beans and peas), peanuts, and seeds.

Melissa officinalis (oil of citronella) possesses sedative, antispastic, and antibacterial properties, and in 1964 was demonstrated to have antiviral activity. Both genital herpes and fever blisters show good response to treatment, decreasing the time of the blisters by almost half as compared to placebo, external application (*Phytomedicine* 1 [1994]: 25–31).

Interferon has been recommended, but sells for $100 for a trillionth of a gram. Vaccines and medication offer little hope (*Modern Medicine*, December 1983, 165).

Herpes Zoster, Shingles

Shingles, a virus infection of the nerves, produces severe nerve inflammation with blisters on the skin in persons who have had chickenpox earlier in life. Most frequently the blisters appear near the waist but can be anywhere from scalp to sole. Only one side of the body is usually involved, and the nerves leading to the eyes, or other vital structures, may be affected. When the eye is affected, the blisters form not only on the forehead and eyelids, but even on the eyeball itself. If the eyeball is involved, it can cause blindness, and it requires professional attention. The affliction often comes when the body resistance is low, and may be preceded by smarting pain, general feeling of indisposition, and/or respiratory or digestive disturbances for two to three days prior to the onset of the blisters. These may persist for a week or two, then dry up.

External pain is rare but occasionally happens, and fever and feeling poorly occur with a few patients. In adults, acute shingles can be followed by pain in the area called "postherpetic neuralgia," which can last for weeks, months, or for life. Treatment with the following natural remedies in the early stages must not be neglected.

Pain is usually intense, burning, knifelike, and punctuated by attacks of greater severity. Pain often precedes and persists after the blisters and rash have subsided. Reduced sensation or increased sensation may occur in the healed area. Sixteen percent of people having chickenpox will get shingles by the ninth decade of life. Patients with malignancies, especially Hodgkin's disease, have been especially prone to shingles.

Outline a physical conditioning program appropriate for the stamina of the patient, with the diet restricted in fats and sugars.

Upon diagnosis, immediately put the patient into a full-body pack, or a heated tub or whirlpool, to induce a fever of 102°F by mouth. Do this daily for three to five days or until the skin eruptions dry up. An early, mild case may subside with three treatments. An advanced, severe case will require more treatments. The treatments have often been completely curative, even when they are not begun until three weeks or more after the onset of the disease.

Give a full body massage once or twice a day for a week or two. Do not open the blisters.

To treat post-herpetic neuralgia, put one teaspoon of red pepper (cayenne or capsicum) in a pint jar with one cup of rubbing alcohol. Let it soak together for two to three weeks, swirling it once a day. Strain the mixture through a cloth and use the alcohol. Paint the alcohol solution on the painful areas six times daily for six days, then two times daily thereafter as long as pain continues. Use a cotton-tipped applicator to prevent contact with fingers.

Charcoal by mouth, and charcoal compresses worn at night over the blistered area can be very helpful.

Administer a cup of golden seal tea four times daily for one week.

Garlic or aloe vera should be taken by mouth, and aloe vera compresses should be worn directly on the blisters in the daytime. (See the *Herbal Remedies* section.)

For discomfort, one can use kava-kava tablets three times daily and St. John's wort essential oil. These can be very soothing for the person who has uncomfortable shingles. The essential oil should be diluted 1 to 10 with olive oil and applied sparingly three times daily. Test the solution by using a small portion of the dilution over about one inch of skin adjacent to the area of discomfort. Leave it on for about half an hour before applying to the entire area. If stinging or itching occurs, you are probably sensitive to the St. John's wort essential oil and should not use it. But if you can use it, you should see good results in a few days. Our most excellent result, however, has been with geranium essential oil. Dilute as with other essential oils and apply directly to the skin.

Case Report

Alice wrote to us that her friend Betty came to her house one night on business looking very sick. On inquiry Betty said she had shingles and was in a lot of pain, was itching, and was not able to sleep. Alice remembered our report of a woman who had shingles in her eye and had applied aloe vera. Betty had just been to see her doctor and gotten some salve, but it was not giving her any relief. She said she would try anything. Alice gave her some aloe vera plant cuttings and told her how to use it. Betty took a blade of the plant, sliced it with a sharp knife and laid the slices on the painful areas, bandaging it on for several hours. She slept all night. She was so happy. She had no more pain, itching, or burning.

Hiccups

Individuals having chronic hiccups (hiccups lasting more than six hours) may have a small foreign body so deep within the external ear canal that the foreign body is resting against the ear drum. Often this foreign body is a bit of trash or even a bit of hair. Persons will usually recover immediately after these foreign bodies are flushed out by irrigation with lukewarm water (*New England Journal of Medicine* 318 [1988]: 711). (See "Irrigation Fluids" in the *Natural Remedies* section.)

The following suggestions may also bring relief: Put some sugar or salt on your tongue. Drink water from the opposite rim of a glass. Bend forward from the waist at a 90 degree angle. Rub the palate with a blunt instrument such as a spoon handle. You may also drink a glass or two of water, gargle with water, lie on the left side 5 to 10 minutes, put pressure from the fist in the pit of the stomach for a minute or two, pinch the upper lip just under the nose and push upward toward the nose sufficient to make the lip hurt, induce sneezing, hold the breath as long as possible then blow it out and hold it out as long as possible. Repeat until the hiccups stop.

Another method of curing hiccups is sipping a glass of water in small swallows through a straw while holding both index fingers firmly in the ears to shut out all sound and make a slight vacuum seal.

Drink water through a cloth napkin. Simply place the napkin over the rim of the glass and suck the water through it. It is most effective.

Another cure for hiccups is gently tickling the hair in your ear canal with the paper end of a match. Try not to touch the flesh of the ear.

Put a spoon in a large glass of ice water until the spoon is cold. Then touch the rounded side of the spoon against your forehead as you drink the entire glass of water.

Try coughing at the exact moment the hiccups come. The reflex to cough is sufficient to repress the reflex for hiccups.

Another remedy is that of drinking a glass of water as hot as you can tolerate without a pause to breathe. Try to relax

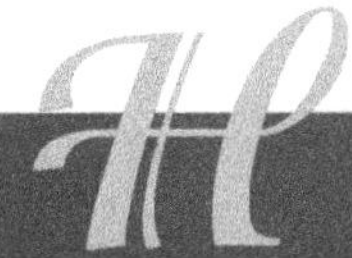

your abdominal muscles at the same time. Usually the hiccups will go away immediately.

Hold your breath as long as possible, exhale as far as possible, and hold it out without taking another breath. The buildup of carbon dioxide inhibits the hiccup reflex.

Hip Pain

Pain in the hip typically causes a pain directly on the front of the hip in the center of the groin, or in the corresponding position in the upper buttock, directly in the back. Pain from nonjoint areas such as the hip capsule usually occurs on the outside or lateral aspect of the hip. Causes of hip pain in childhood may be osteochondritis of the femoral head, separation of the capital femoral epiphysis, or trauma. People with joint involvement of the hip often complain of pain in the knee and front of the thigh. Anyone complaining of pain in the knee should be examined also for hip joint problems.

Pain on the side of the hip is usually because of pain in the joint capsule rather than in the joint itself. Overuse of the joint such as in excessive walking can cause this kind of pain. Injury sustained many years before pain develops can be the cause of capsular pain or pain in the bone or cartilage. This kind of pain often occurs only at a certain point as the hip is being moved, as in walking.

Hives, Urticaria (Acute or Chronic)

Hives are pale or reddened elevated areas with reddish "feet" that stick out in all directions from the elevated patch. Hives are accompanied with painful itching that may be burning and intense.

Stop all milk products at once. Not only is milk protein very allergenic, but dairy products may contain traces of antibiotics to which the person may be sensitive.

Some surface irritant, food, or chemical to which one has been exposed is the most likely cause. A glassful of water every 10 minutes for an hour and an enema may be very helpful to stop acute hives by moving out the irritating substance from the bowel. If the affliction becomes chronic, it is necessary to examine one's diet to determine the foods causing the hives. (See "Elimination and Challenge Diet" in the *Dietary Information* section.)

A shower, as hot as can be tolerated, may halt acute hives progression. Chronic hives can be treated by fasting. Rashes begin to decrease about the third day of the fast and will completely disappear on day 11. The hives may return after breaking the fast, but are usually milder than the previous ones. It may be possible to introduce one food at a time while breaking the fast, taking note of any food that causes a return of the hives and eliminating that food. Return one food at a time every five to seven days and thus determine the food causing the hives (*Dermatology* 19, no. 7 [1992]: 428–31).

Probably the most helpful treatment we have used for hives has been activated charcoal powder. A 47-year-old man with almost intolerable hives of three days duration called for our help. We prescribed two heaping tablespoons of charcoal powder in a glass of water every two hours, a charcoal bath, an enema, and plenty of water by mouth. Within three hours he was well.

A warm starch bath, oatmeal bath, or charcoal bath helps the painful itching.

Herbal teas such as nettles, feverfew, and echinacea are helpful.

Hoarseness, Laryngitis

Hoarseness may be caused by drinking, smoking, speaking, singing, dehydration, a food sensitivity, or a viral infection. Rarely, hoarseness is because of polyps or cancer of the vocal cords. If it persists more than two or three weeks, seek medical care for a diagnosis.

To treat hoarseness, Fill a vaporizer or kettle with hot water. If you like, add a few drops of eucalyptus or wintergreen oil, one or two tablespoons of dried or fresh mint leaves per pint of water, or two to three drops of the mint oil. Set the kettle or vaporizer on a bedside stand or chair. Open an umbrella on a chair or bedside stand, and drape a sheet over it to form a tent. By lying on one side of the bed, the patient can stick his/her head under the tent and breathe the steam. Continue for one-half hour two to three times a day or more.

The effects of the treatment are as follows: warming and soothing for the respiratory tract; relief of nasal and lung congestion; healing for laryngitis or cough; increased blood flow to the respiratory tree; and loosening of secretions making it easier to expectorate.

Drinking a glassful of water every 10 minutes for an hour will often be very helpful.

Add two tablespoons of the Balm of Gilead to one quart of water. Boil gently for 20 minutes. Gargle it for pharyngitis and laryngitis.

One of the best treatments is the liberal use of white oak bark tea.

Huntington's Disease

This disease is the result of a mutation on chromosome IV. As a rule, it becomes expressed as loss of mental and nerve functions by the age of 30 to 50. Vitamin E has been used, but not a lot of good seems to result from it. Antioxidant therapy is easy to accomplish by the use of vitamins C, E, and selenium. All fresh fruit and vegetables, soybeans, whole grains, nuts and seeds have very large antioxidant effects. This dietary treatment may slow down the rate of muscle decline early in the course of Huntington's disease. The earlier in the course of the disease the treatment is instituted the better the case turns out.

Hyperactive Child, ADHD

(See also "Mental Disorders" in the *Conditions and Diseases* section.)

Rich rewards will come from learning some fundamental principles and faithfully following a few basic suggestions in regards to this common disorder. The child should be treated aggressively to promote long-term benefits. School dropout, drugs, and crime are more common in those for whom the cause is not determined and eliminated. The child faithfully trained at home throughout all the formative years does best. The book *Child Guidance* by Ellen G. White provides a wealth of parenting information and suggestions.

Attention deficit disorder (ADD), with or without hyperactivity disorder (ADHD), is a behavioral disturbance usually starting before the age of seven, and lasting at least six months, and in some cases persisting to some degree into adulthood. Intelligence is usually normal or superior, but the victims have symptoms that are observed by third parties who may label the child with ADD or ADHD as a troublemaker. These children may talk excessively, interrupt and intrude upon others, and have difficulty in playing quietly or sitting still. They tend to leave tasks unfinished and shift prematurely from one subject to another. They may be very compulsive, plunging heedlessly into touching, opening, or picking up something they are being told to leave alone. Once the symptoms are well developed, they usually tend to remain constant for that individual, not usually getting much worse. Mild cases will often grow out of it, especially at puberty, but about 10 percent persist into adulthood (*Journal of the American Medical Association* 273 [1995]: 1871).

ADHD has three sub types. The first is inattention with forgetfulness, distractibility, losing things, poor organization, and inability to sustain attention on activities. The second is the hyperactivity, impulsivity type characterized by fidgeting, restlessness, inability to sit still, difficulty waiting their turn, excessive talking, interrupting, and inability to engage in leisure activities quietly. The third type is a combination of the first two.

Brain imaging studies indicate that the brains of ADHD children have certain regions that are smaller in size.

Facts and Treatment

Hyperactivity in children is a common childhood disorder involving 3 to 10 percent of school children in this country. It is a modern societal disease, developing from features in our lifestyle. Boys are affected more than girls—about nine boys to one girl.

Stimulant drugs are often given for this disorder, but need not be used if a proper program for the child is instituted. Often the treatment is worse for the child than the illness, since, under the influence of the drugs, the personality is altered, with many becoming compulsive "goodie-goodies," sensitive to discipline, and incapable of proper use of the mind. One personality problem and physiologic reaction is exchanged for others, without improving the condition of the child, and only giving temporary relief to the parent.

Hyperactive children may be growth-retarded. A large percentage of hyperactive children have a low blood sugar. These children should have a blood insulin level checked by a laboratory. If it is abnormal, the parents should read *Diabetes and the Hypoglycemic Syndrome* by Dr. Calvin Thrash.

In addition to hyperactivity, many of the children are found to have anemia, impaired achievement, and defective breakdown of stress hormones in the body. These all indicate a multiple systems disorder, not just neuromuscular, not just digestive, and not just central nervous system, as many have supposed.

A disordered home life intensifies the child's condition. Family problems are never to be discussed in the hearing of children.

Fathers are needed by children as well as mothers, especially beginning at about age five. Fathers should give some of their leisure hours to their sons in particular. Let your son help you with household chores, building projects, and business transactions with other people, etc.

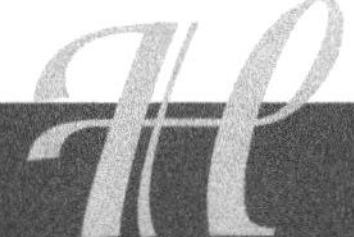

Do not place the child with unfamiliar persons at night. He should go to bed in his own bed every night. Have no other persons in his bed. Sleepovers are fashionable but are unhealthful, both physically as well as socially. Plan some other type of social activity.

He should not be expected to do activities that are beyond his years, such as learning to read early, being responsible for a younger child, etc. Schooling should be delayed until physical maturity indicates that he is able to concentrate for long periods, and the ideal is home schooling. Other children always have an adverse effect on hyperactive children. If the child must be sent to school, the time should be delayed until about 8 to 10 years of age for these children. To start a child earlier usually results in unhappiness for all, and in his forming a permanent mental image of himself as a poor achiever, a pest, a slow learner, and someone who is not liked by others.

Factors now known to be related to the development of hyperactivity are as follows:

- Lead poisoning – 20 PPB are allowed in water. There is 10 to 15 percent absorption in adults and 50 percent in children! Learning difficulties and hyperactivity from lead occur in children. Decreased concentration occurs in adults. Avoid softened water, as you will get more cadmium and lead. There is 35,000 tons of lead put into America's atmosphere per year. Lead absorption is greater if one is fasting. Lead in the food or atmosphere goes to bone, blood, soft tissue, brain, and nerve cells.

  Zinc, iron, copper, calcium, and magnesium deficiencies all cause a greater absorption of lead.

  Lead decreases myelin-synthesizing enzymes, the enzymes that help form a sleeve around nerve cells to improve function. Kidney tubules and blood vessels are damaged. Hypertension is likely. Lead damages the internal structure of the cells' mitochondria. Household sources include moonshine, paint, house dust, soil in the yard and street, newsprint, lead pipes, three-piece cans used for canned foods, drinking water, milk, toothpaste, kettles, and painted glassware.
- Iron deficiency anemia.
- Other factors of malnutrition. These include overnutrition, or selective over feeding of certain nutrients such as white flour and white rice products, boxed cereals, sweet food or drink, and too-rich foods. Oils and margarine are also rich foods that imbalance the diet. Don't use lard, and check the labels as it is often found in homogenized peanut butter, bread, and crackers.
- Certain food colorings, especially red dye II, a common dye used in many red foods from hot dogs to suckers; many food additives, including flavorings, preservatives, and vitamin and mineral supplements, are stimulating to some.
- The overuse of sweets begins in the hospital nursery with sugar water. Breastfeeding is all the baby needs for the first six months. Since certain children are sensitive to eggs and milk, it is worth a strict trial of six weeks without either of these or any of their products. Read food labels carefully. Similarly, since meats have stimulating purine substances in them, eliminate all flesh foods from the diet during the same six-week period. Supply the child with plenty of greens, whole grains, and legumes (beans, peas, and peanuts) in place of animal products.
- Eliminate stomach irritants such as pepper, spices, baking soda, baking powder products, caffeinated drinks, chocolate, and any foods that "disagree" with the child (milk is a common offender).
- The most important vitamin supplements for ADD are vitamin B3 (niacin) and vitamin B6. Niacinamide does not produce a skin flush but is very bitter. The starting dose is 1.5 to 3 grams daily in three divided doses. If the dose is too high, the major side effect is nausea. The earliest sign is a lack of appetite.
- Inadequate external controls in the parental environment, reflected by such things as eating between meals, temper flare-ups, and no set pattern of life, enhance the child's problems.
- TV, comics, radio, stereo, and competitive games irritate the nervous system.
- Noisy home environment and city living make improvement difficult. A quiet home in the country with space to run, explore, and investigate is ideal.
- Improper clothing of the child is a cause of discomfort and hyperactivity. The arms and legs, feet, hands and ears should always be warm. There should be no patches of cold skin anywhere on the body except the face. Tight bands must be avoided. If a band leaves a mark on the skin, it is too tight. There should not be more layers of clothing on the trunk than on the extremities. Similarly, the child should not be over-clothed. When the temperature rises, the clothing should be adjusted. Multiple layers of thinner garments are better than one or two thick garments.

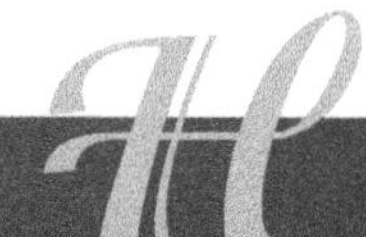

- Inconsistent discipline and unwise supervision lead to poor personal control. Have few rules for the child, but strictly enforce them.
- Disarray and clutter confuse children and lead to poor performance. Keep everything the child's eye rests upon neat and orderly.
- An irregular schedule upsets the natural biologic time-clock. Have set times for all major events: bedtime and arising time, exercise time, mealtime, bath time, story time, etc. Irregularity may seem a small thing to the parents, but it takes a great toll on the child's nervous system.
- Be sure to recognize good behavior because it tends to reinforce it, and gently and briefly disapprove or ignore misbehavior, depending on whether the child is misbehaving to gain attention or misbehaving because of not knowing. If the child knows that the parent does not approve of certain acts and does them anyway, that should not be ignored. A loud or harsh reprimand is harmful. A gentle, soft-spoken disapproval with hope expressed for future behavior is much more effective and encourages cooperation.

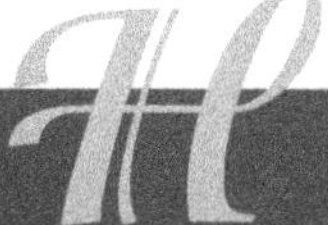

Idiopathic Thrombocytopenic Purpura

This disorder is characterized by bruised spots on the skin because of low platelet count. ITP can be successfully treated using simple remedies.

Case Reports

A lady once came to Uchee Pines Lifestyle Center whose platelets (thrombocytes) were below 10,000. She had been treated in many different ways in standard medicine with only brief success. The treatment program we used consisted of mild fever treatments followed by cold mitten friction. Friction on the skin should be gentle so as not to provoke a shower of petechiae. We gave her barley grass, one teaspoon three times daily; flaxseed oil, one tablespoon twice daily; and licorice root tea, one tablespoon in a liter of water boiled gently for a half hour and administered four doses throughout the day and made up fresh daily. She got sun baths daily, full body massage (done gently and fully clothed to prevent bruising) three times weekly, and a plant-based diet. The plant-based diet is the most favorable diet for healing, although we noticed initially a small reduction in the thrombocytes. She did well on this program, platelets rising to 55,000 in less than a month.

Another patient, a fifty-four-year-old, single, black female office manager, came to Uchee Pines for help because of easy bruising on the right leg; aching in the wrist, ankles, knees, and other joints; severe fatigue; and a platelet count of 6,000. Her sed rate was 99 done in a hospital in a distant city. She had a low grade fever and anemia of 9.6 grams hemoglobin, 28.9 hematocrit. She had been offered a treatment schedule of cortisone, but hesitated and then decided to seek alternative treatment. On arrival at Uchee Pines, her platelet count was 5,000. After one week of warm baths, exercise, and sunning to tolerance, lots of green juices, salads, and cooked greens, massage and other treatments, her platelet count had risen to 11,000, and in two weeks to 23,000. The patient's symptoms improved, and she felt stronger both physically and emotionally after one month.

Her treatment consisted of the health recovery program (see the *Supplemental Information* section), regularity, vegetarian diet, and avoidance of sugar, free fats, and free carbohydrates. Her diet was specifically restricted in the following ways: no night-shades (tomatoes, potatoes, eggplant, peppers, pimento, paprika), or whole wheat, nut butters, or nuts. She could have avocados and olives, flaxseed, and pumpkin seeds, as she wished, but no citrus fruits or juices.

The restrictions even in the vegetarian diet are because of the potential those foods have for causing an adverse immune system reaction. The almonds and walnuts, unless known to cause a sensitivity reaction, can provide essential fatty acids—omega-3 and eicosapentaenoic acids—to stimulate the immune system. Flaxseed has an anti-inflammatory effect similar to cortisone. Pumpkin seeds have a high content of zinc. We sometimes use licorice root tea, white willow bark, hawthorn berry and other anti-inflammatory herbs.

Physical therapy included mild exercise to her tolerance and five weekly fever treatments in a whirlpool. Vinegar was rubbed on a skin rash that was diagnosed as ringworm. She took dandelion tea, licorice root, ginseng, hawthorn berry, and Pau d'Arco tea. She took two charcoal capsules five times daily, and barley green. Upon arrival she could walk about one block without excessive fatigue, but after two weeks she was walking three miles a day. We added licorice root, echinacea, and golden seal, one tablespoon of each, to a quart of water and gently boiled it for 20 minutes. After it was set off the heat, we added yarrow and butcher's broom. It was steeped for 30 minutes. She took this tea daily for six weeks.

This case illustrates the fact that without the use of steroids or other pharmaceuticals a case of ITP can be handled if great care is used and the patient led to trust in the Lord. This patient had a continued rising of her platelet count until within six months she was above a hundred thousand. Five year follow-up showed her to be in good health and traveling to a foreign country for a period of service with a mission board.

Immune System, How to Strengthen

(See also "AIDS" and "Stress" in the *Conditions and Diseases* section.)

The immune system is the most important regulator of our body. Therefore, regularity in all things is essential to keep it strong. The central nervous system can direct the immune system, and is probably the mechanism whereby trust in divine power has a healing function. It is of interest that macrophage activity and cell proliferation in lymph nodes increases toward the end of the dark period of the day, and peaks in the mid to late afternoon, on much the same pattern that the temperature varies.

Calorie restriction retards aging and increases life span, provided the restriction does not result in actual nutrient deficiencies or imbalances. Beneficial changes can occur in the circadian pattern of the immune system by calorie restriction. These changes are not well understood at the present time (*European Journal of Clinical Nutrition* 569S3 [2002]: S69-S72).

When you are sick, you may do several things to get well. Alternate exercise suitable for your sickness with diet suitable for your sickness and sleep or keeping your eyes closed every moment you can. Closing the eyes rests the brain and mind. Healing electrical rhythm starts as soon as the eyes are closed and ceases immediately when they are opened. This rhythm acts as a clearing agent for "negative charges" from the brain. Activity of the eyes retards recuperation and the clearing of these negative forces. Try to get more sleep or closing your eyes.

After activity, the brain grows weary and the physical demand for sleep and/or closing the eyes increases with each hour since the last period of sleep. Nerve cell fatigue or exhaustion can get quite deep-seated and requires a good bit of time to recover. It is the reduction of vital energy in the nerve cells that can lead to a complete physical or mental breakdown.

The weaker the person's body, the greater the necessity to close the eyes and do nothing for a period of time. The person can spend the time concentrating on the characteristics of God or meditating on the Scriptures. Do not allow negative thoughts. When discomfort or depression prevents your from sleeping, simply keep your eyes closed until the pain, discomfort, or depression leaves. If you cannot sleep at night, as long as you continue to keep your eyes closed, concentrating and meditating on sacred themes, you will arise almost as refreshed as if you had slept for that same period of time. To encourage healing of any disease, you should rest your brain and body by keeping the eyes closed, especially during periods that should be devoted to sleep. Open your eyes only to satisfy your needs, whether they be biological, physical, social, economic, or spiritual.

Fasting a day or so can strengthen the immune system. During a fast it is best to have total rest during the major portion of the fast. You can only accomplish total rest by prayer and meditation. Lie down, close the eyes every moment you can. It is the most important thing you can do to recuperate during the time of your fast.

Eating too much polyunsaturated fat produces widespread immunologic defects in laboratory animals, consisting of depressed T-cell responsiveness and lymphoid tissue atrophy. Even mega-doses of vitamin E may inhibit the immune system, although proper amounts of vitamin E enhance the immune response (*Journal of the American Medical Association,* January 1981, pp. 53–8).

Breastfeeding boosts immunity, whereas cow's milk tends to reduce immunity. Mother's milk has a special feature of stimulating the baby's own immune system. Breastfeeding along with its many other advantages appears to protect infants from disease by encouraging the maturation of a child's immune system. Breast milk especially encourages an agent in the immune system called tumor necrosis factor, which is known to bolster the immune system.

To increase the effectiveness of the immune system, or when recovering from an illness or childbirth, use seaweed soup or tea to regain strength. One teaspoon of Savorex, Marmite, or yeast flakes in hot or cold water can be taken as a drink to boost the effectiveness of the immune system.

Eat onions, garlic (equivalent of three cloves or four 500 milligram garlic pills), yellow or green vegetables, red vegetables, or other very colorful fruits and vegetables. Ginger (a half teaspoon twice a day or four 500 milligram pills), turmeric (a fourth teaspoon twice or three times a day or two 500 milligram pills), are both stimulators of the immune system.

A loss of three hours sleep between the hours of 3:00 and 7:00 a.m. can cause a 20 to 30 percent decrease in the activity of natural killer cells. These cells help us to fight viruses, cancer, and other viral disorders. This information was presented by Dr. Michael Irwin at the World Federation of Sleep Research's annual meeting in Hawaii in May 1993.

Exercise and relaxation were found to lower anger-hostility expressions. Blood pressure and heart rate were reduced, and overall benefits were experienced (*Journal of Behavioral Medicine* 14, no. 5 [1991]: 453; *Research Quarterly for Exercise and Sports* 63, no. 1 [March 1992]: A-78).

Elderly persons who regularly attend religious services, have healthier immune systems than non-attenders (*International Journal of Psychiatry in Medicine* 27 [1997]: 233–50). Religious exercises such as Bible study and prayer also have a salutary effect on the biological functions.

It is well known that serious personal problems can increase the likelihood of getting stress of severe enough proportions to cause the immune system to function poorly. Contrary to Freudian psychology, progressive Christian counselors have taught that verbal expression of a known problem could be harmful. Research now provides evidence that Freud was wrong. If a person talks about problems being experienced, the immune system suffers. Natural killer cells are decreased. More hostility is generated by speaking of the troublesome problem, and natural killer cells are more profoundly depressed as hostility rises.

Other systems than the immune system are also harmed—nervous, mental, gastrointestinal, even musculoskeletal—by talking about your problems. It is better to keep one's problems to oneself and to speak earnestly only to the Lord in prayer concerning the matter. When praying about problems, begin the prayer by asking the Lord for control of any hostility (*Psychosomatic Medicine* 58 [1996]: 150–55). Speak to the Lord personally. This is the time to talk about your problems and ask God to remove the stress resulting from the problem. Then rise from your knees, believing that God now has your permission and cooperation to deal with the matter.

The immune system is strengthened by creativity and by responsibility. Writing is a strengthener for the immune system.

- To discipline the mind. Normally thoughts roam about. Writing things down provides a pathway for the mind, gives direction to one's thinking, and helps one to master the faculty of thought.
- Intellectual humility. Writing demands humility. First, I must look at myself as I really am. I must see the vagueness of my thinking, the inconsistency of my logic, and the triviality of my life. This experience can and should be humbling.
- To record graces received from God. We should keep a record of the graces, the power from God to accomplish a task or overcome a weakness, and answers to prayer that we have received from God. We should record when we have received His mercies and when we should have received His judgment.
- To cultivate the memory. By writing down our thoughts and spiritual experiences, we can remember life's experiences.
- To make a moral inventory. The importance of a daily review of one's conduct put in some written form serves three purposes.
  - It shows how serious we are about overcoming our failures.
  - It shows how honest we are about wanting to grow in virtue.
  - It gives us an opportunity to evaluate our progress in the spiritual life.
- To assist in cultivating Christlike speaking. Too often we speak without thinking. The practice of writing will help us to develop the art of speaking according to God's will. James 3:2: "If anyone does not offend in word, he is a perfect man."
- To have something to share. If we keep a record of our experiences, interesting episodes, and uplifting sentiments, we have something to share with others that can be a blessing to them. Each of us has parables that occur in our own lives. We should make a written memo of the parables in our own lives so that we can share them with others for the blessing it will be to them.

To encourage the functioning of the immune system take from 30 to 150 milligrams of CoQ10 daily. Higher doses are taken for more severe cases of weak immune systems (*Biochem Biophys Res Commun* 153 [1988]: 888–96).

Beta 1,3/1,6-D-Glucan is a powerful immune booster from baker's yeast. Herbal immune stimulants include barberry, basil, blue cohosh, burdock, chamomile, echinacea, golden seal, Indian gooseberry, licorice, marshmallow, and nettle are all good for strengthening the immune system. Ginseng, oregano, rue, fennel, figs, gingko, tarragon, thyme, yarrow, grapefruit, and astragalus enhance the immune system and also fight against the development of cancer.

Immunization

The vaccinations for Haemophilus influenza have been suspected in some quarters to be related to an increase in Type I diabetes. In a group of children receiving four doses of the vaccine, the rate of diabetes was elevated by 26 percent after seven years compared to children receiving no vaccine. Immunization against Haemophilus is expected to prevent seven deaths and between seven and twenty-six cases of severe disability per 100,000 children immunized. There are, however, 58 cases of diabetes per 100,000 children immunized, more than would be expected in those receiving no vaccine. Dr. J. Bart Classen published his findings in the May 7, 1999, edition of the *British Medical Journal.* Diabetes also results in an increased death rate and severe disability. It seems best to evaluate taking one's chances with the disease and treating it with natural remedies if it occurs, and pray for God to add His supernatural blessing to His natural remedies.

Two measles vaccines were tested during a major U.S. epidemic of measles in 1989. The researchers failed to mention that one of the vaccines was experimental. Fifteen hundred minority infants in Los Angeles were used in the experiment. A spokesperson for the Centers for Disease Control, to explain why minorities were chosen to conduct an unannounced experiment, said, "A mistake was made; it shocked me." It seems there are many such mistakes made in relation to various vaccination programs and in the production of many vaccines. These mistakes do little to increase the confidence of parents whose children are of the age to be vaccinated. In Africa and Haiti the same vaccines were used, and there was an increased death rate among female infants who received the more potent of two dosages being studied. The vaccination program in Los Angeles was halted in 1991. Very little publicity is given to these mistakes and tragedies involving vaccines, but they serve to cause many parents to fear any substance that is injected into their helpless infants.

Some evidence has been presented that some cases of chronic fatigue syndrome may be related to the rubella (German measles) vaccine. We suggest caution in the use of similar (attenuated) viral vaccines.

Impetigo

This skin disease consists of red spots that may quickly develop into tan blisters. The fluid is infectious and quite contagious. Adults sometime get impetigo, but it is the most frequent skin infection among children in which there are pus-filled eruptions. The blisterlike swellings surrounded by a tiny rim of redness will form a honey colored, crusted lesion in four to six days, and will heal with good treatment in a week or two. It is transmitted either directly from one person to another or by contact with pets, toys, or articles used by an infected person.

If the infection is promptly treated, recovery is often achieved in a week without extensive spread from the original site. The red spots develop one after the other, sometimes within hours of one another, causing a good bit of consternation in parents who witness its rapid spread. The lesions may be intensely itchy, and the child's fingernails should be cut off to the quick and the hands covered with gloves, mittens, or socks, which are secured on the arms by ties or tapes, to prevent nighttime scratching.

Neglect of treatments may allow growth of germs other than those of impetigo, and thus prolong the infection. Removing the crust of the lesions increases rapid clearance of symptoms. Bathe in soapy water every four hours. Use warm compresses. For stubborn scabs, use a little bleach mixture of one teaspoon bleach to one quart of water. Hot compresses and alternating cold compresses may be helpful.

Antiseptic herbs can be used such as garlic blenderized in water and used as moist compresses put on the skin lesions between baths. Comfrey root compresses, golden seal root compresses, and starch compresses are all good direct applications. To encourage the crusts to fall off, bathe four to six time a day, or even as often as once every two hours during the waking part of the day. Put two drops of grapefruit seed extract, such as Nutri Biotic, in one ounce of water or glycerine and apply to lesions directly after soaks.

For impetigo in the scalp make an echinacea and golden seal tincture to be sprayed on with a clean hair spray bottle. This tincture is also excellent for impetigo elsewhere. Be careful to protect the eyes and nose from the spray as the alcohol of the tincture will sting.

Mix flowers of sulfur, obtained from a pharmacy, with liquid hand soap or honey. Use about one-half ounce of the sulfur to two ounces of the liquid soap or honey. Spread it on at night and let it dry. It can be bathed off in the morning. It is also useful for scabies or fungus.

Charcoal baths made by stirring one-half to one cup of charcoal in a bathtub of water, or one-fourth cup in an infant bathtub, can reduce the total germ load. Start by mixing the charcoal and water in a cup, then transfer to the tub. Washing the lesions with chamomile tea is also beneficial.

If the application of poultices between baths makes the lesions spread, the lesions should be left to air dry. Air and sun are antimicrobial. Drying can be encouraged by an electric fan, sunning, or the use of a blow dryer. If the scalp becomes involved, the hair can be plaited rather tightly in small braids, to prevent the necessity of cutting the hair short, making a large number of tiny braids so that the scalp can be more easily treated between the braids.

Change bed clothes and bathroom linens daily, keeping the linens of the patient separated from the linens of the rest of the family to reduce the likelihood of contagion. Add bleach or Lysol to water used for washing clothes. Do not expose other children by swimming, school attendance, doctor office visits, or other visiting.

Use a diet free from refined sugars or refined fats. If lymph glands become swollen, hot baths will boost the effectiveness of the immune system. Use one minute for each year of the patient's age. (See "Hydrotherapy" in the *Natural Remedies* section.)

Impotence

Impotence falls into two categories.

- Physical impotence, which accounts for 90 percent of cases.
    - Nerve damage – mechanical trauma or chronic conditions such as diabetes, alcoholism, or heart disease
    - Poor circulation – hardening of the arteries, severe varicose veins
    - Certain drugs – Propranolol (Inderal); atenolol (Tenormin); serotonin reuptake-inhibitor (SRI); antidepressants such as fluoxetine (Prozac); sertraline (Zoloft); and certain herbs, ephedra, pseudo-ephedra
- Psychological impotence
    - Emotional stress
    - Depression
    - Marital disharmony

Physical Causes

One of the most common causes is diabetes. It can be borderline or extremely mild, but still be enough to affect the nerves to the pelvic area.

Circulatory problems are also very common. These can be generalized or can be localized to the blood vessels supplying the penis. Very large amounts of blood are required for an erection. Researchers are finding that in some cases the scars from an old forgotten injury can cause sufficient restriction of blood flow to prevent an erection.

The male climacteric, or "change of life," though much more subtly in men than in women, can alter a man's sexual function. It is now possible to measure the levels of testosterone in the blood, and if they are low for a man's age, plant sterols from certain herbs and foods may be of great value.

- Herbs high in plant sterols – Alfalfa leaf tea, saw palmetto, licorice root tea, red raspberry leaf, hops, and ginseng. All ginsengs have a lot of saponins, plant estrogens and progesterone in them.
- Foods high in plant sterols – Apples, peaches, carrots, cherries, coconut, garlic, nightshade plants (bell pepper, paprika, pimentos, eggplant, potatoes, tomatoes), olives, peanuts, plums, soybeans, whole grains (barley, corn, oats, rice, wheat), yams, anise seed, food yeast, parsley, sage, and wheat germ.

The use of many different kinds of drugs are notorious, especially those used for high blood pressure. Tranquilizers, alcohol, and the use of tobacco are also common drug causes.

Prevention and Treatment

We advise a totally vegetarian diet free of all animal products that may contain female sex hormones. Make certain you get plenty of fruits, vegetables, and whole grains, and some nuts, seeds, and legumes. This is the most favorable diet. In countries where this diet is used from childhood, impotence is rare.

Avoid sugar or highly refined carbohydrates, molasses, honey, syrups, and white flour products.

Avoid the free fats, margarine, salad oils, cooking fats, fried foods, mayonnaise, butter, peanut butter, and all nut butters until the condition is gone.

Men over 55 sometimes begin to lose their capacity and interest in sex. A lack of exercise and a poor diet may be factors. An imbalanced diet, such as a very highly refined carbohydrate diet or a low-fat diet, can so imbalance nutrients as to cause a drop in testosterone. A balance of nutrients is needed. Use fruits, vegetables, whole grains, and a tablespoonful or so of nuts and seeds at each meal. To raise the level of testosterone, take a short cold bath every morning sometime before noon.

Magnesium should be tried. It can be easily taken in the form of Epsom salts (magnesium sulfate), which is an excellent vasodilator. Start with one-half teaspoon dumped onto the tongue and followed by a glass of water. Do this twice a day. You can go up to one teaspoon twice a day if necessary. Back off if it causes diarrhea (it very seldom does in these low doses).

Exercise should be done daily, out of doors; walking is fine, as are any other good kind of exercise. It should not be violent, just a brisk walk once or preferably twice a day, or the equivalent in gardening, indoor gymnasium workouts, stretching, etc.

Sunning is very important as it produces vitamin D, a precursor of male sex hormones.

Correct any known physical problem such as high blood cholesterol or blood pressure. Thus one suffering from impotence should have a complete physical exam and lab work up.

Correct any possible psychological causes, such as discontent, grief, guilt, jealousy, etc.

Ginkgo biloba can help circulation and act as a potent blood thinner. Use 120 milligrams of ginkgo extract twice a day.

Ginseng, a mild stimulant, can be found in two varieties: Panax ginseng and Panax quinquefolius. Ginseng has been highly rated by the Orientals and is an excellent tonic-type herb. The American, Korean, or Chinese/Japanese ginsengs are all about the same. Drink a cup of the tea three times a day. You can mix one teaspoon of American sarsaparilla with the ginseng if you can find it. These products can be useful in just about any of the causes of impotence.

Yohimbe is also said to be good for impotence, but unfortunately it can raise blood pressure and heart rate, cause anxiety, dizziness, headaches, and tremors. It should be used with care.

Incontinence

Incontinence of urine may be the result of different factors.

- Stress Incontinence
  - Occurring on laughing
  - Occurring on running
  - Occurring on crying or any kind of emotional stress
  - Occurring on sneezing, coughing, or straining
- Urge Incontinence
  - Loss of urine only when the urge to urinate occurs.
  - Loss of urine when the intention to empty the bladder has been received by the conscious brain.
  - Loss of urine when the bladder gets full, sometimes without the knowledge of the person until the warm urine is felt on the skin.
- Weakness of Muscles
  - In old age
  - From trauma as in childbirth
  - From nerve weakness

Women who are overweight, who have undergone a hysterectomy before the age of 45, who have had at least one child or a post-dated pregnancy, who had a labor lasting more than 24 hours, or who were given oxytocin during childbirth are at increased risk of later urinary incontinence. The use of estrogen also increases the risk of incontinence (*Obstetrics and Gynecology* 90 [1997]: 983–9).

Incontinence can be encouraged or caused by allergies, food sensitivities, and not drinking enough water. When one does not drink enough water, urine becomes very concentrated and, therefore, irritating to the bladder. Bladder irritants can cause contraction of the involuntary muscles of the bladder to cause loss of urine. Potential bladder irritants are alcohol and, in some people, apples and apple juice, cantaloupe, carbonated beverages, chili and spicy foods, citrus fruits and juices, chocolate, colas, tea, coffee (including decaffeinated), cranberry and cranberry juice, grapes and grape juice, pineapple and pineapple juice, strawberries, tea (except herbal tea), tomatoes and their juice or sauce, and vinegar (*Internal Medicine News* 29 [May 15, 1996]: 36).

Since urinary tract infections increase the likelihood of having incontinence, these risk factors should be born in mind by women who have incontinence. Marital relations increase the rate of occurrence of urinary tract infections, particularly

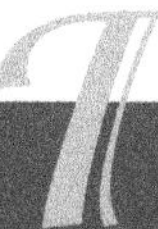

with the use of condoms. The risk is increased by 43 percent as compared to women who are not married and not having marital relations. This percentage can be reduced by simply urinating after marital relations.

Drinking carbonated soft drinks also increases the risk of urinary tract infections. In addition, the use of deodorant sanitary napkins or tampons has been found to increase the risk (*Epidemiology* 6, no. 2 [1995]: 162–8).

The use of estrogen in older women for such disorders as osteoporosis or the menopause syndrome increases a woman's risk of getting urinary tract infections (*Journal of the American Geriatrics Society* 40, no. 8 [1992]: 817–20).

Weakened muscles allow the bladder to slip down, placing the bladder neck and uterus in an improper position. Thus urine can leak out more easily when the bladder contracts. Also, a rectum filled with gas or feces can press on the bladder and encourage incontinence.

For women over 40 stress incontinence affects one woman in five. It is more commonly because of pelvic floor muscle weakness caused by childbirth or aging than by other problems.

Treatment

There are a number of treatment options to try in the case of incontinence.

Foods and Supplements

Many people are sensitive to certain foods or beverages, causing the bladder to become unusually sensitive. Then upon stress or filling, the bladder, being irritable, gets such a stimulus to contract the involuntary muscles that the voluntary muscles are unable to prevent loss of urine. In order to prevent this sensitivity, discover those foods to which one is sensitive and remove them from the diet. Eliminate the following list of foods for 28 days or until the incontinence stops.

The commonest foods causing food sensitivities are in order of their probability: dairy products (causing more than 60 percent of all food allergies), chocolate, colas, coffee, tea, eggs, pork, beef, fish, all flesh foods, legumes, peanuts, soybean products, citrus fruits and juices, tomatoes, potatoes, eggplant, peppers, corn, cornstarch, corn products, rice, wheat, oatmeal, yeast, cane sugar, cinnamon, irritating substances, spices, beer, alcohol, food colors (both artificial and natural), strawberries, apples, bananas, nuts (all kinds), seeds, lettuce, garlic, onion.

As soon as the 28 days are up, or the incontinence ceases, start adding the foods back one at a time every five days until the incontinence returns. Make a list of all those foods causing the incontinence and strictly avoid them. If you are very sensitive, even a teaspoon of the food can cause the problem.

A 59-year-old woman who had had a portion of her stomach removed developed B12 deficiency anemia with urinary incontinence. Her case was further complicated by peripheral neuropathy in all four of her extremities. When she had completed taking 17 milligrams of B12, using one milligram a day, the anemia was relieved, but the incontinence and the peripheral neuropathy continued. Then she was given a single dose of 7.5 milligrams of B12, even though her blood level was 1,180. During the next two months she was entirely cured of the incontinence and the peripheral neuropathy (*Journal of Internal Medicine* 231, no. 3 [1992]: 313–5).

Exercises

Kegel exercises six times daily for one minute each time may help. Practice contracting to the full power of the musculature of the perineum, buttocks, thighs, and lower abdomen for cutting off an imaginary urinary stream. These exercises should follow each other as rapidly as possible to get a full and intense contraction. Then relax fully before repeating the contraction. At least 20 contractions should be done during one minute.

If it is stress incontinence, the Kegel exercises have been shown to be beneficial in all patients who have tried the exercises. A group of 14 women had supervised pelvic floor exercises for four weeks, and all improved. It has been shown that most women, even though they have benefited from the exercises in a four-week period, failed to continue the exercises over a long-term period. It appears that motivation for the exercises is fairly low (*Southern Medical Journal* 88, no. 5 [May 1995]: 547–50.

While passing the urine, after urination has been fully established, practice stopping the urine flow. Then start it up again, and a second time practice stopping the urine flow totally. Then empty the bladder and press the remaining urine from the bladder with a straining action.

Bridging is done while lying on your back on the floor. Support the entire weight of the body on the heels and the shoulders by lifting the hips and thighs, head and arms, off the floor. This exercise should be maintained for three seconds

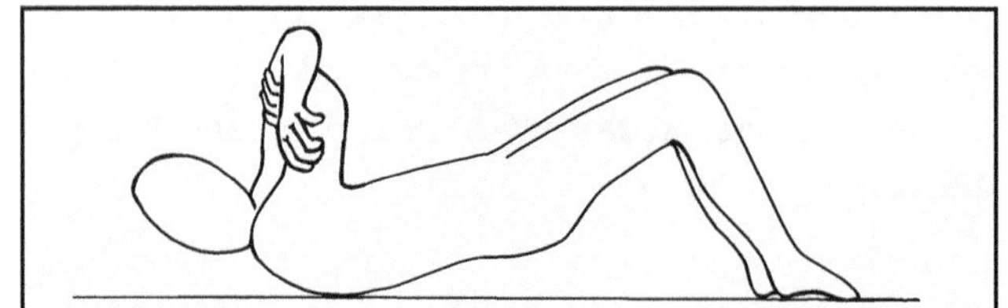

only on the first day. If no discomfort arises from having done the exercise, the second day the time may be doubled. Continue advancing the number of seconds daily up to one minute.

Another exercise is called winging. While lying face down on the floor, lift both the lower and the upper extremities, shoulders and head, off the floor behind your back, supporting the weight entirely with the abdomen. This exercise should be maintained for three seconds only on the first day. If no discomfort arises, the second day the time may be doubled. Continue advancing the number of seconds daily up to one minute.

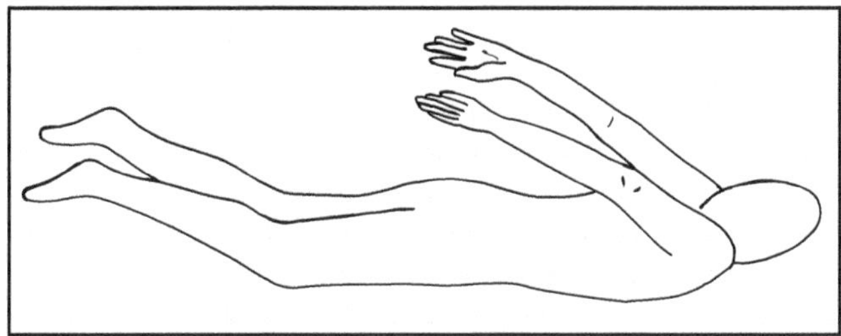

Have the patient schedule a certain time for voiding, every hour at first, trying to abstain from voiding at any other time. After 10 days the person increases the interval between voidings, the goal being an interval of two and a half to three and a half hours.

Positions

Kneel on the bed or floor, bend over to rest head and arms on the bed. Try to actually get your chest on the bed. This position allows the organs inside the abdomen to move toward the head, which promotes good positioning of the bladder and good circulation and stretches the muscles of the perineum, encouraging good tone. Hold the knee-chest position for one to five minutes.

Stand, sit, and lie with good posture. When performing any physical function, whether it be exercising out of doors, chopping vegetables in the kitchen, doing shop work, or sitting at the computer, good posture should always be maintained. If the head and shoulders are carried forward during walking, it can lead to neck or shoulder pain. The skeleton should be entirely balanced, one vertebra held correctly over the one below it as much as possible so that the back and neck are in the "neutral position," that is, the cheek bones directly perpendicular to the collar bones and the knees relaxed, not hyperextended. The shoulders must be back and down, hips slightly extended, and head erect. Mental and emotional benefits, grace, dignity, self-possession, courage, and self-reliance are all promoted by an erect posture.

Practice breathing deeply before sleeping, while sitting at one's desk, working in the house, or exercising out of doors. Every time you go through a door, take a deep breath. Breathe in to the count of four, hold the breath in to the count of seven, and exhale to the count of nine. Tight belts, elastic, or bands around the waist should not be allowed, as they make it difficult to correctly take a deep breath.

Herbal Remedies

Horsetail or shave grass can be made into a tea by steeping one-fourth cup for half an hour in one quart of boiling water. Drink one quart a day in four equal doses.

Corn silk, one-third cup to one quart boiling water, should be steeping for 30 minutes off of the heat.

Buchu tea is made by placing one teaspoon of the herb in a cup of boiling water and left to steep for 30 minutes. Drink one to eight cups daily as needed for soothing the bladder.

Cayenne pepper possesses some desensitizing action because of capsaicin and can be used to treat urinary incontinence. The dosage is one-fourth teaspoon once or twice a day taken with meals (*Life Science* 51 [1992]: 1777).

Boil three cups of water, and when it has reached a rolling boil, set it off the fire and immediately add three tablespoons of St. John's wort and two tablespoons of horsetail. Steep for 30 minutes, strain, and drink half of the tea in the middle of the morning and half of the tea in the middle of the afternoon. Take this on a continuous basis. It will take about two weeks before it begins to be effective.

Juniper berry capsules can be very helpful. Take one capsule a day until the incontinence is better, at which time you can drop down to one capsule every other day, and finally perhaps even one capsule every third day. One woman wrote that taking the juniper berry was quite effective for her. She said, "I do not use any pads any more. I had been having this incontinence since 1989 until 2000." A rare person is sensitive and can overdose on juniper berry, causing a temporary blurring of vision that goes away when the herb is stopped.

Cervical Diaphragm

A recent report in a medical journal indicates that a cervical diaphragm, such as used for contraception, may control stress incontinence in women. It will require fitting by your doctor. Cut away the part that fits over the opening of the cervix, leaving just the ring around the cervix. The ring will press against the bladder neck and control most leakage. It can be easily inserted by the patient. Remove it for thorough cleaning as suggested by the manufacturer's directions on the package. This is very important. Do not neglect this step.

Indigestion

A sense of discomfort over the stomach may be the major sign of indigestion or the feeling that food is not digesting well. Sometimes pain over the stomach is the principal symptom. The following simple treatments should be followed:

- Eat meals at regular hours, within 15 to 30 minutes before or after the scheduled time.
- Avoid large or heavy meals and large numbers of dishes at one meal.
- Eat slowly, take small bites, and chew food carefully.
- Avoid irritating stimulants: spicy or greasy foods, vinegar, and foods known not to agree with you.
- Never eat between meals or at night. Do not lie down within an hour after eating.
- Test and eliminate foods that might cause you to have indigestion. (See "Elimination and Challenge Diet" in the *Dietary Information* section.)
- Avoid alcohol, tobacco, drugs, or other known stomach irritants.

Infections

(See specific types of infections and also "Inflammation" in the *Conditions and Diseases* section.)

If you want to avoid infections of any kind, you should keep physically fit and avoid the overuse of sugar. One study showed an incubation with *Staphylococcus epidermidis* with white blood cells from individuals given 100 grams (about seven tablespoons) of sugar from glucose, fructose, sucrose, honey, or orange juice. It was found that all of these sugars significantly decreased the capacity of white blood cells to take up bacteria. Eating starch or starchy vegetables did not cause this effect. The decrease of white blood cell activity rapidly follows the ingestion of the sugars and reaches its peak at one to two hours after eating, but the values were still below fasting control values five hours after eating. The number of white blood cells was actually not decreased in these studies, but only their function. Fasting for 36 or 60 hours significantly increases the ability of white blood cells to take up bacteria (*American Journal of Clinical Nutrition* 26 [1973]: 1180).

A large number of germs and other organisms can be involved in causing infections in the body. Parasites, viruses, bacteria, protozoa, fungi, and rickettsiae may all cause infections. Fortunately, a group of foods and herbs have antifungal, antiviral, antibacterial, and antiparasitic actions. These include garlic, golden seal, comfrey, echinacea, usnea, astragalus, grapefruit and grapefruit seed, myrrh, and calendula among many others.

Infectious Mononucleosis

This is a viral infection that causes fever, swelling of the lymph glands, changes in white blood cells, and flu-like symptoms such as fatigue, sore throat, headache, and a sense of not feeling well. Sometimes only one or two of the symptoms may be present (sore throat is most consistently present). Some people also experience skin rashes and a swollen liver or spleen. The Epstein-Barr virus is responsible for infectious mononucleosis, but a number of viral agents may unite to cause the chronic fatigue syndrome. (See "Chronic Fatigue Syndrome" in the *Conditions and Diseases* section.)

It usually runs its course in about three to six weeks, but sometimes it hangs on for months or even years with occasional flare-ups.

Treatment

For both the acute and chronic forms of infectious mononucleosis, use hot baths, raising the mouth temperature to 101°F to 103°F. For the acute case, as few as three daily fever treatments may be curative. In certain chronic cases one may need to give a series of 15 once-daily treatments five days a week, with two days rest period, until 15 treatments have been given. Lay off the treatments for one to six weeks, and then repeat the series of 15 with a second vacation of one to six weeks, followed by a third or fourth series of 15 treatments. We have only rarely had a patient with true chronic fatigue syndrome who failed to respond to the prolonged series, even in people who have longstanding symptoms.

Rest, moderate exercise, and patience are the best treatments in the acute phase, along with a very simple diet free from refined sugars, refined fats, or meat substitutes. The purely vegetarian diet is the most advantageous.

Corticosteroids such as cortisone or prednisone have been used extensively to treat this disease, but we have never found it necessary since we have been using hot baths, and we often see dramatic results with none of the serious drawbacks of corticosteroids. Antibiotics fail to influence the course of the disease and should not be introduced into the body.

A large quantity of water should be taken daily, as much as 10 to 12 glasses. Warm or hot salt water gargles or irrigations may be done once an hour for the pain of the sore throat.

Infertility

Causes in Men

Lifestyle has been associated with infertility in men. Some of these lifestyle features are coffee consumption; foods to which the person is sensitive (milk, yogurt, cottage cheese, etc.); alcohol consumption; smoking; sitting posture for work; X-ray exposure; use of tight trousers; low physical exercise; certain types of sports; use of drugs for peptic ulcers, hypertension, and/or mood altering prescription drugs; high socioeconomic levels; certain educational levels; and use of chemicals in agriculture (especially pesticides).

A man who has a job that requires him to sit for more than three hours a day, such as those who drive motor vehicles or who sit at computers, are less likely to father children than those who do not sit for long periods. It is believed that it is the elevated scrotal temperatures that reduce sperm production, thus decreasing fertility.

Overdosage of the antioxidant vitamins C and E interfere with the ability of spermatozoa to move normally and to fertilize ova. All vitamin overdosage can have serious consequences. If you eat well, it is usually safer not to take a multivitamin pill every day than to take one (*Medical Tribune* 36, no. 22 [1995]: 13.

Treatment for Men

Thirty minutes daily of exposure to a 150-watt electric light bulb to the scrotal area produced, after 14 consecutive days, a depression of spermatogenesis followed by rebounds to temporarily high sperm counts. Contrariwise, an ice-bag to the scrotum for 30 minutes cooled the testicular environment by 6.9°F on the average. When continued for 14 consecutive days, beginning not less than 12 days following cessation of exposure to heat, spermatogenesis was stimulated, and increased in comparison to the pretreatment count. When the heating was carried on for 14 days and the cooling for 14 days, oligospermia (deficiency in the number of spermatozoa in the semen) subjects responded to consecutive heating and cooling faster and to a relatively greater degree than did men with a normal sperm count (*Journal of the American Medical Association*, 1968.

Since the gonads (ovaries and testes) are organs on a timed schedule, regularity in all things is essential to combat infertility. Certain fixed events of lifestyle should be on a regular schedule. Times for retiring and arising, mealtimes, exercise times, etc., should all be as nearly at the same time every day as possible. The infertile hopeful should go to bed as early as possible in the evening, as three to four hours of sleep before midnight can go far toward setting these timed organs on a more efficient schedule, and will, of course, increase growth hormones.

Try the short cold bath to increase fertility. Sit in a tub of water deep enough to cover the legs and thighs when they are extended and flat against the bottom of the tub. The water temperature should be at least as low as 85°F, and decreasing down as low as 65°F. Men should sit from four to seven minutes, longer for increased musculature or increased weight.

To raise the level of testosterone, take a short cold bath every morning sometime before noon. Take 30 minute cold baths every day for two weeks to treat male infertility. It has been found that oligospermia is helped, and there is a rise in sperm count and an increase in motility of spermatozoa with the prolonged cold bath. Following a two week treatment for two men, one had a sperm count increase from 12 million to 25 million per cc., and the other from 18 million to 43 million per cc. The first had an increase in motility from 40 percent to 75 percent, and the second had an increase from 50 percent to 70 percent. There are several known factors associated with a low sperm count. Even daily baths in water 98.6°F and higher have been shown to have a suppressing effect on spermatogenesis. Other factors besides hot baths include tight underwear, scrotum supporters, seated occupation, dark tight slacks, standing for long periods by an open fire or a source of heat, and electric blankets (*Journal of the American Medical Association* [1974]).

Causes in Women

"Trans fats increase or cause infertility" is the name of a large report in which 18,000 women were studied. It was found that four grams of trans fats daily (about one teaspoonful) will increase infertility by 74 percent. In order to cut out all trans fats, one must cut out all hydrogenated or partially hydrogenated fats from the diet and avoid animal products (*American Journal of Clinical Nutrition* [January 2006]).

Regular douching reduced fertility in a sample of 840 married women who had previously given birth in King County, Washington. Women who douched were 30 percent less likely to become pregnant than counterparts who did not douche, both groups attempting pregnancy. The reduction is not related to the type of douching solution used (*American Journal of Public Health* 86 [1996]: 844–50).

Mothers who have their babies wear cotton diapers instead of plastic lined diapers are more likely to preserve the full fertility of their sons. The scrotal and testicular temperatures were found to be increased by approximately 2°F while wearing plastic lined diapers. While it is not known whether plastic lined diapers are responsible for the decrease in sperm count and sperm quality of men in recent years, disposable diapers are one possible explanation (*Experimental Clinical and Endocronological Diabetes* 107 (Supplement 1) 1999).

Female infertility has also been associated with having multiple sexual partners (*FDA Drug Bulletins*, 1985).

Treatment for Women

Remove all dairy products from the diet. Read labels and look for casein or lactose in any of its various forms. One physician found four patients who became pregnant three months after eliminating dairy products of all kinds. Each of these delivered healthy babies. In one case the gluten grains were also eliminated as well as dairy. These patients had tried everything to reverse their infertility and had been infertile from four to eight years subsequent to marriage.

Changes in diet, lifestyle, clothing, and other suggested corrections in the mode of living have resulted in a healthier couple, 60 percent of whom conceive within a year of making the changes, and 15 percent additional within the second year, and another 10 percent in the next year. About 9 percent of women in their 20s are infertile, and 27 percent of women in their 40s.

Do not eat of free fats (margarine, mayonnaise, fried foods, cooking fats, salad oils, and nut butters). A diet high in free fats was found to reduce a female rat's capacity to conceive and her ability to maintain her litter both before and after birth of the pups. The high fat-fed female rats did not have the expected reduction in plasma-insulin levels at the end of pregnancy as did the rats fed a normal diet. This indicates that the body's mechanisms for controlling fuel nutrients are not functioning properly while on a high-fat diet (*Journal of Nutrition* 127 [1997]: 64).

Remove all tight clothing that restricts the chest movement and causes shallow breathing (thereby encouraging unhealthful congestion of the pelvis). Belts or bands constricting the waist and pushing the organs down into the pelvis may overheat the trunk and pelvic organs, causing congestion. Chilling of extremities causes pelvic congestion in most women. There are reflexes between the blood vessels of the pelvis and the extremities, so that when one constricts the others do also. Habitually chilled feet, legs, arms, and hands lead to reduced blood flow to the pelvic organs (*Los Angeles Weekly* [1985]).

Another treatment is directed toward decreasing the thickness of the cervical mucus that could make the travel of spermatozoa from the vagina to the fallopian tubes easier. Therefore, drinking plenty of water may be the treatment of choice for those desiring to overcome infertility. Additionally, substances in the vagina that might be hostile to spermatozoa will be diluted by the additional water (Dr. Jerome H. Check, *Associated Press*). Foods known to make mucus thicker must be avoided. Prime among these is milk and dairy products (cheese, ice cream, etc.), salty foods, sugary sweet foods, and animal products, etc.

Exercise should be done daily out of doors; walking is fine, or any other good kind of exercise. It should not be violent, just a brisk walk once or preferably twice a day, or the equivalent in gardening, indoor gymnasium workouts, stretching, etc.

Since the gonads (ovaries and testes) are organs on a timed schedule, regularity in all things is essential to combat infertility. Certain fixed events should be on a regular schedule. Times for retiring and arising, mealtimes, exercise times, etc., should all be as nearly at the same time every day as possible. The infertile hopeful should go to bed as early as possible in the evening, as three to four hours of sleep before midnight can go far toward setting these timed organs on a more efficient schedule, and will, of course, increase growth hormones.

Try the short cold bath to increase fertility. Both men and women may benefit, but men are likely to get the most good. Sit in a tub of water deep enough to cover the legs and thighs when they are extended and flat against the bottom of the tub. The water temperature should be at least as low as 85°F, and down as low as 65°F. Women should sit in the tub three to five minutes, longer for increased musculature or increased weight.

The best hydrotherapy for women is a hot bath every day for five days a week, skip two days, and begin again with five days more, skip two days, and take a final third set of five hot baths for a total of 15 baths, interrupted after every fifth treatment with two days off.

Hot baths have been used in treatment of a group of 115 women who were successful in becoming pregnant after the treatment, in whom ovariogenic (arising in the ovary) sterility had been diagnosed. These women showed anovulatory (no ovum discharged) cycles in 53, hypoluteal (a decreased amount of progesterone) cycle in 54, and ovarian androgenesis (production of an egg containing only paternal chromosomes) in 5, and adrenal androgenesis in 3. The most difficult and resistant to therapy were those having long lasting sterility because of profound ovarian hypofunction (*Gienkologla Polska* [1980]).

Inflammation

A reaction of the tissues to injury or infection characterized by redness, heat, swelling, and pain, regardless of the cause. The redness and heat are because of the influx of blood to the affected area. When germs are involved in the inflammation, the area is said to be infected.

Hot applications to promote circulation of the blood will ease pain and promote healing. Cold applications generally have about the same effectiveness as hot ones, bringing more blood to the area. If used, they should be made quite cold and used for only 5 to 10 minutes. Often alternating hot and cold treatments are more effective than either alone. In that case use three to six minutes of the hot applications followed immediately by 30 to 60 seconds of a cold application. Repeat this exchange three to six times.

For a list of anti-inflammatory herbs, see the "Uses for Certain Herbs" in the *Herbal Remedies* section.

Influenza

(See also "Immune System, How to Strengthen" in the *Conditions and Diseases* section.)

This highly contagious disease, also called the flu or grippe, is worldwide in extent and was probably known even to Hippocrates. After World War I, from 1918 to 1920 a form of severe influenza, "swine flu," spread over more than half the world with devastating results. In some communities four out of five people died of the flu. However, in 1957 an epidemic of swine flu broke out in the Orient as had broken out in 1918 to 1920, and although hundreds of thousands of persons were affected, most cases were very mild and the epidemic was not at all serious. We do not understand this waxing and waning of the seriousness of disease, but have experienced it with a large number of infectious diseases: polio, lobar pneumonia, typhoid, mastoiditis, rheumatic fever, syphilis, leprosy, and tuberculosis among others.

The symptoms of influenza appear rather suddenly from one to three days after exposure. Chills and fever, headache, backache, and extreme malaise are present. The viral infection lowers the resistance of the respiratory tract and exposes the patient to invasion by other germs. Fever lasts from one to five days.

Treatment

For many different kinds of diseases, including infectious diseases such as the flu, there are several simple things you can do to treat yourself. Treatment is aimed at relief of the symptoms and any complications.

- Rest – This is so simple that many people forget to rest when they start getting sick. A 24-hour rest may be enough to alter the course of an illness and put you on the road to recovery.
- Fasting – This old-fashioned remedy is found not only in humans but also in animals. Take in nothing but water or herb teas, and this will allow the body to use the energy usually used in operating the digestive organs for the healing process. A fast of one to three days can make you feel like a new person, resulting in sharper senses, clearer head, and a more energetic body.

  Long-term fasting continued for more than three days can sometimes result in complete remission in ailments resisting all other treatments—bronchial asthma, rheumatoid arthritis, ulcerative colitis, and certain tumors. These fasts should be done very judiciously. It is not wise to have a fast for longer than 10 days without the supervision of somebody knowledgeable in conducting fasts who has access to a laboratory to check blood minerals periodically. Fasts longer than 10 days have rarely been associated with sudden and unexpected death. No such death has ever been reported with a fast 10 days or less.
- Sweating – Sweating is capable of eliminating many salts, drugs, toxins, and even viruses. Be certain to take in enough water. The sweating can be done in a bathtub with hot water. Be certain to keep the head cool, or you may feel weak and dizzy after the treatment is over.
- Steam inhalation – This remedy is excellent for respiratory conditions.

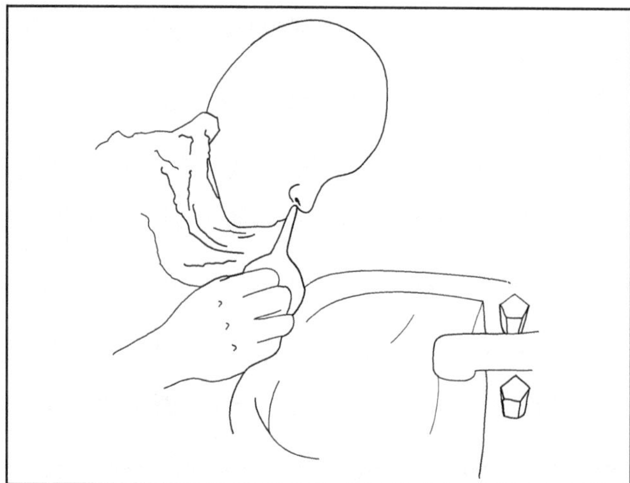

- Nasal douching – This is the practice of rinsing the nasal passages with a salt-water solution, using one teaspoon of salt to one pint of water. Use the salt solution at room temperature. This treatment is good for hay fever, a head cold, and sometimes even for a headache.
- Gargling – There is no better way to speed the healing of a sore throat or to open up congested ears that may accompany the flu than by gargling. Use hot water or hot saline water gargles every hour to relieve pain and promote healing. Charcoal powder can be made into a thick paste and held in the mouth to trickle down the throat to soothe and heal a sore throat.
- Hot and cold applications – Many very powerful responses occur in the body with hot and cold treatments. The blood vessels dilate followed by constriction of blood vessels, which gives a pumping effect. This brings fresh blood laden with healing proteins and carries away wastes and toxins. Cold compresses can be put on bruises, sprains, painful joints and muscles, burns, bites, and stings.
- Massage – The healing touch is practiced in every culture, and on oneself. After an injury the first impulse a person has is to rub the injured area. Several healing properties are brought about by massage—a favorable change of the cellular pH, a relaxation of tight or painful muscles, a quickening of the circulation of both blood and lymph nodes, elimination of wastes, and many other benefits. Back rubs and full body massage may be used for muscle aches and pains.

Antibiotics and corticosteroids should not be used as they are not only not effective but may be quite harmful.

An earache can be treated by holding an ice cube over the ear and letting the water drip off into the ear canal until the canal is filled with the cold water. Then turn on the side to drain the water out. Pain relief will often be dramatic, and the patient may go to sleep and wake up free from the earache. The next day after such a treatment, the ear canal should be filled with ordinary rubbing alcohol and then drained in the same way. Use the little finger with a tissue to dry as much of the alcohol as can be reached with the finger. Do not insert anything into the ear smaller than the little finger.

A humidifier can be used for nasal stuffiness, or a shop lamp with a 60- to 100-watt bulb may be held one to two inches from the nose. The nose can be irrigated by using saline irrigations. Saline is made by combining one level teaspoon of salt to one pint (two eight-ounce cups) of water.

Chest congestion can be treated with fomentations over the chest or hot foot baths. Each of these treatments should be carried on for 30 minutes or more followed by 30 minutes or more of bed rest. Dr. Wayne McFarland tested the pH of the bronchus immediately after this treatment and found a reduction in pH to 6.3, an unfavorable pH for the flu virus to replicate itself. Prevent chilling and fatigue. Have a good supply of fresh air in the room at all times.

Sometimes at the very beginning of symptoms, if they can be caught within the first 20 minutes, a hot bath for seven to eight minutes followed by an enema and a 10-minute deep breathing exercise, breathing in through the nose and holding it for 20 seconds, and out through the nose and holding it out for 10 seconds, can cause the flu virus to fail to develop. It is also a good idea to take a long walk at the very first sign of the flu.

Of course, alcoholic beverages, smoking, coffee, and its relatives, should all be avoided. The diet should be simple, just two to three simple dishes and bread, without free sugars or free fats.

Make a recipe of "Immune Builder Soup." Dice one large onion and boil it in three quarts of water until clear. Add one quart of canned tomatoes and any of the following seasonings: dulse, parsley, dill, salt, and herbs. Set the pot off the heat and press one or more bulbs of garlic into the soup or put a portion of the soup in the blender with the cloves of one entire bulb of garlic and blenderize briefly and return the entire contents of the blender back to the hot soup to continue to heat, but not boil. The heating will make it so the stomach can tolerate the quantity of the soup needed for building the immune system. If this soup is taken for supper it will prevent coughing at night. Do not reheat.

Ingrown Toenails

(See "Skin Diseases" in the *Conditions and Diseases* section.)

Insect Bites and Repellent

(See "Bite Wounds" in the *Home Emergencies* section.)

Insomnia

(See "Sleep" in the *Conditions and Diseases* section.)

Intermittent Claudication

(See "Lameness, Intermittent Claudication" in the *Conditions and Diseases* section.)

Intestinal Permeability, Increased

(See "Leaky Gut Syndrome, Increased Intestinal Permeability"in the *Conditions and Diseases* section.)

Iritis

Iritis is a painful and often serious inflammation of the iris. It may occur because of a virus infection, or it may be associated with such systemic diseases as rheumatoid arthritis or tuberculosis. It has a tendency to recur frequently and to become chronic. It is characterized by pain that is often deep and severe, different from the mild or moderate irritation and burning of conjunctivitis. There is often intense redness and engorgement of conjunctival vessels and photophobia (aversion to light). We have treated severe cases with artificial fever therapy using either the Russian steam bath or heated whirlpool. In every case the acute attack has subsided without complications. The number of treatments has varied from one to six. It has not been necessary to use drug dilation of the pupil as is commonly prescribed with this ailment.

We have also cleared cases of acute iritis by charcoal compresses worn every night until the inflammation stops. The diet should be evaluated for foods to which the person is sensitive if the iritis recurs. Inflammation can be promoted by food sensitivity, as well as by eating too much.

Aloe vera gel, three to four drops three times a day put directly into the eye, benefits some if they are not sensitive to plants of the onion family. Test yourself first by holding a spoonful in the mouth for 15 to 20 minutes to see if any irritation develops. If not, put a tiny speck of the gel inside one lower lid. Wait six hours. If you have no reaction—pain, redness, blurry vision in that eye—it is unlikely you are going to develop a sensitivity to the gel.

Use anti-inflammatory herbs, taken orally, such as wild yam, white willow bark, licorice, chamomile, chaparral, echinacea, flaxseed, hawthorn berry, etc.

Irritable Bowel Syndrome

One of the most common reasons people see a gastroenterologist is irritable bowel syndrome. The principal symptom is bouts of abdominal pain with or without diarrhea or constipation. It has been determined that fermentation is at least a part of the root of irritable bowel syndrome. Foods that ferment rapidly, such as beef, dairy products (read all labels for casein, lactose, whey, yogurt, buttermilk, etc.), and yeast, are among the worst offenders. Coffee can also have an adverse affect on the system. Food sensitivities such as to cereal grains, citrus fruits, and other fruits may also be involved (*Lancet*, October 9, 1998).

A carefully and faithfully done Elimination and Challenge Diet will relieve the condition in more than 95 percent of cases (See "Elimination and Challenge Diet" in the *Dietary Information* section). For pain relief, use charcoal by mouth, fomentations or ice packs over the abdomen, and aloe vera, slippery elm, or catnip tea. (See also "Abdominal Pain" in the *Conditions and Diseases* section.)

Peppermint tea and a peppermint massage oil used on the abdomen can help to ease bloating, gas, and stomach cramps almost immediately. Drink from one to three cups of the peppermint tea at one time, and then one cup every four hours as long as the irritable bowel lasts. Peppermint oil is also very helpful for irritable bowel syndrome.

Itching

(See also "Skin Diseases," "Pruritus Ani," "Women's Conditions and Diseases," and "Hives" in the *Conditions and Diseases* section.)

There are several causes of widespread itching such as liver or kidney failure, dryness of the skin in winter, certain types of malignant diseases, including leukemia, scabies, and jaundice. Another cause that may be associated with sudden and dramatic increase in generalized itching is that of abscesses. These abscesses can be situated anywhere in the body but a good place to look is under or beside a tooth.

For itching that accompanies jaundice, remove the free fats in the diet as well as nuts, olives, and avocados. This can decrease bile acid production and reduce itching (*Hepatology* 13 [1991]: 1084–9). Also, take milk thistle herb.

Activated charcoal may help remove bile or toxic substances or excessive hormones from the body, and in this way charcoal can relieve itching. Persons with kidney failure on dialysis who develop itching should be treated as follows: Use two heaping tablespoons of activated charcoal each day for two months. Two showers daily may help itching of kidney origin.

Exposure to sunlight can relieve itching by stimulating the oil glands and by thickening the keratin layer. It reduces the amount of bile held in the skin. Several days may be required to bring relief.

For itching associated with diseases such as jaundice or diabetes, the use of a tincture of cayenne can be effective in stopping the itch in the same way as it is effective in stopping pain.

Persons who are taking golden seal herbal preparations who develop itching should stop the herb. We have had several cases of itching as a reaction to golden seal.

Jaundice

(See also "Hepatitis" in the *Conditions and Diseases* section.)

Jaundice in the newborn may or may not be serious. If it occurs within the first 12 to 24 hours of life, it is more likely to be serious than if it develops between the fourth and the seventh days of life. The intensity of the jaundice is also an indicator of its seriousness. If the eyes and cheeks only show a yellow color and the bilirubin level is approximately 5 milligrams, it is unlikely to be serious. The bilirubin can only be measured by a laboratory test.

If jaundice reaches the mid chest, the bilirubin level will be approximately 10 milligrams; to the abdomen approximately 15 milligrams; to the feet approximately 18 to 20 milligrams. If the feet are involved, the level is dangerous. If there is a blood incompatibility such as with Rh, professional help will be needed to ensure the safety of the baby.

For prolonged jaundice, more than two weeks from the time it starts, be sure to check the thyroid level as a low functioning thyroid can cause persistent jaundice (after two weeks of age) and is often associated with development of feeblemindedness. Urgent attention needs to be given to this matter as each day counts in the development of the brain during the first six weeks.

Treatment

There are two good home remedies for jaundice of the newborn, even the severe type. If jaundice is visible on the abdomen and not just limited to the head, arms, and chest, treatment must be prompt, continuous, and persistent.

Sunlight exposure, while carefully protecting the eyes, can cause metabolism of bilirubin in the skin, remarkably reducing jaundice. Put a thin blindfold over the eyes, even if the baby is asleep, and expose the total body for 60 minutes, 30 minutes front and 30 minutes back. If jaundice does not fade promptly, acquire "grow lamps" from a nursery or seed company for a nighttime light bath also. The baby is less likely to develop sunburn than an adult because of its hormone production.

Charcoal is quite effective in lowering bilirubin levels. Stir activated charcoal powder into water and administer with a nursing bottle. Stir as much charcoal powder as is possible to get through the nipple. If the baby refuses to take the bottle, it must be administered from a spoon, holding the baby's mouth in such a way that swallowing is mandatory.

Neonatal jaundice is more likely to occur if the mother took certain drugs during pregnancy, labor, delivery, or breastfeeding. These drugs include Valium, sulfonamides, hydrocortisone, gentamicin, oral contraceptives, thiazide diuretics, and others. Jaundice from any cause can be treated in this way.

Jet Lag

People who are hardest hit by jet lag are people over 50, persons traveling eastward, and persons traveling westward for longer than eight hours. It takes one day to fully recover from each hour difference between your home time and your new location time. The following tips will help you deal with jet lag.

Avoid greasy, deep fried, or spiced foods. Every meal should have plenty of fresh fruits and vegetables and plain whole grain breads or rice. Taking bread plain without a spread such as margarine or mayonnaise is by far the best. Avoid cheese and other strong or pungent flavors. Eat at least four hours before bedtime, and avoid sugar, nuts, and chocolate. You will actually be better off if you fast entirely as jet lag can be recovered in a fraction of the time if one eats nothing during the day of the flight.

Bananas are high in tryptophan, a natural sleep inducer and sedative. Take one about four hours before the new bedtime.

Do not self-medicate with alcohol or caffeine. Alcohol is a very poor sleeping potion that does not work well and can give a serious hangover with jet lag, which makes you less alert in the daytime and intensifies the daytime discomfort. Caffeine is a long-term stimulant that may keep you awake too long, interfering with sleep when you would otherwise be able to drift off to sleep. Even decaffeinated drinks can interfere with sleep.

When going from east to west, you should go to bed early the night before to start out well rested in order to stay awake longer, waiting for bedtime in the new time zone. When going from west to east, however, stay up longer in order to be sleepy when the earlier bedtime comes in the east.

Do not begin a trip with a sleep debt. Sleep and eat on your new schedule as soon as you arrive and even in the plane when it is time to sleep at your destination. When you arrive at your new location any naps that are not at the time when everyone else is sleeping should last only an hour or less.

Expose yourself to an hour or so of sunlight early in the day when going from west to east, as sunlight exposure makes one more sleepy about twelve hours later. If you are going from east to west, expose yourself to sunlight later in the day so that you can stay awake later.

Pack ear plugs and eye shades, as well as a machine for making "white noise" such as a tape player or a small electric fan, so that you can sleep easier, no matter what time it is.

While flying, try to drink about eight ounces of water every hour of your flight.

Exercise substantially reduces the time required to recover from jet lag as it eases stress, relaxes muscles, aids digestion, and helps with sleep. If the hotel where you are has an exercise facility, hiking trails, beaches, or jogging tracks nearby, avail yourself of these advantages. Try to get an aisle seat during the flight so you can relax better. Also, stretch and take walks around the plane. If the plane stops and time allows, deplane and take a brisk walk through the terminal.

Kidney Failure and Chronic Nephritis

Nephritis is an inflammation of the kidneys and may be discovered by finding protein or sometimes blood in the urine. Sometimes high blood pressure or swelling of the body tissues signals nephritis. There may be diminished appetite, headaches, sleep loss, or weight loss or gain from fluid retention. Eventually more symptoms will appear such as nausea, diarrhea, vomiting, enlargement of the abdomen and liver, and lung congestion.

As the kidneys terminally fail, a "uremic frost" may occur on the skin, followed by convulsions and coma. The frost represents the attempt of the skin to get rid of toxic wastes usually excreted by the kidneys.

The commonest causes of kidney failure are chronic glomerulonephritis, diabetes, hypertension, collagen diseases, and damage from antibiotics or other drugs or toxins. Treatment should be directed first toward the underlying cause, while at the same time protecting and healing the kidneys.

Treatment

The first thing to do when kidneys start to fail is strictly adhere to the natural laws of health by being very careful to drink plenty of water and eat a plant-based diet with careful elimination of all foods high in protein. A high protein diet is damaging to the kidneys. Even beans and nuts should be eaten in small quantities and chewed thoroughly. The protein found in soybeans is healing to the kidneys—one-fourth cup of cooked soybeans should be eaten every day. Do not use the commercial soy products or purified protein derivatives. The majority of food should consist of fruits and vegetables, which can be eaten freely. Whole grains can be eaten in moderate quantities, but all other foods must be taken sparingly. Depending on the kind of nephritis the person has, and the exact location of damage in the kidneys, various nutrients may need to be withheld, such as salt or potassium. The information from a laboratory can be very helpful in regulating the diet. Avoid those foods high in the mineral or minerals the kidneys are not excreting well.

Fasting is often good for nephritis. Try a five-day fast if you are well nourished and have nutrient reserves. Appropriately break the fast and then eat regular food for three weeks before starting another five-day fast. (See "Fasting" in the *Dietary Information* section.)

Both sucrose (common table sugar) and lard alter the hormonal response of kidney nerve supply according to studies that demonstrated a unique pattern of sympathetic nervous symptoms regulation in the kidney. These foods can be damaging to the kidneys and should be severely limited or eliminated. Fasting was very helpful to the neurologic control of the kidneys (*American Journal of Physiology* 263, no. 4 [October 1992]: F586–93).

Nephritis from lupus can benefit from the high lignin content of flaxseed. It is recommended that those who suffer from nephritis take two to four tablespoons of flaxseed, freshly ground, each day. You can sprinkle it on your cereal, salad, or vegetables, or stir it into juice or soup. Flaxseed has an anti-inflammatory effect (*Clinical and Investigative Medicine* 17, no. 4 [August 1994]: B97, 98). In polycystic kidney disease and interstitial nephritis, flaxseed lowered

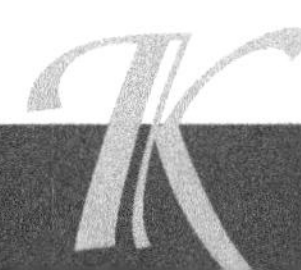

serum creatinine and reduced the rate of progress of renal disease.

In experiments, inositol with choline has been found effective to partially reverse nephritis. Phytic acid, the raw product from which inositol is extracted, is found in corn, rye, wheat, oats, peas, barley, rice, beans, flaxseed, cotton seed, peanuts, and soybeans. These foods become important to those needing more inositol in kidney failure or diabetic nephropathy.

A high fiber diet can increase excretion with the fecal matter of substances causing a high blood urea. What happens is that fermentable fibers increase urea disposal in the large bowel. A 20 to30 percent decrease in blood urea occurs in animals given a diet high in this kind of fiber. Some of the best fiber can be found in the same foods that are high in phytic acid listed above.

A high consumption of dietary protein results in an increased acid load, causing your bones to dissolve, which results in increased kidney stones and osteoporosis.

Lactulose has been reported to depress ammonia absorption from the large bowel and to increase fecal nitrogen excretion. Unfortunately, it causes diarrhea. Oligosaccharides, such as inulin, enhance urea capture in the large bowel and promote excretion without any digestive disturbances, particularly when the level of protein in the diet is moderate (*Journal of Nutrition* 125 [1995]: 1010–16). Inulin is high in Jerusalem artichokes. Other dietary sources are asparagus, bananas, salsify, wheat, chicory, onions, and garlic.

Use herbs that help cystitis. They are generally soothing and nutritive for the kidneys. Use CoQ10 as a support for the kidneys. It can help all internal organs. (See "Cystitis" in the Conditions and Diseases section.)

Soy protein has been shown to reduce protein in the urine, hypercholesterolemia, creatinine, and BUN (blood urea nitrogen) (*Life Sciences* 74, no. 8 [January 9, 2004]: 987–99).

Charcoal compresses worn on the back at night remove toxic wastes through the skin. Soaking in water three to four hours a day at about 96°F to 98°F, being careful to keep the head cool, can remove toxic wastes through the skin. Retention charcoal enemas and charcoal by mouth can assist in removal of kidney wastes through the intestinal tract in much the same way they are drawn through the skin. Use one heaping tablespoon of powdered charcoal in each cup of water taken by mouth.

In one study, one way to help the kidneys get rid of their wastes was found to be deep pool therapy. After 30 minutes with the kidney failure patient standing or walking in a pool up to the shoulders, there is a diuresis of water, sodium, and potassium. The deep pool bath is much preferable to a tub bath in this regard. The slight pressure of the deep pool water against the body tissues increases the effectiveness of the treatment, encouraging the blood to pick up wastes and transport them to the kidney. An hour or two each day can be a sort of natural dialysis (*Zeitschrift Fur Physiotherapie* 37, no. 6 [1985]: 409).

Keep fresh air circulating in the home at all times to assist the lungs in removing toxic wastes. Exercise is helpful to keep good circulation of the kidneys. Echinacea and golden seal have healing properties and are adjuncts to other forms of treatment.

In chronic kidney failure because of diabetes, hypertension, nephritis, or toxic substances, the damage to the kidneys is permanent. The above-noted treatments are helpful but cannot be expected to bring about a cure. Kidney dialysis will be essential for life, but it may be delayed for months or for years. Do not build up unreasonable expectations.

Heavy drinking of alcohol and low physical activity has been found to be closely associated with an increased risk of spilling protein in the urine. It is the spilling of protein in the urine that damages the kidney's tiny nephrons, the filtering units in the kidney. There is also an increased risk of protein in the urine with the number of cigarettes smoked per day (*Japanese Journal of Public Health* 42, no. 4 [April 1995]: 243). There is a close relationship between these three enemies—alcohol, a sedentary lifestyle, and smoking. Someone who smokes is usually less willing and able to engage in strenuous physical activity. With the diminution of sensitivity of the taste buds because of the poisons in tobacco smoke, alcohol tastes better and better. With alcohol use comes a decreased ability to exercise at all. The alcohol lowers the reasoning powers so the hapless human smokes more and more since the body can no longer sense the discomfort the increased load of toxins is causing. And all the while the injured kidneys are trying to process the poisons found in the alcohol and tobacco.

A very helpful laboratory test for kidney function is the creatinine. If the level begins to drift upward, especially if the level goes above 1.5 milligrams per decilitre, you should begin a program to protect the kidney and improve its function. Exercise and diet alone with careful application of the eight natural laws of health can be effective in protecting the kidney from further damage. The most favorable diet is the totally plant-based vegetarian diet. If kidney failure can be discovered before it has caused the creatinine level to rise to 5.0, there is still hope of reversal of the degenerative process.

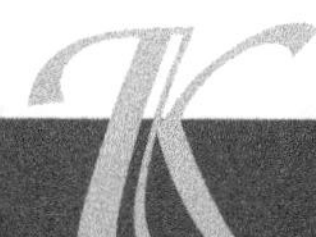

Plant-based Diet Guide for Kidney Failure

Food Group	Include	Exclude
Main dishes Two servings daily Select one per meal	2 tbsp. peanut butter or tahini 3 tbsp. nuts or seeds ⅓ cup lentils/bean 1/6 cup firm tofu or ⅓ cup regular tofu	All animal products, especially objectionable are ham, bacon, corned beef, frankfurters, sausage, kosher meats, frozen fish filets, and canned salted meats
Milk Substitutes One serving daily	½ cup soy milk or nut milk	Chocolate milk or cocoa
Bread, Starch, and Cereals Four servings daily	1 slice wheat bread or ½ English muffin or ½ cup brown rice or whole grain pasta or cooked cereal or ¾ cup whole grain flake cereal	Saltines, self rising flour, quick cooking cereals, and commercial baked products *Note: In late stages of kidney failure, the patient may have to exclude whole grains to prevent blood mineral elevation.*
Fruits and Fruit Juices Three servings daily	½ cup of grapefruit juice or any fruit or fruit juice except for the excluded juice	Dried fruits, bananas, oranges, melons, fresh peaches, and guava
Vegetables Three servings daily	½ cup any vegetable except for those excluded ½ cup potatoes, white or sweet, or ⅔ cup winter squash	Pickles, canned vegetable juices and soups, sauerkraut, beet greens, pumpkin, artichoke, avocadoes, raw carrots, spinach, and tomatoes
Fats and Oils Three or more servings daily	1 tbsp. olive oil, sesame oil, or vegetable oil 6 olives 4 Brazil nuts, 8 almonds, 8 walnuts halves, pecan halves, or 8 cashews	Salt pork and commercial gravies
Fluids 4–6 cups (8 oz.) daily (unless allowed more by Dialysis Unit)	1 cup of any of the following: ice, water, juices, soup, milk	Softened water, Dutch process cocoa, instant cocoa mix, postum, regular or salt-free bouillon cubes or powder, all canned or dehydrated soups, and alcoholic beverages
Miscellaneous Use as desired	Fresh spices and herbs, seasonings, lemon, lime, small amounts of peanut butter, all sauces and extracts, monosodium glutamate, any casserole containing tomato sauce	Seasoning salts, salt, salt substitutes, chili sauce, Worchestershire sauce, soy sauce, and pickle relish
High Calorie Foods		Molasses, brown sugar, candies, sugar, commercial pies and cakes, any bread, cake, cookies, or crackers that are made with baking soda or baking powder

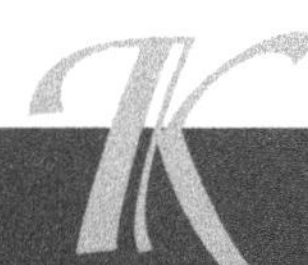

All "bad habits" should be discontinued immediately and good health habits instituted.

Kidney Stones

Men are twice as likely as women to form kidney stones. Stones may be formed anywhere in the kidneys, ureters, bladder, or urethra, or they may travel from the kidney down through the urinary tract. The rapid onset, or even sudden onset, of severe sharp pain in the flank may be the first sign. Associated with this can be nausea, vomiting, blood in the urine, paleness, and sweating. The pain is often of an exquisite nature, and those who have had both say that kidney pain is worse than the pain of a heart attack. The pain of stones is because of either the stretching of the ureter or the kidney pelvis by backed up urine by the stone; or by the actual movement of the stone down the ureter.

Causes

The causes of kidney stones include tumor of the parathyroid glands, too much vitamin D, gout, or leukemia. However, in most cases it is diet related, and is brought on by eating meat, drinking soft drinks, coffee, tea, colas, chocolate, or alcoholic drinks, as well as the failure to drink sufficient water during periods of hot weather to compensate for fluid loss (*Annals of Saudi Medic* 8 [1988]: 108). The risk of forming kidney stones can be greatly reduced by cutting out soft drinks. The phosphoric acid in the drinks is sufficient to put a person at greater risk of forming stones.

Chocolate is rich in sucrose (table sugar), fat, and oxalate. This combination greatly increases one's likelihood of getting kidney stones. The urine after a single chocolate bar contains high levels of both calcium and oxalates, the culprits in increasing the risk of kidney stones (*Hormone and Metabolic Research* 26, no. 8 [1994]: 383–6). Sugar in chocolate increases excretion of calcium in the urine.

Rich sources of oxalates, which cause 70 percent of kidney stones, include chocolate, black tea, beets, figs, black pepper, peanuts, oysters, parsley, rhubarb, spinach, and poppy seeds. Calcium oxalate is the major component of 70 to 80 percent of kidney stones, and it readily forms crystals in urine when urine is concentrated. Furthermore, there must be a "seed" in the urine onto which calcium oxalate can crystallize. This is usually a crystal of uric acid, the presence of which is common in those who eat a lot of meat. In others, especially those who eat a lot of salty food, a sodium chloride crystal serves as the seed. In people with urinary infections, a clump of pus cells may be the seed. There are several types of kidney stones other than calcium oxalate. Many of them are phosphates, or are chemically mixed in nature.

Paradoxically, reducing one's calcium consumption (in an attempt to reduce stone formation) increases stone formation. This happens because, when there is less calcium in the urine, its uric acid content increases, and uric acid crystals are the most common type of seed for stones. Another good reason for not reducing your calcium intake is that, by doing so, you increase your risk of developing osteoporosis and fractures. For individuals who have a genetic or a dietary problem with the use of refined carbohydrates, eating foods high in oxalates will increase their risk significantly for getting kidney stones (*UROL.INT.* 39 [1984]: 165). A high intake of salt increases calcium loss, which may be converted into kidney stones (*Lancet* 2 [February 17, 1990]: 412).

Stone formation is known to be associated with certain lifestyle factors, age, and heredity. As a person gets older the probability of kidney stones increases. As the dietary intake of milk and animal protein goes up, so does the probability

Various Lifestyle Factors Known to Increase Risk of Certain Types of Stones

Lifestyle	Stone Type	Prevention
High protein diet	Uric acid	Low protein diet
Milk drinking	Calcium	Avoid dairy milk (may use soy, rice, nut milks)
Refined carbohydrates	Calcium	Complex carbohydrates
Animal products	Oxalate	Plant-based diet
Alcohol	Various	Use no alcoholic beverages
Vitamins A and C supplements	Calcium	Beware of fortified foods and pills
Worcestershire sauce	Various	No sauce of this nature
Sedentary lifestyle	Calcium	Get up and get out

of formation of kidney stones. Sedentary professions and reduction in total fluid intake can increase stone formation. The risk of stone formation increases by 35 and 37 percent respectively when drinking apple juice or grapefruit juice between meals (*American Journal of Epidemiology* 143 [1996]: 240). Stone formation can be greatly reduced by increasing one's fluid intake. Most people with stones need to double the amount of fluid they drink and avoid soft drinks containing phosphoric acid (*Journal of the American Medical Association* 293 [2005]: 1107, 1158).

Because people lose fluid through sweating in hot weather, kidney stones are more common during the summer. Iced tea contains oxalates that contribute to stone production in summer. In winter sitting in hot tubs or saunas cause excessive sweating. A long car ride or plane trip with inadequate water intake (juices do not count) can start stone development or urinary tract infections. The overuse of magnesium-containing laxatives and antacids may cause a similar problem.

Antacids, such as Maalox, Tums, Mylanta, Di-Gel, Amphojel, etc., can increase one's risk of developing kidney stones (*Aust. NZ Journal of Medicine* 20 [1990]: 803).

Large doses of vitamin C have been associated with kidney stone formation in susceptible individuals.

There is a prevalence of kidney stones in persons who experience extremely stressful life events such as divorce, death, disgrace, or the loss of one's job or home (*International Journal of Epidemiology* 6 [1997]: 1017).

Male marathon runners have a higher incidence of kidney stones than those who do not run marathons (*Journal of Sports Medicine and Physical Fitness* 21 [1981]: 295).

Prevention

To prevent kidney stones, eat a high fiber diet of grain brans and reduce oxalate intake. Protein should also be low as it encourages excretion of excess calcium in the urine. Americans tend to eat much more protein than they need. The high protein weight loss programs are potentially harmful, not only because of what happens to the kidneys but also for several other reasons such as what happens to the bones and to the blood vessels, not to mention the increased risk of cancer.

A person should drink enough water so that almost clear urine is passed four to five times a day. While most people do not need this counsel, drinking more than two gallons of water daily can also be injurious to the kidneys. Diabetes and high blood pressure are two major diseases that harm the kidneys. Certain medications can also harm the kidneys, particularly the pharmaceutical diuretics, pain killers, and some antibiotics that are excreted by the kidneys (*Physician and Sports Medicine* 25, no. 5 [1997]: 123).

Celery keeps stones from forming. Three stalks of celery pureed and taken daily should be adequate. A cucumber every day is also helpful in prevention.

Adequate magnesium in the diet will go far toward preventing calcium oxalate kidney stones from forming. When magnesium supplements are taken for this effect, they do more good when taken with meals than when taken on an empty stomach (*Journal of Urology* 143 [1990]: 248–51). Dietary sources of magnesium include nuts, whole grains, and legumes.

Men prone to developing kidney stones may help to prevent them by drinking orange juice or eating ample quantities of oranges. About one pint per day is as effective as standard drugs for keeping kidney stones from forming. Citrate in the juice inhibits calcification of the stones (*The Journal of Urology* 149 [1993]: 1405).

Seven oxalate-rich foods were tested for their ability to increase urinary oxalate crystal excretion. The analyzed value for oxalate was highest for spinach, chocolate, and tea, and lowest for vegetable juice, cranberry juice, pecans, and orange juice. The urinary oxalate increased by 29.3 milligrams during the eight hours after ingestion of spinach, but rose less than 4.2 milligrams from the consumption of the low oxalate food items (*Urology* 17, no. 6 [June 1981]: 534–8). Calcium and oxalate are two keys to renal stone formation (*Journal of Urology* 123, no. 3 [1980]: 317–9).

Some people are known to form kidney stones on a regular basis. These people should ask a laboratory for an analysis of their stones. They should then pay attention to foods having high analysis of that particular substance of which their stones are made up of, such as phosphates, oxalates, calcium, uric acid, etc.

A diet low in protein is helpful to prevent uric acid stones. Of high calcium foods, milk is especially prone to cause stones, and elimination of dairy products may help prevent calcium stones. Eliminating alcohol is important as it is involved in the production of several types of kidney stones. Refined carbohydrates such as sugar and white flour products increase the risk of calcium stone formation. The elimination of animal products, meat, fish, chicken, milk, and eggs, will decrease the incidence of oxalate stones. (See "Food Sources of Certain Nutrients" in the *Dietary Information* section and look up oxalate, phosphate, and calcium.)

A high potassium diet decreases urinary calcium excretion and tends to be high in alkali, thus increasing urinary citrate. This combination has been found to reduce stone formation by 51 percent (*Comprehensive Therapy* 20, no. 9 [1994]: 485).

After World War II, fats, oils, animal protein, and milk products greatly increased as a reaction to the severe restriction that was unavoidable during the war, and by 1970 kidney stone formation was about three times higher than prior to 1940 (*UROL.INT.* 39 [1984]: 32; *The Journal of Urology* 143 [1990]: 1093).

Although grains are high in phosphorus, they prevent kidney stones because of the fiber content. Three heaping tablespoons of unprocessed wheat, or rice bran, were found to reduce the risk of formation of renal calculi by half. Since animal products are devoid of fiber and also high in fats, it may be in part because of the increase in fiber and reduction in fats that vegetarians have fewer stones than nonvegetarians. It is certain that a low fat and high fiber diet will help prevent the formation of kidney stones.

Eating oranges, lemons, limes, and grapefruit with meals seems to prevent kidney stones, as certain people prone to stones have low levels of citrate in their urine (Dr. Robert J. Irwin, *Your Health*, October 31, 1995, 82). Citrus fruits, although they are acid in the stomach, leave an alkaline residue in the urine. Acid urine tends to precipitate uric acid stones.

We suggest generous quantities of pumpkin seeds in the diet as they have been found to inhibit crystal formation in the urine (*Journal of the Medical Association of Thailand* 76, no. 9 [1993]: 487). Evidence suggests that a vegetarian diet with its plant-based protein is handled more efficiently by the kidneys than animal protein. Individuals who are prone to form stones should maintain a strict plant-based diet. Soybeans contain a protein that is quite favorable for the prevention of kidney stones (*Alternative and Complimentary Therapies,* May/June 1996,168 –72; *European Urology Journal* 8 [1982]: 334).

Lithium can effectively dissolve uric acid stones, although lithium is used in very small doses, such as can be absorbed from mineral-rich water.

The use of aspirin and other pain killers has been shown to increase the risk of renal stones. Most drugs are potentially injurious to the kidneys and should be avoided.

Be as physically active as possible. Lying down or even sitting down alters calcium metabolism and encourages excretion in the urine. Patients who remain in bed for long periods of time are far more likely to form stones.

Avoid dairy products, red meat, excessive salt intake, and whole sesame seeds. Always drink at least 10 eight-ounce glasses of water per day if you have a high risk of kidney stones.

Treatment for an Acute Attack

With the onset of symptoms, the use of one glassful of water every 10 minutes for an hour will often prevent the attack. This water may be made into tea if one has on hand buchu tea, corn silk tea, burdock tea, cleavers, or watermelon seed. A teaspoon of each per cup of boiling water is the recipe for the first four teas, but the last one is one tablespoon of ground watermelon seed stirred into a cup of boiling water. Each of the teas should be allowed to steep for 20 minutes before straining and drinking. Strain all the urine produced through a funnel lined by gauze so the stone can be retrieved and analyzed by a laboratory, if the crystal forming the stone is to be determined.

Maintain a sitting or standing position as much as possible, as lying down (and even too much sitting) slows the production and drainage of urine.

Very large, hot fomentations are needed and should be applied quickly, while the heat is almost unbearable. (Do not blister the skin.) Maintain the hot application, keeping it hot for 45 minutes or more with hot water bottles or a heating pad. Keep the head cool by cold compresses. The application of the fomentations to the back should include from about the level of the shoulders all the way down to the buttocks, and should be applied constantly as long as the patient can tolerate it during the first 24 hours of an acute attack.

Many patients feel more comfortable in a hot bath than with fomentations. The bath should be maintained between 105°F and 110°F, trying to keep the mouth temperature no hotter than 100.5°F to 102°F. Keep the face cool with ice cold compresses and a small electric fan trained on the face. Give cold water as it can be tolerated.

At least three types of herbs should be mixed in a formula for kidney stones with kidney colic. (See herbs below.) Discomfort usually begins on one side of the back and radiates to the abdomen or groin. Nausea and vomiting may occur, and blood may appear in the urine.

One patient told us of having kidney colic and taking three tablespoons of lemon juice and two tablespoons of olive oil, which caused the stone to pass into the bladder. In four or five hours the stone had passed from the bladder. The lemon/oil treatment had been preceded by alternating hot and cold baths and drinking plenty of water.

One tablespoon or more of lemon juice daily helps to prevent or dissolve kidney stones. Lemons are rich in citrate, an acidic compound known to hamper the formation of calcium-based kidney stones, the most common type.

After two months of treatments with herbal remedies for

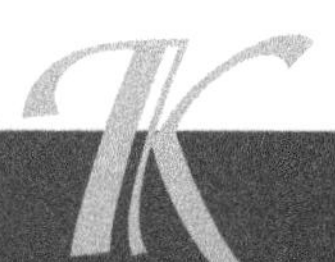

a large kidney stone that you are having difficulty in passing, take a large dose of magnesium sulfate at around 2:00 in the afternoon, about a tablespoon of Epsom salts (magnesium sulfate) in two glasses of water. Follow it by a second eight ounce glass of water. The magnesium sulfate is for the purpose of relaxing and dilating the ureter, alternating with peristaltic action, so that the ureter can more easily carry the stone. During the entire treatment period for difficult stones, the patient should tape two magnets, 3500 gauss each, to the skin of the abdomen, or the back if the stone is known to be nearest the surface there, just over the place the stone is suspected to be in the ureter. The expectation is that the mineral of the stone, as it is softened and dislodged from the stone will be attracted toward the magnet and away from the stone to gradually diminish the size of the stone. The large amount of water will cause the mineral to pass from the body.

(See also "Kidney Stone Pack" in the *Natural Remedies* section.)

Herbs and Teas

Demulcent herbs are those that sooth and comfort the patient with urinary tract pain. Marshmallow root and parsley root fall in this category. Twenty drops of kava kava tincture in a glass of water can be helpful for pain. Castor oil packs over the area of pain, with or without fomentations, can also help.

Lithotriptic herbs are those that soften and help dissolve stones, as well as smooth off rough edges. This would include stone root and gravel root. Some have said apple cider vinegar (with its malic acid) can soften stones. Use two tablespoons in a glass of water. Rinse mouth with water after vinegar use to protect the teeth from the vinegar.

Obstruent herbs tend to clear out the ureters of mucus and increase peristaltic activity. As mucus travels down the urinary tract, it may carry stones with it. Increased peristaltic activity helps with the extrusion of the stone. Lobelia is an obstruent for the urinary tract. Virgin olive oil is also an obstruent. Take two tablespoonfuls every night at bedtime just before lying down.

Take two quarts of water, two tablespoons of gravel root, two tablespoons of stone root, three tablespoons of marshmallow root and boil vigorously for 25 minutes. Take off the stove and add a handful of corn silk or burdock. Allow to sit for 25 minutes. Strain and drink. If the patient is having an acute attack, the two quarts of tea should be drunk in about two hours for best results. For treatment of a stone lodged in the ureter and not giving much trouble, drink two quarts a day until the stone passes. It may take a year.

Another good stone tea is one part stone root, one part marshmallow root, one part parsley root, one part gravel root, one-fourth part lobelia, and one-fourth part ginger root. Of this mixture take two ounces and simmer for 20 minutes in one quart of distilled water. Drink one cup four times a day. Lobelia may make the heart beat stronger and faster. This tea causes the ureter to contract. It encourages mucus formation by the urinary tract. Take a total of 12–14 glasses of teas and water daily, not counting juices, soups or water in foods, until the stone passes.

A special routine with the teas is as follows: At the same time the tea is being taken, the person should fast except for taking unsweetened cranberry or orange juice for three to four days. At the end of the juice fast, four ounces of lemon juice stirred with four ounces of olive oil are taken first thing in the morning. As bowel action increases in the intestinal tract, it reflexively increases peristaltic action in the ureters, as well as the gallbladder.

Case Report

A 38-year-old patient of ours had a kidney stone so large that the urologist said it could not pass. When first observed by X-ray, it was close to the kidney. The urologist said it would gradually pass along the ureter until it got down to the small part of the ureter about six centimeters from the bladder and get stuck. He was correct. The stone lodged right there for 10 months and did not move. Several painful attacks came during those months. Sitting in a bathtub of neutral or hot water for 20 to 30 minutes would give him relief enough to sleep. Sometimes he slept in a bathtub filled with "neutral" water (90 °F to 96°F) as it was the only place he could relax enough to rest.

He occasionally had serious attacks of kidney colic during which he paced the floor, sat in hot water for hours, and eventually would drift off into a short sleep, only to awaken with the same severe, intolerable pain. These attacks would last four to twenty-four hours.

The cost of standard treatment with lithotripsy at that time began at $8,000 and went upward to $21,000 or more, depending on how much treatment was necessary before the stone could be broken up into small enough portions to pass. The patient had no medical insurance.

His mother wrote the following in a letter. "After earnest prayer we decided to do the following routine: For fluids he had from one-half to one and one-half gallons of distilled water daily. He used the following herbs, five or more at a time, during the entire year—cramp bark (urinary antispasmodic), mistletoe (diuretic and antispasmodic), black haw (antispasmodic), fringe tree (antispasmodic), burdock (powerful diuretic), dandelion leaf (the most powerful diuretic), cold pressed castor oil (a peristalsis stimulator), and a liniment made of DMSO, comfrey, and white willow bark rubbed on the skin over the location of the stone and up and down the entire ureter.

"Other measures included jumping on a trampoline, jumping down the steps of stairs, vibration to the back with a hand-held, strong electrical vibrator. Magnets at 3600 gauss were taped over the location of the greatest pain for four months.

"One morning he began early to try to induce the stone to pass by taking two liters of intravenous fluid (his next door neighbor was a doctor and helped him) within two hours with as much herb tea as he could drink by mouth, nearly a gallon in two hours. He took a tablespoon of Epsom salts at the beginning to try to relax the ureter. We rubbed the liniment of the DMSO and herbs on the kidney and ureter area every 30 minutes. This routine was ineffectual in moving the stone. We had spent most of the day in this activity.

"We treated the condition for eleven months total. For 10 months it had not moved from the position at the brim of the bony pelvis. The urologist had continued to tell us it would never pass, that it was too large and too angular, being one centimeter in its greatest diameter. On New Year's Day he assumed an upside down position with his feet almost straight up for a few seconds, with no thought of the kidney stone. Within five minutes he felt a strange sensation in his flank and lower pelvic region, and upon passing urine passed the kidney stone with a clink against the ceramic toilet bowl. The stone was 11 millimeters in its greatest diameter.

"You can imagine the rejoicing the family has had and the seasons of prayer to thank the Lord for His goodness in hearing our prayers that he would pass the stone. Our Father is a merciful God and hears the prayers of His penitent children!"

Knee Pain

(See "Skeletal Problems" in the *Conditions and Diseases* section.)

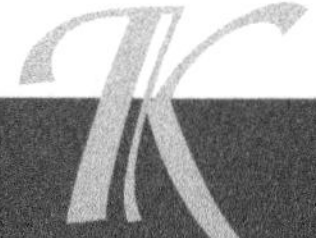

Labor, Childbirth

How to Start Labor

Walking briskly increases the contractions of the uterus. In late pregnancy, walking several miles a day, if possible, can be helpful. It does not need to be all at one time.

Short fasts of 12 to 15 hours, even daily for five days, can often initiate labor. Omit all food from lunch until the next morning at breakfast.

Blue cohosh, parsley, shepherd's purse, and vervain can be taken to encourage the onset of labor.

A "small cold enema,"—one ear syringe of cold water inserted into the rectum and expelled after one minute will increase contractions.

Take one teaspoon of *blue* cohosh tincture followed 30 minutes later by one teaspoon of *black* cohosh tincture followed 30 minutes later by the *blue* cohosh, then the *black*, until you have repeated it four times. Wait to see if you get a response. If not, wait about 10 or 12 hours and repeat the process, continuing for eight doses taken on the same schedule. The herbs can be taken in a little pineapple juice if desired.

Another good remedy is as follows: Two tablespoons of chopped cotton root dried and boiled in one-and-a-half quarts of water for 30 minutes. Give one teaspoon of the tea in four ounces of pineapple juice. If cotton is not grown in your area and the herb cannot be obtained through an herb store, three times the amount of okra root can be used instead. Okra and cotton are close botanical relatives.

Labor Pains and Pain Reduction

Fomentations to the low back or to the perineum can bring great relief.

Firm pressure with the fists into the low back can be very comforting.

Guard against fatigue. Tired muscles make up the major part of the unpleasantness and pain of many a labor that could have been a pleasant experience. A friendly hand to rub shoulders, feet, temples, arms, and legs can banish much fatigue.

Massage of the thighs may be very helpful along with gentle encouragement.

Relaxation with determination from the very beginning of each contraction, along with deep, slow breathing, will eliminate the tightness that causes a large part of the discomfort.

Alfalfa, red raspberry leaf, red clover, catnip, or chamomile are very good for labor pains.

Lacerations, Cuts

Lacerations may be caused by a blunt or sharp instrument, from machinery, or from a fall against an angular surface. If dirt or debris are ground into the wounded tissue, every particle must be removed with scissors or with irrigation or the wound cannot heal. A clean wound requires no trimming.

If there is extreme pain or tenderness in the area, it can be anesthetized by the application of ice directly on the wounded area continuously for three to five minutes. As soon as the wound loses its feeling, the cleansing by lightly snipping off

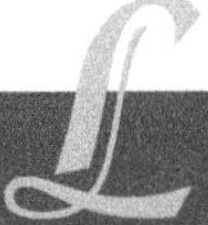

all the dirt particles that cannot be irrigated out of the wound should begin. The anesthesia from ice lasts about three minutes. Work fast for best results.

If the fat is visible, you may see dirt particles, as fat often traps dirt and debris and may need to be lightly trimmed. If a large quantity of fat is removed, however, as much as a spoonful or more from a three-inch wound, it may leave a depressed scar. Therefore, care should be used to avoid removing much of the subcutaneous tissue by too freely snipping or cutting while cleansing the wound, but trim enough to be thorough.

If the wound edges do not fall together by themselves, they should be pulled together by the use of adhesive tape. The wound should not be entirely covered by adhesive as it must have room to drain serum or blood if such fluids should accumulate in the wound. Therefore, the tape may need to be cut more narrow in the midsection, a so-called butterfly, to enable the serum and blood to escape. The tape is anchored in place on one side of the wound while holding it off the skin on the opposite side. Then with appropriate pulling and pushing, get the wound edges as nearly back to their original position as possible. As soon as the wound edges meet, the tape is then brought in contact with the skin on the opposite side, and the laceration is thereby closed. We have seen wounds up to four inches in length closed successfully in this way without suturing. Several thin strips of tape may be required to make the wound edges stay neatly in their original place. Only if wound edges cannot be put together rather accurately by this method, or if bleeding cannot be stopped by continuous pressure for 15 to 30 minutes, do sutures need to be placed.

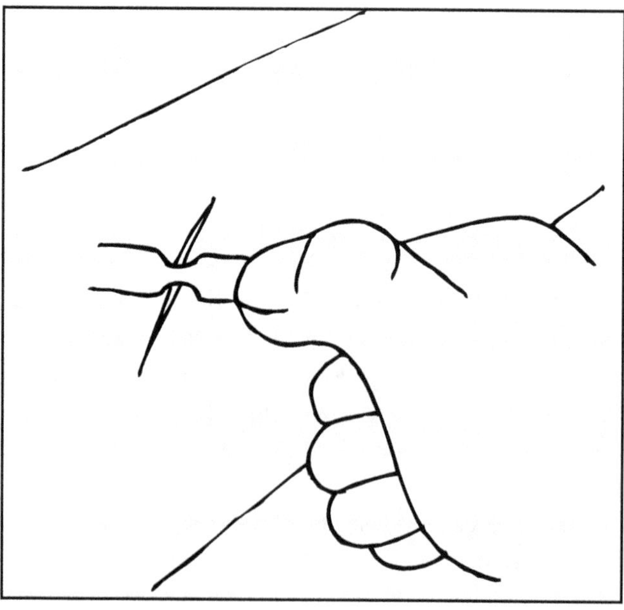

Lameness, Intermittent Claudication

This is the name we give to the lameness brought on by poor circulation to the lower extremities, and it is to be distinguished from poor circulation from the extremities that is caused by varicose veins or inadequate lymphatic drainage. The arteries become blocked, and blood cannot get to the legs and feet. The lameness or cramping pain comes on occasionally along with weakness and tension in the calves of the legs with minor exertion such as walking. When the person sits down there is no pain. It is associated with such diseases as Buerger's disease, arteriosclerosis, diabetes, etc. Walking causes an increased need for oxygen, which cannot be supplied by the blocked arteries, and the muscles begin to hurt.

Treatment

A totally vegetarian diet, keeping away from free fats such as margarine, mayonnaise, fried foods, cooking fats, salad oils, and peanut butter is the best choice. The same instruction given to reduce cholesterol or cure angina will apply here. Use no alcohol or drugs and reduce stress. (See "Stress" in the *Conditions and Diseases* section.)

Use no animal protein of any kind as it has an adverse effect on the blood vessels.

Stop smoking, as you are roughly 10 times more likely to have the disease if you are a smoker.

It has been discovered that in persons with intermittent claudication the blood is quite thick and has a slow-flow condition somewhat like honey on a cold morning. It is not known whether the lameness comes first and causes the thick blood, or whether the thick blood comes first and causes the lameness. We favor the latter position. We believe that too many red blood cells and plasma containing too many nutrients and wastes promotes the development of intermittent claudication (L. Dintenfass and G. V. F. Seaman, eds., *Blood Viscosity in Heart Disease and Cancer* [Pergamon Press, 1981]). If your hemoglobin is above 15 grams, donate blood to the Red Cross if you are an eligible donor and drink plenty of water to keep the blood thin. Thick blood flows with greater difficulty.

Try a series of hot leg baths no more than 103°F for 20 to 30 minutes daily for 14 days. Be cautious. Do not blister the skin as persons with claudication can be more easily injured by hot water. The patient's temperature in the mouth may go up with each bath but should not rise to higher than 102°F.

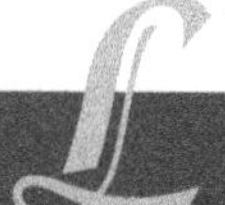

Keep the head cool as soon as sweating begins by placing washcloths squeezed from ice water on the forehead.

Exercise regularly by walking or swimming or simply doing calisthenics. Get some indoor gym equipment if you need it.

The risk of contracting this disease is three times as great in people who have high blood pressure. It is therefore important to treat high blood pressure to decrease this risk.

Control diabetes as it is impossible to control intermittent lameness if diabetes is not brought under good control.

Use one to three cloves of garlic with each meal. It will thin the blood and make it able to perfuse the leg vessels better. Garlic also helps clear arteries of plaques, along with appropriate lifestyle changes.

The long-term use of ginkgo—more than three months—can be worthwhile in the elderly. Taking 40 to 80 milligrams of ginkgo extract three times a day can help intermittent claudication and slow down Alzheimer's disease.

Laryngitis

(See "Hoarseness, Laryngitis" in the *Conditions and Diseases* section.)

Lead, Tin Intoxication

(See "Toxic Heavy Metals" in the *Supplemental Information* section.)

Leaky Gut Syndrome, Increased Intestinal Permeability

Under certain conditions the intestinal tract fails to hold back food particles until complete digestion has occurred, or fails to prohibit certain nutrients, of which the bowel has already taken up enough, from pouring into the bloodstream without a barrier. This condition is called "increased intestinal permeability" or, more commonly, "leaky gut syndrome."

Think of your intestinal tract as a one-way fence with small openings for particles of food to pass through into the bloodstream. In a healthy person the holes are small enough to keep any food particles inside the intestinal tract that would cause harm if they got into the bloodstream before they are completely digested. These holes also do not allow toxic products that may be present in the food to pass through.

Additionally, as soon as any foodstuffs are absorbed into the bloodstream, they must go promptly to the liver through a filtering and detoxifying system. Liver enzymes can transform certain partly digested food products that slip through the intestinal tract into more usable forms. This entire process, however, produces free radicals and oxidation. It is for this reason we need to ingest large quantities of antioxidants and fiber with our food to hang onto toxic substances. When this intestinal barrier is damaged in any way, free radicals can increase and the size of food particles getting into the bloodstream is larger or they are less well-prepared for use in the body and can cause damage in cells and organs throughout the body. Further, toxins can also slip through the leaky gut.

Crohn's disease patients and their relatives may have increased intestinal permeability. One study showed that about one-fourth of all first degree healthy relatives of Crohn's patients have leaky gut (*Acta Gastroenterologica Belgica* 58, no. 1 [1995]: C61).

In 1992 it was discovered in Mexico that certain mushrooms would cause small intestinal damage characterized by flattening of the mucosa, fusing of villi, and other alterations in the cells of the absorptive surface. It is felt these evidences of injury are sufficient to cause abnormalities of absorption.

Increased intestinal permeability can be associated with a variety of problems such as painful joints and muscles, arthritis-like syndrome, allergies, headaches, fevers, food intolerance, gastrointestinal problems, fatigue, just not feeling well, abdominal pain or distention, diarrhea, skin rashes, toxic feelings, memory loss and inattentiveness, shortness of breath, poor exercise tolerance, asthma, and many other problems, many of which appear unrelated to the gastrointestinal tract. There are a number of conditions that have been recognized to promote increased intestinal permeability. A listing of some of these follows:

- Overeating, drinking lots of fluids with one's meals, eating off-schedule, eating too fast or too frequently can all cause a leaky gut, as can germs of various kinds, alcohol, steroids, and too little oxygen from hardening of the arteries or open-heart surgery or shock. Beginning the eating of solid foods too early in life or failure to breast-feed may also cause leaky gut.
- Increased intestinal permeability commonly occurs with certain diseases including inflammatory bowel disease, rheumatoid arthritis, ankylosing spondylitis, asthma, eczema, food allergies, alcoholism, trauma,

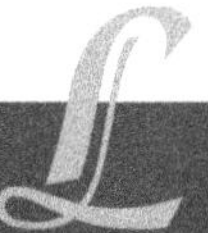

and surgery. Periods of fasting, being very careful never to overeat, using foods high in flavonoids, and avoiding drinking large quantities of liquids with meals, or lying down after eating, can all help in correcting this abnormal permeability (*Alternative Medicine Review* 2, no. 5 [1997]: 330).

- Malnutrition, which may be associated with diarrhea or constipation, can be a cause. This can be corrected by fixing the diet or by overcoming the inability to absorb certain nutrients by giving a dietary supplement.
- The taking of nonsteroidal anti-inflammatory drugs (NSAIDs) can cause injury to the lining of the stomach and small bowel and increase permeability or a leaky gut. These drugs are the most commonly prescribed medications worldwide, and the most common drug side effects in the United States are probably to the NSAIDs (*Nutrition Reviews* 53, no. 1: 13).

Having this clinical disease may mimic or cause a number of other conditons—bowel, joint, kidney or lung infection; food allergy; Crohn's disease; celiac disease (gluten intolerance); dermatological conditions like psoriasis, allergic dermatitis, eczema, acne, colitis; or autoimmune diseases like rheumatoid arthritis, ankylosing spondylitis, Reiter's syndrome (urethritis, arthritis, and inflammation of the bowel, more common in men). These are all associated with increased bowel permeability.

Your doctor can order an intestinal permeability assessment kit to test whether you have leaky gut syndrome.

Treatment

A day or two of fasting per week and eliminating all those foods known to give you a sensitivity reaction is often effective.

Whole grain rice with its gamma oryzenin in the bran has a healing effect on the stomach and small bowel and has a very potent antioxidant activity. It should be taken at least once daily for the first six weeks after the discovery of a leaky gut (*Rephokaido Institute of Public Health* 16 [1966]: 111).

Do not take supplemental forms of dietary fiber in large quantities as too much may increase intestinal permeability (*Journal of Nutrition* 113 [1983]: 2300).

Take flavonoids before eating as they can block allergic reactions that cause, or result from, increased permeability. Catechins, milk thistle, and dandelion root all have very favorable flavonoids for this function as well as that they protect the liver. The use of foods high in flavonoids can help in correcting this abnormal permeability (*Alternative Medicine Review* 2, no. 5 [1997]: 330). (See "Food Sources High in Certain Nutrients" in the *Dietary Information* section.)

Essential fatty acids such as those found in walnuts and flaxseed can be most helpful to protect your body from toxins produced in the digestive tract (*American Journal of Clinical Nutrition* 54 [1991]: 346).

Glutathione (GSH) and N-acetyl cysteine are considered extremely good supplements to use in the leaky gut syndrome. Do not take these if you are taking artemisia or any other parasite medicine. Wait until the herbs for parasites are no longer being used.

Zinc in fairly large quantities, 150 milligrams a day, will sometimes stop the increased intestinal permeability caused by malnutrition (*Gut* 39 [1996]: 416).

"Friendly bacteria," which includes acidophilus, lactobacillus and bifidobacterium, are probiotics and may be helpful.

Use the following:

- Symbiotic with fructo-oligosaccharide (FOS), one-fourth to one-half teaspoon three times a day in water for one year.
- NAG (N-acetyl glucosamine), two pills three times a day for one year. This helps heal the leaky gut.
- If abnormal bacteria are present (dysbiosis), use herbal antibacterials. Most bacteria are sensitive to herb gentian and particularly to grapefruit seed extract.

In addition to protein, fats, and celluloses, chlorella has 3.3 percent glucosamine, which may be helpful.

One teaspoon slippery elm in water half an hour before each meal can be helpful.

If a hidden infection is a probability, use golden seal, echinacea, artemisia, garlic, and grapefruit seed extract as antimicrobial agents. You must chew your food thoroughly to encourage epithelial growth factor from the saliva. Glutamine, an amino acid known to help in the maintenance of intestinal metabolism, can help to heal the intestinal tract (*Archives of Surgery* 125 [1990]: 1040–5).

Food should be prepared with simplicity. You should keep grease out of your food.

What influence does overeating have on the stomach? It becomes debilitated. The digestive organs are weakened and can't take up or keep nutrients out. Some of the symptoms that are known to be the results of overeating include headache, confusion, digestive complaints, malaise (not feeling good), reduced spirituality because of poor thought processes, fatigue, clumsiness, faintness, insomnia, and depression.

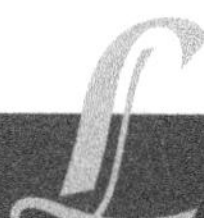

If rats eat half to two-thirds less than they have been accustomed to eating they live 50 percent to maybe 90 percent longer, and some human beings have the same experience too. I believe many of us overeat. Under eating can be a problem too. It can rob you of cheerfulness and cooperation and a sense of well being. Eat enough, but don't eat too much.

Exercise a little after a meal, not hard—just some moderate exercise, like a brisk walk. If you sit down or lie down you are more likely to develop problems with your intestinal tract.

An all-soft diet, like porridge and soups and juices, is not good for us on a long-term basis. We need to chew firm food to break down the food and get it ready for the stomach to digest. There are chemicals in the mouth that help with digestion, and are released by thorough chewing.

Food should not be too hot or too cold.

It has been found that anxiety will increase permeability and make it so that your intestine cannot keep partly digested nutrients out. Take time to eat and avoid anxiety with the meals. If the brain is burdened, reduce the amount of food that you take.

Use two to four dishes of simple foods, prepared in as natural and tasty a way as possible. We find that the diet selected for us by our loving Creator was fruits, grains, nuts and vegetables.

Use no baking soda or baking powder as these upset the chemical balance of the entire digestive tract. Additionally, no milk should be used in bread baking. Just use water. Fermented milk yields unhealthful chemical compounds.

Cook grains a long time. For rice it's about three hours. Corn grits should be cooked four or five hours, or all night in a slow cooker.

Case Report

This is a story that came from the April 6, 1992, issue of *Newsweek*. "Molly's symptoms had baffled her doctors. More than 50 doctors had worked on Molly, many of them at major university hospitals, since mid-November. Why should a cheerful, active, 17-month-old suddenly stop eating? Why would she stop walking and playing when nothing showed up after three days of round-the-clock testing in December? We were sent home with instructions to pop a bottle of milk in Molly's mouth first thing in the morning instead of breastfeeding her, to give her vitamins, and not pick her up as much as we had been. Was this meager advice the best modern medicine could do for my baby? Doctor's advice notwithstanding, I held my baby much during the holidays as she continued to waste away. What was even more disconcerting was her behavior. She wanted nothing to do with toys, books, Christmas, or her two older sisters. 'No,' she yelled, when anybody came close.

"Not knowing what was ailing my child had to be the most frustrating experience of my 38 years on this planet. Doctors, too, were clearly uncomfortable about being unable to come up with a diagnosis for a 17-month-old who had, in two months, dropped from 23 to 18 pounds, and lost all her body fat. Not that they didn't try. Because Molly was so sick so long, she continued to be poked and prodded, sedated, sliced, and scanned for what I started to call the 'Disease of the Week.' Different specialists took turns chasing every possible lead—leukemia, chronic mononucleosis, neuroblastoma (that was another childhood malignancy), infant botulism, neuromuscular disease (like muscular dystrophy), cystic fibrosis, heart disease, and any number of debilitating genetic disorders.

"While drawing her blood one Monday, our pediatrician asked, 'Should we add HIV to the list?'

"'Why not,' I replied, over my baby's screams. I was numb.

"The next hospital stay—this time on the Oncology Ward (that's for cancer)—in late January brought more theories of the hour, but still no answers. It seemed as if everyone we knew had ideas to propose. We relayed every one to the doctors. Then, finally, three weeks later, on our third admission with yet another doctor's name on Molly's tiny hospital bracelet, I heard the magic words: 'We have a diagnosis.'

"The doctors had not figured this out on their own, mind you (that's hard to bear). Just by chance, a colleague of my husband's—not a physician—asked if we had checked for gluten intolerance, a chronic disorder caused by sensitivity to protein found in wheat, barley, and rye. And that was her diagnosis. She had an intolerance to gluten. They removed the gluten grains from her diet and she soon became again the lively, cheerful and sweet tempered Molly."

Leg Cramps

(See "Cramps of Legs and Other Muscles" in the *Conditions and Diseases* section.)

Lice, Pediculosis

These are small wingless flat insects that live on the skin of birds, mammals, and human beings. Three kinds of lice

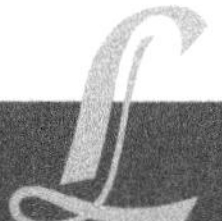

may infest humans and cause irritating dermatitis and carry disease—the head louse, body louse, and crab louse.

Lice infestation was once a condition of those living in crowded, unsanitary conditions. In recent years, however, we have seen a more educated and refined group of lice, and it is no longer a disgrace to have an infestation.

School children are particularly prone to get head lice, a grey insect about one-fourth inch long, which attaches tiny nits (eggs) on the hair shaft close to the scalp. The diagnosis is made by the intense itching and the presence of lice and eggs on the hairs. Head lice are spread by coats, caps, scarves, carpets, upholstered furniture, bedding, combs, brushes, and so forth. An adult louse will live about 30 days, the female laying about 10 eggs per day, producing hundreds of offspring. The intense itching will cause scratching that can result in infection and swelling of the neck glands.

Body lice are comparatively rare and live mainly in the seams of clothing. They move onto the body twice a day for feeding. Typhous and other fevers may be carried by body lice.

Crab lice live principally in the pubic hair, but may also spread to the hair of the chest, armpits, beard, and eyelashes.

Treatment

Since isolated lice of all kinds have a life span of only about eight days without eating, putting clothing into a plastic garbage bag, sealing it securely, and leaving it for 8 to 10 days, will allow plenty of time for the nits to hatch and the adults to die. The clothing may then be laundered.

In the past DDT, benzyl benzoate, Kwell (lindane), and RID (pyrethrins) have been widely used for lice. Lindane has been reported to induce convulsions, cancer, birth defects, nerve damage, and aplastic anemia. Pyrethrins are toxic and irritating to mucous membranes and eyes, and allergic reactions are especially likely to be intense in persons who have a ragweed sensitivity. Since simple measures that are nontoxic and nonirritating are very effective, there seems to be little need for using these toxic agents.

Laundering clothes and drying on the hot cycle will usually kill lice attached to clothing. A soak in very warm soapy water for half an hour will kill lice on the body. Non-washable items may be deloused by sealing in plastic bags for 10 days.

Articles that can tolerate freezing can be sealed in plastic bags and placed in the freezer overnight to kill the adults.

The hair can be deloused by a number of methods:

- Mix equal parts of olive oil and kerosene, sufficient to wet all the hair and scalp. Wrap the head in a towel and leave it on for one to three hours. The hair is then shampooed thoroughly, and the nits combed out with a fine-tooth comb.
- Dousing the hair with kerosene alone and wrapping in a towel for two to three hours has been used successfully for generations.
- Use enough warm mineral oil to completely cover the entire scalp. The oil suffocates the lice in about 10 to 15 minutes. Then the hair can be shampooed and the dead lice combed out. The procedure should be repeated at days 3, 7, and 10 to make certain any new lice hatching out from the eggs attached to hairs will be suffocated. For body lice and crab lice, the same procedure is effective. Sit in a bathtub to avoid drops of oil getting on the floor. Take a sponge bath in ordinary mineral oil, using a cotton sponge or your fingers saturated with the oil, working it into the lice-infested areas quite liberally. Allow it to stay on for 10 to 20 minutes, then wash it all off with soap. The oil coats the eggs and prevents hatching as well as stopping up the spiracles in the lice and suffocating them.
- One bulb of garlic, containing 10 to 20 cloves, blended in sufficient water to wet the scalp and hair entirely, may then be wrapped with a towel around the head for two hours. Make certain the person is not sensitive to garlic before using this part of the remedy. A portion can be applied to the skin on the inside of the arm, fastened there with tape for two hours to see if blistering or a rash occurs at the place of contact with the garlic.
- Pennyroyal oil mixed with equal quantities of alcohol and rubbed with the fingertips into the scalp may be left on for 10 minutes followed by thorough shampooing.
- One tablespoon of rue (*Ruta graveolens*) gently boiled in two-thirds cup of water may be used to wet the hair and scalp thoroughly. Then wrap the head with a towel for two hours.
- Hot vinegar applied directly to the scalp and hair will loosen nits and allow removal with a fine-tooth comb. If the scalp is irritated by scratching, full strength vinegar may burn. The vinegar may be diluted with hot water and the fine-tooth comb dipped into the water as hot as can be tolerated on the scalp and used for removal of the nits by combing.
- A hairy area, such as underarms and eyebrows, may be deloused by thick applications of petroleum jelly for 10 minutes twice daily for a week, followed by combing with a fine-tooth comb.

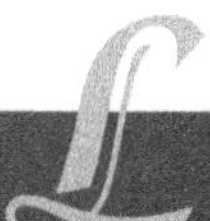

- A paste made of neem oil and turmeric powder and spread over the scalp and hair, wrapping for eight hours or overnight with a towel, and then shampooing, is a very effective remedy.

Lichen Planus

Lichen planus consists of recurring itchy lesions that may be rough, scaly patches. They can occur in the mouth, inside the wrists, the trunk, and genitals. The lesions can measure up to about one-forth of an inch or more and run together to make large, irregular sorts of violet patches with a distinct sheen on cross lighting. Some dermatologists believe food high in iodine may cause these lesions. Also suspected have been dust, cats, gold, latex, perfumes, nickel, plastics, molds, soaps, bleach, medicines, stress, etc.

We recommend a very strict diet be followed for lichen planus. You should eliminate all the foods on the list of the top 10 food groups causing food sensitivities for a period of six weeks. During that time the skin lesions should disappear. When the skin lesions have disappeared, you should then begin adding back foods, one group every two weeks, until each group that you wish has been returned to the diet without the reoccurrence of the lichen planus.

During the first six weeks, take a heaping tablespoon of activated charcoal in a glass of water four times daily (unless on medication). Take a short cold bath daily four days a week, and a hot bath once a week, bringing the mouth temperature up to 101°F while keeping the head cool. (See "Hydrotherapy" in the *Natural Remedies* section.)

Obey all health laws carefully. Get to bed at least two hours before midnight, and preferably three.

Lichen Sclerosis

This is a skin disorder that occasionally occurs on the perineum of older women. It is characterized by flattening of the skin, scarring, loss of hair, loss of elasticity, and sometimes itching or discomfort. It is a chronic condition and considered to be incurable.

Lichen sclerosis is notoriously difficult to treat and that is why most gynecologists simply bypass any simple remedy and proceed directly to the steroids. You can, however, use the simple remedies to control your symptoms and bring about healing as well as with steroids.

Get a shallow pan or a small tub large enough to allow you to immerse the perineum when you fill it with herbal teas and vinegar water. The vinegar water should be used three times a day, and especially just before retiring at night. If you cannot find a suitable tub, you may sit on a plastic sheet in the bathtub with the edges of the plastic pulled up and the vinegar water applied to the perineum by a small face towel.

The vinegar water should consist of one-fourth cup of vinegar to each quart of hot water you put in the pan. You need only enough to be able to touch all the surfaces, the labia minora, the labia majora, the entire perineum, and even the rectal area with the vinegar water. Sit in the vinegar water for 10 minutes as hot as you can comfortable tolerate it. Do not scald yourself, nor try to get it excessively hot.

Two hours later take an herbal bath. It does not need to be hot, but can be hot if you like. Make up this tea by putting two rounded tablespoons of licorice root chips in each quart of water, which you should gently boil on the stove for about 12 to 20 minutes. This makes a licorice root tea that is double strength. You should sit in that for 20 minutes. It can be used three times, so it can be set aside or poured into a jar, kept for four hours, and repeated. Two hours after doing the sitz bath with the licorice root tea, sit in another hot vinegar water tub, again for 10 minutes. Two hours after that repeat the licorice root tea sitz, and two hours after that repeat the vinegar water sitz, etc.

A schedule could run like this:

- 6:00–6:10 a.m.: Hot vinegar water sitz
- 8:00–8:20 a.m.: Licorice root sitz
- 10:00–10:10 a.m.: Hot vinegar water sitz
- 12 noon–12:20 p.m.: Licorice root sitz
- 2:00–2:10 p.m.: Hot vinegar water sitz
- 4:00–4:20 p.m.: Licorice root sitz
- 6:00–6:10 p.m.: Hot vinegar water sitz
- 8:00–8:20 p.m.: Licorice root and vinegar water sitz at bedtime

Between each of the treatments, you should apply a comfrey compress. This can be made by putting a moderately large leaf of fresh comfrey into a blender with sufficient water to enable the blades to turn and blend the comfrey leaf. It should be a paste about the thickness of warm peanut butter when you have finished blending it. Put this paste on a folded paper towel, spread it out, and place it against the perineum with plastic over it before replacing your panties. The plastic will keep your panties from getting green stains from the comfrey poultice. Wear it for one hour just prior to

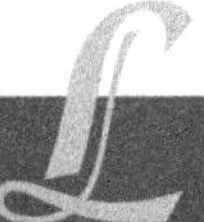

the next fluid treatment. You should be making a treatment every two hours with one of the two fluids, and halfway in between treatments apply the comfrey poultice for one hour. You should not use the poultice more than two or three times before making it up again fresh.

These treatments must be done daily for 30 days. At the same time, you should be taking by mouth several herbs:

- Aloe vera juice or gel: one ounce two or three times daily.
- Licorice root (tea or capsules): one dose four times daily.
- Hawthorn berry: one dose four time daily. This can be either a tea made by gently simmering hawthorn berries for 20 minutes, one teaspoon per cup, or a capsule or tablet used according to the recommended dosage on the package.
- Flaxseed: two tablespoons of freshly ground flaxseed sprinkled on cereal every morning for breakfast.
- Vitamin A: 100,000 IU daily for 30 to 60 days.
- Zinc: 30 milligrams twice a day for 21 days.
- Garlic: one raw clove daily or one globe of garlic lightly steamed or baked, just enough to take away the hot garlic quality.
- Golden seal: for the first week of the one-month treatment period, you should take one teaspoon of golden seal tincture or its equivalent in golden seal tea or golden seal capsules or tablets. The golden seal should be taken four times daily for eight days.

Treatment may be needed for three months, but you should notice a difference within four to six weeks.

Liver Toxicity From Iron

For many decades in America the principle concern of physicians with respect to iron was anemia in women. In recent years polycythemia, or too much iron in the blood, has become an even more serious concern than anemia. Since several life-threatening problems can result from iron overload, it is natural that a greater concern be exhibited for it than for ordinary female anemia, which is not in itself lethal.

Iron is obtained from enriched grains, from nutrient supplements, from iron cookware, and from many ordinary foods such as beans, greens, and grains. One of the principle objections to enriching refined grains, is the problem with iron. Many authorities in the field of nutrition point out that men are more likely to be fatally injured by the enriching programs than women are to be benefited in the small increase in hemoglobin they may get from eating enriched grains.

While iron is essential for life, in excessive amounts it is toxic to body cells. The liver is particularly subject to the toxic effects of iron. It is one of the major sites of storage for iron, and an inherited and an acquired disorder may result in liver cells storing too much iron. A genetic form of iron overload is called hemochromatosis, a disorder of iron metabolism in patients who absorb too much iron from the intestinal tract. It is then transported to the liver where it forms free radicals and peroxidation of organelle membrane lipids. If this mechanism becomes far advanced, it can cause death of liver cells known as sideronecrosis. Liver cell death is followed by the formation of scar tissue, which progresses to cirrhosis. Once cirrhosis is developed in the iron-damaged liver, risk of cancer of the liver increases by 200 fold.

Iron is also harmful because it acts as an oxidant at high levels. Best hemoglobin levels for women range from 10.5 to 12.5 and for men from 12.5 to 14.5. Serum levels of iron should range from about 20 to 85.

Herbs that can be used to treat the liver are turmeric, green tea, licorice, and milk thistle (*Alternative Medicine Review* 4, no. 3 [1999]: 178). Use one tablespoon of any of these per day, made into tea. Also use angelica, anise, barberry, fennel, ginseng, and yarrow.

Liver damage can often be prevented by choline if it is present in proper quantities. The body can make choline, which protects the liver, but in disease there may not be quite enough produced for its protective benefit. Good sources of choline include leaf lettuce, cauliflower, peanuts, whole wheat, and tomatoes. One may be able to get from 0.6 to 1.0 gram of choline per day in the typical American diet and considerably more in a vegetarian diet. Nine patients with severe cirrhosis of the liver were treated with 1.5 to 6.0 grams of choline per day plus other vitamins for several weeks. They had a reduction in edema and fluid retention in the abdomen, had a better appetite, and better sense of well-being. Enlarged livers became smaller, jaundice subsided, and laboratory tests of liver function improved (*Annals of Internal Medicine* 21 [1944]: 848).

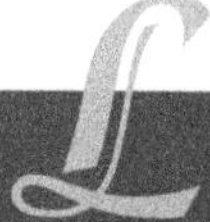

Lung Problems, Respiratory Illnesses

A Canadian study revealed infants whose mothers consumed mercury-containing fish during pregnancy are at risk of delayed lung development. Fish in many areas of the United States are known to be contaminated with mercury.

For people who live or work in very dusty or heavy air, use a few drops of grapefruit seed extract boiled in water on a hot plate or stove as a vapor. People breathe more easily with this vapor in the air, even those who have asthma.

Respiratory illness is linked to gas stoves according to an article in Feburary 18, 1984, issue of *The Atlanta Journal*. Those who have pulmonary problems should rid their homes and work places of any source of fumes.

Cow's milk plays an important role in chronic respiratory disease. Some 2,000 patients were tested and found to be sensitive to milk, many of whom had lengthy histories of illnesses from vomiting, diarrhea, chronic stuffy nose, middle ear infections or coughing blood. Neither the patients nor the physicians who treated them had recognized a milk intolerance as the cause of their illnesses in the great majority of them (*Medical World News*, June 3, 1960, 8).

A meal high in fat may temporarily reduce lung function, persisting up to 48 hours. Excessive fat in the blood impairs lung gas exchange (*Journal of the American Medical Association,* 223 [January 1, 1973]: 15).

Free fats such as margarine, mayonnaise, fried foods, salad oils, and cooking fats should be removed from the diet when there is any lung disease. Get essential fatty acids from whole grains, nuts, avocado, olives, seeds, and legumes.

Lupus

(See "Collagen Diseases" in the *Conditions and Diseases* section.)

Lyme Disease

This disease is caused by *Borrelia burgdorferi*, first discovered in Lyme, Connecticut. The disease usually begins with a flu-like illness, which is often, but not always, followed by a distinctive rash. The initial lesion is a large blotchy red ring that fades in the middle to resemble a target. Weeks or months later it can cause arthritis, almost indistinguishable from rheumatoid arthritis although it will usually improve in one to two years. More serious are the heart and neurological diseases that form a part of this syndrome.

We have treated Lyme disease with a series of artificial fever treatments and had the disease clear up for as long as two years, when we had our last follow-up.

Only 60 percent of tick bite patients get the bull's eye lesion typical of Lyme disease. It occurs within 32 days of the tick bite. Blood should be drawn for antibodies in the serum as soon as the patient becomes sick, and then two to three weeks later to see if the level of antibodies has risen. This procedure can greatly help in identifying Lyme disease. It can mimic many other diseases, and the diagnosis can be very difficult without laboratory confirmation.

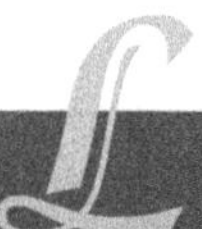

Macular Degeneration

(See "Eyes" in the *Conditions and Diseases* section.)

Malaria

Malaria is caused by plasmodium, a parasite introduced into the bloodstream by a bite from an infected female anopheles mosquito, the one that stands on her head to bite. The parasite enters a red blood cell and multiplies until it forms a whole brood of new parasites and bursts the cell. When the red cells begin to burst, the patient starts having chills, and the fever rises. There is usually backache, muscle soreness, and extreme malaise. When the red blood cells rupture, all the new malaria parasites are set free in the bloodstream, and each one immediately searches for a new red blood cell to inhabit. The patient continues to have a fever while the parasites are free in the plasma. Even a small number of parasites free in the blood are capable of provoking a high fever with shaking chills. Any successful attack on malaria has to be made during this parasite migration phase. In falciparum malaria there may also be blood in the urine, which gives this most serious form of malaria the name of "black water fever."

Cases of malaria are not limited to overseas. The United States has also had cases in such states as New York, New Jersey, Texas, and Michigan (*MMWR* 45 [1996]: 398).

Prevention depends on control of the anopheles mosquito. Swamps must be cleaned out, breeding places eliminated, and water not allowed to accumulate in tin cans, old tires, ditches, etc. These mosquitoes lay eggs only on still water. These mosquitoes are usually more active beginning about one hour before sunset. A heavy application of citronella insect repellant and protective clothing, mosquito screens over the bed at night, and window screens to banish mosquitoes from the home are effective preventive measures.

Hydrotherapy Treatment

The superintendent of the St. Helena Sanitarium in California reported in 1909 that he used hydrotherapy to treat two men with malaria who had been taking quinine unsuccessfully. He used cold mitten friction every two hours with hot and cold to the spine to tone up the nervous system. He reported that the two men were free from the attacks in two or three days and the blood was free of the parasites in one week. Dr. H. F. Rand was a hospital superintendent at that same time and also told of giving cool half-baths (see "Hydrotherapy" in the *Natural Remedies* section) about 10 hours before the next chill came over the patient. He mentions other cold treatments such as cold mitten frictions, cool showers, etc., as successful treatments for malaria, even better than hot treatments in his opinion, as the leukocytes were not hindered in their work of destroying the parasites by the change in blood to alkaline from acid, as will occur with a hot bath. A week of the hydrotherapy was all that was required, and it was successful from the beginning (*Life and Health*, August 1909).

Dr. Paulson wrote about his experience with a patient who had been taking quinine and other medicines but to no effect in the *General Conference Bulletin* in 1907. The doctors told him it would probably be three to four months before he would be well. They knew that the malarial parasites could resist their medicines, and live in spite of them. This case was more serious than the others had been. Finally, the

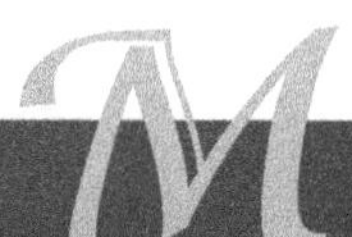

doctors used cold mitten friction, beginning about the same number of hours before the chill was expected each time, and the chills kept coming further and further apart until finally they ceased in about a week.

"Naturally quinine was considered just as indispensable in malaria as morphine was following certain surgical operations. We soon had an abundant opportunity to put our principles in regard to quinine to a practical test. It happened to be a malarial summer in Michigan. During the summer something like 50 cases came to us of all ages and in all stages of the disease. Dr. Kress and I determined we would discover for ourselves what God would help us to do in malarial cases without quinine. It was mutually agreed that as the patients came in, one was to be assigned to the physicians using quinine, the next one to Dr. Kress and myself, so alternating. As he was also a microscopic expert, having taken special training in blood work, every case, not only his own, but ours, was carefully checked up by himself by laboratory work, so there was no chance for guess work.

"We carefully took the temperature every 15 minutes. As soon as there began to be the least rise of temperature, that was a notification to us that the chill was approaching. We at once put the patient into a hot blanket pack, which brought on profound perspiration and thereby, if we had hit it right, we would invariably prevent the chill. The patient would perspire for a time, we would take him out carefully, provided it was the alternate day variety, we gave tonic treatments (hot and cold). The following day we again instituted the temperature taking program. We invariably found that the rise of temperature was much delayed, showing that the treatment was working. We would then go through the same program. Frequently we did not have to do this the third time; the work had been done, and in a week or 10 days the patient was fully restored to health. Sometimes we would miss hitting it just right for several days, so there would be a delay.

"One day an old feeble broken down man came in so loaded with malaria that it seemed he was on the brink of the grave. According to the rotation he belonged to the quinine list. The doctor, after sizing up the situation, said he did not dare to undertake his case, so he was turned over to our list. I will never forget when Dr. Kress and I earnestly told the Lord that His principles were on test, and pleaded with Him to vindicate what He had said. We then took hold of the case. Within a week the man was restored to health."

The results of this experiment were as follows: the blanket pack patients were a total success. Not one case resulted in serious complications or treatment failure. On the other hand, the quinine patients didn't fare so well. Some developed deafness that was irreparable; there were some reversible impaired mentality; and others with numerous minor complications.

Herbal Treatment

Artemisia contains a nutrient from which artemisinin, a very effective antimalaria drug, is extracted. There was reduction of malaria parasites in the blood by 50 percent within nine hours of taking the first dose in a trial of the drug. The body temperature usually fell below 37.5 (99.3 F) within 24 to 25 hours (*Quarterly Review of Natural Medicine* [Fall 1998]: 217).

Dr. Ibraheim Motanya came down with cerebrospinal malaria and was treated with "a lot of hops, rosemary, thistle, cinchona, periwinkle, mint, comfrey, and parsley, along with some garlic and lemon." He also did a stomach cleansing that brought almost immediate relief for the severe headache he had suffered.

In the 1800s a tea made from olive leaves was used as a cure for malaria. By the early 1900s, olive leaf tea was found to be far superior to quinine for treating malarial infections, but quinine was easier to administer. Therefore, quinine continued to be the treatment of choice. In 1957 oleoropine was isolated from olive leaves as the active ingredient. This same compound was found to lower blood pressure, increase blood flow to the coronary arteries, relieve arrhythmia of the heart, and prevent intestinal spasms.

Oleoropine was further purified to yield elenolic acid (as calcium elenolate) and was found to be effective against dozens of different viruses, many strains of bacteria, and several parasitic protozoa. All viruses showed a high susceptibility to inactivation by calcium elenolate except reovirus-3 and poliovirus. These were reduced in activity, but in a lesser degree.

Olive leaf tea not only does not destroy any immune properties, but stimulates phagocytosis (cell feeding). It does not destroy the friendly intestinal microorganisms ("Acute Antihypertensive Effect in Conscious Rats Produced by Some Medical Plants Used in the State of Sao Paulo," *Ethnopharmacol* 15, no. 3 [March 1986]: 261–69; "Vasodilator effect of olive leaf," *Planta Med.* 57, no. 5 [October 1991] :417–19).

A missionary who had been in India takes 12 lemons a day for three weeks to treat malaria. Others raise the temperature in a hot bath three to four hours before the fever is anticipated. Both methods are quite effective. One man told us that when he lived in the tropics, taking one lemon or one lime every day helped him to ward off malaria just as well

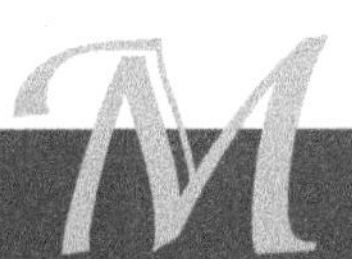

as the drug given to others. It should certainly be tried as the prophylactic drug medication is effective in only about 50 percent of persons taking it and has undesirable side effects.

One study showed a diet high in omega-3 fatty acids and low in vitamin E appears to cure malaria. Vitamin E protects the cell membranes of the malaria parasites, while omega-3 makes them more vulnerable to damage. The nutrients act like a form of chemotherapy. Food sources that are high in vitamin E are wheat, rye, oats, corn, peas, parsley, spinach, carrots, onion, garlic, avocados, hazelnuts, sunflower seeds, almonds, Brazil nuts, safflower nuts, pumpkin seeds, flaxseeds, flaxseed oil, walnuts, olive oil, sunflower oil, and soybean oil. Supplemental omega-3 should also be taken (*Medical Tribune* 34, no. 13 [July 8, 1893]: 3).

A report of constriction of the extremities at the beginning of an attack of malaria was reported in the August 28, 1926, *Journal of the American Medical Association* on page 714. The report said that the treatment was an age-old treatment popular in Russia. Constriction of the extremities at the beginning of an attack would stop the chill but not the fever. The next attack, however, did not arrive. Bind all four extremities snugly with elastic or other bandages.

The following suggestions were made by an Australian man who told us the routine he was using to treat malaria.

- Diet: Become a total vegetarian—no meat, milk, eggs, or cheese.
- Papaya seeds: Take 12 seeds, crack outer shell or chew them, and swallow all of them. They are a bit peppery. Take 12 seeds every second day thereafter. The active ingredient in the seeds has a quinine effect. Malaria symptoms, he said, will disappear within half an hour to an hour after taking the papaya seed, longer in those on a mixed diet.
- Onion: Eat a large, hot onion every day, lightly steamed (just enough to cause beginning transparent appearance and to remove most of the hot taste in the mouth).
- Garlic: Eat one whole globe (10 to 15 cloves) baked in an oven at 250°F for 10 minutes, or just enough to get rid of most of the hot taste and begin appearing transparent.
- Water: Drink around 12 glasses per day.

An excellent treatment with the onset of fever is a hot water enema followed by two quick fomentations of three minutes each to the abdomen. As the second of these two fomentations is being applied, begin a cold mitten friction to the rest of the body, starting with the upper extremities and proceeding to the lower extremities. Terminate the second fomentation with a cold mitten friction to the abdomen and chest. Then turn the patient and end the treatment with a cold mitten friction to the back. Follow this phase of treatment with a rest in bed of one to one-and-a-half hours.

The next portion of the treatment is alternating very hot fomentations with very cold compresses, two quick exchanges to the spine, very hot, and about three minutes, alternating very cold compresses for about one minute. When the fomentations to the spine have been completed, give a hot foot bath with alternating hot and cold spray to the liver and spleen area. The patient may stand in the hot foot bath in the shower while the hot and cold spray are being administered to the midsection. Give the hot spray at about 110°F for two minutes, and the cold spray at about 40°F to 50°F for 20 seconds. Administer these sprays with a lot of water pressure.

Continue the treatment for 10 to 20 minutes. The patient should be quite warm during this part of the treatment. The second phase of the treatment ends with a vigorous cold mitten friction for five minutes while sitting in a bathtub, the water at about 70°F to 80°F. One may substitute a salt glow followed by a cool cleansing shower at about 90°F to 94°F. Treat a debilitated patient more gently than a healthy and vigorous one. At the end of the second phase the patient should again rest in bed for one to one-and-a-half hours.

Another method of treatment for malaria consists of taking the temperature every 15 minutes; at the first sign of an elevation of body temperature, put the patient into a full body pack, a Russian steam bath, a whirlpool, or a hot bathtub to elevate the mouth temperature to about 102°F to 103°F, bringing out the army of white blood cells into the bloodstream to attack the parasites before they can enter new red blood cells. You probably will not catch them all the first treatment, but persevere. Be ready with the heating treatment every time the symptoms appear, whether it is every three days, four days, or at irregular intervals. Used with persistence and proper timing, this treatment will completely eradicate the disease.

Case Report

A 66-year-old man relates his experience with malaria. He was infected with malaria as a soldier in the medical corps in New Guinea in World War II. Atabrine was administered, which had also been used as a prophylactic medication. It did not prevent his getting malaria; instead, it only changed the quality of the disease. The drug produced nausea and vomiting and other toxic symptoms. A tolerance developed. When his malaria flared up, he was given massive therapeutic doses every four hours. He began to get toxic symptoms from the

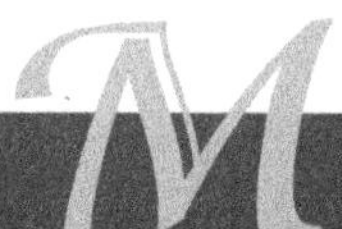

drug. His heart became involved, and eventually he had to discontinue the medication. When he was released from the army, he was visiting friends and had an attack of malaria with a fever up to 104°F. Quinine, a relative of Atabrine, was currently used in the area he was visiting, but remembering his near-death experience with Atabrine, he opted for hydrotherapy.

He received fomentations to the spine, the liver, and the spleen, alternating with short, brisk applications of cold. The treatments were timed to start about one hour before the chill and fever were due, and continuing until the chill was over and he broke out in a sweat. Between treatments he took contrasting hot and cold showers, morning and evening. The attacks, occurring every three days, became worse. His red blood count became perilously low and some felt he would die. He had no choice but to continue with the hydrotherapy. With his very next treatment his fever rose only to 100.4°F instead of above 104°F as had been customary in previous attacks. Three days later, when the next attack was due, no attack came.

He relapsed in three weeks but two hydrotherapy treatments subdued the symptoms and he had a remission of another three weeks. Then he had the worst attack he had ever had. His fever was 105.8°F and the chill was violent. That attack occurred March 6, 1946. His treatment was the same as it had been using water treatments as hot as he could bear, and again his friends had earnest prayer with him. He never again had the slightest symptom of malaria. He lived a good long life and died of a stroke in 2001.

Manic Depression

(See "Mental Health" in the *Conditions and Diseases* section.)

Mastitis

(See "Breast Conditions" in the *Conditions and Diseases* section.)

Mastoiditis

(See "Earache, Otitis Media, Mastoiditis" in the *Conditions and Diseases* section.)

Measles

Common throughout the world, measles are an acute, highly communicable childhood disease. Symptoms resemble those of the common cold with fever and the early appearance of a rash on the mucous membranes of the cheeks and lips, and later over the entire body. Measles is spread through secretions from the eyes, nose, and throat and by droplet infections spread by coughing, sneezing, or talking. It may be transmitted from seven to eleven days after a person has been exposed. The person is most infective just before the rash appears.

If the child has a fever but a rash has not broken out yet, pour three cups of boiling water over one tablespoon of calendula, steep 15 minutes, flavor with one drop peppermint oil, and drink one cup per day (Jude C. Williams, *Jude's Herbal Home Remedies* [St. Paul, MN: Llewellyn Publications, 1996]).

During a measles epidemic, if a child has symptoms of a cold and a fever, check daily for the presence of Koplik's spots, bluish-white spots opposite the first molar or inside the lower lip. They may be pinpoint in size and surrounded by a bright red area. With the appearance of these spots, the child should be isolated. The fever rises steadily to its height with the appearance of the rash, which can be expected three or four days after the onset of fever. It seldom lasts longer than four or five days.

It first appears at the hairline behind the ears, on the neck, and across the forehead. Then it extends downward gradually, covering the entire body. They are tiny red raised spots, becoming larger and redder. They tend to increase and group together, giving the skin a blotchy appearance. Fever may go up to 104°F or 105°F. The skin itches and burns, the face is puffy, the eyes get red and swollen and sensitive to light. A hoarse cough occurs, and the patient feels miserable. After the appearance of the rash, the fever drops readily, cough disappears, the rash fades and dries, and the skin sheds gritty, with brownish scales.

Uncomplicated measles is a fairly mild disease, but since it tends to lower resistance, the patient is susceptible to secondary infections that may involve the ears, nose, sinuses, larynx, and lungs. The most serious complication is bronchial pneumonia or sore eyes (conjunctivitis). For this reason patients should be isolated and protected from chilling, fatigue, constipation, etc. A daily bath for cleansing can be coupled with hot baths to treat fever and to encourage the onset of the rash. The complications are almost always prevented by carefully protecting the patient and by simple treatments.

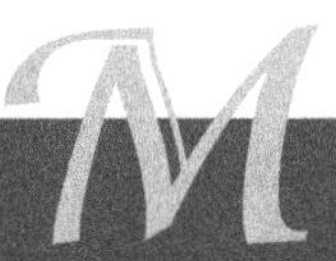

Treatment

Use 10 glasses of water daily, an eight-ounce glass being the measure for an adult, and a four ounce glass for a ten-year-old. A two-year-old would have about a two ounce glass as the measure.

Cool moisture from a vaporizer for the cough; aloe vera gel, hand lotion, or petroleum jelly for itching; saline compresses for eye irritation; and hot baths to relieve fever will generally take care of most problems related to measles. Fomentations to the chest can be used for the cough and hot footbaths for headaches.

Protect the eyes from bright lights. Instead of using aspirin or Tylenol for the fever, simply sponge the child lightly with hot water or give a brief hot bath about one minute for each year of the child's age to draw the blood to the skin for cooling. Repeat every two hours as needed until the fever has finished. The treatment not only cools the blood, but also boosts the immune system. Shelter the patient, particularly avoiding chilling until recovery is complete.

Melanoma

(See "Cancer" in the *Conditions and Diseases* section.)

Memory, Mental Illness, and Mental Alertness

(See also "Alzheimer's Disease" in the *Conditions and Diseases* section.)

Memory

A variety of regions in the brain store different fragments of a single memory and work cooperatively during memory creation and retrieval. Therefore, one part of a memory for an event can be lost such as where and who, but not when or what, as these aspects are all stored in different parts of the brain.

Brain scans indicate that the hippocampus, the sea horse-shaped structure located beneath the grey matter of the brain and nearby tissue, springs into action when a person remembers a previously studied word. Other areas in the front of the brain orchestrate attempts to retrieve the memory of the word prior to its conscious return. Tests now indicate that the front of the brain becomes more involved when the subject matter is difficult to recall and requires an intense effort; whereas the hippocampal area is more active with easily recalled materials. As soon as the material is recalled, the back of the brain close to the vision area then begins to be stimulated.

Stress hormones can cause memory to fail to be recorded or can make it so that the memory cannot be recalled. Thus, stress hormones can be linked with actual memory loss in humans. The highest stress hormone levels in the blood result not from stressful lives but from physiological imbalances such as adult onset diabetes, hypertension, etc. This suggests that memory deficits could be reversed by lowering stress hormone levels, such as through exercise, prayer, and Bible study.

Intelligence enhancement can be acquired by studying music. Certain types of very good music have a priming effect for the IQ that works for a short time, perhaps 10 to 15 minutes. Apparently good music enhances the ability of one part of the brain to communicate with another part. Repetitive music may actually interfere with reasoning.

Outdoor exercise can sharpen the memory of anyone from ages eight to eighty. Exercise helps depression even if endurance capacity and athletic training are not achieved (*Journal Suisse de Medecine* 121, no. 35 [August 31, 1991]: 1254–63).

The first year of brain development can set a child's course for life. This period of time provides the basic building blocks that will determine to a large degree the success or failure of the child. Touch, eye contact, and sensory stimulation actually help the brain to grow. Stressful, neglected, or violent environments negatively affect the formation of the brain and can have lasting effects.

Different parts of the brain are stimulated when a person is simply learning a skill, or is beginning to learn to reduce pauses and errors, and then doing the task faster. The activity shifts from one portion of the brain to the other as each of these steps comes into play.

Essential fatty acids have been found to dramatically improve the intellectual output of children. We can assume they might also do the same thing in adults (*Let's Live*, September 1997, 45). Breast-fed babies show a dose response relation between the proportion of mother's milk in the diet and subsequent IQ (*Lancet* 339, no. 8788 [1992]: 251).

Treatment

Vitamin E is the only antioxidant that appears to prevent memory loss. (See "Food Sources of Certain Nutrients" in the *Dietary Information* section.)

Scientists have long known that adequate sleep is important for the forming of different memories of facts. Memory

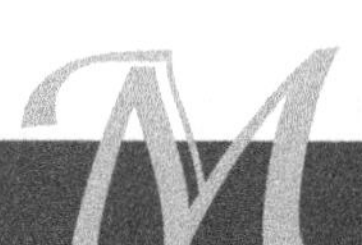

of motor skills, however, had not been studied until recently. Two studies, one at the University of Lubeck and another at Harvard, showed that adequate sleep is important to learning skills from playing a musical instrument to mastering a sport. Students taught either finger tapping sequences or keyboard routines performed 35 percent faster and made 30 percent fewer errors if they had a good night's sleep compared to those who had not slept as well. The tests were reported in *Neuron* in July 2002. The researchers concluded that good sleep cements practical skills as well as memories of facts. Even after both the sleeping groups and the non-sleeping groups had a good nights sleep, those who had had good sleep all the way through had much better performance compared to the non-sleeping groups when retested.

Lead absorption in the body from water, air, cans, and other sources results in learning difficulties and hyperactivity in children. Decreased concentration occurs in adults. (See also "Toxic Heavy Metals" in the *Supplemental Information* section.)

A survey done on 500 children showed that as TV viewing increased so did the incidence of sleep problems. Those having a television set in their bedroom were particularly troubled with sleep problems. The more the child watched TV, the more anxious the child was concerning sleep. The child slept fewer hours each night and was more likely to resist going to bed. They were also slower in falling asleep after going to bed (*Pediatrics* 104 [1999]: 552).

Drugs and chemicals that can affect the memory and cause memory loss include alcohol, sleeping pills, sedatives, antihistamines, blood pressure medicines, stomach medicines, pain pills (including aspirin), arthritis drugs, heart rhythm drugs, antidepressants and even some antibiotics (*American Family Physician* 54 [1996]: 167).

Mental Functioning and Diet

Laboratory rats were given a diet high in free fats, which resulted in a loss of mental ability. Rats given diets high in saturated or polyunsaturated fat had learning and memory defects. Fats from lard and beef tallow were more harmful than diets that had soybean oil (*Behavioral Brain Research* 101 [1999]: 153).

Young healthy men who ate diets low in zinc did poorly on tests measuring memory and attention. Foods high in zinc include popcorn, pumpkin seeds, lentils, peas, whole wheat, oatmeal, lima beans, carrots, garbanzos, and peanuts.

Ginseng, and ginkgo greatly improve learning and memory (*Plantamed* 59 [April 1993]: 106).

Flaxseed, flaxseed oil, and walnuts are high in omega-3 fatty acids. Scientists gave subjects 10 grams of omega-3 fatty acids daily for four months and found that their well-being improved on every psychological test compared to a control group given olive oil. Sleep improved, depression was less intense, and aggression and agitation registered at lower levels. The omega-3 fatty acids are thought to work much like Prozac or lithium to increase the levels of serotonin, a mood regulator (*Tuft's University Health and Nutrition Letter* 17, no. 6 [1999]: 2). (See "Food Sources High in Certain Nutrients" in the *Dietary Information* section.)

Pyridoxine (vitamin B6) is often deficient in the tissues of persons having memory problems as well as in patients taking Prozac or other antidepressants. Cooking and refining foods damage or destroy pyridoxine ("Vitamin B6 Supplementation in Elderly Men: Effects on Mood, Memory, Performance, and Mental Effort," *Psychopharmacology* 109, no. 4 [1992]: 489–96).

Memory Herbs

Ginkgo biloba has known memory-supporting enhancement properties. Both ginseng and bilberry, as well as hawthorn, have cardiovascular benefits that strengthen capillaries and help heart muscles to reduce heart attack risk. These same qualities strengthen memory. Vinpocetine has also been shown to be effective.

Mental Illness

Fever therapy has been found to be quite effective for various diseases of the central nervous system, including most of the diseases classified as mental disorders. About one-third of patients treated with hydrotherapy in some studies have been returned to complete usefulness in the community. Another one-third are useful under protective conditions, with only one-third being found to be resistant to fever treatments.

Other forms of hydrotherapy, such as the continuous flow bath, a specially constructed covered tub through which warm water flows, have been found to produce a quieting effect on patients who overreact. They often drop off to sleep in the tub. Wet sheet packs applied cold, but intended to immediately warm up, will reduce pulse rate and produce a soothing sedation. Various types of showers, both hot and cold, with and without friction, have been used to stimulate individuals who are depressed.

Initiate a program of reeducation by which the patient is helped to leave his/her own private world and again to feel a responsibility and a willingness to fit in with associates,

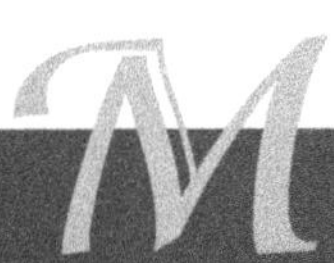

family, and community members. At the simplest level this includes such things as bathing, dressing, eating, sleeping, and so forth. Then the patient advances to exercise, play, work, and creativity. Assignment of duties and occupation, music, orchestras, occupational therapy, physical therapy, and Bible study groups all have their place in mental illness treatment (Edith Stern and Samuel W. Hamilton, *Mental Illness: A Guide for the Family* [New York: The Commonwealth Fund, 1942] 71, 73).

Mental Alertness

Mental alertness follows the same circadian pattern as hormones, pulse rate, and blood pressure. Performance of any work tends to go down as the time increases since the last time one slept or rested. These mental performances include judgment, memory, initiative, creativity, forethought, reason, tactfulness, people skills, job skills, etc. Glucose metabolism in the brain goes down as the length of wakefulness increases. The thought integrative areas of the brain—the frontal and parietal lobes of the brain—are more affected.

Proper evaluation of your own performance is one of the important functions of the brain. As wakefulness increases and fatigue creeps up, the ability to perform this evaluation goes down. You may be driving quite poorly, or correcting your children unwisely, or dealing with a problem neighbor thoughtlessly, all because you have not had enough sleep. Take your sleep very seriously. Guard it carefully. About eight hours sleep should be obtained each day.

One physician reported that on Fridays when he would begin a long weekend of being on call the nurses were competent and very helpful, but by Monday they were definitely incompetent and intolerable. They were miraculously back up to their proper competence on Tuesday after he had had a good sleep Monday night.

Ways to Insure Mental Alertness

1. Eat a wholesome diet, drink plenty of water, and keep a regular schedule in all habits.
2. Get regular and adequate sleep. Most individuals need around eight hours. Some find seven to be all right. Tonight's sleep gives you tomorrow's mental energy.
3. Set healthful priorities.
4. Take a nap *before* you are sleepy in the daytime—best in the late morning.
5. Exercise daily for the best brain performance.
6. Have a regular time for recreation and diversion. It was said by Winston Churchill during World War II that one must have one holiday per week, and one week per year of rest and relaxation if mental efficiency were to be kept high.
7. Avoid alcohol, caffeine, and nicotine as all of these interfere with sleep.

Ménière's Disease

This is a chronic ailment in which the major symptoms are dizziness and sometimes deafness, noise in one or both ears, and nausea and vomiting because of an interference with the function of the inner ear. It may involve the young, particularly women, but is more likely to come on late in life and affect both sexes. The disease may begin with a high pitched hissing, ringing in the ears, generally heard on one side at first and varying in intensity from day to day. The vertigo, a strong feeling of swaying, rocking, or turning, begins abruptly and lasts from a few minutes to several hours. This is usually associated with nausea and vomiting. It comes back at irregular intervals, but complete rest helps to reduce the severity of attacks. Hearing impairment is progressive, and a form of rolling of the eyes from side to side, known as nystagmus may occur.

Treatment

Fast for three days with nothing except water and herbal teas by mouth. Use a low-salt, plant-based diet when you resume eating. Several studies have shown a relationship between Ménière's disease and diet. Dr. Roger Boles of the Department of Otolaryngology of the School of Medicine at the University of California reports that almost 9 out of 10 Ménière's disease patients are greatly improved on a strict, salt-free diet.

Remove all free fats (margarine, mayonnaise, fried foods, cooking fats, salad oils, and nut butters) to improve blood circulation in the tiny capillaries of the middle ear. Eliminate any foods that you are sensitive to. There are reports that allergies to milk, eggs, corn, wheat, and yeast are sometimes the cause of Ménière's. (See the "Elimination and Challenge Diet" in the *Dietary Information* section.)

Hot baths may be of great advantage. Take one daily. (See "Hydrotherapy" in the *Natural Remedies* section.)

Lying quietly on the affected side with your eyes turned in the direction of the affected ear may assist in relieving an acute attack.

Patients should move at their own rate, protecting against sudden moving and jarring as this aggravates vertigo.

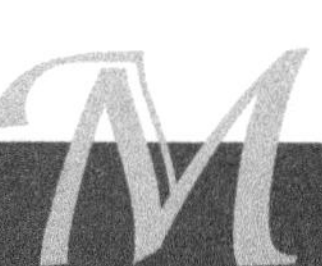

Persons speaking to victims of Ménière's disease should stand directly in front of them so the patient does not have to turn his/her head.

The patient should not try to read and should be protected from bright lights.

Ginkgo, skullcap, valerian root, catnip, and echinacea tea are all helpful. Mix two tablespoons of echinacea, two teaspoons each of skullcap and valerian, and two quarts of water. Boil gently for 30 minutes and pour over two tablespoons of catnip and one tablespoon of ginkgo. Steep for 30 minutes and drink. Make up fresh daily. Ten to 15 eight-ounce cups of the tea should be taken daily.

Ginger root tea should be used generously. It can be made separately and mixed with the above recipe.

Diuretic teas such as watermelon seed, buchu, burdock, and corn silk may be helpful. Asparagus shoots have a diuretic action and may help Ménière's.

Meningitis, Encephalitis

Meningitis is an inflammation of the membranes covering the brain and spinal cord caused usually by an infection of the cerebrospinal fluid by various germs, one of the most serious of which is the meningococcus. Encephalitis is an inflammation of the brain substance. It is usually caused by a virus. These are serious infections and should be treated with the greatest of care. Trained medical attention is required. If you cannot transport the patient to a hospital because you are in a third-world country, diligently use as many of the following remedies as possible.

Observe the patient carefully and be skillful with all treatments. Begin with a hot leg pack with ice neck pack and ice cap to the head and ice bag to the base of the brain and upper spine. After placement of the ice, add fluxion to the spine by using alternating hot and cold packs in a narrow strip down the center of the spine about three to six inches wide. A fomentation should be put on the feet at the same time.

The main objectives of treatment in meningitis are (1) to reduce the cerebral congestion and relieve the cerebral symptoms and (2) to relax the muscular rigidity. Using both the hot water to the lower extremities and simultaneous cold to the head will help with the cerebral symptoms. Do not use ice on the scalp as some will develop a headache. The rigidity can be helped by warm packs or a warm bath at about 99°F.

It has been shown that raising the mouth temperature to 103°F to 106°F for at least 30 minutes daily for five consecutive days in an ordinary bathtub with the temperature of the bath being gradually raised to 110°F causes an increase in the permeability of the blood vessels in the spinal cord. It seems that a greater fluxion and removal of toxins from the brain will occur with fever treatments (*Proceedings of the Society for Experimental Biology and Medicine* 26 [January 1929]: 287, 288).

Neutral baths at 90°F (32°C) were given in two cases of cerebrospinal meningitis with such marked success that it was widely adopted as a therapeutic measure. The effect of the first bath was surprising; the irregular pulse became regular, the temperature fell, and the patient felt much better and requested more neutral baths (*Journal of the American Medical Association* 216, no. 2 [June 21, 1971]: 1926).

Dr. Osler treated meningitis with hot baths beginning at 100°F to 103°F for one minute, then rapidly increasing the bath temperature to 107°F for three to six minutes, the longer period for older children. Use no cold pour at the end unless there is difficulty breathing, in which case use water at 93°F, never colder (*Archives of Pediatrics,* May 1908, 358–67). The hot foot bath with cold compress to the head and neck make a good derivative in inflammation of the brain or meninges, as well as in strokes.

Menopause

Strictly speaking, menopause is defined as the cessation of menstrual cycles at about the age of 50. This event may occur much earlier, even in the 30s, or somewhat later as in the late 50s. Unless the patient's period has disappeared for at least two years, one cannot be certain menopause has occurred. The symptoms sometimes described as representing the menopause syndrome are not actually an integral part of menopause, even though such symptoms are very common among women, particularly in the Western world where a diet high in fats and animal products is the rule.

The great majority of women require no treatment during menopause, as the symptoms are minor and will pass without any particular treatment in a few weeks or months, or at the most two or three years. Since the use of hormone supplements has been associated with such serious problems, it is recommended that the administration of hormones be avoided if at all possible. An increase in breast, ovarian, and endometrial cancer has been associated with the use of estrogens. The Centers for Disease Control issued a report early in 1992 stating that 15 years of female hormones increased a woman's risk of breast cancer by 30 to 35 percent. Even five years of hormones increases the risk. Taking progesterone

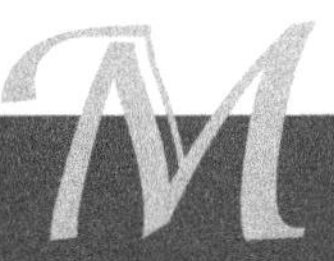

also increases the risk of developing cancer of the breast and cervix. Taking progesterone also increases the likelihood of getting gallstones, hypertension, and intravascular blood clotting (*Annals of Internal Medicine*, May 1, 1992).

Often the time of menopause is a time when a woman loses confidence in herself and her role in life, her usefulness, and her relationships. She should have a physician or counselor who can help her through this time. The counselor should have special skills that can enable him/her to lead the menopausal woman through this period, which may be difficult.

The very act of defining the phrase "change of life" may be able to shift an entire mind-set in this area. Divide it into sides, and view these sides as two sides of a coin, the new replacing the old. This mind-set may help to stop depression or a frantic series of face-lifts.

An understanding of the various stages of life, each with its own set of handicaps, duties and privileges, will assist in the understanding that the change of life is not for the worse, but actually for the better. A woman should pass through menopause recognizing that the change is good and that we have the ability to harness all that is good in order to capitalize on the challenges and rewards.

Try to change the idea that youth has a lot to offer and old age has nothing. Youth has its blessings, and so does the post-menopausal age.

There are changes that occur before menopause as the body prepares for menopause, which involves much more than simply a cessation of menstrual periods. Attitudes change, physiologic processes change, mental and emotional emphases change, and a woman can begin to question even her sanity.

Stresses play a role in exacerbating the problem. The time of menopause is also the time when deaths occur in the family, when older children's behavior can cause a lot of stress, when there may be the loss of a job, the illness of a spouse, or the presence of major repairs necessary on one's home or one's automobile. A woman should be aware of the stress such losses can deliver. She should cultivate hopefulness and expectation, which can help to bring relief without the use of drugs and surgery. Natural remedies for ailments actually carry much more power than medicine to take one through this time, and the end result is far better.

A woman can now begin to assume a role of "the wise woman," a custom that many communities try to continue, selecting those women who have reached a certain age and responsibility. These women become counselors for the younger ones and fulfill a very needed role in the life of the community.

Many doctors remove "spare organs" from women with freedom just because they are now past menopause. These organs have a function, albeit small, past menopause, and there are sometimes complications that may be permanent after surgery.

Women should understand that it is natural to cry. A woman going through menopause often is unusually sensitive to the feelings of others and to change in familiar patterns of life.

Menopause is a natural event being "medicalized" by profit-obsessed pharmaceutical companies and unscrupulous medical practitioners who can increase their revenue. The protective effects once presumed and widely proclaimed from estrogen replacement therapy for the heart and bones did not materialize. The large studies, which have seemed to suggest such an effect, were made by huge selection biases. Lifestyle changes would protect women more than these supposed benefits of hormone therapy, but lifestyle changes are not strongly encouraged by physicians. Taking hormones for more than 10 to 20 years can cause health problems at least as serious as those the medications are supposed to prevent.

Osteoporosis is a major health topic in menopause. (See "Osteoporosis" in the *Conditions and Diseases* section.) It is a condition of 5, 10, or even 40 years in the making, and at the time of menopause, it usually has no recognizable symptoms. The major unpleasant symptom in menopause is hot flashes.

Advice for husbands: Understand that your wife needs extra help during this time. Participate with her in her programs such as exercise program, weight loss program, and stress control program. Understand that she may at times be inconsistent in her feelings. She may tell you to call before you come home if you are going to be late, and then when you call she scolds you for interrupting her. Understand that she may not know quite who she is since she is not needed as a mother anymore, she is not pretty in the same way she once was, she may not be physically up to the same amount of work, and other physical feats she once did easily she may be unable to do. Never comment in a derogatory way about any of the changes taking place. Try to recapture the companionship you enjoyed before having childen. Reassure her of her worth and strength. Be patient. Be compassionate. Believe she will come through this and not be a whining, dependent person. Learn to apologize and to repeat often the words, "I'm sorry." A woman in menopause is unsure of herself. She

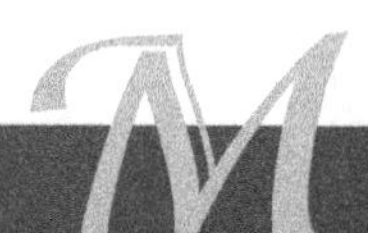

looks to her husband as a mirror. Society can help change the false idea that youth has a lot to offer and old age has nothing.

Following are common symptoms of menopause, many unrelated to hormones:

- Cardiovascular system: Palpitations, high blood pressure, and hot flashes.
- Musculoskeletal: Aches and pains, usually because of the development of food sensitivities. About that time in life, osteoporosis may be discovered, as it is usually symptomless until a fracture occurs.
- Genital: Irregular bleeding, decreased libido, vaginal dryness, and vaginal itching.
- General: Dryness and wrinkling of skin.
- Neurological: Nausea, dizziness, mood changes, irritability, depression, insomnia, numbness, and tingling.

See "Women's Conditions and Diseases" in the *Conditions and Diseases* section.

Hormone Replacement Therapy

Oral contraceptives have been linked to an increased risk of cervical cancer, apparently caused by the sex hormone progesterone. The cervical cancer is particularly likely to occur in women who are infected with HPV (human papilloma virus) (*Science News* 143 [1993]: 38).

Aloe and Dioscorea in a formula extract are very good for menopause symptoms. Usually a woman who is taking hormones for her symptoms can entirely leave them off and be quite comfortable if she takes these herbs.

A vascular surgeon reports that he gets referrals of numerous young women on birth control pills, and menopausal women on hormone replacement therapy who have developed blood clots of the upper and lower extremities, occlusive disease of the arteries, and strokes caused by these drugs (*Cortlandt Newsletter for Physicians*, March 1996, 109).

There are chemicals in our environment that effectively mimic or block the function of estrogen in the body:

1. Although DDT is now banned in the United States, it is still present in our environment, and may be brought into the country on products produced in countries where DDT is not yet banned. It may be helpful to use a heaping teaspoon of charcoal stirred into a glass of water daily for several weeks to see if there is a benefit.
2. PCBs (polychlorinated biphenyls) are industrial compounds that have been restricted in the United States but will continue to linger in our environment for decades to come.
3. Dioxins are chemical compounds produced sometimes during garbage incineration or as a result of paper bleaching. These can be released into the air, water, and soil. Dioxins have carcinogenic properties.

The Heart and Estrogen/progestin Replacement Study (HERS) indicates that hormone replacement therapy for postmenopausal women has no benefit for the heart. Actually, the reverse seems to be the fact; that is women are 50 percent more likely to have a heart attack if they take hormone replacement therapy. A report was published on these findings in the August 19, 1998, issue of the *Journal of the American Medical Association.*

On January 27, 2000, morning newspapers across the country revealed that the commonly prescribed estrogen/progestin combination could increase the lifetime risk of breast cancer much more than previously suspected. The newspaper report was based on a study published in the *Journal of the American Medical Association* showing that 10 years of hormone replacement therapy gives a woman an 80 percent higher risk of developing breast cancer than a woman who has never taken the hormones (*AARP Bulletin,* May 2, 2000, 1).

There is not only no protection from heart disease by hormone replacement therapy as was once thought, but an actual increase in heart attacks, strokes, and blood clots during the first two years of treatment. Hormone replacement therapy does not halt Alzheimer's disease either. Many of the problems of menopause are blamed on hormones but are actually just part of the aging process.

Hot flashes

Soybeans are a great help for hot flashes. Take about one-fourth cup of cooked beans per day. The isoflavones in soybeans are antioxidants—that is, they slow down aging. Whole dry soybeans are inexpensive, and delicious dishes can be made from them. One of the simplest is scrambled soybeans. Soak soybeans overnight, grind them in a blender with an equal quantity of water, boil for a few minutes, stirring until thickened. Turn on low and cover and allow to simmer for about 20 to 30 minutes. Put in some yellow coloring such as turmeric, paprika, or saffron, and seasonings such as garlic, chicken style, salt, etc. You may serve these as you would scrambled eggs.

A larger percentage of overweight women have hot flashes compared to women who are normal weight, suggesting that the known effects of body fat on the production of

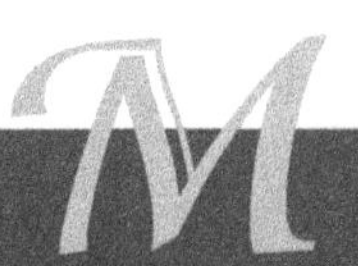

estrogen outside the ovarian tissue is an important variable determining the occurrence of hot flashes (*Obsetrics and Gynecology* 59, no. 4 [1982]: 403).

Physical exercise on a regular basis affects neurotransmitters in the brain that regulate the control of temperature. Thus, highly physically active women have hot flashes in menopause only 5 percent of the time, whereas 16 to 20 percent of women who engage in little or no weekly exercise have hot flashes (*Maturitas* 29, no. 2 [1998]: 139).

An experiment was done measuring the tightening of blood vessels in the skin after applications of ice. Women with hot flashes tended to lack the normal tightening of blood vessels, whereas women who had no flashes or very mild flashes tended to have a more brisk tightening of the blood vessels. There was a significant relationship between the degree of tightening and the severity of the symptoms with the applications of ice. This experiment indicates an abnormal response of blood vessels as the primary cause of the hot flashes. A plant-based diet apparently causes this function of blood vessels to be more normal as women who eat this diet rarely have problems with hot flashes.

Use a short cold bath to help balance the hormones. This measure is helpful to prevent hot flashes and has the added feature of boosting the immune system to fortify against viral infections. Regular bathing in cold or cool water helps stimulate the production of sex hormones such as testosterone in men and estrogen in women.

Treatments

Following are a variety of remedies broken down into different categories.

Botanical Remedies

Menopause symptoms are not so much a result of low estrogen but may be a result of major fluctuations of hormones. Hot flashes are possibly related to temporary elevations of hormones in the body (*Obstetrics and Gynecology* 64, no. 6 [1984]: 752).

Estrogenic effects are observed from the following herbs: foeniculum, angelica, red raspberries, red clover, and Arctium. And a progesterone effect has been observed in glycyrrhiza (licorice), Dioscorea, and smilax.

These herbs can help to balance estrogen and progesterone in women who are imbalanced. Other herbs that have estrogen and progesterone precursors are hops, cramp bark, blessed thistle herb, sarsaparilla, squaw vine, and ginseng. All ginsengs have a lot of saponins in them which stimulate the nerves and bowels. Aloe vera, anise, fennel, and garlic can be used for menopause.

Use one cup four times a day of the following herbal recipe:

- 3 cups boiling water
- 1 teaspoon catnip tea
- 1 tablespoon red raspberry leaf
- 1 teaspoon alfalfa leaf
- 1 teaspoon licorice powder

Licorice root can be very helpful in menopause. One tablespoon of the powder can be simmered in a quart of water for 10 to 20 minutes. Take one cup four times a day. Make it up fresh daily. Do not overdose on licorice as large quantities can cause a retention of sodium in susceptible individuals and can cause the blood pressure to temporarily rise.

For night sweats, use sage (*Salvia officinalis*) as well as ox-eye daisy (*Chrysanthemum leucanthemum*).

Clothing

The clothing should be checked carefully for healthfulness. Girdles and pantyhose are taboo. There must be no band tight enough to leave a red mark on the skin. Perhaps the most important, yet most difficult to attain, is warm clothing for the extremities. Even though there is no sensation of chilliness, the extremities should be clothed. The blood loses much latent heat from a bare skin area. Experimentally there is alteration of the blood flow in the pelvic organs if only one hand or one foot is chilled for more than five minutes. Jumpers are not the best unless warm sleeves are worn to balance the circulation and prevent congestion of the breasts.

Habits of Life

Stopping smoking is a treatment for menopause. Smoking itself leads to a decrease in estrogen levels and increased bone loss at an earlier age.

Alcohol suppresses bone growth, is toxic to the breasts and ovaries, and can cause infrequent ovulation and menstrual irregularities.

Hormones

The following hormone producing organs can be naturally stimulated in order to optimize the physiological processes:

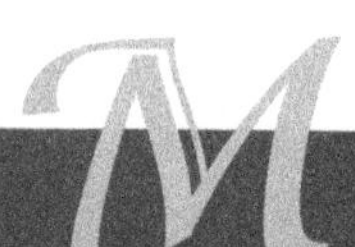

- Adrenal glands – The adrenal glands secrete small amounts of male hormones, some of which are converted to estrogens in the body's fat cells. Stimulate the adrenals as follows:
  - Vigorous tapping over them with the fingertips for two minutes.
  - Administer alternating very hot water applications and very cold water applications, one minute of cold for each six minutes of hot, ending with cold.
  - Repeat one or both treatments daily. Locate the adrenals by measuring about two inches above the waist, and one inch to the side of the spine.
- Liver – The liver can break down estrogen. Relieve the liver by one day of fasting each week, ending the fast with breakfast, never with supper.
- Thyroid – The thyroid affects metabolism. Stimulate by a cool shower each morning, followed by a brisk but brief cold mitten friction for three minutes.
- Hypothalamus – Stimulate the hypothalamus by starting a new intellectual program, such as initiating a Bible study group in your home or organizing a group ministry for a prison or an orphans' home, or take up a new artistic endeavor such as studying a musical instrument.
- Pituitary – The anterior pituitary with its FSH and LH can be stimulated by going to bed and rising at a regular time, taking regular meals, and exercising daily with an hour or more of activity.

Mental Health

Improving one's interpersonal relationships not only makes one more at ease but actually lessens women's hot flashes. The 12-step program is very good for this purpose. (See "12-Step Program" in the *Supplemental Information* section.)

Nutrition

Hot drinks, hot meals, and hot spices can aggravate hot flashes. So can sugar or simple refined carbohydrates. Do not be disappointed if you must go through several months trying to improve hot flashes. If you use a purely plant-based diet without sugar or added fat, the hot flashes will often stop.

The following foods have been found to be high in naturally occurring plant sterols similar in chemical formula to estrogens. Some of these should be eaten daily in liberal quantities if you do not have sensitivities to them. They are anise seed, apples, cherries, coconut, garlic, whole grains (barley, corn, oats, rice, wheat), nightshade family foods (bell peppers, paprika, pimentos, eggplant, potatoes, tomatoes), plums, sage, soybeans, wheat germ, yams, and yeast.

Taking vitamin E by mouth can help to manage hot flashes. You can also puncture a vitamin A or E capsule and insert it high in the vagina each night for dryness of the vagina. The vitamin A or E suppositories have to be used daily for six weeks to get relief. In six weeks drop back to about once or twice a week. The vitamins strengthen the lining of the vagina.

Physical Activity

Exercise is not just a healthful thing to do, it is one of the main treatments women need during menopause. We recommend that a woman over 50 obtain one to five hours of outdoor labor daily, such as gardening or one hour of walking, to stimulate the ovaries and other endocrine glands. Weight bearing exercise is ideal, as it protects against osteoporosis. Swimming one hour three times per week has been shown to increase bone mineral content.

To prevent humpback, several times a day, (at least four), rise up from your work, stand or sit tall, hold the elbows at shoulder height, and try to touch the elbows together, both front and back. Maintain a good posture throughout the day.

Water

An attempt should be made to avoid irritation of all mucous membranes as these surfaces become quite thin following menopause. When the vaginal area is cleansed, the hands should be first washed and then the hands used to thoroughly wash the area. Then more plain, clear water is used to meticulously rinse the area, being gentle and using no soap and no abrasive cloths. Drying of the non hairy portions is done by blotting rather than rubbing. Douching is to be discouraged, as the surfaces are washed free of the light covering of mucus and shed cells. Never use soaps on the genital area of a sensitive or irritated person.

Mental Disorders

In the book *Diet and Disease* by Drs. Cheraskin, Ringsdorf, and Clark, pages 186–207, there is a discussion on the known association between nutrients and blood disorders and psychological disorders. Some of the known associations follow:

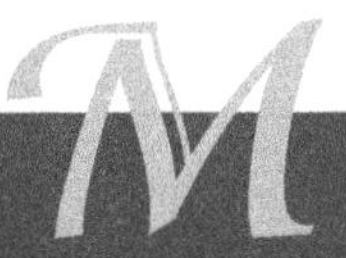

Dietary or Blood Condition	Psychological Disorder Associated
Riboflavin deficiency	Depression
Pyridoxine deficiency	Nervousness or Confusion
Nicotinic acid deficiency	Confusion, Depression, Psychosis
Thiamin deficiency	Agitation, Confusion, Depression, Anxiety
Decreased glycine reserves	Schizophrenia
Low glutamic acid	Schizophrenia
Elevated plasma ceruloplasmin	Schizophrenia
High blood cholesterol levels	Manic Depression
Low magnesium	Disoriented, Delirious
High magnesium	Psychotic Depression, Schizophrenia

Autism

Children with autism generally have abnormal intestinal permeability. This may allow incompletely digested food particles such as peptides into the bloodstream. The influence of these particles on the brain is such that behavioral abnormalities can result (*Acta Paediatriaca* 85 [1996]: 1079). (See "Leaky Gut Syndrome, Increased Intestinal Permeability" in the *Conditions and Diseases* section.)

There is a growing sentiment that early childhood immunizations may be related to neurologic problems in children such as autism, epilepsy, learning disabilities, type I diabetes, SIDS, ADD, and ADHD. Parents should investigate this matter.

Gluten is composed of gliadin compounds. Some 18 or more different gliadin-associated medical and mental conditions have been identified.

After a meal all people take up trace amounts of intact protein. Fragments of these proteins in the bloodstream (called peptides) could cause abnormal thought processes. Information on this subject has not been researched fully, and very little is known about it. It is possible this process may have an influence on autism. Mother's milk can contain portions of food proteins, which apparently the intestinal tract allows to get through into the bloodstream where it is carried to the brain. All individuals have antibodies to certain food proteins, indicating that they have been taken up into the blood from the intestines without complete digestion. Autistics have been found to possess these increased IgG antibodies, especially against the grain protein gluten (*Biol Psychiat* 5 [1980]: 127).

Treatment

Use a totally plant-based diet. The same diet used for cancer patients may be beneficial for autistics. Remove all gluten from the diet. Furthermore, a milk sensitivity may also be present in those who have serious vitamin deficiencies. Milk inhibits the absorption of zinc from the intestinal tract. A trial of no milk for six months may be quite helpful.

Patients with autism given a gluten-free and milk-free diet improved so much so that they could easily complete certain tests while on the diet that they could not complete when they were off the diet. Increased intestinal permeability (leaky gut syndrome) may be a factor both in autism as well as in schizophrenia in adults.

Vitamin B6 is considered helpful for infantile autism. Additional magnesium may also be necessary.

Autism may respond to the services of an allergist using enzyme-potentiated desensitization (EPD).

Stay out of doors as much as possible. The world looks different out of doors, and mental development is promoted by the great outdoors, especially in a natural setting such as a national forest or large wooded park.

Andrew Wakefield and colleagues published in 1998 a paper in *The Lancet* titled "Ilio-lymphoid-nodular Hypoplasia, Nonspecific Colitis, and Pervasive Developmental Disorder in Children." Wakefield's hypothesis was that the immuno oral vaccine causes a series of events that include intestinal inflammation, loss of intestinal barrier function, entrance into the bloodstream of "encephalopathic (producing brain disease) proteins" and consequent development of autism. A new United Kingdom study suggests that some cases of autism could be linked to the measles, mumps, rubella (MMR) vaccine. Researchers at Sunderland University believe at least 10 percent of the cases of autism in their study were triggered by the controversial immunization (*BBC News on Line*, June 27, 2002).

Obsessive-Compulsive Disorder

The diagnosis is made by recurrent and persistent thoughts, impulses, or images that intrude themselves on the mind. They are not simply excessive worries about real-life problems. The person may recognize that these thoughts are a product of his/her own mind and try to ignore or suppress the thoughts but is not able to do so.

A compulsion is a disorder defined in psychology as a strong, irrational desire to repeat certain acts. As an example,

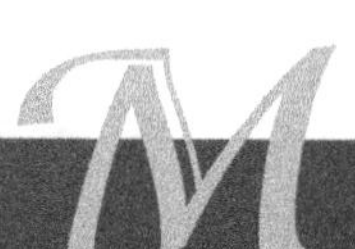

a person may have the compulsion to wash his/her hands every few minutes or avoid stepping on cracks in the sidewalk. Compulsions may be mental acts such as counting or silently repeating words that the person feels driven to perform in response to an obsession or according to rules that must be rigidly applied. One young man had to sit in a chair a certain way, and if the slightest variation occurred, he had to stand up and sit down again until it was perfect or he felt that some terrible thing might happen. The behaviors or mental acts are aimed at preventing or reducing distress or preventing some dreaded event or situation. The obsessions or compulsions are time-consuming, taking more than one hour a day, and interfere with the person's normal routine or work. The severity of the condition is judged by the proportion of the person's day occupied by the obsession or compulsion.

The condition is often diagnosed after a major depressive episode, alcohol abuse, or drug dependence. Tourette's syndrome has also been associated in certain individuals with obsessive-compulsive disorders. Eating disorders, anxiety, tics, and schizophrenia may also be associated.

Treatment

One of the first things to aim at is helping the patient to understand that the condition exists and that it is abnormal. Then the patient should learn to counteract the obsessional thinking and control any ritualistic behaviors without substituting a new ritual for the old. Compulsions may be controlled by the person truly desiring victory by taking a determined attitude and following a plan.

Plan and provide a very simple diet. Follow that by adhering to a regular schedule and getting plenty of sleep. It is also helpful if a godly person takes the compulsive individual under his/her wing and offers guidance and kindness to the compulsive individual.

Compulsions are easier to treat with behavior modifications than obsessions. Thought stopping techniques should be used. These include the following: a brisk walk in nature, singing, playing a musical instrument, working at crafts that require close attention, orderliness in the home, window or car washing, charitable work for the poor, volunteering to babysit for a neighbor, giving a back rub to an invalid, gathering flowers for a sick person, etc.

Certain herbal remedies can be effective such as St. John's wort, catnip, valerian root, gingko, kava, hops, gotu cola, and skullcap. Family support and religious counseling, with prayer and Bible study, can be of enormous benefit in these patients.

The treatment is sometimes short, but may be long-term, and in severe cases individuals may need to change friends and residence, particularly if persons or places are associated in any way with the compulsive activity.

Case Report

We had a compulsive eater come to us for help. She had the compulsion to eat any food she saw, whether she liked the food or not. At meals she ate enough for two people. Because she was extremely active, she was not greatly overweight. But her habit was expensive and time-consuming. She would buy half a gallon of ice cream when she left work, stop behind some new construction on the way home, spend an hour eating and then a quarter of an hour throwing it up. Finally, she sought help.

We paired her up with a godly young couple who prayed with her and invited her to stay with them. The next morning she told them she was well. She went home with a list of the natural (basic) laws of health and instituted a healthful lifestyle at home, removing all snack foods from her home and all money from her purse, keeping only a credit card and checkbook to discourage buying a snack. I saw her years later. She told me she had had a major struggle in the beginning but had not once in all those years given free rein to her appetite.

Another compulsive person we dealt with was a young mother with a hand washing compulsion, not only her own but her child's hands. We used basically the same approach as with the compulsive eater, but with very different results. She had several periods of success for a few hours to a few days, but would slip back into the compulsion. We gave her St. John's wort with good results. Even more help came when we added gingko. She also got a massage twice a week for two months and once a week for two months after that, which gave her much benefit.

Schizophrenia

This severe mental disorder, a major psychosis, involves a loss of contact with reality and a permanent or temporary disorganization or disintegration of the personality. One-fourth of all hospitalized mental patients fall into this category. Speech may be garbled and actions inappropriate. Voices may be heard and visions seen. Metabolic or biochemical factors may be the cause, as some schizophrenics have experienced complete relief for up to six months after a blood exchange transfusion.

Schizophrenia usually develops during late adolescence or early adulthood as a disruption of thought and emotion. It

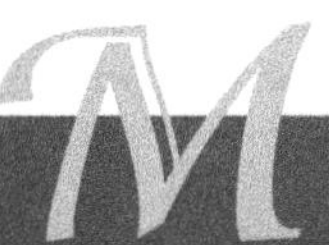

may appear among children who suffer from attention and memory problems, which undermine their ability to communicate with others.

Psychiatric patients generally have shortened life spans, possibly from their diseases, or possibly from the medicines they take to combat the disease. If the patient has a deep religious faith, they have a better chance of recovery and of living a longer life.

Schizophrenics may sometime become unmanageable and, indeed, dangerous to family or friends. In these cases hospitalization, at least until the patient is stabilized, may be necessary.

Possible Causes

After a meal all people take up trace amounts of intact protein. Fragments of these proteins in the bloodstream (called peptides) could cause abnormal thought processes. Information on this subject has not been researched fully, and very little is known about it. It is possible this process may have an influence on schizophrenia. Mother's milk can contain portions of food proteins, which apparently the intestinal tract allows to get through into the bloodstream where it is carried to the brain. All individuals have antibodies to certain food proteins, indicating that they have been taken up into the blood from the intestines without complete digestion. Schizophrenics have been found to possess these increased IgG antibodies, especially against the grain protein gluten (*Biol Psychiat* 5 [1980]: 127; *Annals of Allergy* 48 [1982]: 166; *American Journal of Psychiatry* 136 [1979]: 1306). Furthermore, schizophrenics have increased levels of IgA antibodies against gluten, lactoglobulin (from milk), and casein (from milk).

Since some patients with schizophrenia have a high incidence of celiac sprue, a gluten and milk sensitivity disorder, it is recommended that all patients with schizophrenia be tried on a gluten-free diet. Autism is a form of schizophrenia in childhood.

Schizophrenics have an inability to carry information in "working," or short term, memory. Therefore, they may make illogical or disconnected statements because their memory response is so delayed. Tests have shown that tasks that typically spark surges of electrical activity in one or the other brain hemisphere do not function among schizophrenic youngsters. The right and left hemispheres are not as finely specialized in schizophrenic children. We believe the reason for these phenomena could be the loss of the zinc compounds in seminal and other genital fluids (the same zinc compounds used by the body for fine nerve transmissions). Since masturbation is often a practice that schizophrenics engage in, this could explain the lower zinc compound levels.

It has been discovered that in persons with schizophrenia the blood is quite thick and flows slowly, somewhat like honey on a cold morning. It is not known whether the schizophrenia comes first and causes the thick blood, or whether the thick blood comes first and causes the schizophrenia. We favor the latter position. We believe that too many red blood cells and plasma containing too many nutrients and wastes promotes the development of schizophrenia (L. Dintenfass and G. V. F. Seaman, eds., *Blood Viscosity in Heart Disease and Cancer* [Pergamon Press, 1981]).

Schizophrenia is more prevalent in urban than rural areas, presumably because of the deleterious role of environmental hazards and social factors (*British Journal of Hospital Medicine* 52, no. 4 [1994]: 149, 152).

The central nervous system is a target organ for vitamin D. Dr. J. McGrath proposes that low maternal vitamin D intake may adversely affect the brain of the developing fetus, causing the child to develop schizophrenia. To support this argument of schizophrenia, the author notes there is an excess of schizophrenia in winter births, increased rates of schizophrenia in dark-skinned migrants to cold climates, an increased rate of schizophrenia births in urban versus rural areas, and an association between prenatal famine and schizophrenia (J. McGrath, "Hypothesis: Is Low Prenatal Vitamin D a Risk-Modifying Factor for Schizophrenis?" *Schizophrenia Research* 40 [1999]: 173–177).

Treatment

Diet could play as important a role in helping schizophrenia as it does in controlling disease in diabetics, so says a report from the Medical College of Georgia in Augusta. The dietary culprit could be the same one that increases cholesterol and the risk of heart disease—saturated fat. The outer coat of cells, the cell membrane, is apparently abnormal in people with schizophrenia. These cells may be further damaged by a diet rich in saturated fats—hard fats at room temperature. The abnormal cell membranes occur throughout the body of people with this disorder, and have been found even in developing fetal brain cells, white cells that fight infections, red blood cells that carry oxygen through the body, and in laboratory grown skin cells from these persons or their relatives. The abnormalities have their most serious consequences in the adult brain.

Another important dietary matter for schizophrenics is blood sugar. If blood sugar drops to 40, it could cause the brain to malfunction, and the person would begin to behave

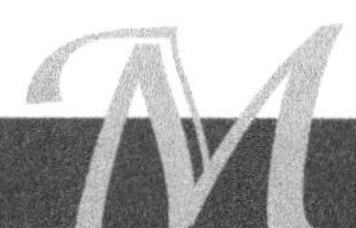

strangely. Perhaps the use of a high fat and high sugar diet from childhood is a factor in later development of schizophrenia. Eat the most healthful diet you can, avoiding sugary and fatty foods.

Use a totally plant-based diet. The same diet used for cancer patients may be beneficial for schizophrenics. Since some patients with schizophrenia have a high incidence of celiac sprue, a gluten and milk sensitivity disorder, it is recommended that all patients with schizophrenia be tried on a gluten-free and milk-free diet. Autism is a form of schizophrenia in childhood. Patients with autism given a gluten-free and milk-free diet improved so much so that they could complete certain tests while on the diet that they could not complete when they were off the diet. Increased intestinal permeability may be a factor both in autism as well as in schizophrenia in adults.

Use magnesium for schizophrenic symptoms. Start with one-half teaspoon of Epsom salts twice a day, placed on the tongue and followed by a glass of water. If no diarrhea results, increase gradually to one teaspoon three times daily. If it is poorly tolerated, use magnesium oxide or citrate capsules two to three times a day.

Niacin deficiency (vitamin B3) is associated with pellagra (a deficiency disease with a mental disorder) and has been linked by psychiatrists to schizophrenia. Using foods that are high in niacin might be helpful along with a daily supplement of niacin.

Some have suggested that large doses of vitamin C should be taken to stop hallucinations. We have had no experience with this treatment, but it would be worth a try. Become acquainted with the signs of overdose before trying it.

It may be beneficial to administer supplements of certain vitamins such as B12, B3, and B6 in high doses for several weeks along with vitamin E, primrose oil, zinc, and manganese.

A study done on schizophrenics showed that red cell fatty acids were deficient in both the omega-6 and omega-3 series. Omega-3 supplements led to significant improvement in schizophrenic symptoms, and correlated with increased levels of omega-3 fatty acids in red cell membranes. Flaxseed oil and walnut oil are high in these fats. Depression has also been associated with low essential fatty acids (*Lipids* 31, no. S [1996]: 157).

Modification of dietary fats and oils should become a part of psychiatric treatments in all patients.

Persons with psychiatric disorders should be given flaxseed oil, one to two tablespoons once or twice daily. In one study, within one to two weeks 8 of 12 patients were significantly helped, and there was a reduction of physical symptoms such as ringing in the ears, dandruff, dry skin, and fatigue. As the flaxseed oil was continued, both emotional and physical benefits occurred, with reduction in cold sensitivity, reduction in food allergies, and better sleep patterns. Another study of 51 students showed that aggression, as measured by psychological testing, dropped significantly with the use of flaxseed oil (*Journal of Clinical Investigation* 97, no. 4 [1996]: 1129).

Allergies and food sensitivities should be identified. (See the "Elimination and Challenge Diet" in the *Dietary Information* section.)

Fasting is most beneficial in some persons and can result in recovery. If they have sufficient nutrient reserves to undergo a five or six-day fast, they may benefit from it. During this time masturbation must be stopped if it is a feature of their disease.

Give daily hot baths for three weeks, keeping the head cool, five days a week with two days off for a total of 15 baths. Each hot bath should be followed by a tepid bath reducing the water temperature to 96°F or 97°F and being sure to have a cold compress to the face, head, and neck. These tepid baths can be maintained for two to six hours if desired to calm an agitated patient.

The continuous tepid bath has a tranquilizing action. The continuous bath was used in Germany in the early part of the twentieth century and resulted in beneficial effects on the metabolism so that the schizophrenic patient could often leave the hospital and return to their professions and have prolongation of useful life for many years.

Massage for the seriously mentally ill can be quite effective. A 30-minute massage, one to five times weekly, can reduce stress (*Journal of Psychosocial Nursing and Mental Health Services* 33 [1995]: 29). If no massage person is available to do the massage, I recommend an oxygenator massager that gently rocks the person by moving the ankles back and forth.

Ginkgo biloba should be given to schizophrenics as it has been shown to improve the function of the brain in schizophrenia (*Psychopharmacology Bulletin* 31, no. 1 [1995]: 147).

Since schizophrenia is often associated with high copper and iron tissue levels, the use of large quantities of garlic or charcoal assist in the excretion of excess copper. Three cloves of raw garlic minced finely and taken with a sandwich three times daily, or blended in tomato juice, would be sufficient. Two teaspoons of dried powdered garlic may also be used instead (*Let's Live,* March 1995, 24). Chlorella or

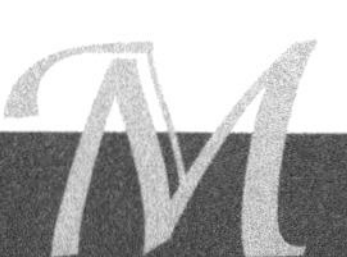

Spirulina and cilantro are helpful to reduce high mineral levels. Use one tablespoon of chlorella or spirulina, and one or two sprigs of cilantro twice daily. These may be blended with juice or water if desired.

A subclinical hypothyroidism may be associated with reduced cerebral metabolism followed by some form of mental illness. One study showed that the level of thyroid-stimulating hormone, a hormone from the pituitary designed to make the thyroid act more briskly, was elevated in a population of patients having mental illness (*Biologic Psychiatry* 40 [1996]: 714). If the thyroid is malfunctioning, one must try to correct this condition. (See "Thyroid Disease" in the *Conditions and Diseases* section.)

Persons with schizophrenia should carefully avoid any organophosphate agricultural insecticides, as they have been found to increase the mental disorder. Important brain chemicals may be upset by the insecticides, including such brain chemicals as serotonin, which regulates moods (*Journal of Nutritional & Environmental Medicine* 5, no. 4 [1995]: 367–74).

A number of years ago a friend started a stamp club in St. Elizabeth's Hospital, Washington, DC, which she understood was the largest mental institution in the States at that time. There was quite a group who came; some probably just to have somewhere to go, but after a while a few really appreciated the exchange of stamps and fellowship it offered. Later she got a couple of letters of appreciation from one of the doctors in charge, stating that two of the patients who really worked with their stamps had been released from the hospital, had found jobs, and were doing well at their jobs. Perhaps becoming more focused and having a goal and a support group could help many a mentally ill person to be able to live independently.

Case Report

A 53-year-old man arrived at Country Life Health Food store to purchase a small item. The cashier noticed cigarettes in his shirt pocket and offered to give him an individual Five-Day Plan to Stop Smoking. His voice was rather dull when he said, "Sure, if you think you can help me."

For two days he came to the store for the sessions. He told the cashier that he had been released from the state mental hospital for a month on leave. He had been diagnosed as schizophrenic when he was 20 years old, but he had maintained a somewhat normal life on medications until age 23 when he got married. The stresses of marriage pushed him over the edge, and he had to be hospitalized three months after the wedding. After a year passed, he got out of the hospital, returned home and tried to get a job. After three months his wife found out she was pregnant and the news again pushed him over the edge and he became sick again. Another year in the hospital, another three month furlough, another pregnancy, another year in the hospital. Most of his life had been characterized by the pattern of being in and out of the hospital.

On the third day of the stop smoking program, he did not show up. The cashier took the materials, drove to his house, and found him sitting on the front porch smoking. He said, "I am hopeless. You can never get me off these cigarettes."

The cashier could not be dissuaded and presented the third day material. The man turned up at the store the next day having not smoked. He said if the cashier cared enough to go to all that trouble he could do his part and not smoke. After the fifth day was successfully finished, the man asked if he could come every day and help out in the store. He did this for five months until he asked if he could move a mobile home to a spot at Uchee Pines Institute and volunteer his services on the farm.

He lived at Uchee Pines for two years, not having one episode requiring even a psychiatric outpatient visit. His wife divorced him one year into his move to Uchee Pines but that did not unsettle him as much as we feared. He moved to Louisiana after a few years and has now been living a productive life for the past 16 years. He is focused, with goals and a support group and no significant psychiatric problems.

Tardive Dyskinesia

Tardive dyskinesia is a muscular disorder caused by antipsychotic drugs such as Haldol and phenothiazides like Thorazine and Compazine. Facial contortions, smacking of lips, and snakelike movements of the arms are principal symptoms. Once it starts, the condition is usually permanent. There are treatments that can reduce the severity of the symptoms, but it is incurable. Nutrients known to reduce tardive dyskinesia include lecithin, vitamin B6, manganese, and niacin. Fever baths should begin immediately after it is recognized. Give three series of 15 treatments over a three- to four-month period.

Mental Health

Depression

The rate of depression has steadily climbed over the past half century, being much more common in those born after 1945 than those born before. The average age of onset is also decreasing, now in the mid 20s, whereas once it was the mid 30s. There is a higher rate of depression in the United States than in almost any other country, and as Asian countries westernize, their rates of depression increase correspondingly. These changes are not the product of individual biochemistry or biogenetics, but pathology within our culture. Information overload is one of those factors. Americans watch between four and seven hours of television every day, having an insidious effect on our culture, one of which is our reducing tolerance for frustration; after all, in "TV-land" any major problem can be resolved in about 30 minutes. TV devotees can lose perspective as to what is reality.

Mental disturbances fall into two general categories: neuroses or simple mental or social discomfort from some kind of emotional or psychological imbalance, which is not usually disabling. The second is psychoses or true mental illnesses with varying degrees of incapacitation. Simple depression has a cause that falls under one of two categories: situational or metabolic.

Situational depression may follow bereavement, a physical illness, a financial loss, etc.

Metabolic depression follows a change in the condition of the internal milieu of the body of such a degree as to influence the mind in a depressive way. The depressed person may complain of a variety of symptoms—headache, facial pain, chest pain, skeleton pain, abdominal pain, digestive complaints, sleep disturbance, constipation, genitourinary, or menstrual problems. (See also "Wilson's Disease, Copper Overload" in the *Conditions and Diseases* section.)

Depression in people over 50 could be from silent strokes because of blockage in the small blood vessels in the brain. These people have no numbness, weakness, or paralysis, but may develop depression (*AARP Bulletin,* May 2, 2000). Men lose brain tissue at almost three times the rate of women, and the brain loss may account for some of the grumpiness in some older men. The loss of brain tissue in the left frontal region of the brain seems to be connected to the development of depression in the elderly.

Fifteen to 30 percent of Americans suffer at least one episode of depression in their lifetime. Only a fraction of these will ever seek professional help. Many depressed persons, particularly youth, may complain of physical problems or appear to be insane.

Fatigue is the most common presenting symptom in any patient with depression. The fatigue of depression usually begins on awakening, when the person is unable to drag himself/herself out of bed. The depressed person may wish to be alone. The person feels sad, hopeless, and sometimes irritable.

Additional symptoms of depression may include poor appetite with significant weight loss or an increased appetite with significant weight gain; inability to sleep or sleeping all the time; anxiety or extreme sedation, restlessness, or extreme motionlessness; agitation or retardation; reduced interest in sex; loss of energy; feelings of guilt; and indecisiveness and inability to think rapidly. Alertness, sharing of experiences, and interests in outside affairs wanes. Work becomes impossible. Preoccupation with regrets about the past and fear of disease, ruin, and death grips the person. Delusion about ill health or financial calamity may occur.

Among the first things to look for in depression is that of a physical cause. Check the diet, the exercise program, whether regularity is observed in sleep time, mealtime, etc., whether fresh air and pure water are used, and all matters dealing with physical health. While one can be depressed because of some situation, the situation is usually recognizable and can be dealt with. Do not allow chronic depression to take hold of the mind, as it can injure not only the mind but also the immune system and reduce the resistance against disease. Once being depressed becomes a habit, the mind defaults into a depression about things over which there should be no cause for depression, such as a beautiful sunset or a newborn baby.

Individuals who attend religious services are less depressed and are physically healthier than those who worship at home or are not religious.

Depression increases one's likelihood of having heart disease. Several studies have shown an association between severe depression and an increased risk of fatal heart disease. Now it has been shown that even mild depression could eventually harm the heart. The Centers for Disease Control recruited 28,000 people ages 45 to 77, none of whom had heart disease when the study began. After twelve years, the rate of heart disease and death was significantly higher among depressed people, about double the rate of those with the most buoyant health. Prolonged depression encourages blood clots and thicken the artery walls (*Consumer Reports on Health,* June 1995, 69).

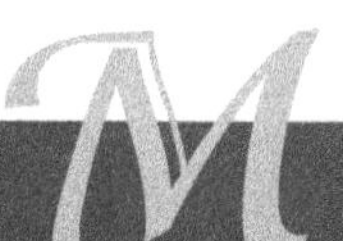

Bipolar State

A manic-depressive psychosis may attack at any age, but is more prevalent between the ages of 20 to 65, women comprising about two-thirds of all cases. In the manic phase the person may have overabundant energy, incessant activity, and exaggerated sense of well-being. Impulsiveness and incessant talking may be pronounced. The judgment and decision-making ability is impaired. Moods may suddenly change to irritability and extreme anger. This is often followed by a painful emotional condition of deep despondency, a sense of guilt over illusory misdeeds and sins. The person may consider suicide. Symptoms such as sluggishness, inability to make decisions, and lack of concentration are pronounced. There may be physical signs such as constipation, sleeplessness or sleepiness, loss of weight, and suppressed intellectual activity almost to the point of stupor.

Bipolar disease often runs in families. It may occur at any age but is rare in childhood and most frequently starts between the ages of 45 to 65. Persons who are rigid, obsessional, or perfectionists are far more likely to become bipolar. Diagnosis is by history, but laboratory tests should be obtained for diabetes, hypothyroidism, and uremia (kidney disease), as these diseases may have symptoms similar to bipolar disease. Get laboratory tests for blood sugar, blood urea, hematocrit, thyroid function, and a battery of chemical tests to determine if a metabolic problem is a factor in the depression. These may be corrected by appropriate dietary and physical changes.

Depressed children and children with bipolar illnesses are more likely than non-depressed children to have alcoholic parents. Children with bipolar disorder are about three times more likely to have alcoholic mothers, whereas depressed children without bipolarity were more likely to have alcoholic fathers (*Journal of American Academy of Child and Adolescent Psychiatry* 35 [1996]: 716).

Treatment for Depression and Bipolar

Diet

Lifestyle and dietary factors are important in treating depression. Coffee, tobacco, alcohol, and drugs (both prescription and illicit) can cause depression. Make changes as needed.

A high protein diet increases one's likelihood of being irritable, having mood changes, and becoming depressed (*Medical Tribune,* April 4, 1996). The most favorable diet for depression is a totally plant-based diet low in free sugars and free fats but containing daily foods from the four basic food groups: fruits, vegetables, whole grains, and nuts or seeds.

Over two hundred drugs have been reported to cause depression, including some that were prescribed for depression. If you are taking any kind of medication, be aware that drugs are a very common source of depression. The antidepressant drugs can have very adverse side effects, including liver damage, dry mouth, constipation, blurred vision, sweating, rapid heartbeat, impotence, etc.

Depression may result because of the wrong kind of fatty acids comprising the cell membranes of nerve cells in the brain. All cells throughout the body are enveloped in membranes composed chiefly of essential fatty acids in the form of phospholipids. The type of phospholipid in the cell membranes of the brain is determined by the kind of fat eaten. If the phospholipid has a component of saturated fat or trans-fatty acids, the structure of the cell will be markedly different than if the membrane contains omega-3 and omega-6 oils. If the cell membranes are stiff, the brain is less likely to function properly; therefore, the diet can impact behavior, mood, mental function, etc.

A case of depression treated with pumpkin seeds, a good source of natural L-tryptophan, was reported in the *British Journal of Psychiatry* in 1990. One and one-half grams of L-tryptophan per day can often abolish depression. About one cup of pumpkin seed will contain about one and one-half grams (500 milligrams) of L-tryptophan (*British Journal of Psychiatry* 157 [December 1990]: 937, 938).

For depression try a phenylalanine intake sufficient to provide at least 30 milligrams, from any of the following:

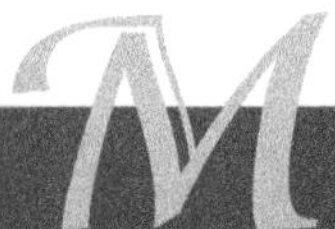

Fruits	
Apricots	8 halves
Banana	1 medium
Cantaloupe	1 cup
Dates	4
Grapefruit	⅔ cups
Lemon juice	6 tablespoons
Olives	6 large
Orange	2 medium
Peaches	2 medium
Pears	3
Pineapple	3 slices, canned
Prunes	4 large
Raisins	4 tablespoons
Vegetables	
Beans, green	6 tablespoons
Beets	6 tablespoons
Cabbage, raw	8 tablespoons
Carrots	8 tablespoons
Celery	3 small stalks
Cucumber	⅔ medium
Lettuce	4 leaves
Potatoes, Irish	2½ tablespoons
Potatoes, sweet	3½ tablespoons
Spinach	3 tablespoons
Squash, summer	8 tablespoons
Squash, winter	6 tablespoons
Tomato	4 tablespoons
Grains	
Cooked whole grain cereals	2 tablespoons (dry)

Coffee, tobacco, and alcohol are causes of depression. About half of the population between 30 and 60 call themselves coffee drinkers, with 450 million cups of coffee being consumed per day. About 30 percent of Americans smoke at least half a pack of cigarettes daily. Cigarettes are also known to be associated with depression. Around 10 percent of Americans are addicted to alcohol, which is also associated with depression. Up to 33 percent of our population consumes more than four alcoholic drinks daily, and one-third of high school seniors are binge drinkers. Thus, we can urge that coffee and its relatives, tea, colas, chocolate, tobacco, and alcohol, be omitted in persons having depression.

Nutritional deficiencies and related factors are also important causes of depression. Hypoglycemia is a common condition among depressed individuals. The deficiency of several vitamins is also known to cause depression. These include thiamin, riboflavin, niacin, biotin, pantothenic acid, B6, folic acid, B12, and vitamin C. These vitamins can all be obtained from fruits and vegetables, particularly when fresh or when gently cooked so as not to destroy the tender vitamins such as thiamin and riboflavin. In elderly people, a deficiency of folic acid may be a part of the whole picture that results in depression (*Nutrition* 16 [2000]: 544).

Vitamin B12 should also be taken as a supplement from a pill, preferably one that can be chewed for two minutes, because there is a salivary factor that activates the B12 (*American Journal of Natural Medicine* 2, no. 10: 10–15). Lithium, magnesium, and iodine may be low in persons suffering from bipolar states. These minerals should be emphasized by eating foods high in them. (See "Food Sources High in Certain Nutrients" in the *Dietary Information* section.)

Tyrosine, an amine acid, can elevate the mood of elderly people, relieve dizziness, normalize blood pressure, and improve the appetite (*Pharmacology, Biochemistry, and Behavior* 47, no. 4 [1994]: 935–41). (See "Food Sources High in Certain Nutrients" in the *Dietary Information* section.)

Even the vegetarian diet must be checked for foods to which one may be sensitive, as food sensitivities are more commonly involved in depression than has been previously realized. Carefully perform an Elimination and Challenge diet. (See "Elimination and Challenge Diet" in the *Dietary Information* section.) Never eat between meals, as eating on an irregular schedule can cause improper digestion, which affects the brain.

Avoid crash diets for weight reduction. Depression often follows such programs.

Some persons with manic-depressive psychosis will require some form of restraint, either physical restraint or chemical restraint. Many have found lithium supplementation to be controlling for the manic-depressive states. When depression and anxiety are quite severe and hospitalization appears imminent, it is often possible to avoid hospitalization by injecting one-half cc of vitamin B12 and one and one-half of vitamin B complex every day. In addition to the injection, certain herb teas such as hops, valerian, and passionflower, in double strength, should be given to encourage sleep. Pray earnestly with the patient.

The use of oats in any way will usually help in depression. Oat groats, oatmeal cereal, oatmeal gruel, broth, or tea may be helpful for some patients.

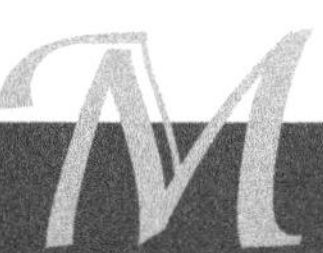

Exercise

Exercise is a most important method of fighting depression. In fact, regular exercise is one of the most important and powerful natural antidepressants we have. Getting plenty of exercise reduces anxiety and tension. Seventy-five percent of persons with depression in a large study showed improvement with jogging. They approached life more optimistically and reported that running gave them more control over their lives. Dr. Keith Johnsgard, professor of Psychology at San Jose University, wrote the report. Even deep breathing exercises carried out twice daily can lift a gloomy spirit.

Hydrotherapy

Cold, wet sheet packs can be very helpful for agitated depression. The single layer wet sheet is laid on a plastic shower curtain on a bed and wrapped around the patient, trying to cover every inch of skin from the collar bones down. (See "Hydrotherapy" in the *Natural Remedies* section.) This treatment can be effective when all other treatment modalities are ineffectual (*Hospital and Community Psychiatry* 37, no. 3 [1986]: 287). Sometimes a wet sheet pack can offer sufficient physical restraint and enough sedation to avoid the use of medications. A continuous neutral bath at about 97°F to 98°F, being sure to keep the head cool, will also calm many an agitated patient.

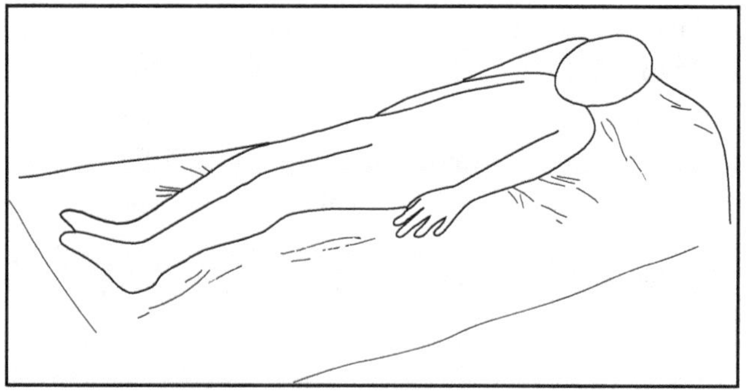

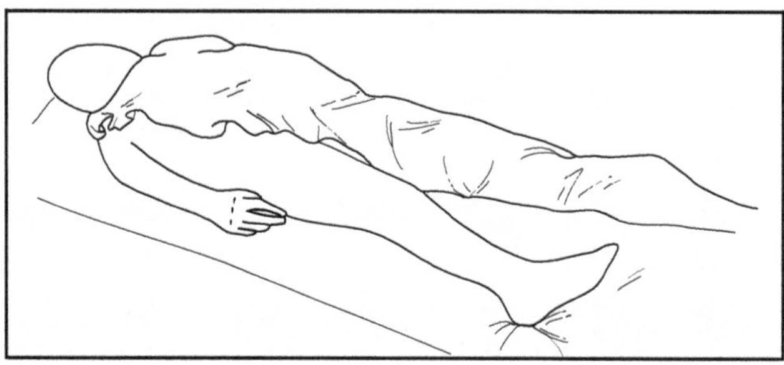

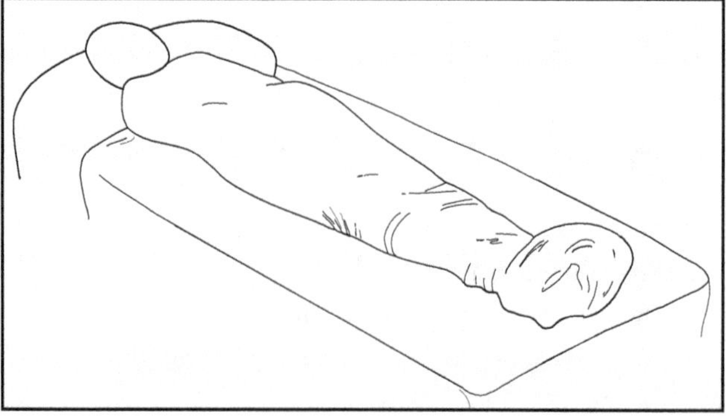

Whole body hot baths can cause a significant improvement in depression (*International Journal of Hyperthermia* 8, no. 3 [1992]: 305). Perform the bath daily for five days, skip two days, and give a second and then a third series of five baths. Get the mouth temperature up to 102°F.

Use skin stimulation with a stiff brush before the daily cool shower. (See "Hydrotherapy" in the *Natural Remedies* section.)

Herbs

St. John's wort and ginkgo have been studied in relation to helping with memory impairment, depression, and anxiety. The research has found that these two herbs are quite effective in the treatment of these and other common psychiatric disorders (*Archives of General Psychiatry* 55 [1998]: 1033). St. John's wort is used for depression the world over. One cup of the tea four times a day can be most effective. It should be kept up, as its effects grow as time goes by. Ginkgo biloba can also be very helpful in treating depression, particularly in the elderly, but also in younger patients. Ginkgo biloba extract or tea contains flavone glycosides and terpenoids that are very useful not only in depression but also in cerebrovascular insufficiency, senility, Alzheimer's disease, impotence, vertigo, tinnitus, peripheral vascular insufficiency, Raynaud's syndrome, premenstrual syndrome, macular degeneration, diabetic retinopathy, and vascular fragility. Many of these diseases are associated with depression, and ginkgo is the herb of choice. It improves the ability of the brain to concentrate and bind serotonin.

St. John's wort can cause photosensitivity in fair skinned persons, and skin will be very sensitive to sunlight. When using it, be careful of the sun.

For postpartum depression, use chaste berry, raspberry leaf, nettles, motherwort, and dandelion leaf and root.

Adrenal exhaustion from stress may represent a portion of the cause of major depression and suicidal behavior. A study done on suicide victims showed hypertrophy of the cortex of the adrenals in suicide victims compared to those dying of other causes. For individuals under extreme stress, the use of licorice root tea might be very helpful as it improves the function of the adrenals (*American Journal of Natural Medicine* 2, no. 3 [1995]: 14). The struggling adrenal under

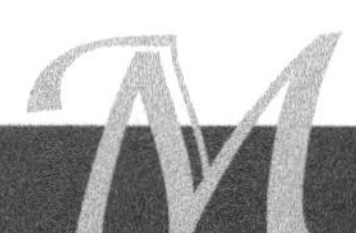

continuous stress overgrows in its effort to keep up with stress hormone needs.

The essential oil lemon balm can sooth agitation and depression in patients with dementia (*Reuters,* August 8, 2002). It can be used in a fragrance diffuser, or a cotton sponge saturated with the oil can be pinned with a safety pin to clothing or a pillow. It may also be rubbed onto the abdomen or shoulders.

The clinical condition of 10 patients with major depressive episodes was improved through the application of citrus fragrances. A reduced dose of antidepressants could be used and a normalization was found of the immune functions (natural killer cell activity and cortisol levels in the urine) (*Japanese Journal of Psychiatry and Neurology* 48, no. 3 [1994]: 671).

Some of the herbal teas such as sage, catnip, mint, or alfalfa can be helpful. Use one cup in the morning and one at night. Skullcap and valerian are very useful on a daily basis. For the acute phase or for severe symptoms, use blue verbena and European mistletoe. The recipe for blue verbena is one tablespoon of the root boiled gently in two cups of water for five minutes; for the mistletoe, use two teaspoons in two cups of boiling water and steep for 20 minutes (do not boil). Use one-half cup of the verbena and one cup of the mistletoe every two hours as needed for control of symptoms.

CoQ10 is good for depressed patients. Use up to 200 milligrams every four hours for one month, then drop down to 100 milligrams three times daily. It is better absorbed if one takes it with meals.

Other Therapies

Bright light therapy was applied to 30 patients of whom 12 experienced improvement of mood during the bright light therapy, while 18 did not improve. The results of an experiment showed a subgroup of patients with major depression making a more pronounced light-associated improvement in heart functions than other depressed patients and controls (*Journal of Affective Disorders* 34 [1995]: 131). The depressed person should be put to bed two to three hours earlier than the usual bedtime; seven or eight o'clock in the evening is probably ideal. The house must be kept quiet and dark. Arise seven to nine hours later and begin some preplanned activity, the best being purposeful labor outdoors. This activity should be in very bright light. If labor is not available or practicable, exercise in a gymnasium. Regularity in all things must become a study. A large part of depression is a sickness of the brain center controlling the circadian rhythm or biologic time clock. Adjusting the hour of bedtime in this way has cured many cases of depression. Get plenty of sunshine. During the day, keep bright lights blazing in the portion of the house the depressed person stays in.

Three to five million Americans suffer from seasonal affective disorders (SAD). Reduced availability of sunlight leads to an imbalance of brain chemicals, resulting in depression. Exposure to high levels of artificial light can restore the balance of brain chemicals in many of these people. Women are three or four times more likely to get this disorder than men. It usually starts after puberty and diminishes after menopause.

Our thoughts are often responsible for our feelings. Habitual negative thinking or critical thinking can lead to psychological disorders such as anxiety, depression, panic attacks, and phobias (*The American Family Physician* 57 [1998]: 2867). The patient can learn to identify, acknowledge, and replace negative thoughts with more positive ones, if necessary. Keeping a daily log to record thoughts and feelings can be a practical way to come to grips with the problem. Through prayer one can recognize a negative thought, identify its cause, and then think of another more positive thought. To have the mind switch to a religious thought such as the home of the saved is a very good way to deal with thoughts that lead to depression.

Depression in both children and adults can be treated with daily massage. It can be curative in some cases.

Eleven manic depressed persons had their amalgams removed and nine subjects with amalgams were given a placebo or a sealant. Depression and hypomania scores improved significantly as did anxiety, anger, schizophrenia, and paranoia, compared to the sealant-placebo group. There was a 42 percent decrease in the number of physical health problems after amalgam removal compared to an 8 percent increase in physical symptoms in the placebo-sealant group (*Journal of Ortho-molecular Medicine* 13, no. 1 [1998]: 31–41).

Volunteer work has a marvelous effect on gloomy spirits. Seek out widows and orphans, the lonely or bereaved, or a homesick student and do something nice for them.

Control sexuality. Many have no extra strength to use in this direction. Masturbation must be strictly avoided.

A Treatment Plan for Depression

The following treatment plan was related to us by Ulrike Gotzinger of Norway.

1. Eat whole foods only. Don't use any refined grains, sugars, proteins, or other refined foods.

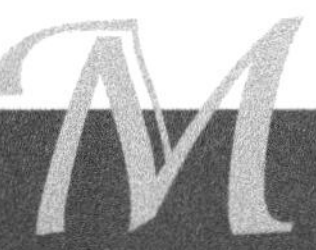

2. Exercise several times daily, quite strenuously for about 10 to 15 minutes. This should be done both indoors as well as outdoors, as some of the exercises need to be done first thing in the morning before it is light, and last thing at night after it is dark outside.
3. Take a daily dose of a B-complex with vitamin B12 for one month.
4. Take an appropriate dosage of Tyrosine for one month.
5. Bolster your spiritual defenses through Bible study and prayer.
6. Use charcoal compresses on the abdomen for the first three days.
7. Administer hot bath treatments every day, bringing the mouth temperature up to 101°F to 102°F.
8. Enjoy a full body massage frequently, preferably daily, but at least once a week.
9. Drink one cup of hops and chamomile tea, or a comparable amount in capsules or tablets, two to three times daily.

Emotional Health in Youth

Teenagers who engaged in regular exercise were tested and found to score higher on happiness quizzes than those who spent much of their time watching the TV program "Beavis and Butt-head." In a separate study of 65,000 teen boys and girls, those reporting regular exercise and participation in sports had significantly higher scores on emotional well-being than their couch-potato peers. Those who reported the least activity of a physical nature reported far more frequent feelings of being upset or other signs of poor emotional well-being (*Lancet*, June 29, 1996).

Boredom is epidemic among children because of computer games, videos, and television. Fast moving stimuli do not give the child a chance to slow down, reflect, be thoughtful, and/or process new information.

If you feel tired after puzzling over a tough problem you have never heard before, there is a reason. The brain has to work harder, and it uses a lot more energy. You may not think of the brain as using fuel although it uses fuel in the same way a muscle uses up fuel. When the task is unfamiliar, the brain uses many unnecessary circuits that require a lot of energy but are not the principle circuits used to solve the problem. With experience one learns to shut off the unnecessary circuits and use only the most essential circuits. Thus the brain saves energy and you feel less tired (*Prodigy,* March 9, 1992). This is the reason you feel more tired the first day on a new job. Many brain circuits are working full speed and using a lot of energy.

Following is a list of nine signs to look for that may be the precursor to impending youth violence:

- Withdrawal and isolation
- Loss of interest in friends and activities once enjoyed
- Suddenly becomes confrontational
- Overreacting to frustrations
- Depression
- Interest in the occult, witchcraft, or Satanism
- Frequent talk or threats of harming people, animals, or destroying property
- Past history of violence or inappropriate behavior toward animals, siblings, or others
- Total disregard for authority and home or school rules

Following is a list of ideas for treating youth who are prone to violence:

- Spend some of your leisure time each day talking and listening to them. Let them know you want them to share their problems with you.
- Help them learn appropriate ways to communicate anger or frustration
- Do not allow them to use hateful or threatening talk to express simple anger. Instead, gently correct them. Teach them to think about what they are going to say before they say it.
- Be a model of appropriate behavior. Try to defuse tense situations or discuss situations if appropriate.
- Avoid the amount of violence children are exposed to through TV, movies, video games, or associates.
- Set standards for your home or family and expect them to respect those standards.
- Tell children to stay away from others who threaten violence and that reporting potential violence is not tattling; it is using good judgment and acting responsibly to protect others.
- Find creative activities or vigorous play that can channel a child's aggressive energy. Gardening, hiking, rowing, carpentry, etc, are all good options.
- If they have problems with self-control, avoid roughhousing. Teach children appropriate ways to seek attention rather than using physical contact.
- Pay attention to changes in behavior or interests that could suggest they are troubled.

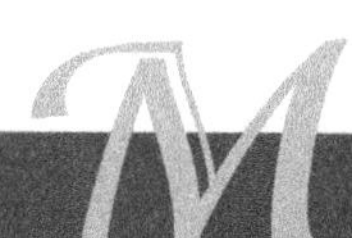

- Offer to help them work through their problems. Offer to get another caring adult they might prefer to confide in. If that doesn't work, get professional help from a school counselor or psychologist within two weeks of believing your child is potentially violent.

Numerous reasons are given for the upswing in violent behavior among children—poverty, poor family structure, television, drugs, and dietary factors such as mineral imbalances. These may all be a part of the total picture. A study done on violent boys, ages 3 to 18, showed elevated copper levels and reduced zinc levels in their blood compared to nonviolent boys. Adults, as well, who exhibit assaultive behavior have significantly higher copper levels and lower zinc blood levels than nonviolent males (*Alternatives* 5, no. 24 [June 1995]).

In order to reduce copper levels, zinc can be taken in quantities of about 30 to 50 milligrams daily for one week and then dropped down to 15 milligrams daily as a maintenance dose. Zinc and copper have a seesaw relationship in the body. Excess lead has been linked to delinquency in boys. A group of boys between the ages of 7 and 11, with high lead concentrations in their bones, displayed attention problems, aggressive behavior, and delinquency. Boys in the same age group with low lead levels showed fewer such problems (*Science News* 149 [Feburary 10, 1996]: 86). (See also "Toxic Heavy Metals" in the *Supplemental Information* section.)

Studying boys even as early as kindergarten age can reveal a tendency to smoke, drink, and take drugs. Personality testing done on 800 Montreal area boys ages 6 to 10 revealed three key personality characteristics if they were later on to develop the unwanted habits listed above. These characteristics were "high novelty-seeking" defined as impulsive, excitable, and exploratory behaviors. The second was "low harm avoidance" or the lack of fear about new things or new situations, even under the recognized threat of possible harm. The third was the "low reward dependence" group expressed as reluctance to be kind, helpful, or sympathetic to others.

If your child has any of these personality traits, there are several things you can do to prevent destructive traits from developing. One is to give the child a structured home life. There should be a time for everything and a place for everything, and the parents must discipline themselves in order that they can insist on an orderly environment. Another thing is to slow down the rate at which the child is maturing by reducing the total quantity of food allowed. There must be a reduction in total calories, particularly those calories obtained from sweets, fats, and all animal products. It is highly desirable to switch to a vegetarian cuisine that will automatically reduce the total number of calories and eliminate the growth-promoting factors in milk products, meat, and eggs. Vegetarians are generally noted for a gentler disposition than others.

Research indicates that infants born to mothers who had complicated deliveries or who were rejected by their mothers early in life were more likely than other children to grow up to commit violent crimes (*Medical Tribune*, October 23, 1997, 16).

The earlier a youngster goes through puberty the greater the likelihood of teenage problems. These problems are delinquency, sex out of wedlock, eating disorders, unwed pregnancies, school dropouts, drugs, drinking, and resistance to authority. Girls who go through puberty after their 15th birthday have fewer problems than their peers who develop earlier. Factors known to reduce the age at which a young girl goes through puberty are as follows: (1) heredity, (2) high protein, high-fat diet, and being overweight, (3) strained family relations, (4) absence of an adult male in the household, (5) psychological maladjustment, (6) exposure to sexuality early or early sexual experiences (*Child Development* 66, no. 2 [1995]: 346–59).

The timing of puberty, as well as adolescent growth and development, is affected by dietary intake and body size from much earlier in childhood. Sixty-seven white girls in Boston were studied from birth during the 1930s and 1940s. Heights and weights were measured semi-annually and diet history was provided by the mothers. The age of their first menstrual period, height, growth velocity, and similar measurements were made at six-month intervals. The girls who ate the most calories and animal protein and less vegetable protein at ages three to five years had greater growth velocity and earlier onset of menstrual periods (*American Journal of Epidemiology* 152 [2000]: 446–52).

Regular times for sleeping, eating, and exercising are essential to developing calmness. Dealing kindly with the youngster goes far toward inspiring kindness in the child. Homeschooling for the troubled child can make a great difference in the demeanor, even if the child does not like being homeschooled.

Many factors in teen problems are believed to be the result of our modern society with its junk foods, stimulating beverages, TV, loss of a strong family structure, and rapid physical maturity. Schools reveal these problems. Teachers complain about the following in students of today:

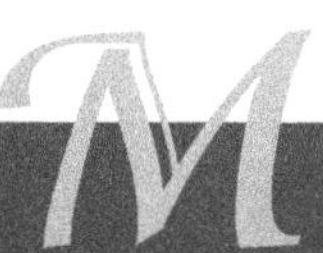

- Are harder to teach than a few decades ago
- Think differently than they once did
- Exhibit verbal resistance, both spoken and written
- Forget directions immediately
- Have a short attention span
- Are easily distracted
- Complain of the workload

There are signs that indicate that a teenager is drinking and/or doing drugs. They are as follows:

- Uses home like a hotel (a place to sleep and eat)
- Suddenly neglects hygiene
- Frequent high mood swings
- Personality changes
- No interest in grades and drops in performance
- Skips class or school for days at a time
- Changes to a different crowd of friends
- Withdraws from the family and becomes secretive
- Sneaks money or liquor out of the house
- Does his/her own activities without regard for the interests of the family

Curiosity and coercion rank in the top three reasons why teens engage in sexual intercourse for the first time (*Family Practice News* 27, no. 19 [October 1, 1997]: 1). Parents can help their children avoid these factors by instructing them to postpone sexual experiences until after marriage in order to preserve the sacredness of the experience. The youngster should be taught that the experience will lose forever a precious quality that can never be regained if their virginity is not protected and saved for marriage only.

Childhood abuse is now implicated as a cause in a number of degenerative diseases ranging from heart disease to cancer. The reason for this seems to be that those abused are more likely to smoke, use illicit drugs and alcohol, overeat, or be sexually promiscuous; all of which are factors for chronic diseases (*American Journal of Preventive Medicine* 14 [1998]: 245; *Medical Tribune*, June 18, 1998, 39).

For nearly a century it has been observed that individuals who mature more slowly have a longer life span. One animal study showed those maturing more rapidly had a shorter life span than similar animals whose growth rate was slower. It is postulated that since females grow more slowly at the critical time of growth spurt, this factor accounts for their longer life span, according to a Cornell University study (*Science Newsletter*, January 6, 1924, 8). Many vegetarians mature more slowly than meat eaters, and vegetarians, as a whole, have longer life spans.

Paralyzing Anxiety and Worry

Inositol is a nutrient fraction of phytic acid. It is one of the best tranquilizers and sedatives on the market today. It also lowers blood pressure and cholesterol, helps the diabetic, provides brain nutrition, and has been used in treatment of obesity and schizophrenia. Some say it can help prevent the loss of hair. There are no side effects, unlike most popular tranquilizers.

Gotu kola is very good to stabilize the nerves and prevent or treat a nervous breakdown. It helps relieve mental fatigue, combats stress, and helps prevent or treat senility. Kava is excellent for anxiety, probably the best herb we have for this disorder.

The use of L-phenylalanine, an essential amino acid, seems to cheer and energize some patients with depression. Vitamin B6 is essential for the metabolism of L-phenylalanine to make II-phenylethyl amine, an internal neuromodulator with properties similar to amphetamine but without the severe side effects. Natural substances contain both the vitamin and L-phenylalanine (*Medical World News*, October 24, 1983). Food sources of L-phenylalanine are avocados, pulses and legumes (particularly peanuts and lima beans), nuts (pistachios, almonds), many seeds, leafy vegetables, and whole grains.

How to Handle Worry

Distinguish between appropriate worry and harmful worry. Good worry encourages planning, action, and solutions to problems. Harmful worry is unproductive, may be paralyzing, and self-defeating.

Put off considering a matter until you can get the facts. Save your worry for real problems. Don't get worried until you know there is truly sufficient information to justify getting worried.

Try not to worry alone. When you share your concerns, they usually diminish. Select the proper person with care—not a gossiper, not a belittler who expects everybody to have all things under control, and not one who will take over your life and make independent moves involving your life apart from you.

Get reassurance and advice. Do not go to persons who merely rubber-stamp your decisions, go to those who think through a problem with you, somebody who expects to and knows how to pray.

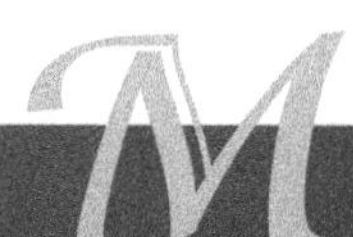

Organize your life. Disorganization in any area increases worry. Structure and order provide security and self-confidence. Once one room in the house becomes organized, it becomes the center from which all other rooms get organized. Give yourself a time frame for completing each section of the task. When each one is finished, go to the next one. Eliminate TV, magazines, and newspapers, as they are full of bad news and potential triggers for additional worry.

Exercise every day. It is one of the best treatments for worry. Pray and meditate. Read the Bible and associate with deeply committed Christians. These practices calm the mind and put everyday problems into perspective.

Keep your house brightly lit except at night when it should be completely dark. Get sunlight both in your home as well as on your person every day.

Do charitable things for the poor, the sick, and the lonely.

Surround yourself with cheerful people.

Listen to recordings of the Bible, to religious music, or recordings about health. Sing along with music as it is difficult to worry and sing at the same time.

Do not fear to cry awhile, but then you should quit crying and plan a course of action if one is warranted.

Do not use drugs, alcohol, caffeine, nicotine, food, gossip, running away, or other crutches as they only create more problems in the long run and do not actually assist you in learning how to better handle problems.

Mercury Poisoning

(See also "Toxic Heavy Metals" in the *Supplemental Information* section.)

Miscarriage

(See "Woman's Conditions and Disease" in the *Conditions and Diseases* section.)

Moles

Count the number of moles on your body five millimeters or more in diameter. Persons who have six or more moles measuring five millimeters and above in diameter have increased risk of developing melanoma. Be sure to also look for and count any flesh colored moles.

There are four key characteristics of melanomas. Monitor your moles by the following acronym: ABCD—asymmetry, border irregularity, color variation, diameter greater than six millimeters. A melanoma one millimeter thick or less as measured by the pathologist, has a 95 percent cure rate. By comparison, if lesions are four millimeters thick the five year survival rate is just 35 percent.

Having just one atypical or dysplastic mole doubles the risk of melanoma. A dysplastic mole is one that changes in appearance. Having 10 or more increases ten-fold the chance of developing the malignancy. Troublesome moles are flat or partially flat, larger than five millimeters (about the size of a pencil eraser), and vary in color with irregular borders or mismatched halves. Small moles are also a hazard, especially if there are fifty or more on your body, in which case you are about twice as likely to develop melanoma than a person with 25 or fewer. Large moles confer a greater risk than small ones. The number and size of moles are not the most important risk factor; family history is by far more important. If another person in your immediate family—father, mother, sibling, or child—has had melanoma, then your risk for the disease jumps by 20 times.

Other risk factors include fair skin, blond or red hair, and blue eyes. People who sunburn easily and never or rarely tan are twice as likely to develop melanoma as people with olive complexions who seldom burn. Blistering and peeling sunburns, especially during childhood and adolescence, make people more susceptible to melanoma later in life. It may take 20 to 30 years from the time of the sunburn to the time you develop melanoma (*Health News* 3, no. 8 [June 24, 1997]: 1, 2). A mole that has changed or grown is an important warning sign.

Moniliasis

(See "Candida" in the *Conditions and Diseases* section.)

Morning Sickness

(See "Vomiting" in the *Conditions and Diseases* section.)

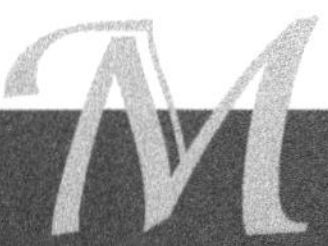

Morton's Neuroma

This condition causes pain in the toes of the foot as a result of an enlargement of the sheath around the nerve because of repeated injury. Standing or walking in shoes with thin soles or high heels causes the nerve to become trapped under the enlarged ends of the foot bones, causing injury, pain, and numbness in a specific spot on the sides of the toe involved. It may feel like a stone moving around under the foot, sometimes causing a sharp snap. This condition tends to worsen over time and repeated injury. As the nerve grows larger, it is more easily injured.

Surgery to remove the neuroma leaves permanent numbness in the toes and ball of the foot and can leave persisting pain in about 5 percent of cases caused by a "stump neuroma." Therefore, following these simple home remedies is recommended.

Treatment

Modify the shoes you wear. A pad in the shoe or an extra wide soft shoe with thick soles is the first step.

Soak your feet in hot water for 30 minutes each night. Cabbage soaks are also good. Cut a cabbage into three sections. Put one section in a foot tub with hot water. Pour boiling water over the cabbage, and when cool enough to soak the foot, soak it for 30 minutes. Use the other sections of the cabbage the next two nights. A single cabbage leaf may be crushed with the hands to release juices and bound to the foot as a compress overnight.

Massage the foot to relax muscles and stretch tendons to relieve the pain.

Use a comfrey compress on the foot similarly to the cabbage leaf compress.

If pain persists, use a red pepper extract poured into melted cocoa butter or beeswax, equal quantities. To make the extract, put a teaspoon of red pepper in a jar and pour a cup of rubbing alcohol over it, seal and set aside for a week or two. Strain, then pour it into melted cocoa butter enough to make a salve. Apply to the skin four times a day for six days, then twice a day for three months.

Standard exercises for the foot not involving standing on the foot can be helpful to strengthen muscles so that bones are held off the nerve because the muscle masses are larger.

White willow bark may be taken for pain. Use a cup of the tea four times a day. It is more effective the longer you take it.

Motion Sickness

Motion sickness affects a variety of people, both young and old. However, there are a number of ways to prevent motion sickness.

Jumping on a trampoline a few minutes once or twice a day will train the balance mechanism of the ear to be in motion and will significantly reduce your susceptibility to motion sickness.

Eat light meals, avoiding all free fats for a few days before a trip. Rich, heavy, and gas-forming foods should not be eaten before beginning a trip. For three days ahead of the trip, if one eats only fruit and dry bread or plain rice, it is less likely one will suffer from motion sickness. Never drink anything alcoholic.

Do not sit in the back seat of an automobile. Raising a car seat so that the eyes can focus on relatively still objects in the distance can avoid or at least lessen motion sickness.

Driving usually does not provoke motion sickness; being a passenger does.

When riding in smaller vehicles, sit low near the center of gravity, which subjects one to as little motion as possible. Sit on the right of an airplane as most turns and banks are made to the left. If motion sickness begins during the flight, slide down as far as possible in the seat and keep the head and neck supported. Lie down if possible, and drink as many fluids as can be tolerated. Keep warm, and get plenty of fresh air at all times. Adequate sleep before and during the trip also helps stave off motion sickness.

If you know you are going to take a trip or be subjected to some kind of movement that will result in nausea and vomiting, take an enema or a colonic just prior to engaging in that motion. If you are on a long sea voyage and get seasickness, try the enema routine to see if it will be effective for you.

Treatment

Mint extract is a remedy for motion sickness. Wet the end of the finger with the mint extract and lick it. It works in less than 10 minutes to stop motion sickness. Repeat every half an hour if needed.

For persons who experience motion sickness, it can usually be treated with ginger root tea. Some of the same treatments used in Meniere's disease can be highly successful for motion sickness. Ginger root is as effective as Metoclopramide in controlling nausea, even sickness that occurs after anesthesia (*Anaesthesia* 90;45(8): 669–71).

A cold cloth to the forehead or across the mouth and chin are very effective for helping nausea subside.

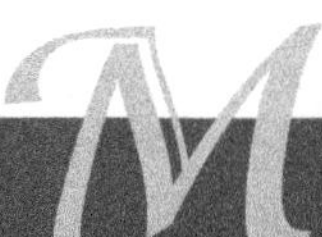

Mouth Ulcers

(See "Canker Sores, Mouth Ulcers, Aphthous Ulcers" in the *Conditions and Diseases* section.)

Multiple Myeloma

Multiple myeloma is a malignancy of the bone marrow involving principally the plasma cells. It can be treated with the remedies described in the "Cancer" entry in the *Conditions and Diseases* section.

In an interview with Dr. Donald Miller, Hematology-Oncologist, at the University of Alabama, I learned that in patients whose bone marrow smears reveal multiple myeloma cells, but who have negative plasma electrophoresis, no Bence Jones protein, are not anemic, and have no signs of renal failure and no hypercalcemia, nothing is to be gained by treating a patient at that stage. It is universally practiced that until patients have symptoms or show blood signs of kidney involvement or hypercalcemia, treatment is not begun.

Multiple Sclerosis

Multiple Sclerosis (MS) is a disorder of the nerves in which the sheaths of myelin surrounding the nerve fiber are destroyed by a process that has, as yet, eluded researchers. The sites most commonly involved are certain areas near the ventricular system in the brain, the optic nerves, and the white matter controlling muscular coordination in the cerebellum.

Human herpes virus VI may play a role in the development of multiple sclerosis (*Medical Tribune, Infectious Diseases*, October 23, 1997, 20).

MS is a common neurological disease that affects approximately 300,000 Americans. Treatment and care of MS patients costs approximately $2.5 billion each year in the United States. Two-thirds of those diagnosed with MS are women. Most researchers believe that MS is an autoimmune disease. The body's reaction to a foreign protein is to destroy the invader with an antibody. In the case of an autoimmune disorder, the antibody then turns upon one's own cells. That is an autoimmune response. In MS, something causes the outer membrane protecting nerve cells, the myelin sheath, to deteriorate. Some believe this to be an autoimmune response.

Some individuals have an accelerated form of MS and will be totally incapacitated within six months of the onset. MS does not appreciably shorten the life span in most patients except those with the accelerated form, unless a serious complication arises. The average age of onset is 29.9 years. There is no laboratory test that confirms the presence of MS, and the diagnosis is made by the meticulous exclusion of all other disorders that could cause the neurologic defects seen. Exactly what happens in MS to paralyze the function of nerves is not yet known. There is some belief that MS is not so much a matter of demyelination of nerves as of deficient function of the synapses, the connections between nerves (*International Journal of Neuroscience* 84 [1996]: 157).

MS is one of the commonest serious disorders of the nervous system. The course of MS is highly unpredictable. Some patients suffer repeated attacks and rapid progression until they are severely crippled within a short time, while others experience a slow progression of the disease over decades. It is recognized that there is no medical treatment for MS that alters the length or severity of the disease. Steroid therapy does not alter the outcome of the disease and should not be used because of its serious complications.

Possible Causes

The cause of MS is unknown, but many factors have been suspected. These fall into several categories: an infectious agent, an autoimmune response of some kind, and a toxic substance, either metabolic or from outside the body.

The increased consumption of animal fat may be associated with MS as there is a greater prevalence of MS in countries with a high average daily per capita consumption of fats, oils, protein, and total calories, especially calories of animal food origin (*Archives of Neurology* 31 [October 1974]: 267). There is a striking correlation between the world distribution and consumption of dairy products and the incidence of MS (*The Journal of the American Dietetic Association,* April 1977, 444; *The New Zealand Medical Journal* 83 [June 23, 1976]: 427). As milk consumption goes up in a population, so does multiple sclerosis (*Neuroepidemiology* 11 [1992]: 304).

The rate of MS is higher than has been previously estimated. As an example, in Canada the previous estimation was 40 per 100,000, but now it appears to be between 110 to 133 cases per 100,000 population in Vancouver. There were twice as many women as men with MS. More than 50 percent of the patients first resided on a farm as compared with 31 percent in a town and 18 percent in a city. These percentages correlate fairly well with the expected exposure to milk-producing livestock and egg-producing poultry between rural and urban population groups, implicating either an infectious or allergic factor.

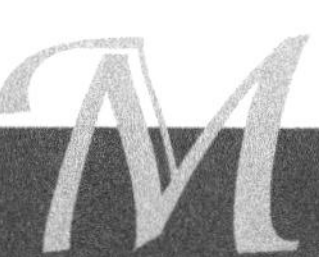

The disease is more common in the colder climates. Those parts of Europe and America north of the 40th parallel have more persons with MS. The location of a person's childhood appears to determine to a large degree the risk one has to develop the disease. This geographical factor may be associated with the greater production of milk and eggs in colder areas.

Something apparently happens early in life to people who live in the tropics so that their immune systems become resistant to MS. Those living in cold climates get the opposite effect on the immune system that makes them susceptible to MS. The immune system can help to reduce over activity in the myelin sheaths of nerves.

Persons habituated to tobacco or those who are exposed to secondhand smoke tend to get more of the central nervous system symptoms of MS.

Development of MS has been associated with many environmental factors, especially occupational exposure to solvents, occupational contact with dogs or cats, leisure-time contact with caged birds, receiving X-ray treatments, and serious previous diseases (*Scandinavian Journal of Work and Environmental Health* 19 [1993]: 399). Another possible relationship is with chlamydia infections.

Viral infections can trigger MS relapses (*Journal of Neurology* 240 [1993]: 417). Perhaps viruses living in animals should have greater attention from researchers. Multiple reports show a correlation between bovine populations, other farm animals, and house pets with MS (*Neuroepidemiology* 12 [1993]: 15; *Journal of the American Medical Association* 238 [August 22, 1977]: 854; *Lancet* 1 [1977]: 980–82). Ninety-two percent of patients with MS had close contact with a house pet in early life, whereas only 48 percent in the control group had similar contact. Especially impressive was the incidence of contact with sick dogs, distemper being most commonly reported in the *Journal of the American Medical Association* study.

MS may be because of a slow virus that acts somewhat after the fashion of polio. Antibodies to distemper virus are found in the blood more in patients with MS than in controls who do not have MS. The distemper virus is related to the human measles virus. Measles virus particles have been found in some individuals with MS, but most authorities believe there is insufficient evidence for accepting the measles virus as the cause. That viruses are involved in the disease, however, seems to be a strong possibility. The use of vaccinations and other sera as a cause of MS has been suggested by the fact that there is often the onset of MS or an exacerbation of MS following the use of a vaccine or some kind of serum.

Inadequate intake of selenium has also been considered in the study of causes of MS. Allergies to gluten and milk have been suspected. The frequent use of NSAIDs in early life, such as aspirin, ibuprofen, indomethacin, etc., also increase the risk for MS. While the highest sources of selenium are seafood and meats, meat is also the primary source of arachidonic acid, which interferes with proper utilization of selenium. Therefore, the best sources are from plants, especially wheat germ, Brazil nuts, apples, red Swiss chard, and oats. Another study showed that eating certain smoked sausages in childhood seemed to increase the risk of developing MS later in life (*Reuters,* June 26, 2002).

People who keep birds as pets are more than twice as likely to develop MS as those who do not (*Ananova,* February 25, 2002). Some wonder if an avian virus could be the culprit.

Some believe that MS is a carrier state of the Sendai virus and that interferon and prostaglandin A-1, along with other prostaglandins, may block the virus replication. There appears to be an immune deficiency in MS so that the virus is not blocked. A young adult who had his tonsils removed as a child is 1.7 times more likely to get MS than a person who did not. Removal of one's tonsils weakens the overall immunity slightly.

Other associated factors have been reported. These include the following: heavy metal poisoning, high-fat diets, low levels of essential fatty acids, overuse of antibiotics, food allergies, childhood infections, carbon monoxide and other environmental poisons, low-level radiation, contraceptive pills, vaccinations, genetic predisposition, and climate and geography.

Symptoms and Signs

The first symptom may be a sudden onset of blindness or weakness of the leg muscles on one or both sides. It may last a week or two and go away, only to reappear a few months or years later. Gradually the leg movements become jerky and spastic, and paralysis eventually occurs.

Another common symptom is slowing of the speech, talking in a monotone with each syllable uttered with great difficulty. The hands tremble, especially on purposeful movement, and the head tends to shake. Eventually such basic functions as sight, hearing, digestion, and control of bladder and bowel movements are involved.

Malabsorption was discovered in 52 patients with MS. A type of sugar called d-xylose was demonstrated to be abnormally low in absorption in 26.6 percent of the patients studied. Fat and meat absorption were abnormal in 41.6 and 40.9 percent, respectively. Stools examined for fat and

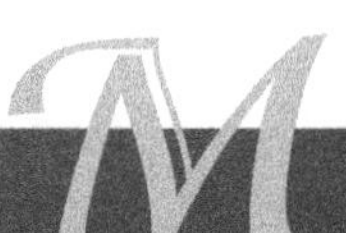

undigested meat fibers were found to be abnormal. Biopsy studies of the jejunal mucosa showed the presence of measles virus antigen in all MS patients studied (*American Journal of Gastroenterology* 68 [1977]: 560–65). It would seem by these studies that a special effort should be made by those with MS to have a healthy digestive tract, to boost the immune system in any way possible, and to ensure proper digestion of fats and absorption of vitamin B12. That would mean eating on schedule, taking two or three dishes only at a meal, using very small amounts if any of watery foods like milk and soup, not eating after about 6:00 p.m., and never lying down after meals. Hot spices and vinegar irritate the digestive tract and should be avoided.

Calcification of the pineal gland has been found in 100 percent of MS patients, and the choroid plexus, a blood vessel cluster in the interior of the brain, was calcified in 72.4 percent (*International Journal of Neuroscience* 61 [1991]: 61).

General Treatment Principles

It is possible to slow down the development of MS. It is not possible with the current knowledge to ensure a cure.

The first line of treatment is to protect a disabled patient from conditions that are especially threatening, such as falling down steps or falling in the shower, etc. Check all the surroundings for safety, going through every room.

On the home remedies front, individuals have claimed benefit or even cure of carefully diagnosed cases from very simple remedies. Unfortunately, many of these home remedies are regarded by some members of the medical profession as useless or even quackery and may be enthusiastically denounced. While I am as opposed to exploitation of a patient under any guise as the most vocal crusader, I have lost the enthusiasm that I had in my youth for fighting harmless "quackery," as I have found through my 55 years of practicing medicine that many things generally relegated to backwoods practitioners when I began in medicine have become main line modes of therapy.

While I would state it differently, I believe as Dr. Michael Halberstam, who states that "among the most precious of patients' rights is the right to make fools of themselves by their own choices." I certainly believe that when dealing with an incurable disease the patient should be encouraged to try any kind of bath, diet, simple exercise, or other non-injurious treatment that he/she feels gives promise of success. No claim of cure or false hope should be held out to the patient, merely a manifestation of interest and assistance.

Certainly it would be well to enhance the immune mechanism by whatever means can be safely applied. A hot bath one to five times weekly, a proper diet, proper exercise, and other important aspects of healthful living are certainly worthwhile. Patients should adjust such matters as clothing, housing, and habits of life to prevent sudden changes in temperature. Changeable weather has been shown to be more important than either hot or cold weather in inducing symptoms. Days with the highest difference between high and low temperatures increase the symptoms. A warm climate and freedom from upper respiratory tract infections coupled with much rest appear to be helpful in the treatment of MS. Very few persons understand that chilling the extremities reduces the defense mechanisms against infection and weakens inflammation and repair. No habitual chilling of skin should be tolerated in a person with MS.

Conventional treatment commonly includes immunosuppressants, immunomodulators, and anti-inflammatory drugs such as steroids. Also used are antispasmodics, anticholinergics (for relief of muscle aches and stiffness), muscle relaxants, antidepressants, and painkillers. Certainly such toxic treatments as methotrexate or cyclophosphamide, which suppress the immune system and cause severe side effects such as vomiting, should be avoided, since the drug is crippling every system that could help the patient.

As many as 30 percent of patients may stabilize with natural treatments after a two-year period and not exhibit a relentless downhill course (*Science News*, April 22, 1989, 135–245). Persons with MS should try a total plant-based diet and fever treatments consisting of fevers going up to 103.6°F daily for five days per week for three weeks, skipping two days after every fifth treatment. They should try taking herbs high in plant sterols including licorice root, red raspberry leaf, black cohosh, squaw vine, ginseng, and ginkgo.

Begin treatment at the earliest warning sign of MS. Persons who experience blindness (optic neuritis) for a few days have a 16.7 percent chance of developing multiple sclerosis within the next two years after experiencing the blindness. With the fever treatments, plant-based diet, and herbal treatments, we expect the percentage to be reduced.

Specific Treatment Suggestions

The first thing to be achieved in a good diet for MS is the permanent and total exclusion of anything that could be considered junk food. The first of these is food high in "free fats," that is, fats not in their natural form, and food containing "free fats." We prescribe a diet entirely devoid of free fats and teach patients how to make the diet palatable with foods

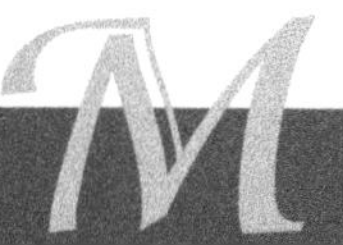

high in natural fats: nuts, seeds, grains, avocados, olives, etc. White sugar has been implicated by several researchers as being a factor in MS. Additionally, anything that can be purchased from a vending machine is almost certainly junk food. TV dinners and similar types of convenience foods should usually be classed as junk foods. There are, however, some foods considered nourishing and good that may not be the best for the person with MS. These will be considered individually.

Beef products, both the flesh as well as dairy milk, should be eliminated from the diet. There is somewhat more than circumstantial evidence for doing so, as MS is higher in heavy beef producing areas. Persons with MS tend to have more antibodies in their blood to beef protein than do persons who do not have MS. Eskimos have very little MS. Perhaps their lack of exposure to beef and dairy products may be helpful in protecting them from a high risk of MS even though they live above the 40th parallel. Of course, since pork is not a good food for healthy persons, all pork and pork products should be eliminated. The most favorable diet is the totally plant-based diet without milk, meat, eggs, or cheese.

The low-fat diet used by Dr. Roy Swank of the University of Oregon Medical School has shown a remarkable benefit for patients, reducing the average number of annual attacks from 1.1 to 0.15 and slowing down the rate at which the disease progressively worsens. Using a modification of Dr. Swank's diet, we have had similar results. We believe that the diet, being simple and easy, is worthwhile. Patients usually lose weight when adopting the diet, but stabilize about 5 to 10 percent below average weight, a good weight for anyone with weak muscles. The diet consists of no free fats (mayonnaise, margarine, fried foods, salad oils, nut butters, and cooking fats) and no heavy natural fats in large quantities (nuts, peanuts, seeds, coconut, wheat germ, etc.) an ounce or two a day being sufficient. The person may take a few olives, avocado, and nuts, but should carefully control the quantity of these items, especially if someone is overweight. Other investigators using a low-fat diet have also reported a reduced frequency of relapses as well as a shortening of the length of the relapses when this diet is carefully followed. Patients with MS should be very careful to avoid rancid foods. Altered fatty acids might have an adverse effect on myelin.

Vegetables and fruit intake should be increased. Patients must be warned against gaining weight and are encouraged to remain lean. Dr. Swank found no severe relapses were ever experienced by a patient who had been on the low-fat diet for as long as one year. The longer the diet is followed the lower the relapse rate. The death rate in untreated MS patients is three to four times higher than in patients on the low-fat diet. The earlier the diagnosis is made and treatment is begun, the greater the success rate.

Linoleic acid, an unsaturated fatty acid present in fruits, vegetables, whole grains, and nuts, appears to improve MS as compared to those receiving oleic acid from olives. Since sunflower kernels are high in linoleic acid, we have at times used a daily portion of one ounce of sunflower seeds for MS patients.

Inositol is a factor especially useful in the early childhood development of myelin. This nutrient is found generously in all fruits and vegetables. It is high in peanuts, cantaloupe, grapefruit and all citrus, whole grains, beans and legumes, yeast, wheat germ, Blackstrap molasses, and nuts. Inositol is almost absent in all foods of animal origin. Some researchers at Vanderbilt University in Nashville, Tennessee, found that turmeric can block the progression of MS (*Reuters*, April 25, 2002). Perhaps its anti-inflammatory features make it helpful. Use one-half to one teaspoon two or three times daily, preferably with meals.

The patient should always maintain a low body weight, which can be figured by allowing 100 pounds for one's first five feet and allowing no more than six or seven pounds per inch thereafter for a man and five pounds per inch thereafter for a women. The patient must exercise daily and follow the eight natural laws of health, which deal with nutrition, exercise, water, sunshine, temperance, fresh air, rest (even taking a nap in the daytime if tired), and trust in divine power.

A low protein diet has been reported by some to improve the general sense of well-being. Adding olives or avocados to the diet may combat dizziness in some patients. A carrot juice fast from time to time may be helpful.

We had one patient who reported that treatment for her candidiasis also helped her MS. Her candida program consisted of being off all salt, taking cold baths, and using all raw foods for three months.

Another patient found that elimination of those foods to which the digestive tract is intolerant resulted in much improvement in symptoms and better general health. This can be discovered by a carefully performed elimination and challenge diet (see "Elimination and Challenge Diet" in the *Dietary Information* section). Maintain the elimination phase for at least three months and preferably six. Then add one food back to the diet every two to three weeks to see if symptoms are worse after adding back the food.

Another study done by Drs. Philip Solomon, Mary Dailey, and Tracy Putnam of Harvard Medical School in Boston City Hospital, and reported in *The American Society*

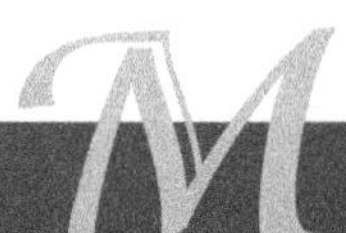

for Clinical Investigation, found that persons with MS had more fibrinogen in the blood than normal persons, which produced a greatly increased clotting threat. MS onset and relapses are often associated with injury, operation, exposure, infection, pregnancy, or high emotional excitement, all of which are known to be associated with an increase in fibrinogen and a slowing of the flow quality of the blood (*Science Newsletter*, May 18, 1935, 315). Therefore, we recommend a reduction in total food intake by about one-third, an increase in outdoor exercise, five ounces of red or purple grape juice twice a day, one clove of garlic twice a day or comparable amounts of capsules or tablets to reduce intravascular clotting and blood viscosity.

Of 144 MS patients who ate absolutely no saturated fat but did eat a small amount of vegetable oils such as olive oil, 95 percent were still alive and physically active at the end of a 34-year study period. In the control group of MS patients who were not on the diet, 83 percent died and most survivors became disabled before the end of the study (*Western Journal of Medicine* 165 [1996]: 320).

Vitamins C and B6, along with zinc and essential fatty acids, such as found in nuts, whole grains, avocados, olives, and various foods from a totally plant-based diet, can assist the immune system. Cold-pressed flaxseed oil is a source of linolenic acid (one teaspoonful per day) and borage seed oil, or oil of evening primrose for linoleic acid, can calm down an inflammatory reaction naturally.

In another study, the addition of only about 8 grams (two and a one-half teaspoons) of saturated fat daily to the diet was accompanied by a very rapid deterioration and by a death rate of 79 percent in MS patients. Persons who follow the low-fat diet very carefully had a death rate of only 31 percent, approximately one-third as high as those not following the diet.

Some have recommended a gluten free diet, which is not difficult to prepare with a little forethought. An article published in the September-October 1952 issue of *Neurology* showed a high percentage of allergic reactions to rye and wheat by individuals with MS. All the gluten grains should be removed as a trial for one to two years. If no improvement is seen, they can be returned to the diet.

Dr. Roy Schwank found small fibrin clots without red blood cells entrapped in small capillary beds. These were associated with inflammation in nearby tissues close to nerve trunks. Since a high intake of free fats, the use of alcoholic drinks, and inadequately cooked grains are associated with a similar response, the proper cooking of grains is recommended for MS patients as well as to other persons to ensure that all has been done possible to prevent the disease. That means boiling rice three hours at a gentle simmer; oatmeal 90 minutes; and millet for three hours. Oven baked grains and waffles need browning on all sides.

It has been suggested that a deficiency of B12 may be linked with MS. A vitamin B12 deficiency was associated in 10 cases of MS. Only two of the 10 patients had pernicious anemia. In the remaining patients the B12 deficiency was unexplained. A B12 binding or transport defect was suspected (*Journal of the American Medical Association*, October 23, 1991, 266 (16:2210). We recommend a plant-based diet which makes the patient require less B12. A supplement of B12 should be given to see if improvement occurs. Malabsorption of B12 was found in 11.9 percent of cases.

Vitamin D may be useful in the treatment of MS. The disease has a very low incidence near the equator, but as the latitude increases northerly, the incidence of MS also increases. Persons living at higher altitudes also tend to have less MS. One explanation is that ultraviolet light intensity is greater at high altitudes, resulting in an increased vitamin D3 synthesis rate. Vitamin D may help prevent, as well as treat, MS. Vitamin D3 in the hormonal form has completely prevented the experimental autoimmune encephalomyelitis that in mice resembles human MS. As a general rule, the MS patient should get as much sun as possible. Recommendations for dosage are that adults should get at least 1,000 IU of vitamin D daily, or a lot of sunlight exposure during the summer, which enables storage of vitamin D for winter use.

Alcohol along with tobacco must be avoided. They are neurotoxins and should not be used.

We believe the group of methylxanthine-containing drinks (coffee, tea, colas, and chocolate) should be carefully eliminated. The methylxanthines have a toxic effect on the nervous system. It is not known if they play any part in the development of MS, but certain serious diseases are associated with their use: mental depression; unsteady balance; cancers of the bladder, ovaries, prostate, and pancreas; and injury to unborn babies, etc. In Scotland where a high tea, high gluten diet is common, the incidence of MS is high.

Use fever treatments in an effort to slow down the progress of the disease. On the other hand, use cold baths to temporarily strengthen muscles, allowing a short period of more vigorous exercise in order to prevent muscular atrophy. In the fever baths, try to achieve a temperature level of 103°F to 104°F rectally, holding for 30 to 60 minutes, three to five times weekly for about 20 treatments.

Use a bathtub of hot water at 102°F to 110°F depending on the vigor of the patient and how well heat is enjoyed. A thermometer is placed in the mouth while the temperature

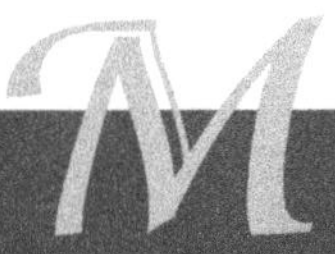

is going up. Someone should be *constantly* with the person since weakness may develop quickly as the mouth temperature goes up and the head could slip down into the water. The mouth temperature may be allowed to rise to 102°F or 103°F, 103°F to 104°F if rectal temperature is measured. This can usually be accomplished in 10 to 20 minutes with a nice soak in the hot tub. When patients have been treated with hot baths and are being returned to their baseline temperature, their performance of muscular tasks at the same temperature is significantly better when the temperature is coming down than when it was going up, indicating some improvement in tolerance to heat, although mainly temporary.

There are certain cells in the brain or spinal cord known as astrocytes that form fibers that make a sort of scar tissue in the central nervous system. These scar cells grow in on a nerve, which has had myelin damage. Heat is believed by some to loosen already formed scar tissue and to reduce the amount of inflammation so that scar tissue formation will be less. This is one reason we use the fever treatments.

The use of cold applications in the management of spasticity or muscle weakness can assist patients to carry out exercise and self-care programs in a more active and functional manner. Techniques for applications of the cold vary somewhat. Moist cold is more effective than a dry bag filled with ice. Heat is not as successful in the treatment of spasticity or in reducing the weakness. Cold applications consisting of crushed ice wrapped in wet towels placed over spastic groups of muscles for 10 minutes should be followed by exercise of the muscles, or groups of muscles, as they will be temporarily stronger after cooling. The favorable effects may last for as long as 12 hours.

Another method of applying the cold is by immersion of an extremity in cold water at 50°F for 10 minutes followed by exercise of the part. Injuries and MS have been successfully treated in this way. To immerse a patient in a tank of water at 80°F for 10 minutes can increase movement and reduce the stretch reflex. Thirty percent of patients derived little or no prolonged benefits from cold therapy, but the remaining seventy percent received considerable help, which could be measured from day to day.

There are some cases of MS that have been thought to start during periods of violent exercising. While the benefits of exercise in the treatment of MS have been clearly demonstrated, we urge patients not to engage in too vigorous exercise when the disease is in an acute stage. With chronic disease, however, moderate exercise must be promoted. Prolonged inactivity in persons with MS plays a large part in the progressive deterioration in muscle strength. Patients should keep active but should not exceed their strength. To go beyond the bounds of reason in exercise is never wise.

A program of exercise improves both the physical condition as well as the mood. Patients doing arm and leg exercises for 40 minutes three times a week for 15 weeks had greater extremity strength, improved blood profiles, and less depression and anger than non-exercisers. Exercising patients have a better long-term outcome of multiple sclerosis (*Annals of Neurology* 39 [April 1996]: 432–41).

Bee venom, using one to 20 bee stings at a time, after building up one's tolerance, has been reported by several naturopaths to be very helpful. I have had no experience with the use of bee venom in MS. Royal jelly has also been thought to help repair the myelin sheaths. Those who have used this type of treatment are so strong in recommending it that I would probably give it a try if I had MS.

External application of magnetic fields has been found to be helpful in some cases of MS, and has even included complete remission. A 50-year-old woman with a 15-year history of chronic progressive MS in whom a magnetic field was applied over her scalp with small magnets received a "dramatic and sustained improvement in disability." It was felt that the pineal gland had an influence on the brain to produce a remarkably effective treatment from a weak magnetic field. The researchers felt that the pineal gland was a key player in the production of MS in the body and that the placement of the magnets over the scalp had an influence on the pineal gland (*International Journal of Neuroscience* 66 [1992]: 237–50).

Since the cause of MS is not known for certain, whether it is an infectious agent, a toxic substance, or an autoimmune disorder, the treatment should address each of these. Charcoal can be given by mouth to prevent toxic substances capable of being adsorbed by charcoal from being free in the body.

Garlic and cilantro taken with meals can help eliminate heavy metals from the body. Use one to three teaspoons of garlic powder and a sprig or two of cilantro with each meal. Echinacea, chaparral, and golden seal tea as well as hot baths will help combat an infectious agent. Autoimmune disorders should be treated by strict adherence to all the laws of health. Childbirth and major surgery should be avoided as much as possible by those suspected of early stages of MS as these have at times been suspected of precipitating the onset of symptoms.

MS and Milk Connection

MS is more common in milk-drinking populations. It is interesting to note that Eskimos and Bantus (50 million living in East Africa) rarely get MS. Neither do those native

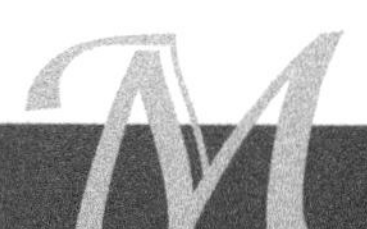

North and South American Indian or Asian populations that consume no dairy products.

Dr. John McDougall cites the British medical journal *Lancet* in pointing out that a diet filled with dairy products has been linked to the development of MS (*Lancet* 2 [1974]: 1061).

A worldwide study revealed an association between eating dairy foods (cow's milk, ice cream, baby formula, cheeses, butter, and cream) and an increased prevalence of MS (*Neuroepidemiology* 11 [1992]: 304–12).

Dr. Michael Dosch and his team of researchers have determined that multiple sclerosis and type I (juvenile) diabetes mellitus are far more closely linked than previously thought. Dosch attributes exposure to cow's milk protein as a risk factor in the development of both diseases for people who are genetically susceptible (*Journal of Immunology*, April 1, 2001; *New England Journal of Medicine,* July 30, 1992; *Lancet,* October 1996).

Dr. Frank Oski reported in his book, *Don't Drink Your Milk,* that a low incidence of MS correlated most strikingly with a relatively low per capita milk consumption. He reports several studies revealing the same findings.

Mumps

Mumps is a swelling and inflammation of the salivary glands, which causes the jaws to round off the corners of the jawbones, a helpful diagnostic sign. Mumps usually attacks children between ages 5 and 15, more commonly in the early winter and spring. The mouth temperature may rise to 101°F to 104°F, and the fever and swelling usually subside within 7 to 10 days. The infection usually comes on an average of 18 days after exposure to a person with mumps, but may come on as early as 12 days, and as late as 26 days. When adults are infected, the complications tend to be more serious and the disease itself is more intense.

Complications, while rare, include inflammation of the testes or ovaries, brain, heart, or other glands such as the pancreas, thyroid, and lymph nodes; deafness; arthritis; kidney disease; and loss of the sense of smell. Type I diabetes is 2.3 times more likely to occur in persons having mumps in the previous six months.

Treatment

Ensure an adequate fluid intake and a very simple diet free from refined sugars, free fats, and concentrated proteins. Spicy, sour, or irritating foods, and those requiring a lot of chewing, should be avoided to reduce pain.

The complications can be reduced and recovery encouraged by giving fever baths, bringing the mouth temperature up to 102°F once a day for five or six days.

A warm tub soak may be used in fevers to redistribute the circulation, reduce restlessness, and diminish pain.

Cold or hot compresses applied to the neck and jaw will also often relieve pain.

Treat inflammation of the testes or other abdominal pain following the procedures in the "Inflammation" entry in the Conditions and Diseases section.

Protect from chilling or excessive exercise.

Muscle Cramps

A magnesium deficiency can cause muscle cramps. A magnesium deficiency can be the result of using refined carbohydrates, drinking alcohol, or an inherited tendency to malabsorption. Food sources high in magnesium are as follows: all nuts and seeds and whole grains, all common legumes, carob, greens, beets, and squash.

Leg cramps, or other muscle cramps, at night or while in bed are not related to circulation but to reflex spasms from chilling, or occasionally from excessive loss of sodium, magnesium, and potassium by heavy sweating.

Cramps in a muscle can be relieved by extending the muscle if it is in a position to do so or rubbing the muscle until the cramp releases. Cramps in the calf that occur at night can be prevented by the following wall-stretching exercise three times a day for 30 days, and then once a week thereafter. Stand facing a wall and step backward about two feet. Brace the hands on the wall at shoulder height and lean the chest directly into the wall while keeping the feet flat on the floor and allowing the hips to sag a bit. Hold that position for 10 seconds, then repeat three times. In addition, wear warm socks or stockings above the knees to prevent a fall in temperature of the legs at night.

For cramps of the abdominal muscles or feet muscles, applications of heat are beneficial.

If these measures are not applicable or not possible, pinch the upper lip close to the nose and push upward into the nostrils for two to three minutes. It must be painful in order to be effective.

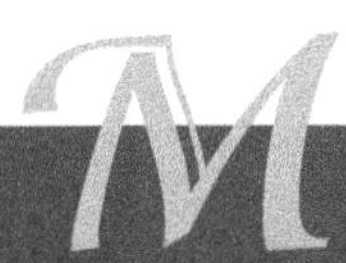

Muscular Dystrophy

This disorder refers to a group of hereditary muscle diseases having the principle feature of relentless muscular weakness. Death of muscle cells and tissue can be expected. More than 100 diseases have similarities to muscular dystrophy. Most types of MD have manifestations in multiple body systems including the heart, gastrointestinal and nervous systems, endocrine glands, skin, eyes, and brain. Mood swings and learning difficulties will be seen at times in some forms of this disease.

While muscular dystrophy has no known cure, there are several things that can be done to slow the progression of the disorder and reduce symptoms such as pain.

- Eat a plant-based diet, low or devoid of free fats. A pastor with another kind of muscle disorder told me he received benefits with a plant-based diet, and it may help the classical Duchenne muscular dystrophy as well.
- Take 300 to 1,000 milligrams of CoQ10 daily. Research done at the University of Texas on 12 muscular dystrophy patients ages 7 to 69 showed an interesting response. They were given CoQ10 for at least three months, and it was found that there was a measurable improvement of the symptoms of muscular dystrophy. It may be that giving 300 milligrams daily would give more marked improvement than with 100 milligrams daily, as given by the researchers at the University of Texas. The administration of CoQ10 may need to be long-term, or even ongoing, process as long as the patient lives (*Biochimica et Biophysica Act* 1271 [1995]: 281–86).
- Braces to keep the spine and ankles straight can be helpful to prevent discomfort and keep the person mobile longer.

Myasthenia Gravis

Myasthenia gravis (MG) is a chronic autoimmune neuromuscular disease characterized by varying degrees of weakness of the skeletal (voluntary) muscles of the body. The hallmark of myasthenia gravis is muscle weakness that increases during periods of activity and improves after periods of rest. Muscles that control eye and eyelid movements, facial expression, chewing, talking, and swallowing are often,

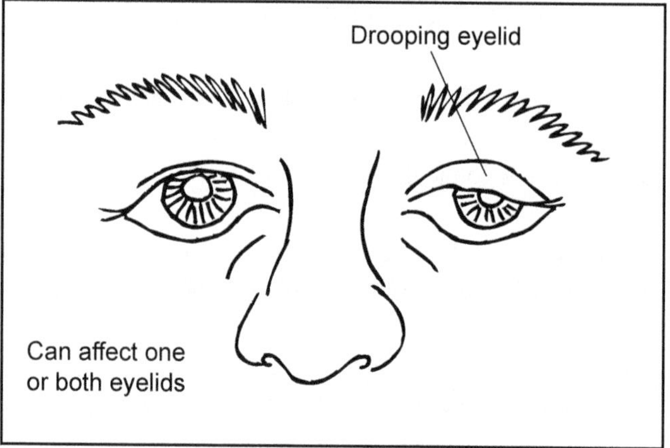

but not always, involved. The muscles that control breathing and neck and limb movements may also be affected.

Myasthenia gravis is caused by a defect in the transmission of nerve impulses to muscles. Normally, when impulses travel down the nerve, the nerve endings release a neurotransmitter substance called acetylcholine. In myasthenia gravis, antibodies produced by the body's own immune system block, alter, or destroy the receptors for acetylcholine. The first noticeable symptoms of myasthenia gravis may be weakness of the eye muscles, difficulty in swallowing, or slurred speech. Symptoms vary in type and severity. Myasthenia gravis is not directly inherited nor is it contagious. The first steps in diagnosing myasthenia gravis include a review of the individual's medical history and physical and neurological examinations. If the doctor suspects myasthenia gravis, several diagnostic tests are available to confirm the diagnosis, including a special blood test that can detect the presence of immune molecules or acetylcholine receptor antibodies.

Treatment

Acceptable treatments include fever baths; plant-based diet, perhaps trying an elimination diet to see if the patient is stronger without certain foods (even a fast might be revealing); massage; anticancer herbal products; anti-inflammatory herbals; and antimicrobial herbals.

Myasthenia gravis can often be controlled by supplements and certain drugs that may improve neuromuscular transmission and increase muscle strength. Some of these drugs may suppress the production of abnormal antibodies. These medications must be used with careful medical follow-up because they are powerful and may cause major side effects.

Thymectomy, the surgical removal of the thymus gland, improves symptoms in certain patients and may cure some individuals, possibly by rebalancing the immune system. Other therapies include plasmapheresis, a procedure in which

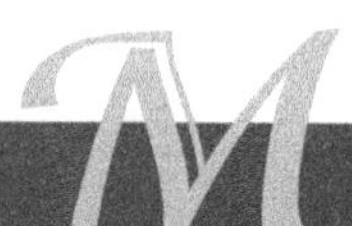

abnormal antibodies are removed from the blood, and high-doses intravenously of immune globulin, which temporarily modifies the immune system and provides the body with normal antibodies from donated blood.

Prognosis

With treatment, the outlook for most patients with myasthenia is bright. They can expect to lead normal or nearly normal lives. Some cases of myasthenia gravis may go into remission temporarily, and muscle weakness may disappear so that medications can be discontinued. In a few cases, the severe weakness of myasthenia gravis may cause respiratory failure, which requires immediate emergency medical care.

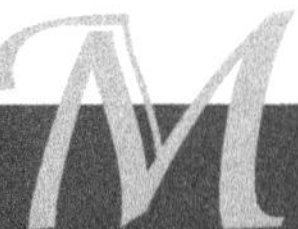

Narcolepsy, Drowsiness

Attacks of uncontrollable sleep may have an association with cataplexy (temporary paralysis of facial muscles and limbs, occurring during emotional states such as laughing, anger, fright, a startling noise, crying, or while one is falling asleep or awakening—the so-called "sleep paralysis"). Men are affected more than women, the condition beginning in late childhood or early adult life. The incidence of narcolepsy is about four out of 10,000 people. Sleep may occur in unusual situations such as while standing or carrying on a conversation. The knees may give way, and the person may fall to the ground without losing consciousness.

Narcolepsy often occurs in persons suffering certain brain diseases or serious head injuries. Some cases are hereditary. While working at something that commands the interest, the person can stay awake, but when left alone or lying down, the person quickly falls asleep. Characteristic of the sleep is that REM sleep occurs almost immediately after falling asleep. Hallucinations may occur during the REM sleep.

Most cases of drowsiness during the day are not because of narcolepsy, but because of chronic loss of sleep, which is cumulative and may require weeks or months to "catch up." Other cases may be because of sleep apnea. About 70 percent of narcolepsy patients have sleep paralysis as well as uncontrollable sleepiness. Attacks may become less frequent with age, and no other neurologic abnormality is associated or develops later.

Treatment

The patient should get a laboratory thyroid panel, a chemistry profile, and hormone tests to evaluate the adrenals. Get a very good laboratory evaluation of your glucose processing. Ideal fasting levels of blood glucose range from 70 to 85. Levels of homocysteine and blood insulin should be obtained. If the homocysteine is above 12 and the fasting blood insulin above 20, a program for treatment of diabetes should be designed. A level of hemoglobin A-1C may also be revealing of an abnormality.

Check your hematocrit. If it is over 42 for a man, 37 for a woman, donate a unit of blood to the Red Cross every six weeks, if you are eligible, until it is below the above figures. Changing the viscosity of the blood might be helpful. Drinking around 10 eight-ounce glasses of water daily will also thin the blood a small amount.

For a trial period of two months, try eliminating all salt and other very concentrated additives—all free fats, honey, malt, meat substitutes, vitamin and mineral preparations, and all chemical additives, including baking powder. A door-to-door book salesperson once told me she became much less drowsy and "foggy-brained" when she left off free fats (margarine, mayonnaise, fried foods, cooking fats, salad oils, and peanut butter). It had become such a problem that she would go to sleep while the people were filling out their checks to pay for the books she sold them.

Try a period of fasting in a supportive environment, without stress or regular work. Break the fast correctly with fruits only in the beginning, taking as many days to break the fast as you remained in the fast. Start with small mono-meals (only one food served), then bi-meals, then non-gluten grains added, and then the gluten grains, and at last soy. Example of the mono-meal would be simply a pear, a bi-meal, pear and kiwi, etc. Give only two meals daily for six weeks.

In some people, food sensitivities cause extreme drowsiness (See "Elimination and Challenge Diet" in the *Dietary Information* section). There are some foods known to be associated with drowsiness—onions, garlic, sugar, fats, too many varieties of food at a meal, etc. Try a mono-diet for two or three weeks—a bowl of peaches at a meal, along with some dried peaches, peach leather, peach butter, a peach frappe, etc. The next meal would be another food in many forms such as rice, split peas, or squash. If certain foods are found to be followed by sleepiness, eliminate those foods for a year before eating them again. A full fast may be preferred, drinking only water for five days. If the sleepiness disappears by the fifth day of the fast, you have shown that a food sensitivity is the cause of the narcolepsy. If this is the case, start adding back only one food at a time as in the mono-diet described above to determine which food is causing the sensitivity.

If overweight, bring the weight to normal or slightly below. Check to see if snoring is a factor resulting in poor sleep at night. A positive pressure machine to eliminate snoring may eliminate daytime drowsiness.

Try to eliminate toxins from the body by breathing fresh air, drinking only pure water, and eating only high-quality foods, up to 80 percent of which can be taken raw. Take a dose of milk thistle four times a day.

Many researchers on sleep pathologies suggest several naps during the day. The best time for naps is probably for 10 to 30 minutes before meals. Get a stop watch or timer with an alarm so you can wake up. Take a 10 to 20 minute nap midmorning, and again in the midafternoon.

Go to bed early and get at least three continuous hours of sleep before midnight. Get seven to eight hours of sleep or more every night.

Go to bed every night at close to 8:00 o'clock if you have a sleep disorder, capitalizing on the good quality sleep that is possible before midnight. Allow little or no deviation in the schedule.

Massage can be considered part of exercise. We would suggest you get somebody to do an experiment for you. Do a tapotement on your back over the adrenals for about one minute each side, followed by cupping or slapping. This small treatment may be capable of eliminating sleepiness for half an hour or more.

The "sick building syndrome" is the culprit in some people's drowsiness. Are you as drowsy out of doors as inside? Sit up very straight and take deep breaths to shake drowsiness. Breathe almost twice as fast as would be usual for a few seconds.

Temperance should be practiced in all your projects, not just in eating and sleeping. Do not prolong time spent in a project for hours unrelentingly, but break every hour for about five minutes of change of activity,—it is best to get a little exercise during the break.

Herbal Remedies

Persons suffering from extreme drowsiness should try all herbs known to have an influence on the nervous system—lobelia, catnip, mint, golden seal, white willow bark, licorice root, gingko, kava, St. John's wort, valerian, lemon balm, rosemary, sage, hops, and skullcap to mention a few. Our reasoning here for using both sedative and stimulating herbs considers the use of amphetamines (one of the "uppers") for their opposite effect in some cases of hyperactivity in children. It might be that in some persons with narcolepsy there would also be a paradoxical reaction.

A naturopath suggests licorice root twice a day, half a teaspoon in a cup of boiling water; allow to cool for 10 to 15 minutes, stir and drink it all. He also suggests liquid kelp, several drops under the tongue several times daily. If it will help, you should see the difference within a week.

I suggest a heaping tablespoon of charcoal powder three times daily for a six-week trial. This substance adsorbs toxins, which can cause sleepiness in some people.

Include in herbal remedies the use of borage, ginseng, gotu kola, and echinacea root. Other herbal remedies to be tried are bee pollen, barley green, and garlic.

Nausea

Nausea is an uneasiness in the stomach that often precedes vomiting, the forcible voluntary or involuntary emptying of the stomach, which is commonly known as throwing up.

A cold compress on the forehead, some fruit juice poured over crushed ice, a juice slushy, or going out on a cold winter morning for a breath of cold air can all quell nausea.

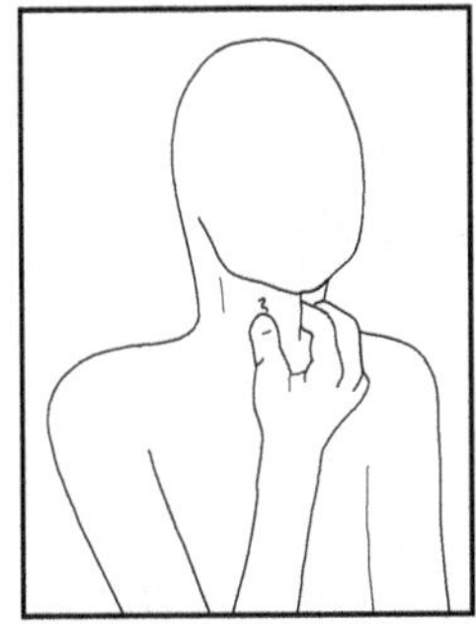

Tilt the head backward and press on the hyoid bone (the U shaped bone in the front of the neck just above the voice box). Press this bone upward but not backward. With the head thrown back, maintain this position for 60 to 90 seconds, and repeat if necessary to stop nausea.

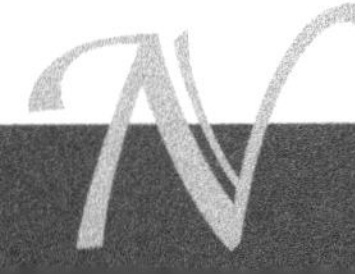

Powdered ginger can be used in quantities not to exceed about one-half to one teaspoon per dose. Measure one teaspoon of the powder into a small cup of water or juice. Take one-fourth of this amount four times daily or until the nausea is gone. Do not use for long periods—more than one to three months—as it may irritate the stomach. You may use it during pregnancy and for occasional use in motion sickness. No side effects have been reported other than an occasional stomachache. It is also effective in controlling nausea after anesthesia or from narcotics. If you want to use fresh ginger, grate or slice about one tablespoon of raw ginger into one cup of water and simmer it for 15 minutes or more. A sip or two may be all that is necessary to quell nausea, or the entire cup may be drunk if necessary.

For nausea, lavender aroma may be very helpful. Moisten a cotton sponge with lavender oil and pin it to the clothing or pillowcase.

Some herbalists say that a cup of red raspberry leaf tea or basil leaf tea will quell even the most violent vomiting and nausea. Other anti-nausea herbs include anise, blackberry, black cohosh, chamomile, fennel, sage, pekoe, etc.

Peppermint or spearmint tea first thing in the morning can be helpful for nausea and vomiting. You can also wet the tip of the finger with mint oil and lick it. This is a very good remedy for nausea and motion sickness. (See "Motion Sickness" in the *Conditions and Diseases* section.)

Peach tree leaves are useful in the treatment of nausea, especially the nausea of pregnancy. Take a double handful of the fresh leaves and simmer gently in two quarts of water. Strain and store the tea in a refrigerator. Use a tablespoon of the tea at anytime nausea is felt. You may take a tablespoonful as often as every 30 minutes, but do not exceed two cups per day as it may cause a stomachache.

Neck Pain

Keep the posture of the head and neck, shoulders and upper back in the "neutral position" while standing, sitting, or lying. Proper posture will go far toward preventing neck pain. Sleep with a pillow that suits your anatomy and sleeping habits. A buckwheat pillow, or similar pillow from a department store, such as used in the Orient, will abolish neck pain for many sufferers.

Do not roll the head around in full circles unless you are certain this will not stress the joint that is causing pain. The best and safest exercises in neck pain are the isometric kind in which your neck muscles are tensed without moving the head. This can be done by standing or sitting upright and pressing your head for 10 seconds against the palm of your hand, first in front, then on each side in turn, and then against the clasped hands in back. The hand is held immobile and not allowed to move with the pressure of the head. Make the pressure as hard as you are able, and hold it about five seconds. Repeat this exercise in all four areas four times daily.

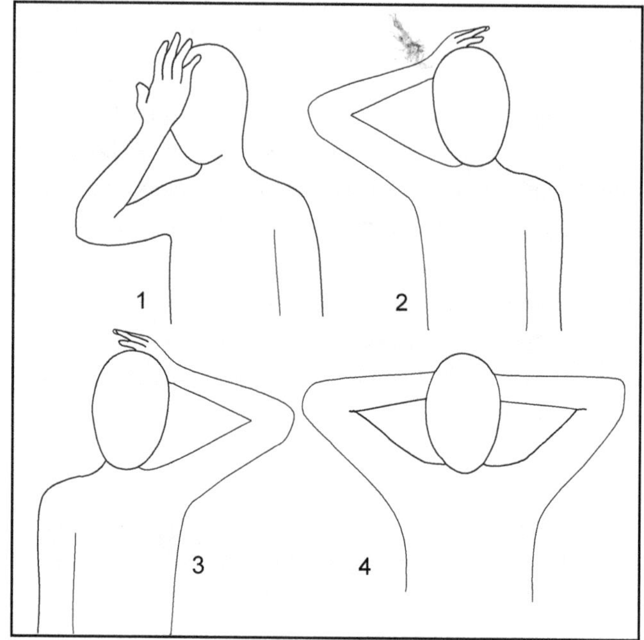

Neurologic Disorders

In a study of 147 patients with different kinds of nerve disorders (53 of which were of unknown origin), some British researchers found that gluten sensitivity was a major factor. In most cases the gluten sensitivity or allergy was undiagnosed previously. Of the 53 with nerve disorders of unknown origin, 30 patients (57 percent) had antibodies to gluten in their bloodstream compared to only 12 percent of persons not having a nerve disorder. Most of these 30 had signs of upper intestinal tract problems, indicating allergies or celiac disease ("Does Cryptic Gluten Sensitivity Play a Part in Neurologic Illness?", *Lancet* 347 [February 10, 1996]: 369–71).

If you have any kind of neurologic disorder, from neuropathy or essential tremor to multiple sclerosis, try a gluten-free diet.

Night Sweats

Night sweats often occur because of improper respiration—heavy snoring, breathing too shallowly, or too infrequently. (See "Sleep" in the *Conditions and Diseases* section for treatment information for sleep apnea and other breathing problems.)

Nosebleeds

(See "Hemorrhage" in the *Conditions and Diseases* section.)

Numbness

There are a number of causes for numbness, such as:

- Excessive and prolonged pressure on nerves caused by the following factors:
    - Posture in bed while sleeping
    - Kneeling for prolonged periods
    - Sitting in such a position that a body part presses on another body part or a part of nearby furniture
    - Constrictive clothing or gear
- Diabetic neuropathy
- Back injury
- Slipped disc

To treat numbness, remove the causes as much as possible. If because of pressure, massage the opposite side of the body while lightly rubbing the area of numbness. In this way a sympathetic reflex increases the circulation and promotes healing.

- Treat diabetic neuropathy by getting the diabetes under control. Good control of diabetes can go far toward curing the numbness. (See "Diabetes" in the *Conditions and Diseases* section.)
- Give myoinositol, a nutrient found abundantly in cantaloupe, beans, grapefruit, peanuts, all citrus, and whole grains.

Nutrient Deficiency

The physical signs listed below are to be regarded as indications that malnutrition may be a problem. The list is presented by specific body parts.

Skull

Finding: In infants, rounded thickenings typically on both sides of the forehead, the sides of the head, or both, usually on both sides, delayed closure of the fontanel (soft spot) later than two years.

Cause: Lack of vitamin D and calcium. May also be caused by syphilis, sickle cell disease, or "sleep position deformity."

Hair

Finding: Dry, wire-like hair, stiff, unkempt, often brittle, or fine, thin, and easily pluckable with some bleaching of normal color.

Cause: Protein-calorie deficiency. May also be caused by low thyroid condition.

Face

Finding: Greasy rash in the crease beside the nose and mouth

Cause: Lack of niacin, riboflavin, pyridoxine

Eyes

Finding #1: Thickened, dull, opaque conjunctivae (linings of eyes). Conjunctivae may appear to be wrinkled, with increased blood vessels, or glazed, sometimes obscuring vision.

Cause: Lack of vitamin A

✦✦✦

Finding #2: Rash of angles of the eyelids.

Cause: Lack of niacin and riboflavin

✦✦✦

Finding #3: Bitot's spots. These are small, rounded, grayish or yellowish, dull, dry, foamy, superficial lesions, most frequently seen on the whites of the eyes. Some have likened the appearance of the rounded spots to lemon meringue.

Cause: Lack of vitamin A

Lips

Finding #1: Rash and swelling of the lips. Lips may be so swollen that the inside mucosa is everted and broken.

Cause: Lack of niacin and/or riboflavin

Finding #2: Cracks at the corners of the lips

Cause: Lack of niacin, riboflavin, iron, or B6

Teeth

Finding: Mottled enamel

Cause: Fluorine excess

Gums

Finding: Spongy, bleeding gums

Cause: Lack of vitamin C. (May also be because of dilantin therapy for epilepsy.)

Tongue

Finding #1: Red, smooth, sore tongue

Cause: Lack of folic acid, niacin, riboflavin, vitamin B12, pyridoxine, iron, or tryptophan

Comment: The tongue is often beefy red, painful, and may be fissured and grooved. There may be serrations on the sides of the tongue or swellings; when swollen, there are tooth impressions at the edges. May have magenta hue in riboflavin deficiency. Symptoms of hypersensitivity of the tongue, burning, and changes in taste sensation almost always occur.

Finding #2: Filiform papillary atrophy

Cause: Lack of niacin, folic acid, B12, chronic iron deficiency. Sometimes seen in well-nourished patients wearing dentures.

Comment: Filiform papillae are low or absent, giving a smooth or slick appearance of the back of the tongue. The appearance remains after scraping lightly with an applicator stick.

Neck

Finding: Goiter

Cause: Lack of iodine

Comment: Endemic in regions lacking iodine in soil and water supply. Incidence is increasing in some localities.

Skin and Extremities

Finding #1: Follicular hyperkeratosis (thickening and roughening of hair follicles)

Cause: Lack of vitamin A or insufficient unsaturated fatty acids

Comment: Skin is rough because of keratotic plugs protruding from hair follicles. More readily detected by touch than by sight. Surrounding skin is dry, distinguishing it from adolescent folliculosis in which skin between lesions is normal or oily. Does not disappear on brisk rubbing or warming.

Finding #2: Hyperpigmentation

Cause: Celiac sprue, starvation; or lack of B12, folic acid, or niacin

Comment: Seen more on hands and face than on trunk. Hairy surfaces of hands darker than palmar.

Finding #3: Scrotal dermatitis

Cause: Lack of riboflavin

Comment: Occurs in protected, moist area, where skin may become slick, red, and wet

Finding #4: Enlarged liver

Cause: Chronic malnutrition

Finding #5: Scurvy, ecchymosis (spots appearing bruised)

Cause: Lack of vitamins C and K

Comment: Occurs at pressure areas. Scurvy, however, is unlikely if the patient has eaten even a limited assortment of vegetables and fruit.

✦ ✦ ✦

Finding #6: Pellagra dermatitis, diarrhea, dementia (the "Three Ds")
Cause: Lack of niacin and tryptophan
Comment: Skin lesions are symmetrical and in areas generally exposed to sun. They are characterized by redness, blister formation, dry, cracking, burnlike appearance, hyperpigmentation, sharp margins, and flaking. Often associated with deficiency of riboflavin and other B vitamins.

✦ ✦ ✦

Finding #7: Bilateral edema of the lower extremities
Cause: Lack of protein. (There are several other causes also of swelling of the legs and feet)

✦ ✦ ✦

Finding #8: Thickening of long bones near their ends (called epiphyses); seen on X-ray
Cause: Lack of vitamins D and C and calcium
Comment: In rickets there is epiphyseal hyperplasia. In scurvy there is tenderness and swelling because of subperiosteal hemorrhage.

✦ ✦ ✦

Finding #9: Rachitic rosary, a string of lumps beside the breastbone on each rib where the rib joins the breastbone at the cartilage.
Cause: Lack of vitamin D and calcium

✦ ✦ ✦

Finding #10: Bowlegs
Cause: Lack of vitamin D and calcium
Comment: Deformity develops when weight is borne by poorly calcified long bones.

✦ ✦ ✦

Finding #11: Calf tenderness found by squeezing calf muscles between thumb and fingers
Cause: Lack of thiamin

✦ ✦ ✦

Finding #12: Absence of vibratory sense
Cause: Lack of thiamin and vitamin B12
Comment: Significant only if absent bilaterally. The way to find this is by striking a large tuning fork and holding it only on the rounded end you are touching. Then feel the vibration on the end you hold, touch this end to the kneecaps, the shinbones, the anklebones, and the big toes. The vibration should be felt in all these areas if it is strong enough to be felt by the fingers and thumb of the examiner, which should be placed on the skin near the place where the tuning fork touches.

✦ ✦ ✦

Finding #13: Absent tendon reflexes, knee jerks
Cause: Lack of thiamin and vitamin B12
Comment: Significant of vitamin deficiency only if absent on both sides

✦ ✦ ✦

Finding #14: Thickened skin at pressure points
Cause: Lack of niacin
Comment: May occur in pellagra or psoriasis. Noted at belt area, over the bones of the seat, the sacrum, and bones on each side of the hips.

✦ ✦ ✦

Finding #15: Spoon nails (koilonychia)
Cause: Lack of iron
Comment: Nails are thin, concave or spoon-like, seen in chronic iron deficiency anemia.

Obesity

(See "Weight Control" in the *Conditions and Diseases* section.)

Osgood-Schlatter Disease

(See "Skeletal Problems" in the *Conditions and Diseases* section.)

Osteogenesis Imperfecta Tarda

(See "Skeletal Problems" in the *Conditions and Diseases* section.)

Osteomyelitis

Osteomyelitis is a bone infection that can occur in tooth abscesses or any deep-seated chronic infection. (See also "Dental Care" in the *Conditions and Diseases* section.) If nutrient reserves are good, do a water fast for three days, followed by a juice fast of 10 days. During the fast, drink the following herbal antimicrobial formula. Mix one quart of water with two tablespoons of echinacea herb and two tablespoons of golden seal powder. Simmer gently for 25 minutes, and give half a cup every two hours. Then get a tincture of the combination of usnea and wild indigo. Use one teaspoon of this tincture along with the echinacea and golden seal. All of these should be given every two hours around the clock. Osteomyelitis is difficult to deal with and must be carefully and faithfully treated. Also put a comfrey root poultice over the area and change every four hours.

Contrast soaks using charcoal in one tub and Epsom salts in the second tub, five minutes in the warm and one minute in the cold, repeated every four hours, can be beneficial. Read the case report below.

Case Report

A 55-year-old diabetic was treated for osteomyelitis and a non-healing ulcer on the foot. It was foul-smelling and non-tender, with no feeling in her feet. We began charcoal soaks immediately in water at 102°F, contrasting with cold at 70°F for one minute. We gave her echinacea and golden seal tea every two hours around the clock for two weeks, along with a tincture of usnea and wild indigo, then reducing the frequency to only daylight hours for two weeks. We continued these treatments for another two months, reducing the frequency again to only four exchanges daily and four doses of the herbs. X-rays at that time revealed no osteomyelitis; the ulcer, however, was still present, but showing gradual healing around the edges. The patient rejoiced that we had not only gotten her diabetes under control but had also saved her from amputation. She lost 50 pounds during this time.

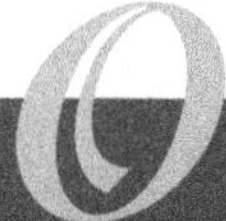

Osteoporosis

Osteoporosis is a thinning of the bones, 90 percent of which occurs in women past middle age. It is a disease of excessive demineralization of the bone, which typically begins in both sexes after age 35.

While men are less affected, by age 75 the gap closes where both genders become equally prone for bone loss. Bone loss increases the chance of breaking a bone, which leads to all kinds of other problems in the elderly. For example, it is estimated that 20 percent of patients die within one year of a hip fracture, 50 percent can no longer walk without assistance, and 25 percent may have to be institutionalized in long-term care facilities.

Bone is composed of two types of tissue, the one being the outside, solid cortical tissue, while the other the interior, the connecting lacework structure supporting the bone marrow, called trabecular or spongy bone. In the early stages of osteoporosis this lacework structure of trabecular bone may already be damaged; however, bone density tests would not show anything abnormal because the bone mass obtained from cortical bone makes it appear to be the same. Trabecular bone has a turnover rate of about 25 percent, in contrast to about 3 percent of cortical bone undergoing remodeling every year. Bone remodeling is a process, in which the adult skeleton undergoes a continuous turnover, and old bone is resorbed by osteoclasts and new bone is formed by osteoblasts.

The United States leads the world in the incidence of osteoporosis, but we also lead the world in the intake of dairy calcium. Although it is taught that calcium makes bones strong, increased calcium intake from milk has been shown in some studies to be associated with increased osteoporosis. The American Dietetics Association guidelines and Minimum Daily Recommendations are set based on pressures from various commercial concerns. The currently recommended 1,000 to 1,500 milligrams of calcium per day is two to four times the calcium that most of the world consumes every day. Actual daily calcium intake does not need to be more than 250 to 350 milligrams, and some doctors claim that it can be as low as 130 milligrams Saying that one should take 1,000 to 1,500 milligrams almost mandates that a person overeat or take calcium supplements. Usually only about 30 percent of the calcium we eat is absorbed. But when needed, as for bone repair after a fracture, we can double or nearly triple the absorption. The calcium supplement industry is a hundred-million-dollar-a-year industry. One can see why pushing calcium supplements can have such power.

Many individuals rely on extra amounts of calcium plus vitamin D when trying to treat and/or prevent osteopenia (early stages of bone loss) or osteoporosis, and when unsuccessful, they generally resort to using drugs specifically formulated to stop the progression of this disease. These drugs possess serious potential for side effects. The long-term effect of many of these medications is still unclear since increased bone mass doesn't always translate into increased bone strength. On the other hand when analyzing individual reasons for developing osteoporosis, it becomes clear that most factors can be resolved through a change in lifestyle or through *individually*-tailored nutritional supplementation.

Some recommend estrogen treatment for osteoporosis. We do not do so, as the Centers for Disease Control in early 1992 issued a statement that if a woman takes estrogen for as long as 15 years, she has a 30 percent increased risk in developing breast cancer. There is also a 5 percent increased risk of getting hypertension, and a two-fold risk of getting gallstones. "Since women lose trabecular bone in their 20s and 30s, a time in life when estrogen is plentiful, it is difficult to see that bone loss is caused by low estrogen" (*Archives of Internal Medicine* 143 [1983]: 657).

Vegetarians who reach approximately 69 years of age appear to suffer no further decline in bone density, whereas in meat eaters, bone loss continues.

Hip Fractures Worldwide

Women of:	Rate/100,000	Daily Dairy, gm/day	Protein, gm/day
USA	102	462	106
New Zealand	97	480	112
Israel	70	315	105
Singapore	15	113	82
Bantu	5	10	47

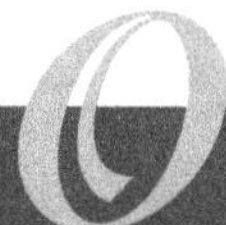

Calcium Overload

Calcium overload is a serious threat to many women. As calcium is moved into the blood from the food, into the bones from the blood, and out in the urine because of too much protein, many body cells are potentially injured by these transfers. Too much calcium can cause constipation and stomach upset. It may block the absorption of other critical minerals, especially zinc and iron. The kidneys can be damaged by too much calcium and can also cause formation of kidney stones. Men who take a high calcium intake are more prone to prostate cancer (*Newsweek,* August 14, 2000).

There are a number of concerns over taking calcium supplements:

- It increases the risk of kidney stones.
- Many calcium supplements also contain vitamin D supplements, the most toxic of the vitamins in over dosage. To prevent over dosage, add all the vitamin D you get from all foods to which it is added and all supplements you take that contain Vitamin D. Avoid a total intake of more than 2,000 to 4,000 i.u. per day.
- When you double the amount of calcium, there is actually decreased bone strength, as has been shown in studies with pigs at the University of Chicago.
- Induced internal bleeding. Vitamin K should always be given with calcium supplements to enhance calcium absorption.
- Calcium carbonate causes constipation and calcium gluconate causes diarrhea.
- Oyster shells are common sources of calcium supplements. Oyster shells are sometimes added to soy milk. You must read the labels in order to protect yourself.
- Calcium supplementation decreases iron absorption. This same seesaw relationship occurs with supplementation of many nutrients.

A woman taking orange juice, cereal, milk, muffins, and margarine for breakfast, plus a Centrum Complete multivitamin and a Viactive Calcium Chew may get as much as 2,400 milligrams of calcium at that one meal. Since some women take a supplement of 1,000 milligrams or more, a woman can quickly become overloaded.

One of the dangers of long-term estrogen therapy is increased cancer risk. Contraindications for taking estrogen include such side effects as endometrial cancer, phlebitis, weight gain, high blood pressure, jaundice, vaginal candidiasis, depression, skin rashes, hair loss, nausea, vomiting, abdominal cramps, cysts, and many more.

Causes

Causes of osteoporosis include a decrease in osteoblast function, a change in parathyroid activity as a compensatory factor for decreased calcium absorption, and usually a combination of either less sun exposure and/or a decreased ability to synthesize vitamin D, or insufficient dietary intake of vitamin D. Additional causes include sedentary lifestyles, which play a significant part, and there are less-common genetic factors, while insufficient sex hormones and body weight (anorexia), various drugs, (glucocorticoids, caffeine, alcohol, etc.), hyperthyroidism, and kidney disease are also contributing factors.

A number of hormones, including thyroid, parathyroid, sex hormones, vitamin D3, and others exert their influence on bone remodeling and interact with immune system proteins such as interleukin-6 (IL-6). Their production in turn is inhibited by estrogen and testosterone, so there is evidence that the balance of sex hormones and interleukin-6 affects trabecular bone loss. Research also implicates the same mechanism as a potential cause of some forms of hyperthyroidism, hyperparathyroidism, rheumatoid arthritis, Paget's disease, multiple myeloma, and others.

Stomach acid is another very important aspect with osteoporosis through its implication on calcium and magnesium levels, whereby high acid levels encourage calcium loss and low levels promote excessive calcium storage (calcification, spurs, etc.), resulting in bio-unavailability of calcium. Both extremes—too much or too little stomach acid—have an unfavorable impact on osteoporosis.

Treatment

Diet

In 119 elderly women 26.9 percent were found to be vitamin D deficient. Following a gluten-free diet for five years, individuals who already had the diagnosis of osteoporosis improved bone mineral density significantly. Celiac disease patients respond more briskly.

The plant-based diet is the most favorable diet for both prevention as well as treatment of osteoporosis. It is naturally high in all those substances needed for good bone health such as zinc and calcium, and is naturally low in those substances causing osteoporosis such as protein, aluminates, phosphates, and purines. A study showed that neither cortical nor trabecular bone density in post menopausal women suffered because

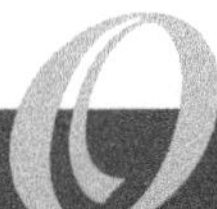

of the vegetarian diet (*American Journal of Clinical Nutrition* 56, no. 4 [1992]: 699–704).

Peak bone mass occurs at between the ages of 25 and 35. After that bones begin to get lighter gradually throughout life, accelerating at about the age of 50. In assessing whether one has osteoporosis, bone mass per se is less important than whether the person has been having fractures. The best way to ensure against fractures is to ensure adequate bone growth and peak bone mass during the time the bone mass is being accumulated, up to the age of 35. For daily calcium intake, one cup of cooked broccoli, or any of its relatives, or tofu (four ounces) have enough calcium to meet your needs.

Certain vegetables have been shown to reduce bone resorption in laboratory rats. Onions, ordinary and Italian parsley, lettuce, tomato, cucumber, garlic (cultivated and wild), and dill were all effective in slowing bone resorption (*Nature* 401 [1999]: 343; *Journal of Clinical Investigation* 95, no. 4 [April 1995]: 1933–40).

Prunes seem to have a positive effect on bones in postmenopausal women by increasing the bone mineral density.

Eat a low protein diet, as the kidneys excrete large amounts of calcium through the urine to balance and neutralize the high sulfuric acid from protein. A significant treatment for osteoporosis, as well as preventive maintenance for any person, is a low protein diet. Many clinical nutritionists are now recommending the low protein diet for problems other than osteoporosis. Low fat means eliminating almost entirely, or even completely if the weight demands it, all free fats such as margarine, mayonnaise, fried foods, salad oils, and cooking fats. Eliminate nut butters until the weight is desirable. This diet is most helpful in menopause, both for the hot flashes and preventing osteoporosis. Low fat consuming women who eat no animal protein or animal fat whatsoever, do not have evidence of essential fatty acid deficiency and have a very low rate of osteoporosis.

A salty diet can be a cause of osteoporosis. The National Academy of Sciences regards 1,800 milligrams of sodium (3,600 milligrams of salt) to be the safe upper limit for daily consumption. More than 1,800 milligrams of sodium daily can endanger your bones and cause you to get osteoporosis (*Lancet* 350 [1997]: 1702). A surprisingly large amount of salt can be found in items that do not taste salty—cakes, desserts, breakfast cereals, soft drinks, tomato juice, processed meats, etc. It usually surprises people to learn that depending on commercial foods almost always leads to excessive salt in the diet. The best way to prepare food is "from the ground up," so that you know just how much salt, sugar, etc., has been used in the diet.

The bio-availability of calcium from vegetable sources is greater than from milk in many, if not most, instances. A study of the absorption of calcium from kale revealed 40.9 percent as compared to the absorption from milk of 32.1 percent. Calcium bio-availability depends on the following factors:

- The forms and the quantity of calcium contained in the food eaten.
- The losses from the bowel such as can occur when there is an increase in phosphorous, protein, sodium, etc.
- The metabolic losses because of the use of tobacco, caffeine, acid diet, etc.
- Oxalates and phytate-rich grains have only a minimal effect on calcium levels in humans. The human intestine is not the same as animal intestines on this matter. Lactose is not a determinant of calcium absorption as was once thought. Calcium from greens, vegetables, fruit, and beans is absorbed as well as calcium from milk.

If a calcium supplement is taken, it may decrease the availability of copper and increase cholesterol. Calcium supplements also decrease iron retention, increasing the risk of iron deficiency anemia.

While she was a medical student at Loma Linda University, Susan Hall did a study on 800 postmenopausal women, which revealed that those whose diets contained high levels of vitamin C had denser bones. For each additional 100 milligrams of vitamin C taken in the diet, bone density increased 2 to 2.5 percent. A three percent increase in bone density reduces the risk of hip fracture by 50 percent. Taking calcium supplements does not produce the same effect.

The following list of foods shows the amont of calcium in a one cup (8 oz.) serving. For comparison, one cup of dairy milk contains 288 milligrams of calcium.

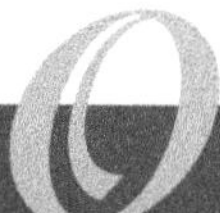

Source	Calcium (mg/serving)
Seaweed	**1,000–3,500**
Sesame seed	**2,100**
Turnip greens	**450**
Collards	**360**
Bok choy	**330**
Almonds	**330**
Tofu	**290**
Chinese cabbage	**250**
Spinach	**250**
Kale	**200**
Parsley	**200**
Mustard	**180**
Dandelion greens, raw	**150**
Okra	**150**
Figs	**78**
Bread	**50–90**
Soy sprouts, raw	**50**
Lettuce, raw Romaine	**40**
Strawberries	**31**
Alfalfa sprouts, raw	**25**
Beans and peas	**20 for split peas to 130 for soybeans**
Lettuce, raw head	**10**

A study done at the University of North Carolina showed vegetarians maintain strong bones in later life better than non-vegetarians. No statistical differences were identified between bone mineral mass in lacto-ovo-vegetarian and omnivorous males in any decade of life examined (ages 20 to 79). There is an indication that some factor associated with meat consumption increases bone mineral loss in postmenopausal females without observable effects in males (*American Journal of Clinical Nutrition* 37 [1983]: 453–56).

Gamma linolenic acid (GLA) and eicosapentaenoic acid (EPA) are both known to increase calcium content in bones (*What Doctors Don't Tell You* 6, no. 12 [April 1996]: 1–3). Food sources for gamma linolenic acid are spirulina and hemp seed.

Boron is one of the minerals essential for strong bones. Boron helps to prevent calcium loss by assisting in the conversion of cholesterol to vitamin D3, which stabilizes calcium.

Boron supplements have been used by some to increase the deposition of calcium in the bones. It also stimulates the production of very tiny amounts of estrogen, even in women who have gone through menopause or who have had a hysterectomy. Take 2 or 3 milligrams per day.

Magnesium is needed to stimulate the absorption of calcium into the bones and is as important to bone strength as calcium. Taking a magnesium supplement of 365 milligrams daily or more slowed down the bone turnover and bone loss that is associated with age-related osteoporosis (*Journal of Clinical Endocrinological Metabolism* 83, no. 8 [1998]: 2742–48).

One of the isoflavones found in soybeans is called ipriflavone and is most effective in treating osteoporosis. It increases the activity of osteoblasts (bone-building cells) and decreases the activity of cells that break bones down (osteoclasts). Bone density can actually be increased by taking soybeans daily. Eat one-fourth cup of cooked soybeans per day.

Soybeans increase the density of bone, even after osteoporosis has been diagnosed (*Integrative Medicine Consult* 1, no. 5 [1999]: 43). The beneficial factor appears to reside in the protein, but the more refined the protein, the less likely it is to be effective. Soy products that contain only purified protein derivative and a lot of sugar and fat will not be effective and may even be harmful.

Source	Boron (mg/100g)
Raisins	**4.51**
Almond	**2.82**
Hazel Nuts	**2.77**
Apricots (dried)	**2.11**
Avocado	**2.06**
Peanut Butter	**1.92**
Brazil Nuts	**1.72**
Walnut	**1.63**
Beans (red kidney)	**1.40**
Prunes	**1.18**
Cashew Nuts (raw)	**1.15**
Dates	**1.08**
Lentils	**0.74**
Chick Peas	**0.71**
Peach	**0.52**
Celery	**0.50**
Grapes (red)	**0.50**
Honey	**0.50**
Olive	**0.35**
Apple (red)	**0.32**
Bran (wheat)	**0.32**
Pear	**0.32**

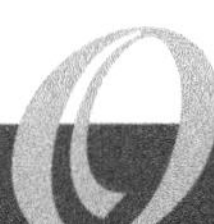

Source	Boron (mg/100g)
Broccoli	0.31
Carrot	0.30
Orange	0.25
Onion	0.20
Potato	0.18
Banana	0.16

Zinc and copper are essential to good bone health and can be found in whole white potatoes. As the quantity of whole dried white potatoes increased in the diet of experimental rats, the levels of zinc and copper increased linearly. High levels of vitamin D3, however, can interact with white potatoes to decrease levels of zinc and copper.

Manganese deficiency is a greater problem now than in the past and may be one of the most important causes of osteoporosis, diabetes, and infertility. In addition, vitamin B6 is an essential factor in bone production. (See "Food Sources of Certain Nutrients" in the *Dietary Information* section.)

Exercise

Get plenty of exercise. Every time a muscle is moved, it puts a bit of stress on a bone. The bone then sends a signal to the intestinal tract to absorb more calcium. That calcium is then deposited in the bone that was moved. The bones of every post-menopausal woman need a daily shakeup. Following are special exercises that can prevent humpback.

- The elbow touching exercise at shoulder height, both in front and in the rear.
- Maintenance of good posture by holding the head high, having the cheek bones directly over the collar bones, and keeping the shoulders in place.
- Strong back extensor muscles can help prevent vertebral fractures in women with (*Mayo Clinical Proceedings* 71 [1996]: 951). Strenuous exercise helps in remodeling mature bone. Even after osteoporosis has developed, strenuous exercise can be of help in strengthening the bones (*Journal of Experimental Biology* 170 [1992]: 1–18).

Older people fall more and get hurt more often. It is believed that taking medications is one of the causes of loss of balance. Failure to be physically fit is another cause of loss of balance and falls. The best preventive measure for osteoporosis is still exercise. It greatly reduces the risk of falling. The determinant for osteoporosis is the amount of exercise the person has had. Daily exercise at a moderate rate, outdoors if possible, for 30 to 60 minutes is minimal.

Sunlight

Sunlight exposure strengthens the bones. Every day at least 10 minutes of sunlight exposure should be obtained, even if the body is fully clothed. The benefits of sunshine are stored, making it unnecessary to get sunshine on consecutive days.

Herbs

Red clover tea, containing calcium and a good form of phosphorous, strengthens bones and teeth. A nice cup of red clover tea three or four times daily would be good for osteoporosis.

Grow or gather wild pigweed to provide an easily digestible source of calcium. This herbal plant is tasty when steamed, in the same manner you would prepare spinach, and it has a high calcium content to strengthen your bones. Nutritionists suggest that getting vitamins and minerals from our diet is the most effective method of nutrient absorption.

Use dried horsetail as a tea, or fill capsules with the herb and take two to four daily. Research indicates that horsetail, which contains silicon, protects bones from calcium loss.

Gather some dandelion leaves and add them to steamed cabbage or steam them alone. Dandelion greens contain high levels of boron, known to strengthen bone density. Make a daily green smoothie to boost your overall health and provide bone-enriching nutrients. Combine alfalfa leaves with the previously mentioned herbs. Mix everything with a littlerapple or pineapple juice.

Fracture Risks

Women who have five or more of the following risk factors, regardless of bone density, have a 10 percent chance of breaking a hip in the next five years, while those with two or fewer risk factors have only a 1 percent chance of doing so.

- Taking tranquilizers or sleeping pills
- Smoking
- Having vision problems such as poor depth perception
- A past history of having an overactive thyroid gland
- Being tall, especially if also thin and blond
- Being unable to get out of a chair without holding onto the arms
- Having a high pulse rate (above 80)

A 1996 panel discussion by the National Women's Health Network found that low bone density is not a good

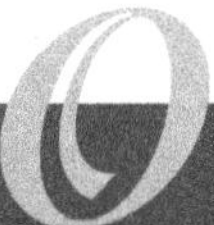

predictor of bone fractures. Better predictors are advanced age accompanied by poor muscle strength or the use of regular medication of any kind. The benzodiazepine drugs, such as Restoril, Versed, Halcion, Xanax, and Valium, have, in fact, been found to increase the risk of hip fracture by up to 70 percent (*Journal of the American Medical Association,* 1989, abstracted in *New York Times*, April 12, 1996).

Eskimos have the highest rate of osteoporosis in the United States. Yet they take between 1500 to 2500 milligrams of calcium per day, but they also take in 250 to 400 grams of protein per day, which increases excretion of calcium. Each gram of protein in the diet causes the body to lose 1.5 milligrams of calcium. Foods that are high in protein include all animal products (meat, milk, eggs, and cheese), protein concentrates such as meat substitutes, and artificial milk powders using soy protein isolates.

The massive Harvard Nurses' Health Study, including 77,761 women ages 34 to 59, followed for 12 years, showed that those who drank more dairy milk actually had slightly more fractures of bones compared to those who drank little or no milk (*American Journal of Public Health* 87 [1997]: 992–7). A similar study done in Sydney, Australia, showed that individuals with the highest dairy product consumption had approximately double the risk of hip fracture compared with those with the lowest milk consumption (*American Journal of Epidemiology* 39 [1994]: 493–503).

In addition to a high intake of protein, there are other well known causes of osteoporosis. A high phosphate intake is one. Foods that are high in phosphates are those using baking powder (half of the baking powders sold in the United States are phosphate based, and the other half are aluminate, also a cause of osteoporosis), processed meats, red meats, brewer's yeast, detergents, instant soups, soft drinks, and processed cheeses. All dairy products are high in phosphate.

Another known risk factor for fractures is that of the use of coffee and its relatives—tea, colas, and chocolate. One or more cups per day of any of these beverages will cause a woman after the age of 50 to lose up to 1.4 percent of her bone calcium per year. From age 50 to 60 she could lose 14 percent of her bone calcium from this one source.

Other foods that encourage osteoporosis are those high in sugar, salt, and purines (which cause an elevation in uric acid, a known cause of osteoporosis).

Medications can cause osteoporosis, as can the use of alcohol, any form of steroids such as cortisone and prednisone, heparin, birth control pills, and the unnecessary use of thyroid hormone supplement. The high intake of vitamins A and D by supplementation can also cause osteoporosis. For every milligram increase in daily intake of supplemental vitamin A, the risk for hip fracture increased in one study by 68 percent (*Annals of Internal Medicine* 129, no. 10 [1998]: 770).

Other fracture causes are subtotal gastrectomy, smoking (causes 1 percent loss of bone substance per year past the age of 50), pancreatic disease, liver disease, high cholesterol or triglycerides, Gaucher's disease, Caisson's disease, and having a diet deficient in zinc, boron, or magnesium.

A study of 500 Australians 65 or older demonstrated that smoking, being overweight at age 20, underweight in old age, and having a high consumption of dairy products at age 20 all increase the risk of hip fracture in old age. Previous studies had identified risk factors as being caucasian, physical inactivity, taking many medications, drinking caffeinated drinks, smoking, and ingesting a high amount of calcium from dairy sources instead of plant foods (confirmed by at least seven earlier studies) (*American Journal of Epidemiology* 139 [1994]: 493–503).

If by your 40th birthday more than half of your hair has become gray your chances of developing osteoporosis increase four fold (*Cutis* 55, no. 3 [1995]: 145). That puts a premium on getting plenty of exercise and having a plant-based diet.

Starting menstrual periods at an early age increases the likelihood a woman will develop osteoporosis prior to menopause (*Journal of Bone and Mineral Research* 8, no. 1 [August 1993]: S340). This research calls into question whether having menstrual cycles has a true influence on osteoporosis. Perhaps surgical menopause, which causes a slight increase in the rate of osteoporosis development, is because of the forced immobilization from surgery, and the postoperative slump in athletic activities, which is often permanent.

A study done in London showed that women with osteoporosis tended to have low levels of alkaline phosphatase, an enzyme necessary for bone formation. Women with the lowest levels of alkaline phosphatase were, interestingly, women who were on hormone replacement therapy (HRT). Fluoride inhibits formation of alkaline phosphatase, and magnesium is required to activate alkaline phosphatase. Two groups of women were given either HRT or magnesium supplementation for nine months. Their bone densities were compared, and it was found that the magnesium supplemented women showed an 11 percent increase in bone density, while those on HRT showed none.

Taking large quantities of cider vinegar has been associated with osteoporosis.

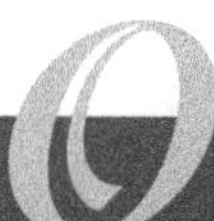

Alum in foods such as baked goods, pickles, and aluminum salts from any source can leach minerals out of the bone, and are an important source of lost minerals.

Antacids containing aluminum, as well as tetracycline type antibiotics can cause osteoporosis.

Thyroid supplements, even average levels of thyroid hormone replacement have been associated with significantly less bone density in the hips, pelvis, and arms of women taking the hormone than those not taking it (*Journal of the American Medical Association* 265, no. 20: 2688–91). Unless a woman is distinctly below normal in thyroid function, she should not be given a supplement. (See "Thyroid Disease" in the *Conditions and Diseases* section.)

Cadmium, a contaminant in refined carbohydrate foods and in tobacco smoke, displaces calcium from the bones. Exposure to environmental cadmium is a significant predictor of bone fractures, osteoporosis, and height loss. For women, a two-fold increase in cadmium excretion in urine gives a 73 percent increased risk of fractured bones. Very low levels of cadmium exposure are sufficient to bring about such a result (*Lancet* 353 [1999]: 1140). One place of cadmium exposure are areas bordering on zinc smelting plants. Refined grains and junk foods also have significant cadmium as a contaminant of processing.

People with iron overload will deposit iron in the bones as well as in other tissues, especially the heart and liver. The iron in the bones causes calcium loss and osteoporosis (*British Medical Journal* 319 [1999]: 1432).

Anorexia nervosa is notorious for causing osteoporosis.

Low sodium in the blood can cause a significant loss of surefootedness and falls with fractures. It should not be overlooked when a person falls that the cause of the fall may have been low sodium in the blood which cases unsteadiness, attention deficits, and potential falls (*The American Journal of Medicine* 119, no. 7A [July 2006]: S83).

Side Effects of Fosamax

Fosamax is a major drug used to treat osteoporosis, but it has a number of drawbacks, one being that the drug must be used for a long period of time to gain the supposed maximum benefit, possibly as long as 20 years. Long-term side effects of the drug and its long-term safety are completely unknown. At least some of the drug stays in the bone as long as the woman lives, even if the drug is stopped. No one knows what that does to bones. No studies are available on patients taking Fosamax for a long period of time. Following are a number of side effects:

1. Irritation of the esophagus and stomach in some cases with ulcer and esophageal stricture
2. Increased blood levels of the drug to the level of toxicity if there is reduced kidney function
3. Patient must not smoke or use alcohol, as tobacco and alcohol react with the drug
4. Glandular tumors and thyroid adenomas have been reported as well as mutations in hamster ovary cells
5. There is an increase in fetal deaths and reduced weight gain in rat pups with delayed delivery of pregnant rats, and an increase of maternal deaths in rats
6. Nausea and vomiting, dyspepsia, gas, constipation, diarrhea, acid regurgitation, difficulty in swallowing
7. Muscle pain or cramping
8. Headaches, dizziness, taste perversion, and other neurologic difficulties
9. Skin problems including rash and hives
10. Inflammation of the eye
11. A softening of the lower jaw sometimes occurs in those taking Fosamax and is greatly feared by dentists who find complications of dental work done on women taking Fosamax may be more frequent

Otitis Media

(See "Earache, Otitis Media, Mastoiditis" in the *Conditions and Diseases* section.)

Ovarian Cysts

(See "Women's Conditions and Diseases" in the *Conditions and Diseases* section.)

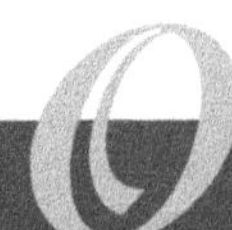

Pain Control

Pain is a problem influenced by many factors simultaneously. The fact that deep frontal lobotomy, surgically cutting across the front lobes of the brain, will block pain is evidence that the frontal lobes of the brain are somehow placed right in the middle of pain perception and are able to influence it greatly. This explains how martyrs can think, sing, and even preach right up to the very last breath. Their frontal lobes can disconnect if the spiritual stimulus is strong enough.

Bear in mind that pain is closely tied in with many body systems—immune, endocrine, cardiac, blood-making, stomach and bowels, mental, and chemical—therefore, physical fitness helps significantly in dealing with pain. The modalities you have available are heat, cold, total body immersion in a neutral bath, a hot foot bath, a cold mitten friction to the extremities, massage, and herbal remedies.

It is the work of Satan to cause pain in the world. He frequently provokes others to be his agents to increase pain. When Peter denied Christ, he caused Jesus great pain. And on the cross when He had taken our sins on Himself, the feeling of rejection by His Father caused Jesus intense anguish. The addition of mental anguish to physical pain causes a patient who develops a sense of rejection to believe the trials are more than can be tolerated, and the whole situation is expressed simply as an increase in physical pain. Jesus is a perfect example of dealing with pain, as well as the solution for pain and for sin. "The first thing to be done is to ascertain the true character of the sickness and then go to work intelligently to remove the cause" (Ellen G. White, *The Ministry of Healing*, 235). Reassurance is needed that one can bear the pain and that God loves him or her.

Relatives and friends can influence pain. If the patient is kindly and tenderly regarded by members of the family, if special efforts are put forth to make everything comfortable that can be comfortable, even the painful part will seem to give less pain. If family members are unsympathetic, incommunicable, or indifferent to the needs of the patient, the parts of the brain that sense discomfort will go into high gear, and pain may become unbearable. Everyone should plan thoughtful little remembrances for the patient.

Pain always carries an associated ministry, both to and from people who have it. Those who are in pain must learn to be patient and kind even when the mind is distracted and the energies have been depleted by long-continued discomfort. There is never an excuse for irritability or harshness. The patient can make nursing duties more pleasant by making a thoughtful effort to consider the feelings of those who perform the duties.

Adverse Reactions to Aspirin

We have become known as the chemical society. Many of our prominent diseases are intimately associated, often in a way that we do not realize, with our exposure to chemicals of various kinds from kitchen detergents and exhaust fumes to powerful drugs like cortisone. Our exposure to chemicals is so common that we do not recognize that a number of these chemicals are causing us injury. We become so accustomed to contact with chemicals and drugs that we have idiomatic expressions in our language such as "harmless as aspirin" using a common chemical as a prototype of harmless things.

We should not regard any exposure to a chemical that is not native to the body or the natural environment as being

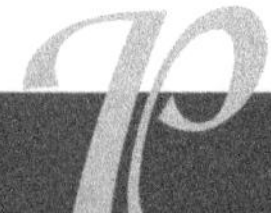

harmless or to be used safely without restraint. Aspirin is particularly harmful, and should be looked on with strong suspicion. About 10,000 Americans each year lose their lives because of taking NSAID's such as aspirin. These deaths are entirely separate from accidental overdose. Aspirin is the common name for acetylsalicylic acid. The naturally occurring salicylate in herbs, methylsalicylate, does not cause toxicity unless taken in a very concentrated form called oil of wintergreen. This form is toxic in large quantities (two tablespoons for a child and six for adults.) There have been no recorded toxicities to methylsalicylate despite its widespread use as far back as records go in the Alabama Poison Control Center. At the same time, hundreds of cases of aspirin poisoning have occurred.

Approximately 17,500 tons of aspirin are used for pain relief and fever each year, to the tune of $600 million a year. Acetaminophen (Tylenol) is used similarly, but contrary to earlier advertising, it appears to be even more toxic than aspirin. I agree with the many physicians who feel that aspirin should be a controlled prescription item, not an over-the-counter drug.

Approximately 5 percent of persons taking aspirin will have heartburn after a single dose. Bleeding in the stomach and ulceration may follow and is the affliction that results in most of the deaths from aspirin. Nearly 70 percent of persons taking aspirin daily show a daily blood loss of one-half to one and a half teaspoons from the bowels, and 10 percent of patients lose as much as two teaspoons of blood daily. Aspirin may double the time necessary for human blood to clot, increasing the likelihood of hemorrhage. In the elderly, taking aspirin can result in a major brain hemorrhage, a disabling stroke, or death.

One of the most adverse reactions to aspirin is asthma. Attacks of asthma are often caused by very small amounts of the drug and may be accompanied by swelling of the larynx, abdominal pain, and shock. In an occasional case (in less than 0.2 percent), death may occur within minutes.

Aspirin is a major cause of drug death in American children up to 6 years of age, accounting for more than 500 deaths each year. Reducing childhood fevers artificially with drugs results in longer absence from school and more complications. The immune system is weakened by the drug. One should never consider any drug, whether over-the-counter or prescription, to be totally safe. No one, and especially not children, should be exposed unnecessarily to any drug. And, if possible, never expose the unborn baby to drugs, no matter how mild, including antacids used for heartburn, antihistamines for morning sickness or motion sickness, or any other drug or chemical. This point cannot be emphasized too strongly as many infants are marked for life because of a small exposure to a drug that the mother took while she was pregnant. Often the defect in the child is of a biochemical nature rather than a deformity. For example, the baby may not be able to make a certain enzyme needed to digest a particular nutrient or make an essential blood component.

Even with all the risks noted here, many people continue to take aspirin every day, thinking that it's worth taking these risks because of believing it protects from heart attacks and stroke. It is ironic that more and more research points to the fact the taking aspirin every day can actually increase the risk of heart attack or stroke in up to 40 percent of the population. Because certain people actually have faster clotting time on aspirin than without it, making them more susceptible to heart attacks and stroke. The research on this was done by Dr. Michael Buchanan of McMaster University in Hamilton, Ontario.

Alternatives to Drugs

Research reveals that endorphin (naturally produced morphine) levels are lower in chronic pain sufferers, indicating that, either they are low producers, or the endorphins are used up in the pain process. Since endorphins work to modify pain and reduce its severity, it would be well for chronic pain sufferers to try to increase production of endorphins by exercising, fasting, engaging in social activities, being creative, and working to help the poor and needy. Avoidance of certain foods known to reduce endorphins—high fats, alcohol, caffeine, and excessive quantities of salt—also helps. The use of anti-inflammatory herbal remedies, such as feverfew, ginger, flaxseed, and hawthorn berry; going to bed at the same hour around 8:00 to 9:30 p.m.; getting eight to nine hours of sleep at night; and a short nap (five to fifteen minutes) about half an hour before lunch, and again in the midafternoon, can also help raise endorphin levels.

Try one thing after another. Don't be disappointed if one thing doesn't work because another will. The pharmaceutical pain-controlling drugs eventually lose their effectiveness, more and more of the drug being required until no amount works short of anesthesia, and then the patient merely becomes hysterical with as much pain as at the first. At this point, the simple remedies may not be as effective to overpower the drugs and the patient is not in control of the body or emotions. If this possibility can be avoided, it is well worth a lot of effort.

Check yourself for food sensitivities, which increase pain, especially caffeinated beverages, spices, and the

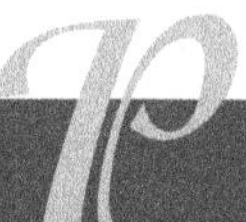

nightshades (solanine is the offending chemical in these foods and is found in tomatoes, potatoes, eggplant, and peppers).

Twenty cherries contain between 12 and 25 milligrams of anthocyanins, a dose more effective than aspirin in relieving pain, especially in gout (*Nutrition Week* 29 [March 12, 1999]: 7).

Never overeat, as overeating intensifies pain.

Massage is a very good remedy. It is more beneficial than most people understand. It is comforting, soothing, and gives the sense that someone is near who can help (*Applied Nursing Research* 3 [1990]: 140; *Lancet* 334 [1992]: 1514). Be as kind and affectionate as it is appropriate to be, paying tender attentions to the person. If a patient has a cancer you can see or feel, do not massage it directly, as squeezing might cause the cancer to spread.

A foot rub is helpful. Work especially on any areas where there is tension or tenderness. The feet are often tense when another part of the body is in pain, and a foot rub will relax these areas.

Try ice massage. Freeze a disposable foam cup with water in it. After it has become solid take it out of the freezer and peel off the bottom end of the cup to expose the ice. Use the top part as an insulated holder. Block off the area with towels to catch the runoff water. Move the ice over the area making small circles, and tearing off more of the cup as the ice melts. Massage for 12 to 20 minutes.

Some people get good relief even from the pain of kidney stones, cancer, or sciatica, by lying for hours in a warm bath. If relief is not obtained, try increasing the temperature of the water. Put music on and listen to something enjoyable to help you pass the time. Kidney pain can be relieved by a heating pad.

Blocking pain in nearby tissues by a cold compress or ice applied over a nerve will also relieve pain, as will helping the patient to understand what is being done, what his pain means, and what is being contemplated.

Water itself has good pain-relieving properties. One glassful every 10 minutes for an hour is very helpful for backache, knee pain, and the pain of childbirth (*American Journal of Obstetrics and Gynecology* 64 [1991]: 1277).

When all else fails, take a plain, hot-water enema. It can give several hours relief and can help you sleep. The water should be no hotter than water you could drink.

If you are able to, walk. Exercise is good for many types of pain because it releases natural pain relieving endorphins. If you cannot walk outside, lie outdoors in an area protected from the wind and where the sun is not too hot. Sunshine penetrating through your clothing into the painful area can bring relief. Sunbathing on bare skin is also an excellent pain remedy.

Counter-irritation can relieve pain. The drugstore has a topical ointment called Zostrix made from capsicum, red pepper, or cayenne pepper. Use it six times a day for pain relief. There is a substance in it that ties up P-substance, the neurotransmitter that sends pain messages to the brain. It may take 5 to 10 days of applying it before you experience pain relief. As soon as you get relief, you can start using it only two times a day. You can make similar product at home with the same active ingredient and good effect. Here is the recipe: Make a tincture by putting a cup of rubbing alcohol in a pint jar with one teaspoon of cayenne pepper. Swirl it once daily for three weeks. You may start using it immediately, however. Rub it on the areas where pain is felt six times a day for the first six days, then twice a day thereafter. As long as you keep using it, the pain will stay away.

For phantom pain after surgery or injury, try rubbing the painful area with DMSO to which you have added cayenne pepper, about one teaspoon to the pint, or one-half teaspoon to a cup of DMSO. Make it the same way as the alcohol extract.

To control pain, use heat or cold, or alternating applications of both, applying the heat or cold by a variety of different methods—heating pad, hot water bottle, ice cap, an ordinary fruit jar filled with ice or hot water and wrapped in a towel. Other methods include a hot tub bath, a hot shower, a "short cold bath" (30 to 120 seconds in cold bath water of 50°F to 65°F). Usually, hot water applied directly to the part, if practicable, is the most effective, the temperature of the water being from 105°F to 110°F, depending on the health of the individual and the part to be treated, but the easiest method should be tried first. Generally, the hot applications should be as hot as can be tolerated and the cold applications should be as cold as you can get them. Alternating hot and cold packs may be applied to the chest, to the abdomen, or to any part for aches and pains. Wring a towel from hot water and place it on the painful part for three to six minutes. Replace the hot compress with an ice-cold compress for 30 to 60 seconds. Alternate, in this fashion, for three to five changes.

Hot applications or massage to the spine can alter the central nervous system's ability to "hear" pain sensation. These simple treatments can be used even when the pain is in the legs, arms, or head, and not in the back.

If headache relief is needed, put the feet in hot water for 30 minutes. The headache will seem to "dissolve" into the foot bath! Of course, if one is a severe diabetic on insulin or has known blockage of arteries to the legs, this treatment

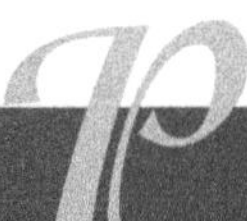

should not be used, for even ordinary temperatures can sometimes cause blisters in these persons because of poor circulation.

Common fevers can easily be treated by sitting in a hot tub bath from 102°F to 108°F until the skin is quite red and profuse sweating occurs. After the first five minutes, put an ice-cold cloth on the forehead, or from the beginning, if the fever starts out over 101°F. Take a cup of hot water or hot herbal tea when sweating begins. When the skin is red and sweating profusely, after 10 to 20 minutes, finish off the remedy as follows: (1) work fast to take a brief spray of cool water over the entire body from the chin downward; (2) then a quick friction rubdown with a coarse towel; (3) wrap a bathrobe around you, jump into bed, and sweat for half an hour; (4) arise, take a brief, cleansing shower if needed to cleanse the skin and relieve a sense of chilliness after sweating, and (5) re-dress.

When one finishes the hot soaking bath, if the treatment has been a good one, a sensation of weakness may develop after a minute or so of standing, because of the transfer of blood from the interior of the body to the exterior, much as in a sunburn. This is normal, because of the extensive reddening of the skin.

Music can relieve pain in recovery rooms of operating suites. Within minutes of listening to soothing music a 32-year-old cancer patient who had been racked with pain that could not be relieved by drugs felt relaxed, and her respiration deepened and became regular. Her hands relaxed, and she fell into a deep sleep. Playing soothing music in the coronary care unit promotes rest and reduces elevated blood pressure and heart rate. The need for narcotics and sedatives was decreased by playing soothing music.

Pain pills disable the alarm system of immunity, making it less possible to resist disease. A massage, however, releases endorphins, which assist in pain control, and enhance immunity, increasing resistance to disease.

Maintain proper weight, optimum nutrition, and obey the eight natural laws of health—proper nutrition, exercise, water (ten or more glasses daily), sunshine, temperance, fresh air, rest, and trust in divine power.

Keep in good physical condition. That will go far toward preventing distress from chronic pain. Exercise at least 20 minutes each day to release the natural pain relieving endorphins.Engage in walking, swimming, gardening, etc., five times a week. Stretching exercises also help.

Do push-ups to strengthen arms and shoulder muscles. Begin at any angle you can, starting with your kitchen counter. After you can successfully perform 5 to 10, progress to the next level: first counter level, then couch arm level, then couch seat level, building up to 50. Then start push-ups on the floor, pushing up off the toes if possible, building up to 30 repetitions. If you are not able to do the push-ups from your toes, you may do them from your knees.

Strengthen forearms and wrists by using a commercial hand gripper, available in easy, medium, and heavy strength. Chose one you can squeeze only three to five times. Do not use the thumb to squeeze but partially close the gripper to fit in the palm between the fingers and the base of the thumb. Squeeze the gripper rapidly a distance of one to two inches with each hand once or twice a day, building up to 10 times more than before strengthening began.

Maintain excellent posture, keeping cheek bones perpendicular to collar bones (use mirror), shoulders back and down, no excessive spinal curves, knees relaxed, feet not pronated (turned in).

Keep your feet comfortable. Wear proper shoes to maintain correct foot posture. Enjoy warm water soaks and foot massages, which will help one to deal with pain in any part of the body.

Vigorous, light friction or rubbing of the skin, or vibrations with a mechanical vibrator for 5 to 45 minutes helps some. A 10-minute back rub may help.

Trigger point pressure or stretching may help. Administer 5 to 10 seconds of pressure on each trigger point, or stretch the muscle group involved, for chronic skeletal pain, for that same period of time.

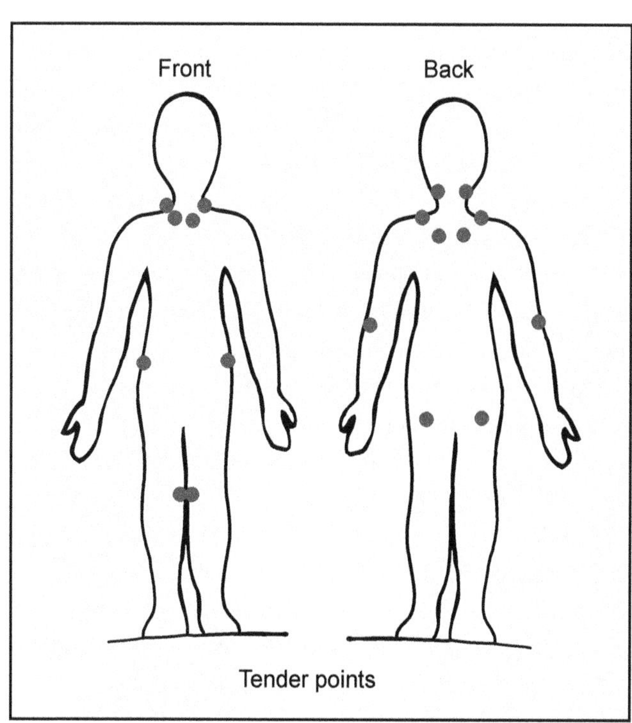

Tender points

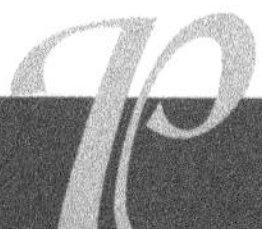

In Europe mud baths have been found to be an effective therapeutic measure in the treatment of soft tissue rheumatism, giving better relief from physical pain than standard physical therapy (*Phys Rehab Kur Med II* [1992]: 92–97). The mud used for full body baths contained potassium polysulfide, sulfur, and huminic acids. The patients treated had osteoarthrosis and nonarticular rheumatism. Other countries have utilized clay to much greater advantage than we have in America. (See "Clay Bath, Mud Bath" in the *Natural Remedies* section.)

Get enough rest since fatigue makes pain seem worse, and use relaxation techniques to reduce stress. Stress is an important enhancer of pain, causing it to appear much worse. To reduce stress, practice long, slow rhythmic breathing. Continue up to 20 minutes or more.

Apprehension, discontent, over-breathing, noise, irritating music, fear, or agitation can enhance pain by lowering the pain threshold. Create a loving and peaceful atmosphere, as social support is very important in pain control.

A "gate" in the spinal cord controls the amount of sensation that can be received through the nerves into the brain. That puts a limit to pain. Interfering sensations such as might arise from some other parts of the body (heat, pressure, cold, rubbing, vibration, elevation, manipulation) or an interfering emotion can influence and modulate the spinal gate control system.

Herbs for Pain

You may grind white willow bark and add some of it to DMSO, about as much bark powder as is required to make a medium paste. Use it to rub onto painful areas on the same time schedule as for the alcohol extract or with the cayenne extract already discussed.

Use arnica rub. It is an oily herbal extract. Rub it on three to four times a day. Make it by putting a pint of olive oil in a double boiler and adding dried arnica flowers, about as many as will loosely pack into a two-cup container. Boil for two hours, strain, and put the oil in a bottle.

Herbal teas for pain: White willow bark, Boswellia serrata, feverfew, devil's claw, myrrh, ginger, wild yam, licorice root, flaxseed oil (two teaspoons three times daily), skullcap, and wild lettuce. These herbs are good for pain and for inflammation. You may need to use the herbs several days before getting relief. Try the following formula: 1 tablespoon white willow; 1 tablespoon valerian root; 1 tablespoon wild lettuce; and 1 quart water. Boil the first two ingredients together gently for 25 minutes. Set off the fire and add the third. Steep 20 minutes and take one cup per hour as needed for pain.

The herbal remedies we have used with considerable success are white willow bark, wild lettuce, hops, and catnip (for sedation). Also, try a combination of hops, meadowsweet flowers, valerian root, black cohosh, blue cohosh, skullcap, and St. John's wort. Use a tablespoon of each of the herbs, except for the black cohosh, which should be one to two teaspoons. Put these herbs in a quart of water and simmer gently for 20 minutes. Strain and drink throughout the day. Make fresh daily. This mixture is quite relaxing and can often turn the tide in dealing with pain.

Make a tea of white willow bark and wild lettuce daily. White willow is the source for methylsalicylate. Its effects are cumulative in the system, so keep drinking it on a schedule whether or not you feel pain at that time, and you will experience better pain control in persistent pain relief.

Instructions for making the tea: Simmer one tablespoon of white willow bark in one quart of water for 20 to 30 minutes. Then set it off the heat. If you wish, add two to three tablespoons of wild lettuce and let it steep 30 minutes. Some get better results from mixing one or more pain-relieving herbs. Remember also poplar buds, black cohosh, meadowsweet, partridge berry, or others. Strain and drink. Make it daily and drink the entire quart spread over a day's time.

Use slippery elm tea or peppermint oil (only a lick of a finger) for stomach or bowel pain. Use one teaspoon of slippery elm in one cup of water.

Oil of cloves and allspice both contain eugenol, a mild local anesthetic that can be used for toothaches and other small areas of pain. Try not to swallow much of the oil as it can cause nausea and vomiting. The oil of tarragon also contains eugenol. Fresh tarragon leaves may also be chewed for toothache, or they may be crushed and applied to ant bites, bee stings, and painful scrapes and bruises. If you have the tincture, use one-half to one teaspoon three to four times a day.

Make a decoction of black haw for menstrual cramps, fever, headache, and general aches and pains. Use three tablespoons of the dried black haw bark per quart of water and boil for 10 to 20 minutes. Take three to four cups per day. You may also make a tincture with one ounce (about two tablespoons) per cup of ethyl alcohol or vodka. Two teaspoons, three times a day of the tincture may be used. Do not use during pregnancy as muscular movements of the uterus may be altered.

Take one-half to two teaspoons, three times a day of meadowsweet. This herb can be used as a digestive aide

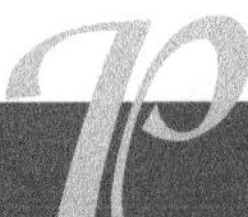

and in inflammation of the bowels. Use for pain, fever, and inflammations.

Red raspberry is useful for painful menstruation, labor pains, and infant diarrhea. May also be used for morning sickness, threatened miscarriage, and menopause symptoms. Raspberry has also been useful in diabetes management, reducing blood sugar when elevated.

Cayenne (red pepper, capsicum) may be used for chronic pain, You can rub a tincture of red pepper into the skin to treat muscle and joint pains. (See "Directions for Making a Tincture, Extract" in the *Herbal Remedies* section.) Capsaicin, the active ingredient in hot peppers, ties up the P-substance, a chemical produced by nerves to send pain messages to the brain. Shingles, diabetic foot pain, and cluster headaches—for each of these the preparation of red pepper must be applied four to six times daily, expecting no pain relief for the first 5 to 10 days. For cluster headaches the red pepper preparation can be rubbed inside the nostril on the affected side, or a tincture can be atomized or squirted into the nostril. Burning nostril and a runny nose will last only a few minutes at first, but will stop occurring usually in about one week, or at least will become much more tolerable.

Vervain can be used for pain, inflammation, laxative, headaches, and fevers.

The Psychology of Pain

Our past failures in managing pain may be because of the fact that we have concentrated on the physiology and on pharmacotherapy, while entirely ignoring the psychology of pain. We have used drugs, surgery, and even physical therapy exclusively. There are other aspects of pain that must also be controlled.

Pain responses can be learned. The way we respond to pain is always a learned matter. As small children, we are taught to be stoical or expressive about pain. Some children with the very same pain inflicted express the matter altogether differently. A professional boxer learns not to exhibit pain while in the boxing ring. A professional speaker shows no sign of physical discomfort while presenting very intricate matters from the platform.

Anyone can learn to experience pain in new ways. One way to experience pain differently is to interpret pain differently than previously. If you believe the pain will result in serious injury or disability, it is more likely to appear painful than when you understand the pain does not reflect some deterioration, malignancy, or injury in the body. Also, pain experience appears more painful when one gives over to thinking about the pain and oneself. If the attention is distracted and the pain is ignored, it will be less painful. Pain control is a skill like any other skill to be learned, such as flying a plane or playing a piano; the more you practice the skill, the better you will be at it.

Expect improvement, but make it realistic. If one expects complete abolishment of sensation in the part, you may be certain of disappointment, and discouragement will follow. A realistic goal is that the pain will no longer interfere seriously with one's daily duties.

Persons having pain will experience a more mild reaction if the surroundings are congenial, affectionate, or kind. Soft music helps many pain sufferers. Studying nature out doors goes far toward making pain tolerable.

Throw yourself entirely into an exercise routine for one hour each day, distracting the thoughts so that pain is ignored and forgotten.

Never stop work or stay out sick or quit a job because of chronic pain. One may need to make adjustments, such as getting transferred to a job in which the painful part will not be especially exposed to injury. You may rest or apply heat or massage to the pain, but it is not recommended to miss work because of sickness. Try to make it a priority that you never miss an appointment or a day of work because of sickness or pain.

Make life a study in regularity, especially sleeping and eating. Pray earnestly for control of the entire life, but do not focus on the pain. Focus on seeing the Savior, the home of the saved, and one's duty. For a clear picture of these matters, read the book *The Desire of Ages* by Ellen G. White, for more complete understanding of God's love.

Never talk of your pain. Even in talking with God, try to avoid focusing on your pain. Pray for victory in the life, and concentrate on subjects other than your pain.

Learn to relax. Prolonged muscle contraction or tension depletes muscles of oxygen and nutrients, necessitating a buildup of toxic substances that result in pain. One must put forth personal emotional energy to experience pain or muscle tension, both leading to fatigue and an increase in pain. Learn to stop several times daily to take a deep breath and relax. If you explosively vocalize on exhalation with a long "Paaa, Paaa," repeating the syllables several times on each exhalation, it will encourage the taking up of a few more oxygen molecules on each exhalation, reducing pain. Relaxation and bed rest are not synonymous, as one can relax while sitting or standing, even walking. While one is relaxing, take consecutively deep breaths, exhaling on the "Paaa, Paaa, Paaa, Paaa" syllable.

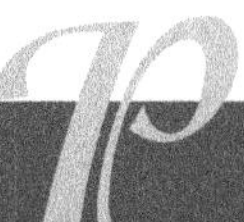

One can easily learn muscle relaxation, and the more one practices, the easier it becomes. You may wish to lie on a carpeted floor or mat in as comfortable and relaxing circumstance as possible, having drunk a large glass of water and emptying the bladder just prior to the exercise to encourage relaxation in the autonomic nervous system at the same time. Focus your attention on the particular muscle being relaxed. Start with the face and relax the scalp, face, chin, jaw and neck, then progress to the hands. Proceed to arms and trunk. Go through the muscles of the lower extremity. Concentrate especially on shoulders, abdomen, feet, and hands. Some people find it helpful to contract the muscle expected to relax immediately prior to relaxing it such as making a tight fist, then relaxing entirely. One may do this without moving the part, simply by thinking of contracting the muscle in the arm, the thigh, the abdomen, or the shoulders.

If some worry or tense thought is occupying your mind, you may try certain techniques to relieve the thought such as counting backward from 10 or listening to a tape of the Bible.

Whatever medications you may have unwisely taken for control of chronic pain, begin tapering those off until you have quit altogether. A good tapering program for medications is to reduce the daily dosage by one dose for one week or by one-half dose if only one dose is taken daily. As an example, if you take pain medication four times daily, omit one dose each day for one week. As you get better control of your life, you will be able to reduce medication by two doses each day; shortly, by three doses; then taking one dose every other day, and eventually taking none at all.

An age old law of life known to humankind since antiquity has to do with doing good to others. Do not allow others to serve you unless they also are sick and need an outlet of charitable feelings for themselves. Learn to serve others. Seek out the widow and the orphan, and minister to them. The biblical principle of self-sacrificing love given hundreds of years ago is a law of life and will result in success.

Referred Pain

The nerve impulses received from certain body parts enter the spinal cord at the same point as the nerve impulses from a diseased organ. This relationship may cause referred pain in the healthy part rather than in the diseased organ. Very often pain in one area of the abdomen actually originates in another part of the abdomen and is referred. Irritation of the diaphragm gives referred pain over the shoulder blade; distention of the bile ducts or gallbladder refers pain to the right sub-shoulder blade area; acute pancreatitis refers pain straight through to the back; an acute heart attack or pleurisy may refer pain to the abdomen or to either arm; pain in the rectum or uterus is referred to the low back; pain in the ureter radiates all the way down from the flank to the same side external genitalia; pneumonia often refers pain from the chest to the lower abdomen.

If the bowel is inflamed, there may be loss of appetite, nausea, or diarrhea. If the urinary system is inflamed, the patient may have pain on voiding, blood in the urine, or pain in the flank. Consider also that abdominal pain may be because of hardening of the arteries, sickle cell anemia, diabetes, kidney failure, intestinal parasites, allergies, ulcerative colitis or Crohn's disease, peptic ulcer, and diverticulosis. Drugs may also be a cause of acute abdominal pain, as may alcohol and cortisone-like drugs.

You may simply watch and wait with the patient with abdominal pain rather than considering an acute surgical abdomen if there is a history of any of these diseases or severe hypertension; or if the pain is relieved by taking a teaspoon of charcoal in water; or if there are signs of viral illness; or if the urine indicates an infection of the bladder; or if there is the presence of swollen lymph nodes; a rash in young children; or the pain can be expected to be ovulation; especially if the person has a good appetite and normal bowel movements. If none of these is present, and the patient is quite ill or has a fever, then a white blood cell count may be helpful to determine if the pain is from a serious problem such as appendicitis or acute salpingitis.

Pancreatitis

This inflammation of the pancreas is caused by chemical irritants or viral infections as from mumps. Alcoholic beverages are famous for causing pancreatitis and should be strictly avoided. Stress can increase the likelihood that a person who is susceptible to pancreatitis will develop a very severe case (*Gastroenterology* 98, no. 6 [June 1990]: 1682–8).

Proper hydration is important in pancreatitis, as the pancreatic glands holding pancreatic secretions dilate and allow the pancreatic fluid to stagnate. This is a common finding by pathologists at autopsy in cases of dehydration. Alcohol, ingested and those produced by fermentation during digestion, should be avoided as they severely damage the pancreas. Alcohols produced in the intestine, resulting from improper digestion, can be avoided by careful attention to proper eating habits—meals on time, chewing well, nothing between meals, avoiding overeating, and limiting the menu to two or three dishes along with bread and spread.

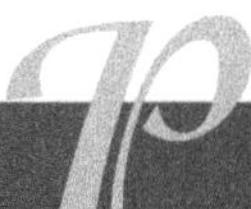

Chew your food well to take a load off the pancreas in digestion. Avoid all caffeinated drinks—tea, colas, chocolate, and coffee. They stimulate the pancreas in an unhealthy way.

Treatment is with hot fomentations across the midsection of the abdomen, charcoal by mouth as well as by compresses over the abdomen at night. Supportive measures, such as saline retention enemas may be essential in severe cases to maintain hydration.

Herbs to use for pancreatitis and diabetes are cascara sagrada and chai. Use one teaspoon of cascara sagrada in a quart of chai tea daily. If the laxative effect of the cascara is too great, cut the dosage in half. Not only is this remedy good for the pancreas and diabetes, but also for gallbladder and liver disease. For visual problems associated with diabetes, this formula is also quite useful.

Case Report

A woman in her 50s who had been having pancreatitis for some years started taking 1200 to 1600 micrograms of selenium daily. After a few weeks she was entirely well, eating well, gaining weight, and feeling stronger, physically, as well as mentally and emotionally.

Panic Attacks

(See "Anxiety Attacks, Panic Disorders, Agoraphobia" in the *Conditions and Diseases* section.)

Parasites

The human intestinal tract is prone to host a number of parasites, from one-cell ameba to long tapeworms. Treatments for different parasites overlap to some degree.

Antiparasite Formula

Use the following formula to deal with parasites. One part thyme, half part fennel, one part black walnut, half part cascara sagrada or buckthorn, one part wormwood, and half part slippery elm powder. Powder any herbs not already powdered and fill capsules. Take four capsules three times a day.

Blastocystis hominis

To treat Blastocystis, use the following program. Take the following three times a day one hour before meals for four weeks:

- 3 cloves of minced garlic blended in hot tomato juice
- 1 ounce pumpkin seed, chewed thoroughly
- 1 capsule ginger (or one-fourth teaspoon of the kitchen powder)
- 1 capsule turmeric (or one-fourth teaspoon)
- 2 capsules walnut hulls
- 2 tablets artemisia annua
- 1 heaping tablespoon slippery elm bark in one-fourth to one-half cup grape juice

During the last two weeks take three to four "garlic enemas" two to three days apart. Use the solution suggested for vaginal douches as the enema solution. Ficin, the fig enzyme, is also a good cleansing agent for intestinal parasites.

Tests show that feeding garlic to humans or dogs infested with hookworms or pinworms significantly reduces the number of larvae grown. Perhaps the dosage needs to be one to six cloves of raw minced garlic daily taken with food. We have found it to be quite effective, especially when used in conjunction with artemisia (wormwood).

For worms and ameba, we recommend that you take quite a lot of garlic on a daily basis for 10 days. That would mean taking the larger portion of an entire globe of garlic, approximately 10 to 20 cloves chopped finely or blended with an orange or a tomato as a smoothie. I suggest you swallow them relatively fast with a little water, and then drink a full glass of water afterward. You may have to split the dose at 10 minute intervals to prevent nausea. One hour after taking the garlic, take four tablespoons of activated charcoal stirred into a glass of water. At the same time take one artemisia capsule three times a day.

At the beginning of each day make up two to three quarts of water with each quart containing 24 drops of grapefruit seed extract. This can replace any water you must take, including that for swallowing the garlic. At least two of the three quarts should be drunk every day, and three if possible.

Foods That Assist in Expelling Worms and Other Parasites

Pomegranates may be eaten for pinworms. Try to eat an entire fresh pomegranate daily, chewing and swallowing the seeds as well.

Eat one to two cloves of garlic with each meal, chopped finely into foods or blended with an orange or a tomato as a smoothie.

Take two or more tablespoonfuls of pumpkin seeds once or twice daily; chew thoroughly.

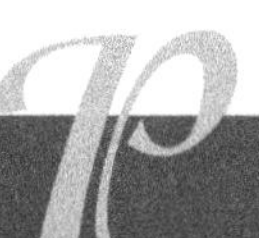

Cabbage, carrots, garlic, and onions contain a sulfur compound that helps expel parasites and worms.

Cloves, oregano, turmeric, flax seed, and slippery elm are also good for treating parasites.

For one cell parasites such as *giardia ameba* or *blastocystis*, use one or more of the following:

- *Artemisia annua*, one pill three times a day for 40 days. Some may require two to three months treatment.
- Aged garlic liquid, one teaspoon three times a day for two weeks.

Drinking water should be checked if it comes from a well. Do not drink from a stream when hiking or camping. They may be contaminated by animals who are carriers for parasites (e.g., beavers carry *giardia*).

Golden seal is very good for *Giardia lamblia*. However, artemisia is probably the treatment of choice.

Black walnut, cloves, cramp bark, fennel seed, pumpkin seed, gentian root, thyme, grapefruit seed, psyllium seed, and golden seal are all good herbs for intestinal parasites. Cloves also increase the circulation of the blood to the intestinal tract, and promote digestion. Cramp bark is helpful as an antispasmodic. Fennel seed helps to curb the appetite. Gentian root also helps weakened muscle tone in the digestive organs. Thyme is a good antiseptic and antifungal as well as antiparasitic. It is especially good for skin parasites. Grapefruit seed extract is also antifungal.

Parkinson's Disease

Also called the shaking palsy or paralysis agitans, Parkinson's is a degenerative disease of the aging central nervous system. The two principal symptoms are resting tremors and stiffness of muscles. The tremor is an involuntary rhythmic movement, and the rigidity consists of difficulty in relaxing a muscle, even during sleep. Eventually difficulty in swallowing both foods and liquids ensues. The person may have muscle rigidity, drooling, loss of appetite, stooping, shuffling gait, and tremors. The speech may be impaired, and there may be a fixed facial expression. The disease more frequently starts with a tremor of the hands while at rest, or in a single extremity.

The cause of Parkinson's has not been fully delineated, but for West Indians there are several suspects: environment, consuming a lot of paw paws (another name is papayas), custard apples, and herbal teas made from the leaves, seeds, or bark of these plants. Similar symptoms have been reported in Guam and Guadalupe. It has been thought that a slow toxin in the islander's traditional food was the culprit in these instances as well as the high incidence of Parkinson's disease in Afro-Caribbean and Indian immigrants to England who continue to eat their own ethnic food (*Lancet* 354 [1999]: 281).

Prevention

Reducing the intake of animal fat and sugar, avoiding exposure to metals such as aluminum, iron, manganese, mercury, cadmium, and copper, and ensuring plenty of antioxidants from fruits, vegetables, whole grains, nuts, and seeds, and by the use of CoQ10, Parkinson's disease may be prevented, or its progress greatly slowed.

Work-related exposure to certain metals over a period of two to three decades appears to increase a person's risk of developing Parkinson's disease. Exposure to certain combinations of metals (lead and copper, lead and iron, iron and copper) has been associated with a much higher risk of Parkinson's. Pipe fitters, electrical workers, chemists, and fire fighters are all in jeopardy from exposure to metals. (See "Toxic Heavy Metals" in the *Supplemental Information* section.)

Industrial exposure to pesticides, as well as head injuries and a low intake of antioxidants such as vitamins C and E, selenium, and fruits and vegetables have all been implicated in the development of Parkinson's. Predisposing factors for Parkinson's are diets high in animal fat, vitamin D (notably milk), vitamin A supplementation, diet low in folic acid (fruits and vegetables), and simply eating too much food over a lifetime might be an intermediate or contributory risk factor for Parkinson's disease because of the potential overload of the antioxidant system. None of the researchers seem willing to state definitely that overeating causes Parkinson's, but merely suggests that there is an increased risk for Parkinson's disease caused by excessive intake of calories and certain nutrients, and relatively less of antioxidants and other nutrients (*Neurology* 49, no. 1 [July 1997]: 310).

Iron supplementation may set the stage for some of the known causes to be more operative in causing Parkinson's.

Organophosphate insecticide poisoning leads to acute Parkinson's, but it is reversible.

Treatment

Keeping the symptoms under control is primary in the treatment plan for the patient. Following are suggested practices under specific categories.

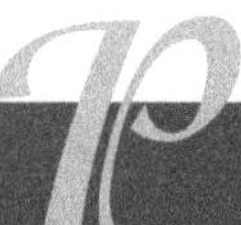

Diet

More and more is being learned about diet and its relationship to Parkinson's disease, such as:

- A low protein diet improves tremors and reduces slowness in walking.
- Food restriction, even in thin patients, may do as it does in animals, increase the lifespan and decrease the neurodegenerative diseases such as Parkinson's, Alzheimer's, and Huntington's disease. Alternating days of feeding with days of fasting helps animals and may help humans as well.
- A diet high in antioxidant foods, especially vitamin E, protects against progression of neurodegenerative diseases.
- Some nutrients that are believed to be helpful include magnesium, niacin, pyridoxine, phenylalanine, tryptophan, and essential fatty acids taken as a supplement, as well as taking some nuts or olives and avocados.
- CoQ10 is believed to be helpful in doses of 250 to 300 milligrams daily. CoQ10 at 300 milligrams, 600 milligrams, or 1200 milligrams was administered to 23 patients with Parkinson's disease. Those on the highest dose had a 44 percent slower decline in mental function, movement, and ability to perform daily living tasks compared to the placebo group. By eight months into the study the differences were clear. The study was continued for 16 months. Research was supported by the National Institute of Neurological Disorders and Stroke.
- It may be that the disease can be slowed down by using large doses of antioxidants, especially vitamin E. As much as 2000 units a day of vitamin E has been recommended. We recommend less than this as a general rule, perhaps 400 to 800 IU as this dose is better for long-term maintenance, as vitamin E can interfere with blood clotting. Use the natural form of mixed tocopherols rather than synthetic alpha tocopherol.
- Avoid long term zinc in any supplement as it may encourage neurodegenerative diseases like Parkinson's and Alzheimer's. Eat foods that are naturally high in zinc. (See "Food Sources High in Certain Nutrients" in the *Dietary Information* section.)
- Do not overeat, and avoid eating freely of heavy foods such as nuts, free fats, and concentrated proteins. Make sure the patient is not overweight, as being overweight has been seriously implicated in Parkinson's.
- Don't eat rancid foods or free fats (margarine, mayonnaise, fried foods, cooking fats, or salad oils), ready prepared mixes with eggs, or mono or diglycerides.
- Eat one-fourth cup of cooked fava beans or velvet beans daily as these legumes contain naturally occurring L-dopa.
- Vitamin B found in uncooked brown rice polishings (two tablespoons per day) should prove helpful in many cases.
- Taking soy lecithin for two months out of every year can be helpful.

Massage

Massage is helpful for Parkinson's. Use the following routine:

- Neck, shoulders, and head massage.
- A relaxing foot rub before or after a soak in warm water to assist in reducing pain and inducing sleep. Even if the bath is not taken, the massage is very helpful.
- Massage to the lower limbs to normalize gait, improve sense of balance, and minimize problems encountered when trying to rise from a sitting position.
- Stretching, traction, and range of motion can help reduce the rate at which weakness and stiffness occur.

Herbs

Taking 750 milligrams daily of any magnesium salt may help to relax the rigidity. Vitamin B6, up to 1,000 milligrams, and vitamin C, up to 3,000 milligrams, may be helpful in the initial stages of Parkinson's. Start with a small amount of the vitamins and build it up slowly. If diarrhea occurs, reduce the magnesium salt to 500 milligrams or less.

Use aloe vera capsules and take 6 to 10 prunes with breakfast. Fresh aloe vera, one and one-half inch squares, may also be used, peeled, and blended with the prunes if preferred.

For spasm and rigidity of the muscles, use *Atropa belladonna*. The root of the *atropa* plant is recommended in all forms of Parkinson's disease, but the dosage must be reduced for a time if dryness of the throat develops.

Boil five cups of water. Then add one tablespoon black cohosh. Simmer gently for 25 minutes. Pour into a container with two tablespoons of St. John's wort and two tablespoons of skullcap. Add one-fourth cup peppermint tea leaves for flavoring the otherwise harsh flavors, if desired. Let steep for 30 minutes, strain, and drink in five doses throughout the day. Make fresh daily. Black cohosh is a muscle relaxant, even for

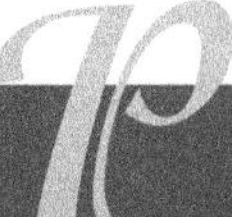

smooth muscles, but it can dilate blood vessels in the head to cause headache because of its muscle relaxing qualities. Cut the dosage of black cohosh in the formula to one teaspoon if one tablespoon causes headaches.

Kava kava is contraindicated in Parkinson's disease. Although no side effects have been reported, kava is believed to interfere with dopamine production and thereby worsen Parkinson's disease. Until this issue is cleared up by research, kava extract should probably not be used in Parkinson's disease.

Other herbs that can be used include *Corydalis cava* to reduce tremors. Harmine (*Peganum harmala*) is also useful for tremors. It should be noted that *corydalis* and harmine recommended for Parkinson's disease can be toxic. It is probably best to use the commercial preparations that have been standardized unless you have sufficient familiarity with these herbs.

Other Measures

Patients who have difficulty walking will often have great improvement of the speed and length of stride, with decreased numbers of times in which they are temporarily unable to move, by using an ordinary musical metronome to help them "keep time." They should try to put the foot down with each click of the metronome. These can be purchased from a music store. (*Lancet* 347 [May 11, 1996]: 1337).

Parkinson's has been related to viral infections, such as the flu, toxins and drugs, and excessive use of polyunsaturated fats without sufficient antioxidants. There is actual death of cells in brain centers, such as could be expected from toxins or viruses. When these conditions begin to develop, treat yourself vigorously with heat, exercise, diet, herbs, and massage to minimize the damage from the agent.

The patient's determination and faithfulness in exercising will go far toward slowing the progression of the disease. Muscles will not freeze up as long as they are kept active. When walking let the heel touch first, and the toes be brought up with every step. They should take large steps and lift the feet as though stepping over objects on the floor. Swing the arms forcefully when walking. Practice rising and sitting at least a dozen times daily. Exercising to music or a metronome, marching, clapping and calisthenics, will all help overcome the slowness of motion typical of Parkinson's.

Singing lessons and speaking or reading out loud are helpful to maintain voice control.

A two-week cleansing program may be tried:

- Fast three days, drinking two quarts of warm water every morning.
- Continue the fast with the water, but add day by day the following meals:
  - First day – one raw food, only take this one food in the one meal.
  - Second day – two raw foods, one in each of two meals.
  - Third day – three raw foods, two of which are at breakfast, and one at lunch.
  - Fourth day – four raw foods, two at each meal.
  - Fifth day – gradually return to a regular diet. A plant-based cuisine is the most favorable diet for Parkinson's.

The patient should never lie down after a meal or do any kind of heavy work—either physical or mental. There should be some light work or light exercise immediately after the meal. The person should not eat a large evening meal. A bit of fruit would be all right, although it must be taken at least two to four hours before going to bed.

Chew all food to a cream before swallowing. This is more important than one might think as improperly chewed food may cause the loss of brain cells.

Check the transit time to see if it takes more than 30 hours to empty the bowels after eating. Constipation should not be allowed, as this condition makes both rigidity and tremors worse. Constipation sends to the brain impulses that signal a disorder, and they act as irritants and cause tremors and rigidity.

In this condition there may be many unpleasant sensations, especially burning of the skin, as well as the tremors and rigidity of muscles. The use of the continuous bath (a hammock bath in a tub of continuously running or intermittently drained water) can relieve symptoms remarkably. The patient does not need to be removed from the bath to urinate, but time urination with the draining of the water. Begin the bath at 92°F in a well-ventilated and cool room. Some patients may want a warmer room than others, and may want the bath water at 95°F or even 98°F. The comfort of the patient should be consulted. Maintain the bath for about two hours and follow it with a light general massage or alcohol rub. Give the baths five to six times a week.

During the first half hour of the bath a slight fall in blood pressure and increase in pulse and respiration can be expected. Very quickly the burning and other unpleasant sensations

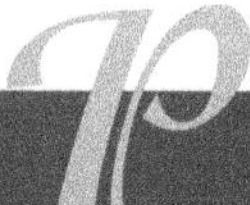

cease. The tremors diminish or stop while in the water. Some patients are enabled to stop all medication and make permanent improvement.

Others are helped only while they are actually in the bath. For these, it is quite permissible to continue the baths beyond two hours, even 12 to 15 hours as availability of personnel permits. The beneficial effect of the bath is the soothing of a barrage of nerve impulses from the skin that reflexively produces a calming influence to reduce the tremors and rigidity. Anything that will quiet nerve impulses from any part of the body will have a beneficial effect on Parkinson's disease—keeping the extremities warm both summer and winter, relieving skin problems, avoiding minor illnesses, and keeping the bowels cleansed and freely functioning (*Medical Record*, August 26, 1916, 367, 368).

Use hydrotherapy and massage as well as wet sheet packs every other day for one month, then one per week. A hot bath or sauna should be helpful, as well as the fomentations.

Take a salt glow with each daily shower. (Salt glow is also very good for arthritis and rheumatism.) The salt tends to draw out acid through the skin from one-eighth inch depth.

Do an olive oil rub, whole body (or at least the extremities), two times a week.

Do not sleep with anyone, as both your sleep and theirs will be disturbed.

Be as independent as possible.

Pure and positive thinking, trust in divine power, and an attitude of forgiveness and trust toward others can have a very positive effect on Parkinson's disease.

Paronychia, "Runaround"

An infection at the bottom of a fingernail begins with a little tenderness, then swelling and redness, and pain and throbbing. This should be treated with the first recognition of its presence by soaking the entire hand and wrist in hot water for half an hour. Often one treatment will stop the runaround without further help, but if it continues, the half-hour hot soak should be repeated every four hours until pus appears. At that time a clean needle can be used to lift the cuticle off the nail, which will usually release pus from the infected area. Continue the hot soaks until all indication of inflammation has disappeared.

Prevention includes care of the cuticle and hangnails, avoiding dirt, chemicals, and grease on the hands, and avoiding dishwashing unless using rubber gloves lined with cotton.

Pelvic Inflammatory Disease

(See "Salpingitis, 'Infected Tubes,' Pelvic Inflammatory Disease" in the *Conditions and Dieases* section.)

Peptic Ulcers

(See "Ulcers—Peptic, Duodenal, Gastric, Pyloric, Stomach" in the *Conditions and Diseases* section.)

Phlebitis and Thrombophlebitis

Phlebitis involves inflammation of a vein accompanied by swelling and pain. The vein can usually be felt with the fingers under the skin as a tender, firm rope-like strand.

Where there are signs of inflammation (heat, swelling, pain, and hardness) along the course of the vein, the thrombus (blood clot) is almost always very firmly adherent to the vessel walls by the time these signs develop so there is essentially no danger of its breaking off and going to the lungs.

Give a diet of very simple foods having no free oil or sugar, since both of these refined nutrients tend to reduce the phagocytic activity of white blood cells, thereby slowing dissolution of the clot. Also take horse chestnut to reduce inflammation in the vein.

One physician notes that two of his patients got phlebitis when they ate fish and citrus fruits. Other triggering foods, chemicals, and inhalants have been observed. Apparently this phenomenon occurs in many patients whose phlebitis is only a part of a more generalized and severe blood vessel inflammation (vasculitis). Ten patients treated in an environmental control unit (ECU) revealed that their symptoms could be reproduced by giving the relevant challenge (in this case it would have been fish and citrus fruits). Avoiding the triggering agents allowed all 10 of these patients to return to work, whereas only 10 percent of patients who did not remove their triggering agents were able to do so (Jonathan Brostasf and Stephen J. Challacombe, *Food Allergy and Intolerance*, London Bailliere Tindall, 1987).

The same researchers found that other spastic blood vessel phenomena such as migraines, vascular headaches, angina, Raynaud's disease, lupus, rheumatoid and other collagen vasculitis, and such disorders as Henoch-Schonlein purpura,

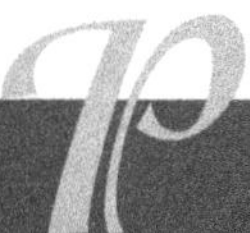

cardiac arrhythmias, and nontraumatic phlebitis may all have a basis in triggering agents such as foods, inhalants, drugs, etc.

In a case control study, 185 patients with recurrent venous thrombosis and 220 controls had serum homocysteine levels measured. The patients had more than three times the risk of having an elevated serum homocysteine level. If the laboratory reveals a high homocysteine level, take vitamins B12, B6, and folic acid.

Heat and elevation are the mainstay for phlebitis. Place a standard steam pack lengthwise under the affected limb and lay another over the limb. It should stay effectively hot for about 30 minutes, and it may be renewed if desired. Wrapping with a plastic sheet helps to prevent heat loss—a garbage bag can be used quite effectively. Follow it with a hot and cold water bath. (See "Hydrotherapy" in the *Natural Remedies* section.)

Phlebitis in a leg may be made comfortable by elevating the foot of the bed a few inches with bricks and putting a cradle over the legs to prevent the weight of the bed clothes from causing discomfort in the painful leg. The cradle can be fashioned by folded pillows on each side of the leg with the sheets and blankets spread over the pillows in such a way that neither the pillows nor the bed clothes touch the leg. Moderate exercise is usually helpful, but standing still is often a source of increased pain. Recovery usually occurs in 10 days with good treatments.

Massage the remainder of the body and use passive exercises and range of motion for various joints other than joints that cause pain when moved. Do not massage the affected area.

Use a charcoal compress over the painful or swollen areas each night until the tenderness is gone.

Tight workout pants can initiate dangerous blood clots in the legs. One 25-year-old man developed such a blood clot in his left leg after riding a stationary bike and lifting weights while wearing midthigh-length pressurized pants made of neoprene and nylon. The clot extended from the calf to mid-thigh where the pants leg began.

A similar case occurred in a woman who was a frequent clinic and seminar guest at Uchee Pines Institute, a 33 year-old-woman who had had repeated bouts of phlebitis for the previous nine years. She came into our office wearing a pair of skin-tight white pants. It had never crossed her mind that tight pants could be a problem with recurring phlebitis. We suggested she replace tight pants with loose fitting clothing. Her comment was, "Oh, well, I guess I will need to buy an entirely new wardrobe, since I have very few outfits that do not include tight pants." Three years later the patient returned to our clinic for another disorder and reported very joyfully that she would never wear tight pants again, since she had not had a single episode of phlebitis since she began to wear loose fitting clothing. She had also adopted a plant-based diet for three years and left off free fats. Her changed lifestyle had also included increasing her water intake. We believe all of these factors played a part in keeping her free of phlebitis.

There is no hard and fast rule about ambulation, but vigorous walking should be discouraged until the tenderness subsides. For superficial phlebitis in varicose veins that are visible, there is no reason to stay off the leg except for pain. In which case, strolling may prove to be less painful than standing; therefore, standing should be discouraged as it encourages pooling of blood in the affected vein with a possible extension of the phlebitis.

Pilonidal Cyst

This skin affliction develops at the end of the spine from an improperly formed gland that contains hair follicles, shed skin flakes, and secretes skin oils and other fluids that have no outlet, so that a cyst is formed. Pilonidal cysts occur most frequently in men between the ages of 20 and 45, especially those who sit for long periods in trucks, cars, planes, or tractors. They may become as large as an egg. They can become hotly inflamed. The result of the hair of that region growing inward through the dilated pores that some people are born with causes a cyst to form.

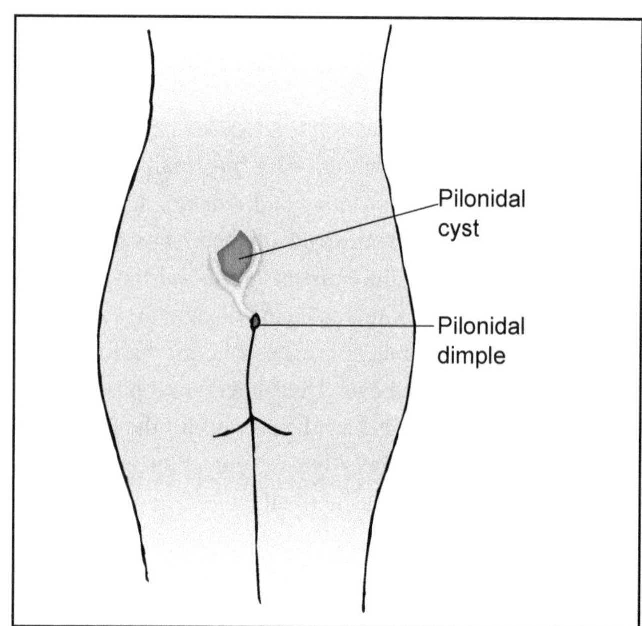

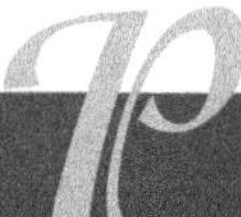

Treatment

Sitz baths and opening the cyst with a needle may give temporary relief, but if the cyst is blocked with hair, dirt, and body secretions, it may eventually require surgery to completely eradicate it. If you are adventurous, you can painlessly insert a very slender crochet hook into the tiny opening and pull out the loose ends of hair. The cyst may be three-fourths inches deep by one-half inch wide, and one to two inches long. It is possible to open the cyst wide enough so that it continues to drain to the outside.

If you are *very* strong in courage, you can deftly slit the edge of the opening with a sharp, thin razor blade. Firmly fix the clean blade with gripper-lock pliers so it cannot move. Make a quick, firm, cutting stab to slit the opening vertically (toward the head or feet—not side to side) about half an inch. No vital structures are near. You can get good anesthesia by holding an ice cube on the cyst for five minutes. That will give you almost three minutes of a fair quality anesthesia. With healing of the edges of the cyst, a process called "marsupialization," a pouch is formed. Keep the fresh wound clean with frequent bandage changes. While this does not eradicate the cyst, it can eliminate inflammation and enable the patient to easily tolerate the condition.

Pink Eye

(See "Conjunctivitis, Pink Eye, Sore Eyes" in the *Conditions and Diseases* section.)

Pinworms

(See "Parasites" in the *Conditions and Diseases* section.)

Plantar Fasciitis

(See "Skeletal Problems" in the *Conditions and Diseases* section.)

Pleurisy, Pain with Breathing

The pleura is the membrane that covers the lung and lines the chest cavity. The pleura over the lung is insensitive, but the pleura over the chest wall is plentifully supplied by pain fibers. The first sign is pain and is felt in the skin supplied by the same nerves that supply the chest wall. The front of the abdomen is also supplied by the same nerves and may be involved in the pain.

In pleurisy, spasm of the intercostal muscles may be a factor in the pain. It is sharp, superficial, and aggravated by deep breathing, hiccupping, or coughing. Breathing in may be abruptly halted by the pain, with respiration then becoming shallow. Holding the breath out will usually relieve pain completely, as may a change of posture in bed. Listening to the chest while breathing may reveal a friction rub, a creaking, rasping, or grating sound that can be heard by placing the ear against the chest over the area of pain. Pleurisy of the lung next to the diaphragm is typically referred to the shoulder, and not felt in the chest.

Cause

Pulmonary infections, lobar pneumonia, tuberculosis, influenza, blood vessel lesions such as an infarction, and lupus erythematosus can all cause pleurisy. The commonest cause, however, is the Coxsackie virus.

One should remember that in the elderly, pleurisy is sometimes associated with more serious underlying disorders such as pneumonia, pulmonary embolism, tuberculosis, or cancer. Only rarely is cancer present in the young. If the patient does not respond rapidly to the measures described, a search for other disorders is mandatory.

Pleurodynia (Bornholm disease) is caused by a Coxsackie virus. The pain of pleurodynia may be extremely severe, like an iron grip around the rib cage, with fever coming on quickly, along with headache and feeling sick. Recovery usually occurs rapidly, but relapses are frequent and may continue for several weeks.

Trichinosis (a parasitic disease obtained from eating pork) can settle in the intercostal muscles and can also produce pleurisy, but it is usually associated with swelling around the eyes or generalized swelling and by an increased eosinophil count in the blood. Splenic infarction from blockage of blood vessels may cause pleurisy. Hodgkin's disease and similar conditions can cause splenic pain referred to the pleura.

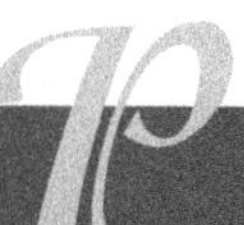

In recent decades, bacterial pneumonia has had a much lower incidence than viral pneumonia, and most of the time when pleurisy occurs it is the result of a viral infection. Therefore, a shaking chill and a sharp stabbing pain in the side may be the first symptoms.

Treatment

The application of heat will usually relieve pain. Once in a while it is necessary to strap one side of the chest to limit movement in order to eliminate pain. This is done by taking broad tape, such as two-inch tape, and placing it horizontally immediately over the place where the pain is, the tape strips being about 8 to 10 inches long or longer for a very large person. A second piece of tape the same length is put on top of the first, allowing the second to overlap approximately one-third of the width of the tape. Another one is placed above the first one, again about one-third overlapping allowed.

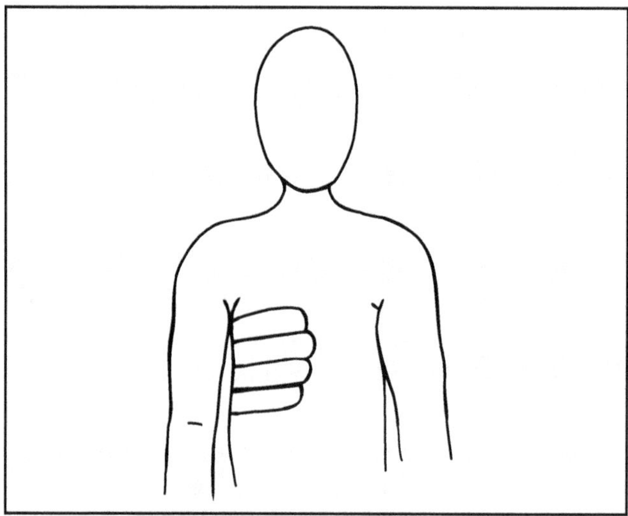

Hot baths can be very helpful both for the underlying disease process as well as to relieve pain and promote healing. Fomentations, very hot and very prolonged, with hot foot baths will also help. Hot foot baths alone can be effective for pleurisy. (See "Hydrotherapy" in the *Natural Remedies* section.)

Do not give cold applications in pleurisy following fomentations or at any other time.

If pleurisy persists, obtain x-rays and blood work for diagnosis of the underlying cause.

As in bronchitis, place the patient in a chest heating compress with a long sleeve shirt or sweater to completely cover the arms. Blood must be equally distributed between the trunk and extremities. Then place a double fomentation pack crosswise over the chest and well down both sides under the arms. Cover with plastic to retain heat for 20 minutes. Remove and place a second pack (no cold between) for 20 minutes, then a third. Finish with a warm shower, a warm friction sponge bath, or an alcohol rub. Use a heating compress to the chest at night.

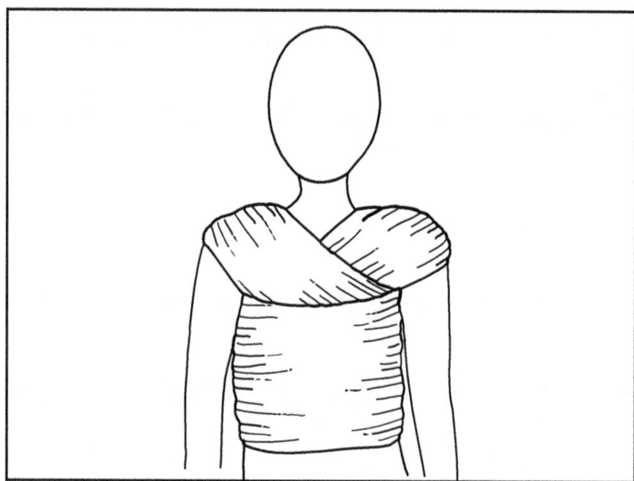

Pneumonia

There are several different kinds of pneumonia, depending on the germ causing the lung infection. The location of the infection will determine if it is lobar (in a lobe) or bronchopneumonia (infection around the bronchi). Bacterial pneumonia is of such a serious nature that complete home care should not be undertaken without the help of a physician, unless one is unavailable as in a mission field.

Despite antibiotics and sophisticated testing and supportive equipment, the mortality for pneumonia and other pulmonary infections has not changed since the 1940s (*Annals of Internal Medicine* 111 [1989]: 232–37). Similarly, there has been no change in the mortality for ARDS (Adult Respiratory Distress Syndrome) despite all our sophisticated drugs and machines such as PEEP (Positive End Expiratory Pressure), etc.

Treatment

The daily program of natural treatments should include one full treatment in the morning. No special attempt should be made to cause perspiration after the first treatment, especially if the patient is very weak, but the reaction of redness should be expected and sought for. Subsequent treatments should be quite hot, but not prolonged beyond the comfortable endurance of the patient. Each hot treatment should be concluded with a cold mitten friction. If the patient is very ill, the afternoon treatment may include only a hot foot bath,

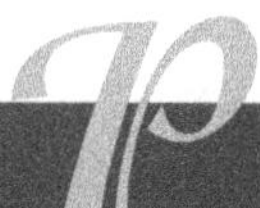

fomentations to the upper chest for cough, and a massage or an enema if needed.

Grapefruit boiled in water can be used for pneumonia, bronchitis, and hay fever. Take a tablespoonful or two several times a day. Place one grapefruit, scrubbed thoroughly and cut into eight pieces, in one-half gallon of water and boil gently for half an hour. For people who live or work in very dusty or heavy air, use a few drops of grapefruit seed extract boiled in water on a hot plate or stove (as a vapor). People breathe more easily, even those who have asthma, when they follow this routine.

For pneumonia, bronchitis, asthma, coughing, etc., sip honey, lemon, or crab apple juice, comfrey, or mullein leaf tea, soy oil, asparagus, grape juice, cranberries, or garlic for free and easy breathing.

Do not allow the development of constipation or gas, as irritating intestinal gases are excreted via the lungs. Inhalations of medicated steam are often helpful. Delirium may occur with fever over 103°F. Cold compresses to the head are helpful in delirium. Dehydration should be studiously avoided by urging water drinking many times daily. Keep a record of intake and output of fluids. Remember that about two quarts of fluid are ordinarily needed by a healthy person, and a person with a fever or receiving sweating treatments will need more. Count on two quarts plus an equal quantity for all that is lost in urine and vomitus. Chapped lips indicate dehydration. Prevent severe cracking from fever blisters by using petrolatum. Hot water to drink may be better than cold if there are abdominal complaints. All treatments should be given with attention to avoiding fatigue. Do not discontinue treatments too soon; they should be continued at least two or three days after the fever has subsided, though tapered in length and frequency.

Vinegar and Turpentine Compresses

For pneumonia, bronchitis, chest congestion, or laryngitis, create a vinegar and turpentine compress.

Boil a gallon of vinegar. Then add six ounces of turpentine, which can be obtained from a paint store. About four cups of this mixture will be required to start with. Fold a bath towel until it is square and thick. Pour the mixture into the folded towel. Wring it out in the scalding solution, then lay it on the front of the chest over the area of congestion, using care not to burn the patient. Cover it quickly with a thick plastic garbage bag and a towel. When it has cooled, wring it out again and apply as before. Continue the process for 20 minutes. Then turn the patient and apply the vinegar pack for 10 minutes on the back of the chest, behind the area of congestion. Keep the vinegar and turpentine solution hot during the entire treatment. Wait two and a half hours and repeat, continuing around the clock. Keep this up until the fever drops. In bronchial pneumonia the fever will usually drop in 24 hours or less. In lobar pneumonia the crisis will usually occur in 36 hours. In bronchitis, usually two packs are sufficient to clear up acute infection in the bronchial tubes.

Garlic and onion blended with olive oil applied in a thick layer on the very bottoms of the feet can be helpful. Then cover the feet with cloth, then with plastic bags. Garlic and onion are likely to blister the feet without the oil. However, some people are sensitive to garlic and may blister even with the oil. Therefore, we recommend that only a small patch be applied to the sole of the foot at first. A thick layer should be used on this small patch, covered with a cloth or a sock, and then a plastic bag applied to prevent evaporation. Leave the garlic compresses on at first for one hour only. Examine for redness, itching, blistering, etc. If there is no reaction in 12 hours after removing the garlic, put a second compress to one-half of the same foot. Again let it remain for one to two hours. If there is no reaction in 12 hours, both feet may be treated with the garlic and onion compress. Be careful not to blister the feet, especially of persons with diabetes or other forms of impaired circulation to the lower extremities. The garlic-onion compress works by reflex action to increase circulation to the lungs. The very same process may be used on the chest.

Garlic taken by mouth is also very helpful for pneumonia. Make a smoothie of one glassful of tomato juice blended with two cloves of uncooked garlic. Drink slowly to prevent nausea.

In 1927 a treatment for pneumonia was given by Dr. James M. Anders of Philadelphia who described it as consisting of sponging the sides and front of the chest, as well as the extremities, with a cold friction mitt wrung from water at 70°F, the temperature lowered two degrees with each subsequent bath, until 50°F had been achieved. He indicated that he had seen cases of bronchopneumonia, particularly among children, successfully treated in this way. Each treatment was finished off by toweling to induce reddening of the skin (a friction toweling with a dry terry cloth).Cover each part after sponging and rubbing to avoid chilling. He stated his preference for the cold mitten friction over any form of drug treatment in severe bronchopneumonia in young patients. The patient should be warm before the treatment begins, and should be warmed by a hot foot bath after the treatment if there is

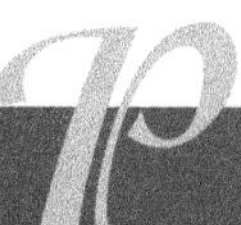

any sensation of chilliness. This kind of treatment may be most helpful where there is no physician.

Lobar Pneumonia

This type of pneumonia can be particularly prostrating and weakening. The pneumococcus is usually the infecting organism. Temperatures may run as high as 105°F to 106°F. Chilling is one of the most significant factors in lowering body defenses and producing the pneumonia. Once one of the common causes of death in young adults, it rarely occurs today, except in those who are immunocompromised. That would include those with AIDS, those who have been on cancer chemotherapy, alcoholics, and elderly people. Three successive stages of pneumonia are recognized: congestion, exudation of blood, and blood products into the air sacs, with subsequent consolidation caused by the coagulation of the blood products. Rational treatment should be directed toward relieving the congestion and producing fluxion of the area to prevent consolidation or facilitate the removal of any consolidated material already formed.

Combine the treatment of a hot foot bath with fomentations to the chest, cold to the head, and a fomentation to the spine, followed by cold mitten friction, repeated once or twice daily. Persistently, carefully, and properly done, this is an effective method of treatment for lobar pneumonia (*Physical Therapeutics* 47 [February 1929]: 89–91).

With the patient lying in bed, give a hot foot bath, fomentations over the part of the chest in which pain is located, a fomentation beneath the patient, and a cold cloth to the forehead. Only the first treatment should be prolonged to the point of profuse sweating. A hot drink may be used to enhance sweating. When profuse sweating has occurred and the feet and skin of the chest are thoroughly reddened, the treatment is then terminated by a cold mitten friction.

The following points are unusually important in lobar pneumonia:

- The room should be warm but never warmer than about 72°F. It is better to be between 65°F to 68°F, as breathing very warm air is not good for the lungs.
- Avoid chilling any part of the patient during the treatment or at any subsequent time (*Physical Therapeutics* 47 [February 1929]: 89–91). It is especially important to avoid the slightest or most brief chilling of the feet; avoid even touching the bare feet to a cold floor.
- Applications must be quite hot. Fomentations should be large and thick, but should not be a heavy weight on the patient, which will inhibit free breathing. And changes should be made very quickly without exposure.
- Cold mitten friction should be energetic, brisk, and to only one small part of the body at a time, the hot applications being removed only as that part of the body is reached during the cold mitten friction at the end.
- Remember to dry the skin thoroughly and handle sweating by repeated drying of the skin. Sweating always endangers the patient to chilling and should be dealt with promptly. It is worthy of repeating that no patch of skin on any part of the body be allowed to become chilled in a patient who has pneumonia.
- Use an assistant to support the patient during any part of the treatment requiring physical exertion beyond the strength of the patient. This is especially important in a weakened patient.

Poison Ivy

(See "Skin Diseases" in the *Conditions and Diseases* section.)

Poisoning

(See "Poisoning" in the *Emergencies and Hazards in the Home* section.)

Poliomyelitis

Polio is a highly infectious disease caused by the polio virus, which invades the nervous system and can rapidly spread to cause total paralysis in a matter of hours. It can strike at any age, but affects mainly children under three (over 50 percent of all cases), and most of the rest are under five years of age.

The virus enters the body through the mouth and multiplies in the intestine and is capable of spreading disease for several weeks after the infection. Fecal contamination of water or food leads to human disease. Initial symptoms are fever, fatigue, headache, vomiting, stiffness in the neck, and pain in the limbs. One in 200 infections leads to irreversible paralysis (usually in the legs). Among those paralyzed, 5 to 10 percent die when their breathing muscles become immobilized. Although paralysis is the most visible sign of polio infection, less than 1 percent of polio infections ever result

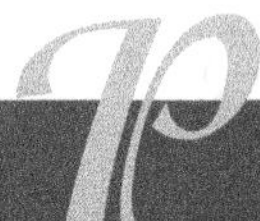

in paralysis. Poliovirus can spread widely in a community before cases of paralysis are seen, as most people infected with poliovirus have few signs of illness, and most are never aware they had polio.

Polio is quite rare in the United States now, with most cases occurring as a complication of vaccination. However, it is still occurring in Third World countries.

It is urgent to begin treatment immediately after symptoms appear. The patient should be given a full body pack twice a day. If there is pain between treatments, use a heavy spinal fomentation for 30 minutes. This extra treatment will relieve pain and reinforce the regular treatments. Hot applications may prevent the development of paralysis.

Back in the 1950s when polio was common, two 14-year-old boys went swimming after school in a polluted canal in Southern California while a polio epidemic was in progress. Late in the afternoon a few days later, both boys began getting sick with a sore throat, fever, and muscle aches and pains. The parents of the boys recognized the ominous signs. One boy, whose father was a physician, was hospitalized and put to bed with the standard pharmaceutical treatment of that day. The other boy's widowed mother was too poor to consider hospitalization, but she gave him hydrotherapy treatments at home all through the night. He was much improved the next day, and well in about one week. The other boy, who received no hydrotherapy, developed paralysis, stayed in the hospital three weeks, and had some permanent weakness in his right leg. He limped the rest of his life.

The Kenny packs are simply hot, thick fomentation packs used over the paralyzed part. Place one hot pack after the other for 30 minutes. Then use a very cold pack for one minute. Repeat these packs in this 30-minute pattern for two hours, ending with the fourth cold pack. Pause for two hours, then repeat four more 30-minute sessions. Pause again for two hours, and apply the third series. Pause for eight hours and begin another day as the 10-hour day yesterday. Continue daily until the patient is entirely well and extremities are free of weakness.

Post Polio Syndrome

Persons who were paralyzed from poliomyelitis in their youth perhaps as long as 50 or more years before may begin experiencing muscular weakness again. This is particularly discouraging since years of training of muscles paralyzed by polio may have resulted in victory years ago, only to find the discouraging situation arising again. The person may have difficulty swallowing with regurgitation and choking on food or drink, may have difficulty breathing, and may have generalized muscular weakness. Once the condition recurs it appears to be permanent. Changes in posture while eating, modifying the diet to more appropriate foods, perhaps softer but not liquid, can help some persons overcome difficulties in swallowing. Postpolio syndrome is not usually progressive, which is good news, but tends to plateau in severity. Victims generally benefit from specially planned nonstressful exercises for the affected parts of the body.

A study on 29 post polio patients showed that 76 percent of the participants had relief of pain when magnets were placed over the most sensitive spots. Dr. Robert R. Holcomb at Vanderbilt University, and the polio center in Warm Springs Georgia, have reported that magnets are quite effective when used in groups of four magnets together, arranged so that positive and negative poles are in an alternating pattern.

Polycythemia

Almost everyone is aware that a low hemoglobin is associated with fatigue, but it is the rare person who understands that rich, heavy blood can also cause fatigue. Pushing around the heavy blood is a strain on the heart and arteries, uses up energy, and results in fatigue.

There are several forms of this disease in which the production of red blood cells in the bone marrow is greatly increased. The condition adds to the viscosity or thickness of the blood, and in its severest forms affects blood flow to the brain and other parts of the body. Symptoms may include dizziness, headaches, feeling of fullness in the head, sometimes fainting, numbness, tingling in the hands and feet, and a feeling of irritability and sluggishness. There may be spells of amnesia. There also may be constant ringing in the ears. The skin sometimes has a purplish red cast because of the prominence of small veins filled with excess blood. There is an increased tendency to form blood clots, and, of course, to have heart attacks and strokes.

The most severe form is called polycythemia rubra vera. Very high levels of hemoglobin, over 17 grams, may represent polycythemia rubra vera and should be investigated by a physician as it is quite serious.

A second form, not as severe as the first, is a reaction to such factors as living at high altitudes, pulmonary or cardiac disease, and most commonly, from stress. Polycythemia is so commonly related to stress that it is often referred to as "stress polycythemia." It probably occurs from excessive diuresis because of stress, alcohol, caffeine products, smoking, and inadequate exercise.

Everything that will reduce stress will eventually bring the hemoglobin down. One should get plenty of exercise, eat

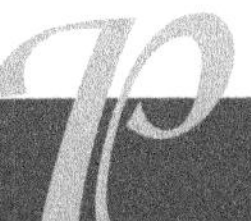

more fruits and vegetables prepared simply or eaten raw, and eat less of all rich or concentrated foods. The ideal levels of hemoglobin where people function best, for women living at sea level to about 1500 feet elevation, are probably around 10.5 to 12.5, and for men from 12 to 14.5, not up to 16 grams for women and 18 grams for men as carried on most laboratory reports. In our opinion this is much too high for an ideal level. Above or below the ideal may result in fatigue, weakness, inability to concentrate, headaches, dizziness, and blood vessel diseases. As the hemoglobin goes up, there is greater and greater likelihood of these symptoms and more serious complications such as an increase in the risks of heart attacks, cancer, and strokes. High blood iron levels act as a pro-oxidant and require a high intake of antioxidants, higher than most people take, in order to balance them.

The size and number of red blood cell clusters or clumps fluctuates depending on the flow speed and friction qualities of the blood and blood vessels. The higher the hemoglobin, the higher the viscosity. The more protein in the blood, the higher the viscosity. The lower the rate of flow, the larger the aggregates formed of red blood cells. This accounts in part for the desirability of remaining active following meals. Heart patients and cancer patients usually show higher degrees of aggregation than well persons. The more clumps or aggregates, the greater the viscosity. An increase in blood viscosity usually comes before the appearance of symptoms. Cigarette smoking increases blood viscosity as does chronic anxiety (L. Dintenfass and G. V. F. Seaman, eds., *Blood Viscosity in Heart Disease and Cancer* [Pergamon Press, 1981]).

Treatment

Use a diet high in fruits and vegetables and low in all other substances, so that for breakfast three servings of fruits are taken to one of grains, legumes, nuts, or any other food. Three servings of vegetables for lunch would be taken to one of any other food.

Diets rich in soybean products can help to reduce iron content of individuals having polycythemia or high serum iron or ferritin levels.

Do not overeat, especially of concentrated foods such as animal products, nuts, seeds, fats, and concentrated sugars. Overeating causes stress on the chemistry of the body and can produce stress polycythemia.

Drink adequate quantities of water to keep the blood as thin as possible. Smoking, alcohol, and the use of caffeine beverages and drugs are potent causes of chronic dehydration. They must be strictly avoided.

Reduce stress in every way possible. The stress hormones increase diuresis, which can lead to relative dehydration. The fluid content of the blood is decreased, with the red blood cells staying constant, giving an increase of red cells per unit volume.

Get adequate exercise for your age and physical condition. For otherwise healthy adults, to build up to one hour of walking or other vigorous outdoor exercise daily can be most helpful.

Practice daily devotions, trusting in God to keep your affairs and your body in good functioning order. Learn to handle the unavoidable stresses through prayer and trust in God.

Frequently donating blood may be very helpful in both kinds of polycythemia, although in true polycythemia it will be done under supervision of a physician.

Polymyalgia Rheumatica, Temporal Arteritis

These two conditions are usually associated and are probably the same disease, possibly one of the collagen diseases. It is a "modern society disease" and generally said to be of unknown cause, but we have seen apparent association with food sensitivities as well as contact with various factors in the environment. Most cases occur in persons over 60 years of age, becoming more common as the population ages.

A host of diseases have been described in the past 50 years that have never been recognized previously. This disorder is one of those, which consists of pain and stiffness in the shoulders and hips, in the thighs, and sometimes in other areas. Women are most usually afflicted. The woman may have great pain when raising the arms, rising from a chair, or getting out of bed. Muscle tenderness may be present, and many of these patients are anemic. Fever and elevated sedimentation rate are the rule, and a giant cell arteritis is found in the temporal artery on biopsy. The artery may be tender to touch, and may show nodular areas along the course of the artery. Headaches, sore tongue, drawing of the side of the mouth, and a generalized sense of not being well usually accompany this disease. In a severe case, if giant cell temporal arteritis is found, there is an increased risk of blindness. The diagnosis is made by the typical history of the pain and tenderness, and by an elevated sedimentation rate. The onset may be sudden or gradual. It may start with something resembling the flu. Generalized muscle stiffness, aches, and pains are the most important single symptom. Also present may be loss of appetite and weight loss. The headache, if present, may be on

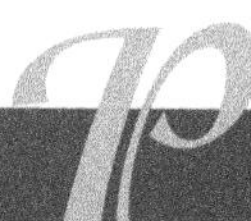

one or both sides, severe, throbbing, and with redness, swelling, and tenderness in the temple, along the temporal artery. There may or may not be a pulse in the artery. Serious complications may occur, including loss of vision, stroke, or heart attack.

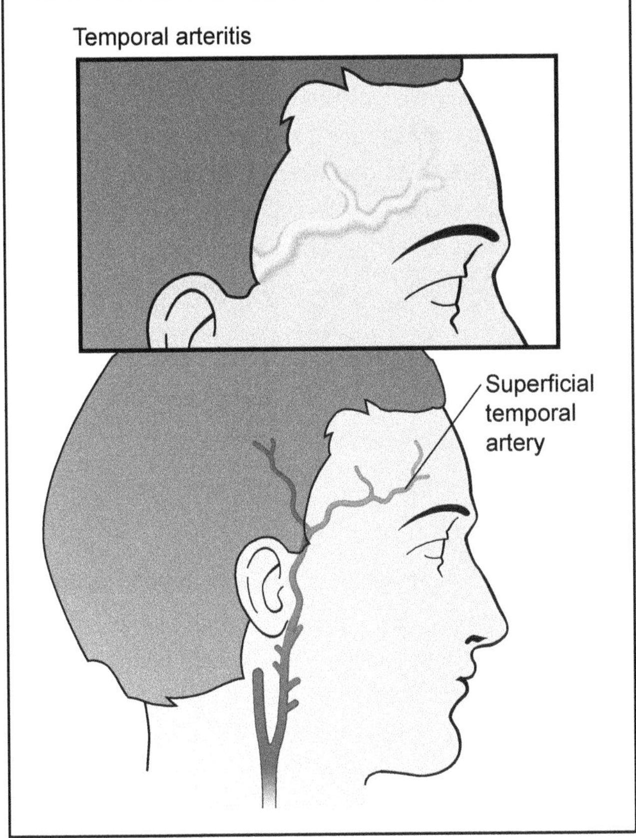

Treatment

The most favorable diet is a plant-based diet, with no contact with any animal products.

Remove with meticulous care all the following for a period of 40 days: dairy products, coffee, tea, colas, chocolate, citrus products, wheat, corn, oats, tomatoes, potatoes, eggplant, peppers, bananas, apples, strawberries, nuts (except walnuts), seeds (except flaxseed and pumpkin), dried legumes, sugar, honey, syrups, malt, all classes of fermented foods, including vinegar and soy sauce, salt, head lettuce, all additives, colorings, flavorings, spices, yeast, and alcoholic drinks. When the symptoms are better, start adding grains, vegetables, fruits, nuts, seeds, and legumes back one at a time every five days. Keep a diary all through the test of what is eaten and the symptoms for that day to see if a pattern develops after eating any food. If any food worsens the symptoms, that food must be eliminated for a year. Then test it again.

Do not eat more than two or three items at any meal, and do not mix fruits and vegetables at the same meal. The "leaky bowel" syndrome may be a part of polymyalgia. In this syndrome the intestinal tract allows macromolecules from incompletely digested food to enter the bloodstream, causing sensitive tissues to react with inflammation. (See "Leaky Gut Syndrome" in the *Conditions and Diseases* section.)

Use anti-inflammatory foods: two tablespoons of walnuts or two tablespoons of ground flaxseed, ground fresh daily should be adequate. Take one to three teaspoons of flaxseed oil daily for two months.

If your general strength will allow it, engage in a total fast of three to five days. If not strong enough for a total fast, have a fresh fruit and fresh juice fast for 5 to 10 days, determined by your strength. Fasting often relieves symptoms remarkably.

Exercise to tolerance daily. Do 15 minutes of stretching exercises every morning before taking outdoor exercise. Walking, gardening, etc., are recommended.

As a test, use all cotton clothing, using old-fashioned soap rather than modern detergents as a laundry aid.

Take a series of 15 fever treatments, five a week for three weeks. Take a break for one week to three months, and repeat with 15 more. May be repeated the third time if needed, then once a year thereafter.

Rub an extract of red pepper (two tablespoons of red pepper soaked for three weeks in a jar with three ounces of rubbing alcohol) on painful areas, beginning four to six times a day until pain relief occurs (about 5 to 10 days), then drop down to only two applications a day. If preferred, you may use a commercial extract such as Zostrix.

Apply hot compresses for 15 minutes to the temporal arteries twice daily. End with an ice cold compress for one minute.

Wear a charcoal compress on the temple each night as long as the temporal artery is inflamed.

Place one-half of a teaspoonful of licorice in a cup of hot water morning and evening. If that dosage is not adequate to improve symptoms, double it. Too much may make you retain sodium, causing a temporary rise in blood pressure. If, after a few weeks of taking it, you begin to see such a rise, reduce the dosage to the level not causing this problem. Licorice has anti-inflammatory properties. Wild yam should also be used as it has the same properties and will enhance the action of the licorice root.

Take two to three Kyolic capsules, or two to three garlic cloves minced or blenderized, with each meal. Garlic is also anti-inflammatory.

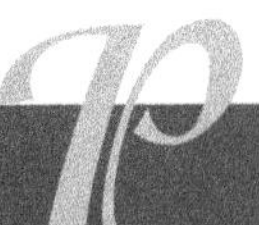

Precocious Puberty

Precocious puberty is defined in textbooks as any indication of beginning puberty before the age of 8 in girls and 9 in boys. We believe, however, that precocious puberty should be defined as puberty coming before age 12 to 14 in girls, and 13 to 18 in boys. In 1997, 7 percent of white girls and 27 percent of African American girls began developing breasts or pubic hair by age 7. Many pediatric endocrinologists believe the suspected precocious puberty epidemic is because of the extraordinary increase in childhood obesity occurring today. Fat cells produce leptin, a protein known to help trigger puberty. There is a premium on keeping children free from overweight.

Premenstrual Syndrome (PMS)

(See "Women's Conditions and Diseases" in the *Conditions and Diseases* section.)

Prickly Heat, Heat Rash

Prickly heat is an acute inflammatory skin rash that itches and consists of tiny elevations containing watery fluid. It is caused by a failure of the skin to adapt itself to an increase in temperature and humidity. The sweat secretions are too thick and the scales on the skin don't shed fast enough. Newcomers in a hot climate often cease to suffer heat rash when they adjust to the new environment. It affects children more often than adults.

Prevention

- Take only small quantities of heavy foods, emphasizing fruits and vegetables.
- Drink lots of water and other liquids.
- Avoid heavy clothing.
- Take frequent cool baths with a one-quarter cup of vinegar in each bath.
- Use a dusting powder, especially in areas where skin often meets skin. Starch powder is best. If powder is inadequate for the amount of moisture produced on the skin, place a folded cotton handkerchief or similar strip of cotton fabric between the two surfaces to minimize the amount of moisture that accumulates.

Treatment

- Cool the skin with cool packs, fans, and air conditioners.
- Take frequent cool baths or showers, every hour or two, with one-quarter cup of vinegar in each bath.
- Dust the skin with cornstarch.
- Avoid soap and skin cosmetics.
- Avoid scratching, which will further damage the skin. Keep fingernails of children short.
- Apply "wet dressings." Use a single layer of thin cotton fabric dipped in cool water to which a few spoonfuls of vinegar have been added. Keep the cloth refreshed every three to four minutes. Continue the treatment for 20 to 60 minutes. It may be repeated as often as necessary.
- Salt should be restricted.
- If the person is overweight, losing weight will help to diminish the chance of getting heat rash.

Prostate

Studies strongly support the idea that diet and sun exposure are the primary controllable factors both in prostate cancer getting started and in attempts to control it by natural means (*The Prostate* 42 [2000]: 243). A plant-based diet is the most favorable diet for health of the prostate, low in free fats, sugars, and salt. Sun exposure should be daily for at least 20 minutes and up to two hours for conditioned skin.

Three common problems may arise with the prostate. Most men develop some degree of benign prostatic hypertrophy (also called hyperplasia), many develop prostatic cancer, and some develop prostatitis. We will briefly discuss these three conditions.

Benign Prostatic Hypertrophy, Hyperplasia

The gradual enlargement of the prostate in men over 50 will first be recognized because of increased difficulty of urination, starting the stream, dribbling, and getting up more often at night to urinate. Urine tends to remain in the bladder, which may irritate the bladder and cause cystitis. Because a man has these symptoms does not necessarily mean his prostate must be removed. He should institute treatments and hope to avoid surgery.

Stinging nettle (*Urtica dioica* or *Urtica urens*), the common weed growing through most of the temperate regions of the world, is a very good treatment for benign prostatic hypertrophy. The nettle root is best for this purpose.

The passage of a no. 17 French catheter may be necessary if urination is impossible. Many patients or their wives learn to do this procedure when necessary. Often after treatment, it becomes unnecessary. The catheter can be kept on hand for emergency use.

Use foods high in zinc. All whole grains, all legumes, pumpkin seeds, most kinds of whole grain corn, especially popcorn, and many nuts and seeds contain zinc.

Benign prostatic hyperplasia has been treated with supplements of plant sterols similar to those used in the menopause routine. In one study there was significant improvement in symptoms and urinary flow with a supplement made from plant sterols by a good herbalist (*Lancet* 345 [1995]: 1529). (See "Food Sources High in Certain Nutrients" in the Dietary Information section for more information about plant sterols.)

Be very temperate in sexual activity as congestion of the prostate may follow and result in stagnation of secretions, one of the suspected causes of benign prostatic hypertrophy.

Exercise vigorously outdoors as activity accomplishes massage of the prostate. Avoid bicycling, horse back riding, or any activity that injures the perineum.

Squeezing and relaxing hip muscles can improve blood flow into the area. The exercise may be performed up to 50 times three times daily. Another exercise done while sitting is stretching the right leg over the left, touching the floor with the big toe, and repeating on the opposite side. As many as 50 repetitions may be performed to encourage a continuous exchange of blood through the prostate.

A hot charcoal retention enema will reduce congestion and promote healing. To one cup of hot water, stir one tablespoon of powdered charcoal and insert into the rectum with a bulb syringe. Pinch the buttocks together to encourage holding the enema until the urge passes and retain overnight.

Use saw palmetto berry tea or the palmetto berry extract capsules two twice a day.

Pygeum (*Pygeum africanum*) bark and stinging nettle (*Urtica dioica*) root act to improve symptoms in benign prostatic hypertrophy. The two herbs used together are quite potent in the treatment of the prostate (*Nutrition and Healing*, February 1999, 3).

A rye grass pollen extract known as ProstaBrit, and known in Europe as Cernilton, is a good treatment for the prostate. Prostate symptoms improve with daily treatment with the pollen extract, two tablets twice a day (*Complimentary Therapies in Medicine* 4 [1996]: 21).

Prostatitis

Prostatitis, or inflammation of the prostate, may occur as a similar picture to acute cystitis in women. There may be vague pain or discomfort in the lower abdomen, groin, or around the seat, rectum, testes, penis, or perineum. There may be the sensation of a "hot potato in the rectum." Upon examination, the prostate feels boggy and tender.

This affliction may be acute or chronic. The acute forms can have pain which may feel hot, tender, and congested in the pelvic area. There may be fever and chills. Urinary urgency and frequency with pain, may also characterize this problem.

Along with hydrotherapy, essential to recovery is an improved body chemistry achieved through diet correction and exclusion of harmful substances that irritate the genitourinary tract. These include tobacco, caffeine, alcohol, chocolate, vinegar, spices, synthetic food additives, and drugs.

Take a hot sitz bath morning and evening for 20 minutes, ending with a cool shower. The hot sitz bath, with or without an alternating cold sitz, is the mainstay of hydrotherapeutic measures for the prostate. Sit in a bathtub with about six inches of water as hot as tolerated. The knees should be pulled up out of the hot water, but the feet should be kept in the small tub of water which should be very hot.

The hot foot bath may be used alone as a good treatment. It increases the flow of blood to the prostate and its neighboring structures. Hot foot baths should not be given to those with severe hardening of the arteries such as insulin-dependant diabetics.

Use also thick fomentations across the lower abdomen and pubic area for 15 minutes. Remove, rub the red area vigorously with a cold sponge, and replace with a fresh hot pack. Repeat four times. Finish the treatment with a cool shower, cold mitten friction, or sponge bath.

A small, hot, retention enema, with water temperature at 108°F to 112°F, is quite helpful. Repeat the enema using eight ounces of hot water each time, every three or four hours.

For urinary retention or inability to void, place a very hot pack on the spine for 20 minutes. Always urinate as soon as the urge is received.

For chronic and subacute prostatitis, massage of the prostate gives a great deal of relief and can be easily performed by someone in the family. The person should be trained to lubricate a gloved finger, insert it into the rectum and massage the prostate, which is located on the front of the body

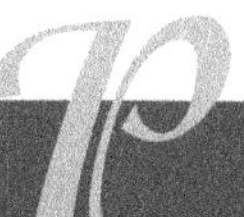

just under the pubic bone. Have the patient bend over a table. The person doing the massage stands behind the patient with the palm of the hand toward the floor.

Reduce stress in the life. Exercise has a neutralizing effect on stress. Prayer and dependence on God reduces stress.

Avoid chilling of the extremities.

Do not sit for long periods unrelieved. It is best to sit on a hard chair or bench, and interrupt periods of sitting by standing every 30 to 60 minutes for a minute or two. Walking will often relieve congestion.

Avoid constipation and gas by appropriate measures.

Increase fluid intake to ensure the bladder is healthy.

Eliminate all known irritants such as tobacco, alcohol, coffee, tea, colas and chocolate; spices such as ginger, cinnamon, nutmeg, cloves, black and red pepper; and all foods made with spices. Also eliminate nuts, vinegar, and drugs containing pilocarpine, atropine, and the antihistamines as a trial to relieve symptoms.

Echinacea, golden seal chaparral, and grapefruit seed extract are useful for accute infections.

You may use equal amounts of spearmint, comfrey, plantain, and catnip. Steep in freshly boiled water for 20 minutes. For one quart, use one tablespoon of each of the herbs. Drink one quart per day in four divided doses for three weeks. The patient may repeat in one month if necessary. This remedy also helps prostate cancer.

Use saw palmetto berry capsules or tea. The capsule should furnish 80 to 160 milligrams two or three times a day. The tea is made from dried berries. Use two tablespoons to a quart of water. Simmer for 15 to 30 minutes. Take one quart of the tea daily in four divided doses.

Prostate Cancer

(See also "Cancer" in the *Conditions and Diseases* section.)

The use of saturated fats in margarine, butter, cheese, milk, eggs, meat, and hardened vegetable fats have been demonstrated to have a causative role in the development of prostate cancer (*Journal of the National Cancer Institute* 87 [1995]: 652).

Take estrogen supplements (used for the menopause syndrome and for cancer of the prostate) such as wild yam, black cohosh (binds to hormone receptors on the cells), licorice tea, angelica, and burdock. A progesterone supplement herb, chaste tree, is also very good for prostate cancer. The same herbs used for cystitis can also be used for the prostate.

A device for putting a hot water balloon next to the prostate for benign prostatic hypertrophy has had good success. Twenty-seven men scheduled for surgery because of benign disease or because of adenocarcinoma of the prostate underwent water-induced thermotherapy. Lidocaine gel was the sole means of pain control. Only mild treatment discomfort was reported. There was death of prostate tissue at a distance measuring from 7 to 11 millimeters from the urethra, up to half an inch. The procedure is well tolerated and gives relief for these patients (*Urology* 56 [2000]: 76). The devices can be purchased for home use in many conditions—thrombosed hemorrhoids, anal fissures, proctitis, etc.

Pruritus Ani

This condition is characterized by itching around the anus, which is most commonly caused by a food sensitivity in adults and by pinworms in children. It may also be caused by seborrheic dermatitis, eczema, psoriasis, infection, inadequate hygiene, liver disease, diabetes, and contact dermatitis to such articles as dyed toilet tissue, soap, deodorants, dyes in underclothing, or detergents used for laundering, etc.

Treatment

Do a test to find foods to which you may be sensitive, called an Elimination and Challenge diet. (See "Elimination and Challenge Diet" in the *Dietary Information* section.) You may start with the following list of foods to eliminate: alcoholic beverages, milk, coffee, tea, colas, chocolate, citrus fruits and juices, tomatoes, chocolate, nuts, popcorn, and highly seasoned or spicy food. When the symptoms go away, start adding back one food per week until symptoms return.

Avoid gas-forming foods as they can often intensify the itching. (See "Gas, Flatulence" in the *Conditions and Diseases* section.)

Do a perineal pour each time you go to the bathroom. The pour should consist of a quart of hot or cold water into which one to four tablespoons of vinegar have been stirred. While sitting on the commode, use care that the water bathes down across all the perineal structures, particularly around the anal area. The fingers may be used to open all the folds around the anus.

Avoid the use of drugs of any kind, either by mouth or the local anesthetics often used in ointments for pruritus ani, as they can cause a severe sensitivity reaction. Avoid the use of mineral oil as a laxative as it may cause sensitivity on the skin.

Use a high bulk laxative such as psyllium seed for complete bowel evacuation daily. Immediately after a bowel

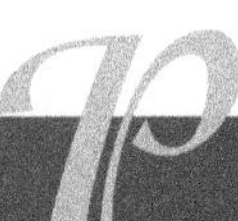

movement, the area should be thoroughly cleaned, but soaps of all kinds should be strictly avoided. A small piece of cotton may be placed against the anus to absorb moisture.

A hot sitz bath morning or afternoon can be helpful to relieve symptoms. Use a cup or so of vinegar in the water.

Do not use soap, toilet tissue, or any kind of cosmetic or chemical on the area. Cleanse the skin with plain water. After a bowel movement, the area should be wiped with a wet paper towel or a wet piece of cotton cloth rather than toilet tissue if toilet tissue irritates the skin.

A bit of aloe vera gel put on a thin pledget of dry cotton may be helpful in reducing itching. The same can be done with a golden seal tea bag moistened in water. It has a dramatic healing effect in many people.

Scratching is very bad for the perianal skin and can convert a temporary problem into a chronic one.

Sweat is an enemy in this area as bacteria can breed in the warm environment. In hot, humid climates, it may be necessary to take a cool shower two or three times a day.

If itching is severe and cannot be controlled by the above measures, try using Solstice (available in most drug stores and supermarkets). It has menthol and other soothing substances in a vanishing cream base.

It is easy to develop a superficial fungus infection in the irritated areas, which will keep the condition going. This can be treated by a quick spray of diluted vinegar. Simply put vinegar and enough water to prevent burning in a well-rinsed, empty spray bottle and give one quick spray to the area every time the area is wiped or cleansed. (See "Skin Diseases" in the *Conditions and Diseases* section.)

One patient reported instant relief after making a powder from rolled oats in a seed mill or blender. Mix the powder with water to make a paste. Spread this paste on the anus, or on the perineum, for itchiness or erosions. The patient reported immediate relief with the application of the paste.

Psoriasis

(See "Skin Diseases" in the *Conditions and Diseases* section.)

Pterygium

A pterygium is a benign growth of the thin covering of the eye, the conjunctiva, which most often grows from the nasal side of the eye over the sclera. It is associated with, and thought to be caused by ultraviolet-light exposure (e.g. sunlight), low humidity, dehydration of the conjunctiva, and dust.

This affliction is usually treated with surgery, but in the early stages it can be treated in a way to make it shrink, or possibly even go away. Use aloe vera gel directly in the eye. There are certain commercial preparations of aloe vera that have a small amount of ascorbic acid added. This is best, but do not use the preparation if it burns. Therefore, if at all possible, test the solution in your eye before purchasing it.

Drink borage tea. Put one heaping teaspoon to a cup of freshly boiled water and let it steep for 30 minutes. Also, you can use eyebright strained and filtered through a gauze or unbleached coffee filter, and used with an eyecup every two hours. You may also use witch hazel leaf (or bark), one heaping teaspoon in a pint of water. If it is the leaf, steep it for half an hour, but if it is the bark, boil it for 25 minutes. Filter and cool. Use it with an eyecup, or put drops directly into the eye every hour or two. Discontinue use immediately if pain or burning develops.

A golden seal tea infusion can be strained through unbleached coffee filters and used for pterygium eyewash.

Instill in the eye with a dropper, four to five times each day, one of the following formulae:

Recipe #1

- Four to five parts aloe vera liquid (buy from a health food store; make sure you get a brand that does not cause burning when introduced into the eye)
- One part of vitamin A oil

Shake together vigorously and refrigerate until ready to use. Once it has been shaken, it is ready to be dropped into the eye.

Recipe #2

- One-half teaspoon golden seal powder
- Two teaspoons eyebright
- One-half quart water, recently boiled

Let the mixture steep for 30 minutes and filter through a coffee filter. The drops should not burn when dropped into the eye.

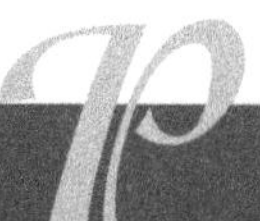

Pulse pressure

What is the significance of the spread between systolic and diastolic blood pressure readings? Mayo clinic hypertension specialist Sheldon Sheps, MD, explains that the numeric difference between your systolic and diastolic blood pressure is called your pulse pressure. For example, if your resting blood pressure is 120/80, your pulse pressure is 40—the difference between 120 and 80. Certain conditions can increase your pulse pressure. These include aortic valve disorders, severe anemia, and overactive thyroid (hyperthyroidism). But by far the most important cause of elevated pulse pressure is stiffness and reduced elasticity of the aorta, the largest artery in the body. This may be because of high blood pressure or fatty deposits on the walls of the arteries (atherosclerosis). The greater the difference between your systolic and diastolic numbers, the stiffer and more damaged the vessels are thought to be.

Evidence suggests that pulse pressure may be the strongest predictor of heart problems, especially in older adults. In adults older than age 60, a pulse pressure greater than 60 millimeterHg is abnormal. Treating high blood pressure usually reduces pulse pressure as well (*Archives of Internal Medicine* 165 [October 10, 2005]: 2142–47).

Pyelonephritis

This disease is a serious inflammation or infection of the kidney, both the kidney pelvis and the functioning portions of the kidney, usually resulting from a germ traveling from another part of the body by means of the bloodstream and filtered out in the kidneys. High fever, tenderness in one loin, and a high white blood cell count, are characteristic. The urine may become cloudy, or even bloody.

Treat the disease diligently with a hot fomentation over the back as one would treat kidney stones. (See "Kidney Stones" in the *Conditions and Diseases* section.) Apply the applications for 45 minutes and repeat every three to four hours until the fever drops below 100°F. These patients may become very sick. Give plenty of fluids, but do not overload the sick kidney. Follow other measures used for other inflammations and infections.

Pyorrhea, Periodontal Disease

(See "Dental Care" in the *Conditions and Diseases* section.)

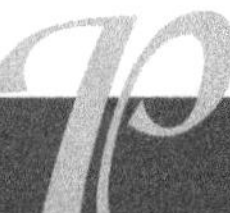

Quinsy, Peritonsillar Abscess

Pain in the ear may be the first sign of peritonsillar abscess. The person may have great difficulty swallowing and talking, having a pronounced nasal sound to the voice. The senses of taste and smell may be almost lost. A low grade fever is typical, though it may become high and spiking. It can be life-threatening because of obstruction of the airway or spread of infection to the brain. For this reason, it is very important to try to control the infection before abscess formation occurs.

Treatment

Patients with quinsy must not be left alone, as their breathing passages may become blocked in extreme cases. If gargling is impossible, irrigate the mouth and tonsillar area with the person lying on one side, holding a basin under the jaw. Use a bulb syringe or water pick, the irrigation fluid being hot garlic water, or hot charcoal water. (See "Hydrotherapy" in the Natural Remedies section.) Continue the irrigation for 10 minutes.

Keep the patient well hydrated. If unable to swallow, irrigate the throat with the above solutions. Give water rectally by small retention enemas, four ounces via bulb-syringe every hour, or about 64 ounces of water and/or the above tea daily.

Mild fever treatments in a bathtub may be carried out every four hours if the patient can tolerate them. Use continuous fomentations (hot steam packs) to the neck on the involved side when the patient is not in a fever bath. A half-filled hot water bottle draped on one side of the neck or a cravat style electric heating pad are also quite acceptable. If the patient becomes weary, a heating compress may be applied to allow the patient time to rest. A charcoal compress, covering the ear, the neck, and the jaws can also be very helpful. The compress can be kept warm with a 100-watt bulb in an ordinary shop lamp fastened to the bed just above the compress.

If the patient can swallow, use echinacea-golden seal tea; one cup every hour, or the tincture, one teaspoonful every hour. Garlic capsules or tablets may be used if they can be swallowed. Use grapefruit seed extract, 10 drops in a glass of water every four hours. If the patient cannot swallow, the echinacea-golden seal tea can be given freely by rectum, but use care with the grapefruit seed extract or garlic, as these herbs may irritate the rectum. If irritation develops, discontinue promptly.

If breathing becomes labored or difficult, you must provide an airway. Even the empty elastic shell of a ball point pen can be carefully slipped into the trachea by pressing past the swollen tonsil and palate. Try to get the patient to emergency medical care immediately, as a tracheostomy (emergency opening in the trachea) may become necessary. While this is a rare complication, it has been reported and should be planned for.

Case Report

A 28-year-old woman who was extremely sensitive to antibiotics, called one Tuesday morning to get assistance with a sore throat. Her voice sounded nasally, somewhat like that of one with a cleft palate. I asked how long her throat had been sore, and she said, "Since Sunday." Her sore throat had gotten worse daily. I suspected a peritonsillar abscess. I

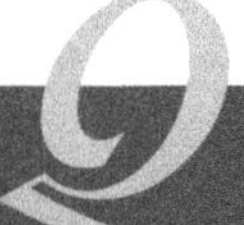

inquired if her right ear were painful. She said it was and that swallowing was almost out of the question. Even trying to swallow her saliva was too painful most of the time, and she simply spat it out, or wiped it from her mouth. When I examined her throat, I saw a large swelling around the right tonsil and extreme redness of the throat on both sides, but there was little if any swelling on the left. It was a failure of the palate to meet the tongue all the way across the back of the mouth that caused the nasal quality of the voice.

We treated her with hot irrigations using a water pick and salt water as hot as she could tolerate. We began using echinacea and golden seal tea as much as she could tolerate as a retention enema. We used a charcoal compress around her neck, on her ear, and on the side of her face. This charcoal compress gave her more pain relief than any other measure. She took hot foot baths every two hours, and a gentle fever treatment up to 102°F mouth temperature once a day, followed by a dry friction rub. She tried to swallow charcoal paste, but usually could hardly hold it in her mouth. A full body massage was given daily. A responsible person was with her continually to report to me any difficulty breathing and to give her treatments. When all other treatments had been done, we gave her a foot rub.

On Friday morning when I visited her, she told me with the same nasal voice that she was exhausted, that she was no better, had not slept since Monday night, and still couldn't swallow without extreme pain. Even though she gave me this discouraging report, on inquiring, I found her ear pain had disappeared, and she had been able to take one-half cup of applesauce and some whole wheat bread soaked in soy milk. We had earnest prayer. By noon she was still in pain. We gave her a hot bath with friction while she was still in the bath, and ended the treatment with cold mitten friction. She fell asleep at 4:30 p.m. for the first time in four days, and slept until 7:00 p.m. When she woke up she was feeling much better. We thanked the Lord for answering our prayers. The next day she was out of bed, had a good voice, good appetite, but was 12 pounds lighter than a week before.

The abscess dissipated without the necessity to drain it. Immediately she was able to go back to work, as she did not need to recover from the harmful effects of heavy doses of antibiotics on the gastrointestinal system and general constitution.

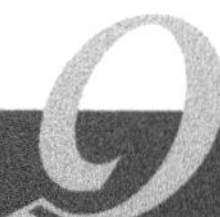

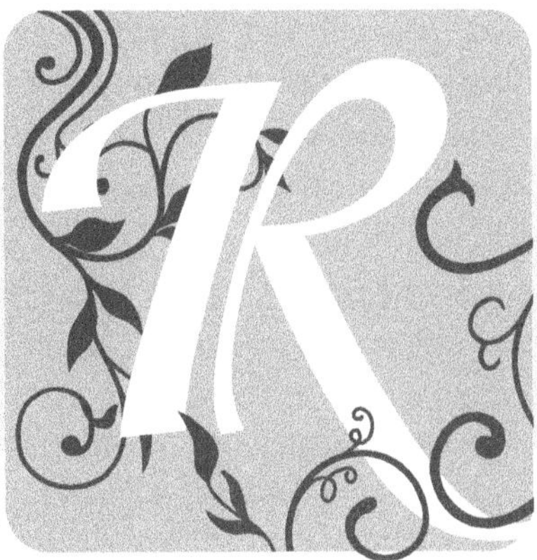

Raynaud's Phenomenon

In this disease, the arteries of the fingers and hands go into spasm when exposed to vibration or cold, turning white, feeling cold, lifeless, and painful. The decrease in blood flow to the skin is usually only in the hands, but the feet, toes, nose, cheeks, ears, and chin may also be involved. The parts initially feel numb and cold, then unpleasant tingling, swelling, and pain begins. When the blanching time is over, the part may turn bright red.

This condition may be because of systemic disorders, or to no recognizable cause, in which case it is called Raynaud's disease. Raynaud's disease is most common in women beginning in the teens or early 20s, or at any time throughout life. Mild attacks last only a few minutes, but severe attacks may persist for hours. Between attacks the skin looks normal until the disease is advanced, at which time the tissues may atrophy, or become swollen and the skin discolored, shiny, taut, and smooth. Nails may become clubbed, or deformed, sensation may decrease, and the ends of the fingers may turn dark as the tissues begin to die and dry up. The loss of the ends of the fingers can occur in rare, severe cases.

Prevention

It has been discovered that in persons with Raynaud's the blood is quite thick and has a slow-flow condition somewhat like honey on a cold morning. It is not known whether the Raynaud's comes first and causes the thick blood, or whether the thick blood comes first and causes the Raynaud's. We favor the latter position. We believe that too many red blood cells and plasma containing too many nutrients and wastes promotes the development of Raynaud's (L. Dintenfass and G. V. F. Seaman, eds., *Blood Viscosity in Heart Disease and Cancer* [Pergamen Press, 1981]). We suggest that all should keep a close watch over the annual laboratory blood report. (See "Blood Viscosity" in the *Supplemental Information* section for methods of getting the hemoglobin and hematocrit levels down.)

Arginine deficiency may be a cause of Raynaud's disease.

Use a fat-free, sugar-free diet with no concentrated proteins. The plant-based diet is the most favorable. Use no highly seasoned foods.

Keep well hydrated, drinking plain water between meals.

Avoid tobacco smoke, even secondhand smoke. Avoid the use of drugs and alcohol, especially the ergot, beta blocking, cytotoxic drugs, and birth control pills.

Keep all rooms in the house approximately the same temperature to avoid sudden changes in skin temperature. Avoid contact with cold objects, even for the briefest period. Use mitts to remove cold items from the refrigerator or freezer. Use tepid or warm water at the sink.

Sleep in a heated bed.

A vigorous hand, wrist, and finger massage every evening prevents attacks for many people.

Avoid machines that vibrate the hands. People who use chainsaws and similar equipment sometimes develop Raynaud's.

Sun baths with the body fully clothed help in general physical resistance.

Dress warmly at all times, using the very best fit and quality underclothing, footwear, and mittens.

Stress should not be allowed, and should be neutralized by vigorous outdoor exercise every day.

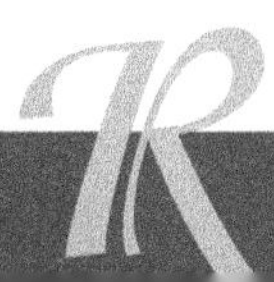

Treatment

To stop an attack, a warm drink may help provide relief within a couple of minutes.

Immerse the affected part in warm (not hot) water, or any warm liquid. Start warming the backs of the hands, the upper chest and backs of the shoulders first, with the use of heating pads, hot water bottles, or warm cloths applied to the area—then lay these aside and immerse the part in warm water.

When the attack comes on, whirl the arms, driving the arterial blood into the capillaries by centrifugal force. The whirling movement should not be performed until the arm and shoulder have been warmed up by a gentle range of motion movement, after the fashion of a soft ball pitcher warming up. If the shoulder is painful, the movement can be simulated by an exaggerated movement of the arms as in walking, reaching as high in front and slinging the arm downward and backward as far as possible, swinging back and forth with as much force and speed as possible until the arterial blood has driven the blood vessels open. The maneuver can be done with the hands held down in front and side to side, rather than all on the side back and forth if there is pain on the backward movement. This maneuver will usually stop the pain in a matter of seconds.

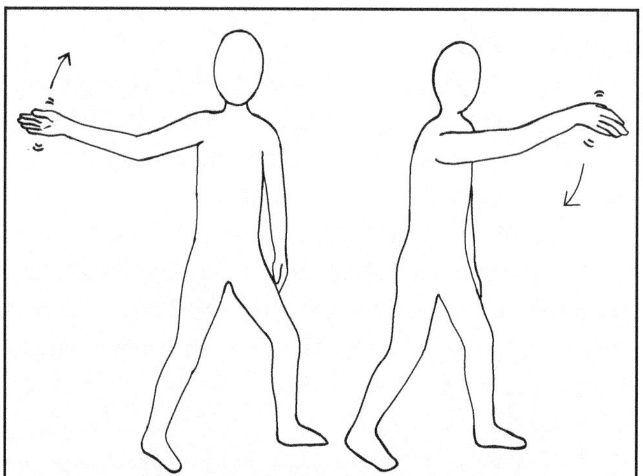

Another way to relieve an acute attack is by putting pressure on the center of the forearm two finger widths above the wrist crease.

One study shows an association of *Helicobacter pylori* infection with Raynaud's phenomenon (*Lancet* 348 [October 5, 1996]: 966). (See "Ulcers, Peptic, Duodenal, Gastric, Pyloric, Stomach" in the *Conditions and Diseases* section for treatment of *Helicobacter pylori*). A trial treatment for one month might be helpful for Raynaud's disease.

Massage makes the condition better. Try rubbing in a dilute suspension of cypress essence in 10 percent jojoba oil, 20 percent wheat germ oil, and 70 percent grape seed oil. The essence should constitute no more than 2.5 percent of the total (about three drops to every very full teaspoon of base oil). Essence of cypress can be obtained from any shop selling essential oils.

Cold weather and cold climates make the problem worse. Those having Raynaud's problem should seek to live in warmer climates.

Carefully perform an "Elimination and Challenge Diet" in the *Dietary Information* section. Many people are sensitive to foods that have blood vessel reactions.

Along with hydrotherapy, essential to recovery is an improved body chemistry achieved through diet correction, and exclusion of harmful substances which irritate the body systems. Become a vegetarian by eliminating all foods that come from animals. Avoid free fats, spices, vinegar, and all foods known to disagree with one.

Magnesium supplements and omega-3 fatty acids (found in walnuts and flaxseed among other places) can help relieve the symptoms of Raynaud's phenomenon. Magnesium deficiency has been linked to Raynaud's phenomenon because of its role in stabilizing blood vessels and preventing cold-induced constriction of blood vessels (*American Journal of Natural Medicine* 3, no. 8 [October 1996]: 21). Omega-3 supplementation can be helpful to decrease the likelihood one will get the whitening response to cold in persons who have Raynaud's phenomenon (*The American Journal of Medicine* 86 [1989]: 158).

We have found that astragalus is a very helpful herb to abolish the symptoms of Raynaud's disease.

Another herb that should be given is ginkgo. It improves circulation. One patient taking astragalus (three capsules per day) and ginkgo (three capsules per day) for one month had a remission of all symptoms that had been unrelenting for eight years.

Rectal Fistula

A fistula is an abnormal connection or passageway between two organs or vessels that normally do not connect. The rectal fistula is an abnormal connection between the interior of the rectum and the skin beside the anus or on the buttocks. It often results from an abscess next to the rectum that burrows into the rectum and outward onto the skin. Persistence is required to treat them successfully, but this can be done if you are patient.

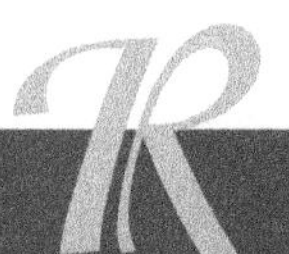

Causes of fistulas include diseases such as inflammatory bowel diseases like Crohn's disease and ulcerative colitis. These are leading causes or anorectal, bowel loop to bowel loop, and bowel to skin fistulas. Radiation therapy can lead to a fistula between the urinary bladder and the vagina.

Use four ounces of coconut oil and two tablespoons total of herbs, one-third of which is golden seal, one-third witch hazel bark, and one-third comfrey root powder. Boil gently in a double boiler for four hours. Refrigerate, and when just beginning to gel, dig out by one teaspoon size portions and roll each into a thin pencil. Refrigerate the pencils until quite hard. Insert one of these about three times per day into the fistula tract if it can be penetrated, or into the rectum as close to the fistula opening as possible. If the cocoa butter does not fully melt, a heating pad or hot water bottle can be placed against the area until it melts.

Another good treatment is a very hot sitz bath (just enough water to adequately cover the opening of the fistula) into which two cups of triple strength witch hazel tea and two cups of triple strength golden seal tea have been poured. Sit for 30 minutes in the hot sitz bath two or three times daily until it shows signs of healing. A small tub, only large enough for the person to sit in, is desirable, such as a baby bathtub or any small plastic tub.

Case Report

A 27-year-old man called us with the beginning of his second fistula from the rectum to the skin. For weeks he had been developing increasing disability while walking or sitting because of pain and bulging opposite the area where his first fistula had been surgically removed. His doctor recommended a second surgery. He did not have the $3,000 for another operation as they had just added another child to their family. We suggested the following routine in an attempt to avoid surgery.

Fast with water for only two days. Then eat only fruits for two days. When resuming a regular diet, he ate a plant-based diet for six weeks, avoiding gluten (we suspected Crohn's), spices, vinegar, coffee, tea, soda, and chocolate. He also used the sitz baths and the herbal pencils. Within five days the fistula opened to the outside, the bulge, discoloration, and pain immediately subsided. Then began the long healing process. He continued the diet for five weeks. Every day brought more improvement until he was completely healed. He saved about $2,900 in out-of-pocket expenses and avoided having to miss work because of the surgery. He rejoiced in the simple remedies.

Reflex Sympathetic Dystrophy, Causalgia

This diagnosis is given to individuals who have pain, discoloration, or decreased range of movement or weakness in a limb following relatively minor trauma or an operation on a limb. The symptoms usually worsen after exercise involving the affected limb. Tremors often develop in the limb as well as muscle incoordination. There is often atrophy of muscles, involuntary movements, muscle spasms, and paralysis that comes and goes.

Treatment

Taking 500 milligrams per day of Vitamin C helped to relieve symptoms of reflex sympathetic dystrophy (RSD). This dosage was given to individuals with wrist fractures, reducing the percentage developing RSD from 22 percent to 8 percent (*Journal of Bone and Joint Surgery, British* 81-B [1999]: 166).

Researchers reported in another study 127 persons with fractured wrists, and of those that received 500 milligrams of vitamin C per day, only 7 percent developed RSD after surgery or trauma, while 22 percent of the control group developed RSD over the course of a year (*The Lancet* 354 [1999]: 9195).

For the pain, put one-half teaspoon of red pepper (cayenne) in a pint jar with approximately one cup of rubbing alcohol. Swirl it around and let it settle. Dip a cotton-tipped applicator into the alcohol and rub it on a test area over the place where you feel a lot of pain. After it has dried, rub some DMSO over the same area. It is likely to burn quite a great deal after the first few applications. Having a fan blow on it can be helpful. It will not cause any injury, and the burning should last no more than 15 or 20 minutes. If it is too unpleasant, the area should be wiped with rubbing alcohol to remove both the DMSO and the red pepper extract. Capsaicin in the red pepper depletes the substance P in the skin, which is essential for the transmission of nerve impulses. If you can tolerate it, put it on six times a day for six days, then twice a day thereafter. You will observe that day by day the intensity of the burning reduces somewhat until it is quite tolerable after about 6 to 10 days. If you prefer not to make up the red pepper-alcohol extract, you can purchase the same material in cream form from a drug store under the name of Zostrix. However, it is quite expensive.

Several people have obtained pain relief by sleeping on a magnetic mattress. This mattress has ordinary magnets placed

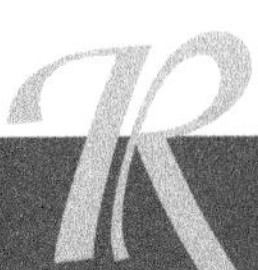

in such a position that it balances nerve impulses according to engineers who have been involved in researching the matter. If you are interested in the magnetic mattress, you should get in touch with a rehabilitation department in a large hospital and ask for a company in your area selling the mattresses.

Case Report

A 66-year-old man with Dupuytren's contracture had surgery to correct the contracture. During surgery there was a malpositioning of the arm. The surgery healed well, but the arm was painful after the surgery and was immobilized for a few days. Immobilization seemed to increase the symptoms, and pain developed in the fingers and along the forearm. He lost about 60 percent of muscle strength in the arm and fingers and continued to have pain. After about five years, his pain began to subside and his gradual loss of strength slowed down. Now, seven years after surgery, he is in a stable condition, almost never has pain, and the weakness is not noticeable.

Restless Legs Syndrome

Nearly five percent of the population is affected by restless legs syndrome. A majority are middle aged or older. Most of the victims have only a mild case. Persons may discover they have it only after their spouse protests of being continually kicked.

Symptoms of restless legs syndrome include strange feelings in the legs such as "creepy, crawly sensations," tiny worms working through the leg muscles, numbness, tingling, pins and needles, and the feeling that walking is a must no matter how tired. Leg twitches may occur every 20 to 40 seconds during sleep, and sometimes during wakefulness. Other signs are depression, muscle or intellectual fatigue, depressed ankle jerk, diminished vibration sense in the legs, stocking-type reduced sensation, and long lasting constipation (*Modern Medicine*, February 15, 1977, 69).

The following symptoms must be present to make a diagnosis of restless legs syndrome:

- A disagreeable, crawling, or tightening sensation in the legs.
- A feeling of needing to move the legs to relieve the sensation.
- Symptoms are the worst during the evening and nighttime hours.
- After lying down the symptoms worsen or you become more aware of them.

Causes

The condition may be triggered by food sensitivities anemia, circulatory problems, diabetes, alcoholism, pregnancy, antidepressant drugs, diseases of the kidneys, nerves or muscles, the use of caffeine, calcium channel blockers, several other types of drugs, folic acid deficiency, or iron deficiency.

The condition tends to run in families, and the familial types tend to be the worst cases. Sudden remissions lasting months, or years, may occur, followed by relapses, many times without recognizable precipitating factors.

Drugs prescribed for the disorder are of little or no benefit, including aspirin, Ibuprofen, other pain killers, sleeping pills, tranquilizers, muscle relaxants, antidepressants (some of which aggravate or even cause symptoms), vitamin or mineral supplements, quinine, and allergy drugs. People have also tried hypnosis, deep massage, acupuncture, thermal baths, meditation, and an alarming array of drugs to no effect.

Treatment

Relief can be obtained by walking, massaging or stretching the muscles, using hot or cold compresses, doing slow, deep knee bends, or working the legs in a bicycling fashion.

Folic acid eases the restless legs syndrome (and some cases of restlessness in Alzheimer's). Foods containing folic acid and vitamin E are most helpful in preventing attacks. Folic acid is found in all beans, especially kidney beans and lima beans; potatoes; dark green leafy vegetables, especially spinach; broccoli; asparagus; peanuts; beets; cabbage; lettuce; avocados; and whole wheat bread. Reflexes improve and IQ goes up with folate. Birth control pills and dilantin interfere with the utilization of folic acid. Vitamin E is found in wheat, all whole grain breads and cereals, wheat germ, broccoli, leafy vegetables, and vegetable oils.

In some instances, restless legs are because of a lack of potassium and magnesium in the diet. Bananas are just one of many foods high in potassium and magnesium.

There are some foods that have active properties in them which may be helpful to activate certain neurotransmitters in the brain and nerve tissues. These include dark leafy greens, parsley, onions, applesauce, and beets.

Use a low-salt diet with no free salt being added to the diet—none at the factory, none at the stove, and none at the table.

Carefully perform an elimination and challenge diet. It is often a fact that much restlessness is associated with

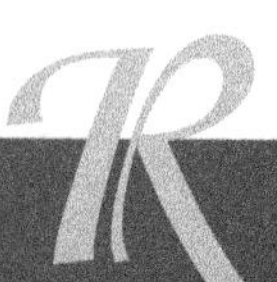

a food sensitivity. It may be that eliminating those foods to which you are sensitive may help you treat the restless legs syndrome without using medication. (See "Elimination and Challenge Diet" in the *Dietary Information* section.)

Take 500 milligrams of rutin and 25 milligrams of vitamin B2 each night at bedtime. For some people this simple supplemental routine has been curative.

A woman in her early fifties reported that she started taking 1200 units of vitamin E daily (400 units three times a day) and that the restless legs syndrome, along with burning feet, went away. The restless legs were completely healed in about three weeks of taking the large dose of vitamin E.

If you wake up during the night with restless legs and can't return to sleep, take some tryptophan capsules. You should be able to obtain tryptophan from a compounding pharmacist. You can also obtain tryptophan from foods high in this nutrient. (See See "Food Sources High in Certain Nutrients" in the *Dietary Information* section.)

In some cases, supplementation with zinc, 30 to 50 milligrams daily, has been helpful.

Entirely eliminate all coffee and its relatives—tea, colas, and chocolate—even if decaffeinated. Avoid tobacco in all its forms, even secondhand.

Be certain to sleep in fresh air, having a current of fresh circulating air in the bedroom at all times. Do not sleep in an electric field such as in a water bed or under an electric blanket. The heating pad should be kept out of the bed until it is needed. Simply turning electrical appliances off does not entirely stop the electrical field around the appliances, it only reduces it.

Do not take medication as drugs are likely to require long-term usage, and most of the medications usually used for restless legs syndrome have serious side effects. Try diligently to find some form of physical therapy to control the uncomfortable sensations so that you can avoid the side effects of medicines.

During the day, keep your extremities, particularly the legs, very warm. This means that during cold weather you may need to wear from two to five layers of warm long-johns, if necessary, in order to keep your legs warm. The thighs must be kept warm. The feet may need only a single pair of socks or tights in order to keep them warm, as the blood coming down from the thighs and legs will keep the feet warm if the blood has warmth to impart.

Put a heating pad near your bed so that when you have the waves of unpleasant sensations you can turn the heating pad on high. If you wear socks and pajamas to bed, the heat can build up substantially before the skin feels it has taken all the heat it can bear.

Before going to bed take a neutral bath, putting the bath temperature at about 98°F and sitting in it for perhaps 30 to 45 minutes. The neutral bath will do wonders for some people.

Your regularity must be impeccable. You should arise at the same time each day and go to bed at the same time each day. Schedule all fixed events of life at the same time—meal times, exercise times, study periods, daily devotionals, etc., so that the circadian rhythm can set itself.

Avoid overusing the legs. Daily regular exercise is helpful in building up the legs so that overuse becomes less likely.

Disorders that interfere with circulation are often present in patients who have restless legs syndrome, resulting in pooling of blood in the legs. This congestion of blood in the legs may be what is responsible for the restless legs. Wearing socks or stockings having a light elastic support to bed may improve the sleeping habits of these individuals markedly. However, for some, wearing support stockings or tight pants may actually cause restless legs. Proper foot and leg gear may prevent the stagnation of blood in the lower extremities. Avoid narrow pointed toes and high heels, garters, and tight waist bands. Use elastic stockings, or ace bandages, to prevent blood stasis in the leg veins. Do not cross the legs. Elevate the legs periodically during the day.

Rotating the feet at the ankles for a few minutes may relieve symptoms.

Cold sponging of the legs, using a coarse washcloth, will often bring relief.

When the legs are recognized as being restless, lying face down can enable the person to go to sleep in many instances.

The following herbal remedies may be helpful: hawthorn berry, white willow bark, skulleaf, licorice root, valerian root, and feverfew. Use one tablespoon of each of these herbs and simmer them gently in one quart of water. Drink the quart throughout the day. Then, have an additional cupful beside your bed so that you can take it during the night if you awaken.

Take wild lettuce and catnip tea. Put one tablespoon of the wild lettuce and one teaspoon of the catnip herb in a cup. Pour one cup of boiling water onto the herb and let it set for 30 minutes. Drink the tea before going to bed or have it ready for use if you should awaken.

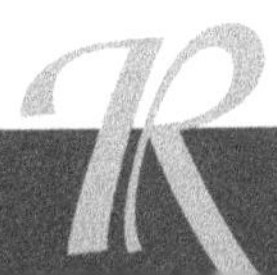

Reye's Syndrome

Reye's syndrome is usually diagnosed in children up to age 25. It has features of encephalitis, starting out with what may appear to be a childhood fever.

A form of aflatoxin appears to be related to Reye's syndrome in some way. It appears that Reye's syndrome is the result of multiple interrelated factors. Aspirin is widely blamed as a principal actor in producing Reye's, which is commonly given to children to bring down fevers. We recommend no aspirin be given to children as it is hazardous to their health (*Pediatrics* 64 [1979]: 71–5.

Six of 58 cases of Reye's were associated with chicken pox. Several cases occurred also with influenza-B, more than with influenza-A (*American Journal of Epidemiology* 101 [1975]: 517).

Rheumatic Fever

A disease of fever and joint pains that migrate from joint to joint. The joints involved are those most subject to stress and strain, generally only one or two joints being affected at any one time. Joints may swell because of inflammation and the accumulation of fluid.

Pain may be quite severe, subsiding in several days from those joints and moving to others (migratory arthralgia). When the inflammation goes away, there is no scarring or damage to the joint. After about five to six weeks the inflammation entirely subsides and patients may recover fully.

The disease attacks young people between the ages of 6 and 20. It comes on after streptococcal infections of the nose and throat, or with ear infections, scarlet fever, or chorea (St. Vitus' Dance). Rheumatic fever is one of those diseases that has greatly reduced in incidence beginning about 1955, followed by slightly increasing incidence since about 1980.

About one in five cases of rheumatic fever has some degree of heart involvement from very mild and self-limiting to severe heart valve deformity. Rheumatic fever is more likely to strike young people whose health is neglected and who live in overcrowded, underprivileged conditions. Treating sore throats and earaches faithfully with natural remedies greatly reduces the likelihood of rheumatic fever developing later. If the heart becomes involved, restricting the activity to only that which is essential for caring for bodily functions is the most conducive to recovery without development of serious scarring.

Treatment

Reduce physical activity to only sitting in a chair half an hour twice a day for meals and getting up to use the restroom.

Being regular in all one's habits, drinking plenty of water, and following a diet low in concentrated foods are all helpful.

Avoid exposure to upper respiratory tract infections, overcrowding in the home, particularly in bedrooms, and unhealthful conditions in the school and community.

Cold baths or cold packs are considered by some to be the best hydrotherapeutic measure for rheumatic fever (*Journal of the American Medical Association* 27 [December 26, 1896]: 1130).

Others, however, use the artificial fever. Dunn and Simmons commented on 15 cases of acute rheumatic fever treated by fever therapy. Fourteen patients became symptom free. Three had relapses, and one showed moderate improvement, although there were still some rheumatic manifestations three months after completion of 48 hours of fever treatments in which the mouth temperature was taken up to between 103°F and 105°F. Fever therapy promptly reduced the symptomatic activity of rheumatic fever and the leukocyte counts, and sedimentation rates became normal in the 14 patients who responded (*Annals of Internal Medicine* 11 [March 1938]: 160).

Simmons points out that of nine cases of acute rheumatic fever with active endocarditis, the disease in six became inactive in an average of 24 days, following an average of five fever treatments (*Journal of the American Medical Association* 109 [September 11, 1937]: 904; *Klinische Wochenschrift* 7 [September 30, 1928]: 1899–1901).

Ringworm, Tinea

(See "Skin Diseases" in the *Conditions and Diseases* section.)

Rosacea

(See "Skin Diseases" in the *Conditions and Diseases* section.)

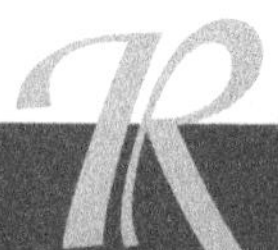

Rubella, German Measles

Rubella is often called "three-day measles" and is generally a more mild form of measles than red measles (rubeola). It does have one more serious feature in that it may result in birth defects in infants born to mothers who are infected during the first three months of pregnancy. Rubella is less contagious than rubeola. Many children escape the disease, entering young adulthood without immunity; thus resulting in contracting the disease during pregnancy. Incubation period is from 14 to 21 days.

Rubella epidemics often occur in the spring. One bout provides lifetime immunity. Newborns seem immune to rubella, but by the age of one year lose their immunity.

Adults have relatively mild symptoms, including malaise, headache, joint stiffness, and lack of energy. Mild irritation of the nose and throat membranes may be present. Lymph node enlargement may occur. The rash, which begins on the face and neck and spreads to the trunk and extremities, may be the first indication of rubella. The rash lasts about three to four days and rarely itches.

Treatment

1. Use abundant fluids and a light diet free from added sugars and fats.
2. Saline applications to the eyes may be soothing, as may darkening the room (Henry K. Silver, *Handbook of Pediatrics* [1959]: 460, 461).
3. Salt water or just plain hot water gargles may be used for sore or irritated throats.
4. Isolate the patient to prevent further spread of the disease.
5. Steam inhalations are useful if a cough is present.
6. A hot half-bath may be used every two hours for fever or itching.
7. If itching is present, a starch bath is often soothing. Add about one cup of starch to a small amount of slightly warm water, diluting in very hot water to form a creamy liquid that is in turn added to about four inches of water in a bathtub. Glycerin may also be added to the bath. The patient may sit in the tub for 20 to 30 minutes and use a cup to dip the water onto the body parts not covered by the bath water. Pat dry to leave as much starch as possible on the skin.
8. Ice bags may be applied to swollen neck glands for 5 to 15 minutes every hour if discomfort is severe.
9. Herbal teas may be helpful: catnip tea for itching or irritability, mint tea for a stimulant if lethargic, and red clover tea as a general tonic.

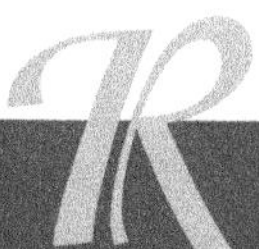

Salpingitis, Pelvic Inflammatory Disease

Salpingitis is an inflammation of the fallopian tubes, which form the connecting link between the uterus and the ovaries. It may be because of common infectious germs or sexually transmitted diseases. It is estimated that 70 percent of fallopian tube infections are because of the gonococcus. In the acute stage, symptoms can resemble acute appendicitis with an elevation in temperature and white blood cells and tenderness of the abdomen to touch and movement. The infection may become chronic without acute manifestations, causing long lasting ill health and eventual sterility.

Treatment

Acute pelvic inflammatory disease requires a vigorous derivative such as a hot hip and leg pack, combined with ice bags to the suprapubic region. When preceded by a copious hot vaginal irrigation (douche), the results in relief of pain usually come within the first 10 minutes of the 30 minute treatment. The treatment can be finished with a cold mitten friction. This treatment may be done in an alternative fashion: (1) with the patient reclining in a bathtub, drain open, administer the copious hot vaginal irrigation (douche)—about one to three gallons of hot douche solution at about 110°F to 115°F; (2) then close the drain and fill tub with hot water to the level of the top of the pubic bone; (3) place ice bags to the low abdomen just above the pubic bone. Try to get the mouth temperature up to 102°F. All treatments should be followed by 30 to 60 minutes of bed rest. Treatments can be repeated twice a day until acute inflammation subsides.

Avoid sexual relations during the time of treatment.

IUD's should be removed as they increase the risk of pelvic inflammatory disease.

A cold enema may be used to relieve pain and pelvic congestion.

Sarcoidosis

This disease is characterized by nodules in many systems often beginning in the chest. If the onset of sarcoidosis is acute with fever, uveitis, and so forth, there is a good likelihood that the sarcoidosis will have a spontaneous remission. The slow onset sarcoidosis, with skin involvement and lymph node involvement, has a less positive prognosis for spontaneous remission. Therefore, treat the sarcoidosis early to try to reverse the disease.

Hydrotherapy should be used freely. A heating compress should be worn each night for four to six months. Three times a week a 30 minute hot foot bath should be given just before bedtime to decongest the chest and encourage healing. Three times a week, alternating days with the hot foot bath, a series of fomentations, and hot and cold treatments should be given in the evening. Once a week a fever treatment should be given, bringing the mouth temperature up to 101°F to 102°F. These measures should be persistently given for four to six months.

Mullein, comfrey, licorice root and aloe vera are all good herbs for sarcoidosis. Mullein is a demulcent, and helps the alveoli to have proper lubrication. Comfrey is a general healing agent. Licorice root has beneficial steroid-like properties

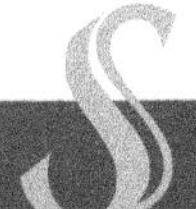

but without the side effects. Aloe vera is a general healing agent.

Golden seal and echinacea should be given in a three to six month course. Other herbs can be chosen to help with specific symptoms in the case.

Sandalwood has been used for scarring in the lungs and may be helpful in sarcoidosis. Its use would be long term, and indications of its benefit would be difficult to assess since sarcoidosis tends to speed up and slow down in its progress. It should be used as an adjunct to other treatments.

Case Report

A book salesman from Florida who sold books door to door was diagnosed with sarcoidosis. He was short of breath and had pain in his chest and sometimes down his arms and in his neck. The diagnosis of sarcoidosis was confirmed by biopsy and was seen in his chest X-ray as increasing the width of the shadow made by his breastbone, heart, and lymph nodes in the mid-section of his chest.

He was anointed by the brethren in his church according to the scriptural instructions in the book of James. He began to take some herbal remedies, a very sparce plant-based diet, and much vigorous outdoor exercise in his garden. The first day he was tired and had much pain in his chest. Day by day as he continued the physical exercise out of doors and reduced the time he spent going door to door, with the stresses it entailed, he observed that he felt much stronger, and his pain gradually went away. Four months later he could walk five miles with no difficulty whatsoever. The Lord had blessed him with healing.

Scabies, The Itch, "Seven Year Itch"

(See "Skin Diseases" in the *Conditions and Diseases* section.)

Scarlet Fever

This is an infection with a scarlet skin eruption occurring most often in the fall and winter in children between the ages of 5 and 12. About three days after coming in contact with an infected person, a painful sore throat, chill, nausea, and vomiting, with a fever as high as 104°F, and headache may develop, indicating the onset of the disease. At first the rash is pinpoint spots of bright red, usually on the chest and neck, which gradually cover the rest of the body. The rash fades in two to three days, but a week or more is required for the skin to regain its normal color. The skin begins to peel in 10 to 14 days in scales and sheets. The tongue may turn strawberry colored.

It is usually a mild infection but can be followed by complications in two to three weeks, the same as strep throat.

Milk can transmit the disease. The *streptococcus* is the cause of the disease, the same as in strep throat.

Treatment

Give a fruit and grains diet as long as the fever lasts, followed by vegetables, nuts, and dried fruits, foods rich in vitamins, minerals, and moderate in protein. Avoid animal products.

Drink plenty of water to place as little burden on the kidneys and heart as possible and to protect them from the toxins.

Avoid chilling, even to the slightest degree, as that encourages complications. About three weeks are required to recover.

For sore throat use gargles of hot salt water or herbal tea such as golden seal, chaparral, or echinacea.

Treat the disease carefully as the complications in untreated cases can be serious.

Schizophrenia

(See "Mental Disorders" in the *Conditions and Diseases* section.)

Sciatica

(See "Skeletal Problems" in the *Conditions and Diseases* section.)

Scleroderma

(See "Collagen Diseases" in the *Conditions and Diseases* section.)

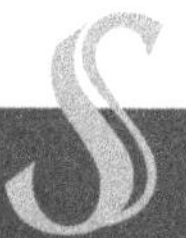

Seborrhea

(See "Skin Diseases" in the *Conditions and Diseases* section.)

Shin Splints, Leg Pains

Shin splints are a common problem among athletes who participate in sports involving repeated jarring impact to the leg. Pain typically centers around the tibia, the shin bone. Unconditioned people who begin a new running or jumping activity, or even conditioned runners who alter their routines and increase pace or distance, may get shin splints.

After especially heavy physical exercise, a day or two of rest from exercise is quite beneficial. It should be kept in mind that, beyond a certain level, additional exercise carries no additional benefits to the health but may weaken the immune system. Exercise at a moderate level has many health benefits.

Treatment

1. Stop the activity that caused the problem.
2. After one week the patient can gradually resume training at about half the previous level of intensity. To prevent recurrence, work on flexibility, particularly heel cord stretching exercises.
3. Pay attention to the warm-up and cool-down phases of the workout, doing stretching exercises before and after the activity. (See "Exercise" in the *Supplemental Information* section.)
4. Wear shoes with a well cushioned heel and insole that absorbs the impact.
5. Run on softer surfaces.
6. Return gradually to the desired level of intensity.

Shingles

(See "Herpes" in the *Conditions and Diseases* section.)

Sickle Cell Anemia

Sickle cell anemia is more common in dark skinned races and is caused by a special type of hemoglobin that becomes elongated and actually curved like a sickle when it loses its oxygen and takes up carbon dioxide. The sickle shapes damage the capsules of the red blood cells and make them more subject to breaking up. It is an hereditary disease. It can be severe enough to be life threatening or mild enough that the person barely knows it exists.

Treatment

Positively avoid all salt in food, much the same as when treating high blood pressure, as salt tends to make the blood cells have less plumpness and to break up more easily. Sugar, honey, syrup, and other concentrated sweeteners must also be avoided, as they too, cause the blood cells to shrivel and break more easily.

Avoid chilling, as that makes the blood move more sluggishly and lose more oxygen, which forms more sickles.

Do not allow any reduction in fresh air in the bedrooms at night, or poor circulation of warm air, or the "sick building syndrome," as poor air causes more sickles. The abnormal hemoglobin does not form when the blood is well oxygenated.

Avoid all cortisone-like products—Prednisone, Ilosone, etc.—as these weaken the already struggling immune system and promote the development of disorders that are life threatening.

Sinusitis

A food sensitivity should be the main cause for consideration for chronic sinusitis unless proven otherwise, such as an air pollutant, a tumor, an ulcer, a foreign body, or a malformation, etc. With the mucosa overloaded by the food sensitivity, germs more readily grow in the sinuses. The germs, however, are not the cause; they are just opportunists.

A study done at the Mayo Clinic on 200 cases of chronic sinusitis revealed that fungi, rather than bacteria are the responsible germ in 95 percent of cases. Antibiotics, therefore, would do little good in treating this kind of infection of the sinuses. The best course of treatment is golden seal, echinacea, and garlic, as they have strong antifungal properties as well as antibacterial. Even better than treating chronic sinusitis is preventing the openings of sinuses from becoming swollen, making them unable to drain into the nasal passages. The best way to do that is by inhaling nasal saline. This must be done several times daily during the season when colds and sinusitis are common. This is a simple yet effective remedy.

Treatment

Fasting for two to four days can be followed by the Elimination and Challenge diet with various foods added

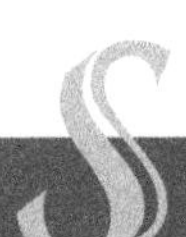

back one by one. (See "Elimination and Challenge Diet" in the *Dietary Information* section.) Begin adding back with a mono diet in which only one food is eaten that day. The next day, if the first food was tolerated without a return of the sinusitis, add another food from the allowed foods on the list. Day by day one food after another can be added, making careful note of any food causing a return of the sinusitis. The diet is usually sufficient when carefully done to turn up those foods that are involved.

Drink lots of fluids as water keeps the mucus moving and the secretions thin.

Keeping the nasal passages open by hot saline irrigations will relieve much of the discomfort. Saline nose drops from a dropper, a vaporizer or steam machine, heat from a desk lamp, heating pad, or hot towels may all clear the nose. Some people prefer cold applications to hot, and for these, crushed ice may be used in a plastic bag and wrapped in a slightly moistened towel.

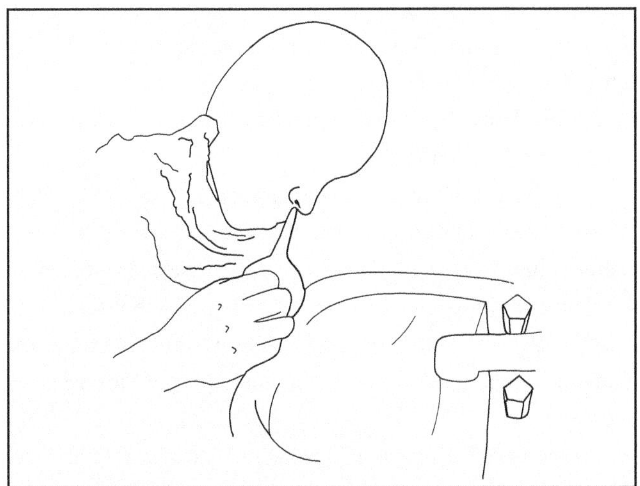

A warm foot bath followed by a firmly done foot rub, giving special attention to the toes, will give relief to many cases of acute sinusitis.

A hot foot bath will relieve congestion in the sinuses and cause the headaches, which are often a symptom of sinusitis, to abate. Similarly, a hot bath can give remarkable relief. Simply sit in a tub of hot water.

Massage over the sinuses and the hard palate, using the thumb to massage the hard pallet. Also, mechanical vibrators over the face or midline of the forehead usually bring pain relief.

If one nostril is more obstructed than the other, lying with the unobstructed side down can encourage drainage.

Avoid all nasal irritants such as cigarette smoke, swimming and diving, fumes, perfumes, cooking odors, chilling, air conditioning, and forcible blowing of the nose.

Avoid nose drops as they always cause a rebound nasal stuffiness.

Antihistamines are ineffectual for cure and are harmful. Antibiotics are not helpful and may cause serious systemic disease and are almost never effective for chronic sinusitis. Over-the-counter nose drops should not be used as they produce a rebound phenomenon, making the sinusitis worse.

Garlic tea—four cups of boiling water with one or two blenderized garlic cloves added—will usually relieve nasal stuffiness.

Peppermint tea, by mouth or as compresses, breathing through a hot towel, or spending some time in a steam inhalation tent, will help most people.

Taking bromelain, an enzyme from pineapple, increases the rate at which healing occurs. In one group 87 percent of patients receiving bromelain cleared with good to excellent results compared to 68 percent of those on placebo (*Headache* 7 [1997]: 13).

Grapefruit with skin boiled in water can be used for hay fever. Quarter a whole well scrubbed grapefruit. Boil gently in two quarts of water for 30 minutes. Take a tablespoonful or two several times a day.

Dissolve one 500-milligram vitamin C tablet in one-quarter cup warm water. Put directly into the nostrils with an eye dropper using one-half dropperful on each side two times a day (Jude C. Williams, *Jude's Herbal Home Remedies* [St. Paul, MN: Llewellyn Publications, 1996]).

Skeletal Problems

Back Pain

One of the commonest complaints seen in doctors' offices today is that of back pain. It is one of the commonest causes of absenteeism from work, and it affects most people at one time or other. Ten to 60 billion dollars are spent each year; six million people are off work any one day because of musculoskeletal pain. The primary cause for most back pain is muscle tension. Lifting a heavy object or other physical strain can bring on the condition, but many authorities believe that muscle tension was present long before the apparent event occurred that was believed to have caused the backache.

Postural tone and movement of the trunk are two important functions of spinal muscles. The sense of balance ordinarily keeps the back in proper alignment. If this postural reflex fails, then voluntary muscles must be used to maintain

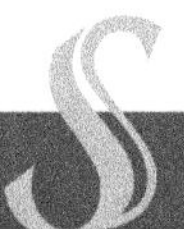

good posture. Fatigue results from faulty posture, and backache follows promptly. Proper posture is one of the most important aspects of avoiding backache, and it goes far toward maintaining the health of bones, joints, tendons, muscles, and nerves, to say nothing about the proper function of heart, lungs, great vessels of the chest, and organs of the abdomen and pelvis. Since the suspension of pelvic and abdominal organs is by means of ligaments attached to the back, any malalignment of the back or disease of the discs can cause abdominal or pelvic pain.

Backache may be acute, chronic, sharp, stabbing, mild, or excruciating. It may be caused by abnormal function or structure of some back component, including bones, ligaments, blood vessels, or nerves. The precipitating causes should be sought. Those who want to avoid exposure to X-rays and expensive procedures should note carefully the following observations:

High technology testing such as imaging of the spine is probably a waste of money and may even be counterproductive to proper diagnosis of back pain. In one study of normal participants, 36 percent turned up with "disk abnormalities" although they had never had a history of serious back pain. More than 50 percent had a bulge in at least one disk. At least 27 percent possessed one herniation, a disk splaying out beyond the vertebrae. The high rate of disk findings in "normal" symptom-free individuals suggests that pain may not be the result of disk problems but simply occurring at the same time (*Science News* 146 [July 16, 1994]: 39).

A reduction in blood flow to the muscles, joints, ligaments, and discs caused by hardening of the arteries supplying oxygen and nutrients to these structures is almost never suspected, but is a very common, perhaps the commonest cause of backache. Then the starved tissues are very easily injured. Therefore, every backache should be investigated by getting laboratory levels of cholesterol, triglycerides, sugar, and homocysteine. Hardening of the arteries can cause not only heart attacks, strokes, and impotence, but the impaired blood supply to the spine can be a major reason for degeneration of the disks between the vertebrae. The arteries that supply the spine usually develop hardening before other arteries in the body. Over 17,000 persons were examined at autopsy for early signs of blockage in the spinal arteries as they arise from the abdominal aorta. Changes began as early as age 10, and by age 20, one in 10 people has advanced blockage. Poor posture is one of the causes of advancing artery hardening, but so are high blood cholesterol and triglycerides. Those persons with the most low back pain were found to have the most advanced hardening of the arteries (*Lancet* 346 [1995]: 888, 889).

The most common injury resulting in disease of the back is a compression fracture of a vertebral body. This fracture occurs with injury such as forceful sitting down or falling down in the upright position. Stepping off a curb or bending over will be sufficient in some very elderly individuals to cause fracture, even though the trauma was trivial. Pain is relieved by bed rest and gradually diminishes in one to two weeks. Pain can be elicited by placing the thumb over the spine of the vertebra receiving a compression fracture, and giving moderate pressure. It is quite sharply localized and may be accompanied by muscle spasm with associated pain in the surrounding muscle.

Osteoporosis itself does not cause pain. When pain occurs with osteoporosis, there is an indication of micro-fractures that have been sustained in the interior of vertebral bodies. Such individuals may gradually develop humpback (kyphosis) or ankylosing spondylitis (poker stiff spine). Those with any kind of abnormal curvature of the spine often have muscular backaches because of the extreme fatigue resulting from the muscular effort to maintain posture. Lying down for a few minutes relieves this kind of pain. Serious but rare disease of the back such as tuberculosis or malignancy may also account for back pain.

The intervertebral disc is the largest structure in the body without blood supply. The facet is the joint between two vertebrae. Fluid from the blood and lymph vessels is responsible for the nourishing and cleansing of the disc. The fluid moves by seepage. Therefore, the worst thing we do is maintain the same position of the back for a long time, which reduces seepage.

Intervertebral discs are semi-fluid structures, not solid like blocks of bone, but an internal structure more like toothpaste with a capsule of fibrocartilage and ligament around the outside. With weakening or deterioration of the capsule, the semi-fluid substance of the interior of the disc can be pressed outward in much the same way that toothpaste is pressed from a tube. This material can then push on nerves and blood vessels adjacent to the discs or vertebral bodies. Ordinarily, the disc is a cushioning device with the pasty central portion.

A severe pain may begin suddenly with a slipping or snapping sensation, which occurs during stooping, lifting, or raising up from a sitting or lying position. The pain is usually midline, and often the patient cannot straighten the back because of pain and muscle spasm. Sneezing or coughing may initiate or aggravate the pain. The soft disc has suddenly squirted out between bundles of the ligament that held it in place. The disk may sometimes be returned toward the normal central position by correcting faulty use of the back and

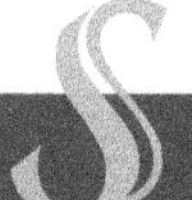

by manipulation. When it is returned to its normal position, the pressure on the adjacent ligaments and nerves is relieved, eliminating the pain.

Poor posture, incorrect use of the back, and often repeated but faulty body movements can all cause back pain. Proper posture includes the proper position of the head, neck, shoulders, back, hips, knees, and feet. If in both sitting as well as standing a proper position is maintained, much backache can be eliminated. Many people with a low-grade backache have a defect in posture that puts a strain on the entire back. If one has proper posture, one can maintain the upright position for several hours without fatigue or pain. Improper posture can cause pain that may persist for days or weeks. Having sway-back (lordosis), hump-back (kyphosis), or having a side to side curvature of the spine (scoliosis) all may cause pain.

Incorrect use of the back includes lifting incorrectly, twisting with heavy loads in hand, and sitting for long periods with the back in a C-shape.

Sitting puts more pressure on the disc than standing, as sitting puts the spine in flexion, which reduces the space between vertebrae. However, standing, bent from the hips, puts pressure of flexion on the discs, and also the pressure of the erector spinae muscles, which contract in order to keep one from falling forward. A forward head does the same thing with the neck. To balance an upright umbrella in the hand is not difficult, but to hold an umbrella at a 45-degree angle lets you see how much the umbrella truly weighs. If the head is at a 45-degree angle with the neck, the head puts a big strain on the neck muscles, promoting neck and upper back pain.

Being overweight, or even overeating with an increased weight in the abdomen, puts a disproportionate load on the back because of excess pull of gravity out front. This can cause back pain. Then a voluntary contraction of the muscles of the back must compensate for poor posture, which leads to fatigue and back pain. The habit of carrying a case or any object in one hand several hours weekly, or repeatedly for short or long periods can cause back pain.

Emotional factors and nervous tension are also common causes of back pain. Any form of nervous or emotional excitement, pleasant or unpleasant, may cause a backache. Often such tension originates in the work place, in the home, or between neighbors. A painful psychological problem should be faced squarely, an attempt should be made to resolve it, and if no resolution can be satisfactorily worked out, there should be a studied attempt to place the matter in the hands of the Lord and not allow it to be uppermost in the mind. Fill the mind with heavenly themes. It is often discovered that the banishment of psychological tension banishes backache.

Smoking and coffee drinking have been implicated as major causes. These must be stopped promptly. Caffeine can cause the development of chronic backache (*Archives of Physical Medicine and Rehabilitation* 78 [1997]: 786). Even secondhand smoke can cause a backache.

Flat feet are a cause of some backaches. Foot exercises can be very helpful. Flex the feet up and down, then the entire leg flexed upon the hip, coordinating with the foot movement. Alternate with walking tiptoe on a carpeted surface, simultaneously stretching the arms high overhead. Continue the exercises from one to five minutes, and repeat four to six times daily. Shoe inlays have been curative of a certain percentage of low back pain, perhaps as much as 20 percent. Wear low heeled shoes most of the time. Do not wear heels higher than one inch more than four hours per week.

An improper bed is a common cause of back pain. The bed should be firm but not hard. To accomplish firmness a piece of plywood can be placed between the mattress and springs to support the back. Flexing the knees over a pillow or folded blanket will straighten the lumbar curve, making the back feel better. Avoid sleeping face down as that causes twisting and exaggeration of the curves of the back.

Avoid repeatedly making a one-sided twist to do common tasks, such as reaching for toilet tissue, getting out of bed, or reaching for the telephone. Change your furniture around to avoid a constantly repeated twist to the same side. Do not make a habit of sitting toward one arm rest of a sofa or couch. Pain often develops in the side away from the arm rest. To get up from a sofa, move toward the front edge, lean forward from the hips while keeping the lower spine slightly hollowed or arched backward, putting as much room between the chest and the knees as possible.

Do not consistently sleep on one side of the bed for many years. One should change from side to side of the bed, and while sleeping on the side should make certain that you do not start off sleeping on the same side each night. You should also change the posture that you use during dressing, bathing, or any other daily experience. A good practice is to lean backward at the waist every time you stand from the bed, chair, toilet, sofa, or car, rather than bending forward to begin to stand erect.

Avoid sustained flexion of the back as stooping to cook, write, or drive a car. Avoid long periods of sitting. Do not put your hamstrings (large muscles at the back of the thighs) on a prolonged stretch, as in sitting while the knees are straight in front of you such as sitting on the floor with the legs in front. Sitting slouched with the back in a bent C fashion such as

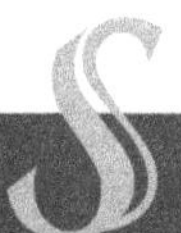

from reading in bed at night, driving in a bucket seat without a "lumbar roll," riding a lawn mower or tractor, sitting long periods on a toilet seat, and reclining in a lounge chair or a chair recliner.

Mothers with small children can make a habit of bathing, or changing, or lifting the child while the hands are held at a distance from the trunk. It is better to bathe a child at the kitchen sink rather than kneeling beside a bathtub. Never reach across a low table, such as a coffee table, to put your child onto a sofa, or remove him from the sofa.

Men at work must avoid any work posture that keeps the waist bent for long periods. You may do an occasional forward bending motion, but you should precede or follow it by a lean-back motion with your hands on your hips, thumbs toward the back.

Before removing objects from your car or your trunk, bend backward with the same posture you have with your hands on your hips. Learn to hip bend not waist bend.

A person who stands on hard pavement all day without rest will often lose a full inch in height between the beginning of his work and bedtime. Rest and good hydration permits the spine to spring back to its full normal length by the next day.

The sacroiliac joint is in the pelvis between the sacrum and ilium. Pain often results because of instability of the joint caused by strain, high emotional tension, lying in bed for long periods, poor posture, weak back muscles, etc. Persons with acute low back pain can be made worse by extended bed rest. Perhaps a day or two of bed rest may be well, but beyond this, the back pain will probably get worse. Those who feel like getting up and moving about should be allowed to do so (*Lancet* 354 [1999]: 1229).

Low back pain that occurs after lifting or reaching over to raise a stuck window is because of sacroiliac strain. Pain in the low back or thighs in a teenage or young adult male brings a suspicion of ankylosing spondylitis. In the presence of psoriasis (a skin disorder), a diagnosis of psoriatic arthritis may be the correct assessment.

Suggestions for Sitting

A lumbar roll or a book in the middle of the back can be helpful to keep a slight extension for the back. This is especially important while driving or flying.

Don't sit flexed too long or extended too long, but emphasize the latter rather than the former.

Lean back after sitting. Place the hands on the hips with the thumbs in the middle of the back at the waist and gently lean back. This should be done after arising from the sitting position, especially from bucket seats of automobiles.

Treatment

Stress and emotional tension are the causes of a large percentage of back pain. Getting rid of emotional tension by the means that are most simple, such as walking, facing one's problems with decision and prayer, and making things as orderly in the life as possible.

Keep the back more in extension (leaning backward) than in flexion (leaning forward).

Use a lumbar roll for prolonged sitting, such as a small rolled towel or a couch bolster tucked behind you at about the waist.

Do not lift heavy loads, stoop long at jobs such as vacuuming, or sit in a slumped position.

After vigorous exercise relax the back with good posture and appropriate stretches or exercises that put the back in some degree of extension.

If you need to cough or sneeze, you should try to stand upright and bend backward if you are subject to low back pain.

Treatment in water for 10 minutes a day or a 20-minute massage was highly effective in reducing back pain (*Clinical Pearls News* 9, no. 3 [March 1999]).

Strains from long sustained positions, sitting, lying, or standing may be relieved by the "pelvic glide" in which a standing posture is exaggerated by leaning backward while bracing the hands on the upper hips with the thumbs placed inward and pointed upward toward the waist.

A "cervical glide" may relieve neck pain. It is merely tucking the chin in, using an exaggerated military stance for a second, then relaxing. Repeat the cervical glide four or five times, not forcing any position.

Do not allow the extremities to get chilled. Wear low heeled shoes. Sit in a chair with your feet on a stool so the legs may be brought up high enough to lift the thighs off the chair seat. Use a straight chair. When driving move the car seat or use padding to maintain the normal spinal profile, not curved in a C-shape or having the legs stuck out directly in front of one. Do not stand or sit for long periods without shifting the weight, changing the position, or placing one or both feet on a foot stool. Even while standing in one place for a long time such as while ironing, a foot stool can be used to good advantage.

Do not bend over to pick up a heavy object. Squat beside the object, maneuver it close to the body and try to support it with your elbows and arms on the knees, then slowly rise to the standing position while keeping the back straight. The strain of straightening up with the load must be on the leg muscles, not on the back. Be very careful not to twist the back

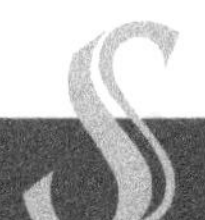

while holding a heavy load in the arms. Turn the feet as well as the back.

Do not repeat the same activity of daily life again and again in exactly the same position.

In one group of people with backache it was found that avoiding bed rest and maintaining ordinary activity, as tolerated, led to the most rapid recovery. While it may not be as comfortable as bed rest, determine to follow all the instructions given here while doing as much as possible of your accustomed activity providing it is not too taxing.

Have work surfaces at a comfortable height.

Use a chair with good lower back support.

Exercise

Even when back surgery had already been scheduled, a group of patients were aggressively treated with a 10-week exercise program for the back. The majority of the patients improved sufficiently that they did not need the back surgery (*Archives of Physical Medicine and Rehabilitation* 80 [1999]: 20).

Sixty-one percent of backache sufferers take care of their own backs rather than seeking help from a doctor. This can be done by various postures, lying flat and stretching, and a number of exercises, including extensions that can reduce the pain of a herniated disk.

Walk on the heels and the toes to improve the general strength of the feet, legs, and lower back.

Put your hands on your hips with your thumbs in the sacroiliac joint behind in the low back, bend forward to see if the thumbs move up equally. If not, try to correct a short leg by sitting on a "lift" under one hip or other, to make the sacroiliac joints approximately level. Do not overcorrect, as that is certain to cause pain to develop. The lift may be a thin magazine or a small folded towel.

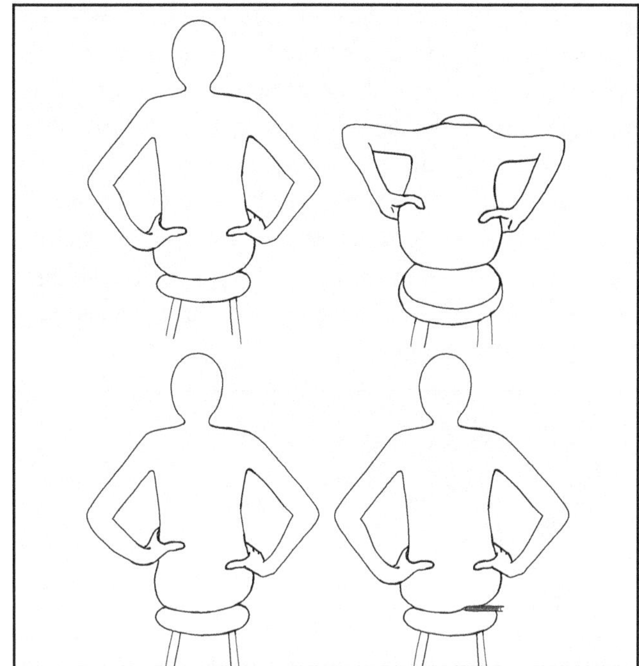

Lying face down puts the back in some degree of extension, and then raising yourself up on the elbows increases the degree of extension. Then, while pushing up with the hands puts the back in extreme extension, which can be very helpful for low back pain.

Lie on the back, raise a leg straight up and hold it three inches above the floor for three seconds. If it feels exceptionally weak, strengthen it by raising the leg 20 times to begin with, increasing gradually to 40 times, three times a day. Repeat with the opposite leg.

To help the back feel better, flex the knees and hips, curling the back by bringing the forehead as close to the knees as possible.

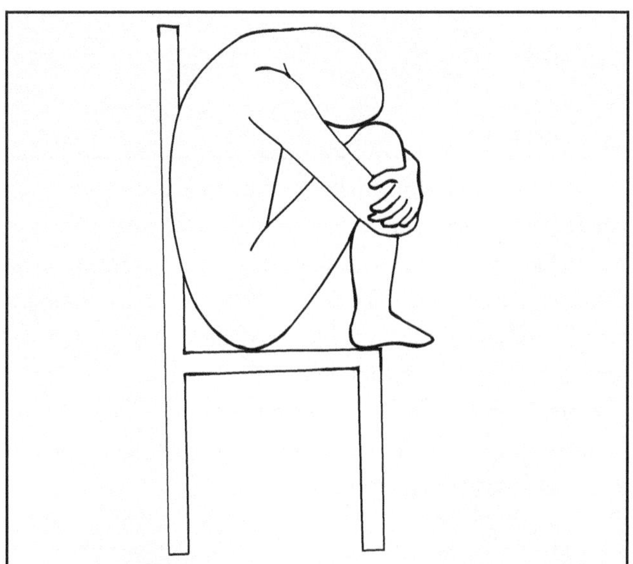

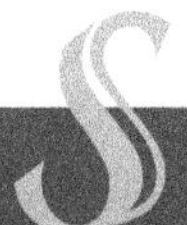

Strengthen the back ligaments and muscles by the bridging exercise. Lie on the back and lift the midsection of the body, supporting the weight on the heels and shoulders. Hold for three seconds, building up gradually to 20 seconds, three times a day. "Winging" is done by lying face down on a surface and lifting the head, arms, and legs off the floor behind you. Hold them off for three seconds the first day; then increase daily until you are doing the exercise 30 seconds three times a day. The winging and bridging exercises are also very helpful for chronic backache.

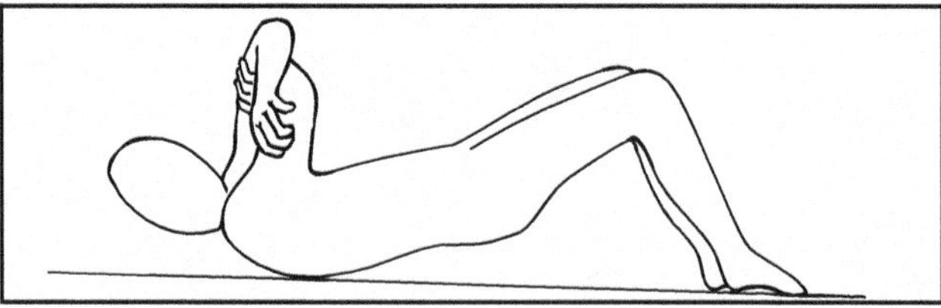

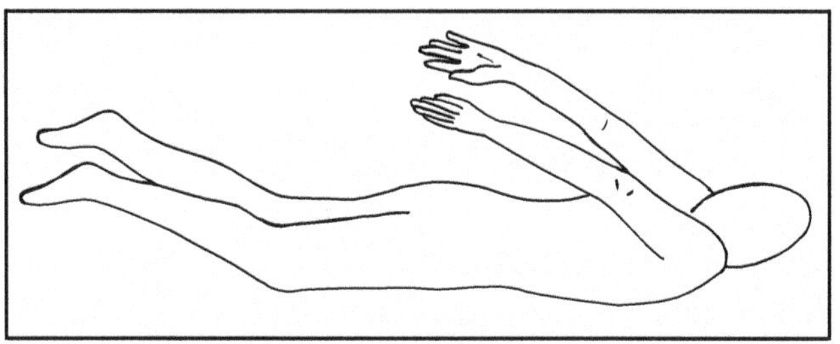

A half-pushup is also good. Lie flat on the abdomen with the palms on the floor near the shoulders, and slowly push your shoulders up, keeping your hips flat on the surface, letting the back and abdomen sag. Hold five seconds. Increase the repetitions as you are able.

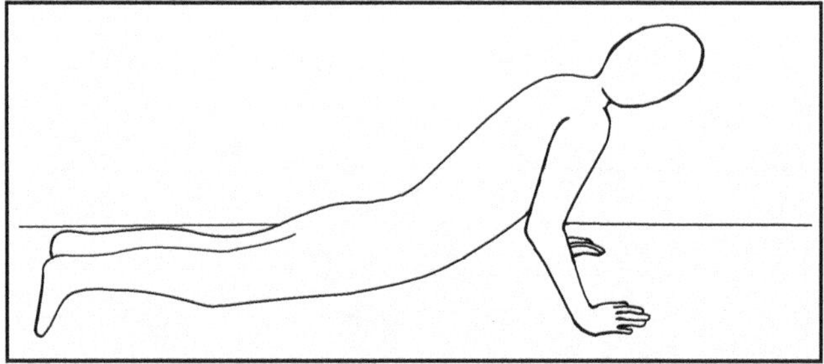

Another back strengthening exercise is done by placing one foot on a knee-high surface such as a chair, the other foot flat on the floor. Bend over to put the chest on the thigh, with the hands clasped under the thigh at the knee. Slowly straighten up, pulling against your clasped hands while you are straightening up, using the muscles in your low back until you are in an arched-back position. Hold five seconds and increase the number of repetitions as you are able. Repeat with the opposite foot on the stool.

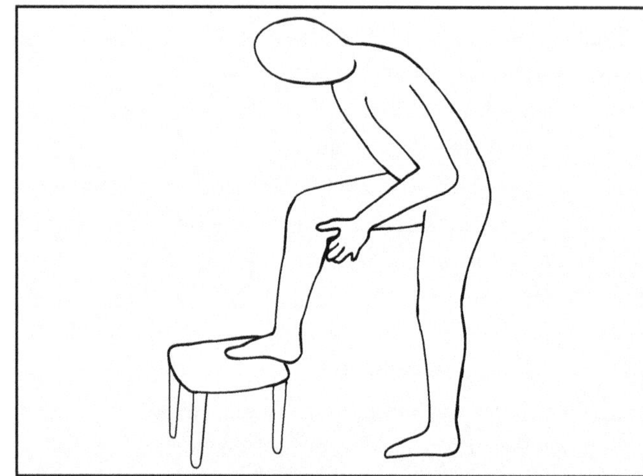

Elevate the feet on a low stool while sitting. If one is driving, push the car seat forward to raise the knees higher than the hips.

If bicycling is your type of exercise, do not have the seat too high or the handlebars too low or the neck could arch backward, creating an ache in the neck. A mountain bike with straight handlebars, and a frame that allows the rider to sit more upright, and bigger tires, which do a better job of soaking up road shock, may be the very best bicycling tips. To determine the position of the handlebar, place your elbow against the tip of the saddle and the tips of your extended fingers should barely reach the handlebar. The seat height can be determined by the fact that the rider's leg should almost be able to straighten when the cycle is stationary.

If swimming is your exercise, dog-paddling is the very best for the back.

Don't underestimate the importance of well-padded shoes when walking. Walking and running are high-impact, and forces develop as much as four times the person's body weight. These pressures can damage the disks and other structures.

Strengthening the lower back muscles can prevent back pain. Very little effort brings big results. Abdominal strength is the key for stabilizing the spine while gluteal and thigh strength helps you crouch without excessive swaying of the lower back. Any exercise intended to increase strength should be performed slowly to maximize the gain you will get and decrease the potential for an injury from exercise. There should be no jerking. A daily stretching program decreases back pain in just two weeks. Not just the back should be stretched but all the muscles, particularly the hamstrings (back of the thighs), as tight hamstrings can pull the pelvis out of place and alter the back alignment.

You're never too old to improve your flexibility. Even 5 to 10 minutes of some type of exercise a day in persons over

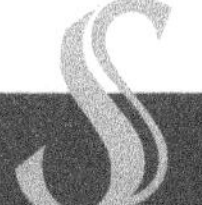

age 72 can improve both back flexion and extension. You should be able to speak comfortably during exercise without panting. When you can do this you are ready for the next step.

Herbs

Anti-inflammatory herbs such as licorice root, flax seed oil, hawthorn berry, etc., can be used along with physical exercise.

Hydrotherapy

For acute low back pain stand in the shower with legs slightly flexed, hands placed just above the knees with the upper body partly resting on the arms. Direct a needle spray of hot water, or the shower with as much force as possible, onto the painful area while performing a gentle exercise as follows: lower and tuck in one hip, then the other. Next raise and push back one hip, then the other. The hip is lowered by allowing the leg to drift forward, and raised by letting the leg drift backward. Repeat these gentle exercises 30 times two or three times a day to loosen up a tight back or eliminate backache.

The crick in the neck or back may be because of wrong positioning or a cold draft while sleeping, but may also be because of a viral infection that causes an inflammation in a muscle. A hot bath is the treatment of choice for a crick. This may then be followed by a good massage with a massage oil such as arnica oil or an alcohol rub, firmly rubbing out sore spots in the back, but avoiding causing injury to an already inflamed muscle by too rough massaging before the muscle is nicely warmed up by gentle rubbing. The patient can tell you how much pressure is too much when giving a backrub.

Ice treatment is the treatment recommended most often for acute low-back pain with or without sciatica. Bed rest has fallen into disuse as a treatment for backache. Use ice in acute back pain or sciatica for the first 72 hours unless it makes the pain worse; then, heat treatments are the treatment of choice.

Block out the painful area with towels, then rub the area with ice, covering about two inches beyond the painful area on all sides. After about one minute of the ice rub, pain develops in the skin, but it stops after about two to four minutes. Stop the massage after 12 to 20 minutes. Many a case of acute back strain will be cured after a single treatment. If not, continue for the first 72 hours, then switch to alternating hot and cold compresses. In between the ice massages, which may be taken as often as every two hours, you may also use a heating pad placed in the bed for the person to lie upon. This kind of treatment often abolishes acute back pain in a day or so. With chronic back pain, a heating pad can bring about excellent pain relief.

Massage

For acute backache, go to a door facing and lean against the corner of it, rubbing the back sideways and up and down. It will often substitute for a nice back rub.

Rubber balls about three inches in diameter can be laid on the floor or braced between the back and the wall in a place where the back hurts. Lying on them, or leaning against them, will give relief. This can be done for a painful area noticed just as one is trying to go to sleep.

A thorough rubbing of the painful back using a good massage oil will often be curative. Make the massage oil from one pint of olive oil and two ounces of dried arnica flowers. Cook in a double boiler for two to three hours. Strain and, if you would like, add a couple of ounces of beeswax or the paraffin used in canning preserves. Use more or less of the wax depending on how stiff you like the massage oil.

Stretching for Backache and Sciatica

An effective but gentle stretching exercise is done by sitting away from the back of your chair with the knees separated slightly and the feet flat on the floor. While keeping the back straight, bend forward and place the right forearm on the right thigh. Extend the left arm up toward the ceiling and, while exhaling, turn and look up toward the left hand. Hold for three breaths, and repeat with the other side. To increase the stretch even more, bend forward and place the right hand along the outside of the left foot. Then continue as above.

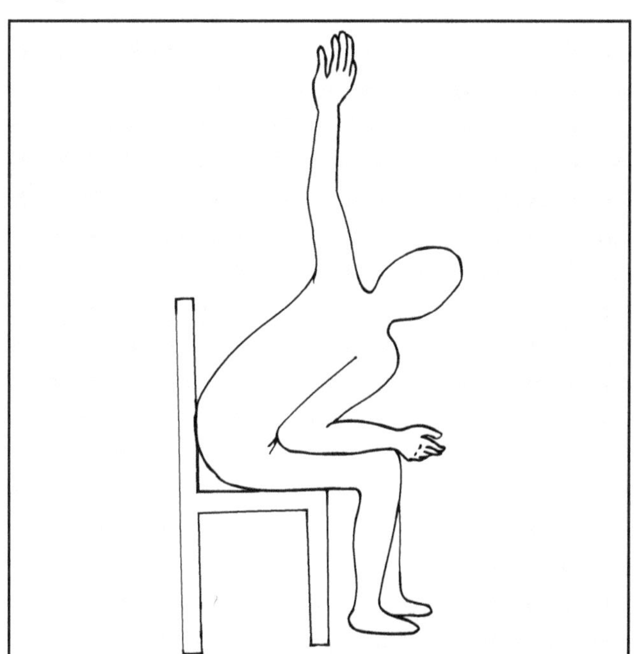

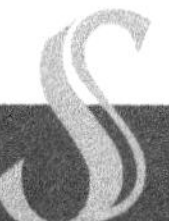

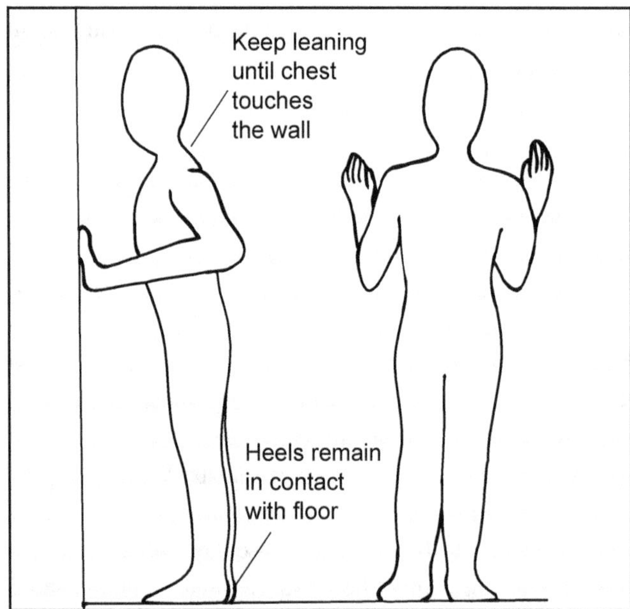

Plant your feet two feet away from the wall. Then lean forward until your chest is resting on the wall in front of you while your feet remain flat on the floor. This is helpful for backache, both to treat and to prevent.

Carpal Tunnel Syndrome

Carpal tunnel syndrome is caused by swelling beneath the carpal ligament, a band of connective tissue that stabilizes the tendons of the hand at the wrist. The condition is often the result of overuse of the hands. The risk of getting carpal tunnel syndrome is increased by the use of caffeinated beverages and alcohol. It is also made worse by being even slightly overweight; and the greater the person's weight, the greater the likelihood of getting carpal tunnel syndrome.

Blood vessels, nerves and tendons must go through this circular ligament. Any reduction in the space inside this circle can reduce blood flow to the nerves and can cause pain. Carpal tunnel syndrome has risen since the increase in weight of women and the use of computers, which require people to hold the wrists bent in an unchanged position for long periods of time. It is also prevalent in electricians who are repeatedly turning screw drivers, anyone doing a job requiring repetitive bending of the wrist, as well as people who sleep with their wrists bent down on the forearms. All of these types of individuals are at risk of developing carpal tunnel syndrome.

Diagnosis

Carpal tunnel is often a complex syndrome, and one of the first challenges is making sure the diagnosis is correct. Many medical conditions, such as diabetes, overweight, arthritis, or food sensitivity, can cause soft tissue or tendon swelling under the carpal ligament, which compresses a nerve inside the wrist, resulting in numbness, tingling, or pain of the forearm and fingers. The thumb and first three fingers are most often involved but the outer two fingers and half of the middle finger may make the diagnosis also. Weakness may follow as well as atrophy from disuse. The knuckles may hurt, and pain may shoot on the undersides of the fingers and up the forearms.

On the hand involved put the tip of the little finger and thumb together and press with all your might. A helper separates the two fingers, making note of how much effort is required. Then while you squeeze your wrist and base of your hand with your opposite hand, the person again separates the finger and thumb. If it is much more difficult to separate them the second time than the first time, that is a good indication that the person has carpal tunnel syndrome.

Prevention

An analysis should be made of the work site to determine the correct posture and the optimum force and repetition of each movement. Changing the height of the keyboard and screen, purchasing keyboard wrist rests, making sure chairs are well suited to the job can help some computer operators.

Losing weight or taking care of any other medical condition that might contribute to the syndrome is important.

The use of vibrating tools has been found to be strongly associated with carpal tunnel syndrome. Tools with protective equipment should be selected for those who do repetitive jobs requiring bending the wrists and using some force.

Following is a list of some potential dangers to your wrist that can be easily prevented:

- Long nails that force the fingers to extend to press keyboard keys.
- Pushing a heavy object repeatedly, such as a door, or opening a difficult car window repeatedly.
- Opening jars with excessive force or even a single straining may initiate the problem. If one such effort results in painful strain, do not repeat that activity for two or more days.
- Holding a telephone with the wrist at an angle for long periods.
- Any repetitious job done by assembly line and clerical workers, food preparers, and packagers, grocery checkout clerks, and computer operators.

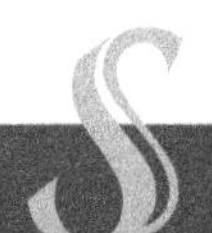

Treatment

Far too many operations are being done on those who have carpal tunnel syndrome. More conservative methods should be applied first, as they are very likely to be effective with some persistence. The first objective is removal of all potential causes.

- Excessive weight, even five pounds, can precipitate carpal tunnel syndrome in some people. The presence of fat deposits in or under the carpal ligament adds tension to all the nearby tissues. (See "Weight Control" in the *Conditions and Diseases* section.)
- A food allergy is a frequent cause of swelling of tissue, and the tissues beneath the carpal ligament may swell in response to food sensitivity. A carefully done Elimination and Challenge diet (see the *Dietary Information* section) will often help in discovering foods to which one is allergic that can cause this kind of swelling.
- Prepare one glass of grapefruit juice and add four tablespoons of lemon juice concentrate. Drink one glass per day for four days. One man who had severe carpal tunnel syndrome took a glass of the mixture every day for four days and had a complete clearing of an acute flare-up of carpal tunnel syndrome.
- Carpal tunnel syndrome may be treated by daily soaks in ice water for six minutes or an ice massage. The soaks must involve the hand, wrist, and arm up to the elbow, and the ice massage should be over the painful area.
- Since a bent position of the hands while sleeping will cause carpal tunnel syndrome in some people, wearing a brace to prevent extreme flexion of the hands during sleep can prevent or cure many cases. You can purchase a splint or make your own. Prepare a splint by wrapping a stiff object, such as a strip of metal or heavy cardboard with a small towel or adhesive tape to make it comfortable. Bind it with a cloth bandage, roller gauze, or a bandage onto the palm surface of the hand and forearm to about halfway up to the elbow. Wear each night.
- One patient received remarkable relief by wrapping an electric heating pad with a towel and pinning it carefully to form a splint for her hand and lower arm. She slept with that warm splint on her arm, wearing gloves at night to prevent the slightest chilling. She did this for years and had almost normal use of her hand with very little pain.
- Firm rubber bands, large enough to put all five fingertips into, can be used to strengthen the fingers and encourage the reduction of swelling in the wrist. The fingers are separated as widely as possible by stretching the rubber band. They should be separated at least an inch. If one rubber band is not sufficient to give a strong resistance, use two or three rubber bands. The exercise should consist of 15 to 20 repetitions every three to four hours throughout the day for one to two weeks (*The Physician and Sports Medicine* 22, no. 9 [September 1994]: 29). Exercises that strengthen the hand and upper arm muscles, like squeezing a hand gripper or swimming, may help avoid the disease or avoid an operation.
- We have not had success with high doses of B6, although there are still those who believe it is helpful. Our best success has come from night splinting, specific exercises, and weight loss.
- Hot and cold compresses to the lower arm (three minutes hot and 30 to 45 seconds cold for four or five exchanges) can be helpful, as can the use of the hot paraffin bath.
- If it is very acute, the use of a charcoal poultice wrapped around the wrist and lower arm every night may be helpful.
- Application of a cayenne extract such as Zostrix or a homemade alcoholic extract using one teaspoon of red pepper to eight ounces of rubbing alcohol (soak for two weeks) may help. Any of these cayenne pepper extracts should be applied four to six times daily for six days. When the pain goes away, only two daily applications need be made.
- Herbal pain relievers may be used such as white willow bark tea and wild lettuce tea. Tablets or capsules may be used if you prefer. The following herbs are also anti-inflammatory and may offer relief: hawthorn, flaxseed oil, turmeric, or licorice powder. A good formula is as follows: A heaping teaspoon of licorice powder and a heaping tablespoon of white willow bark in one quart of water, simmered gently for 25 minutes. Strain and drink throughout the day. Make it fresh daily. Take it without missing for four to six weeks.
- Massage firmly inside and outside of the hand with thumb and fingers for two minutes or more, three times daily. Use a good hand lotion as a massage lubricant.

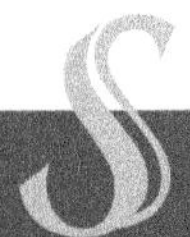

Exercises

Following are specific exercises that may be followed to treat carpal tunnel syndrome:

- Resistance and stretching exercises are good. Resist pushing all four fingers back from the inside of the palm with the opposite hand for five seconds. Repeat at least 20 times during the day.

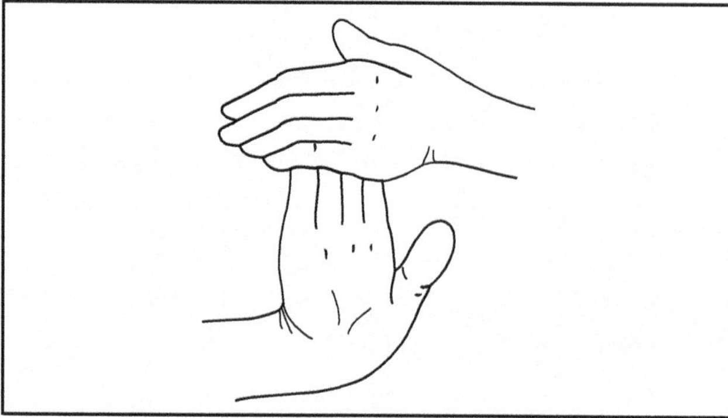

- Gently pull the thumb back toward the hairy part of the forearm until you can feel the stretch. Hold five seconds. Repeat at least 20 times during the day.

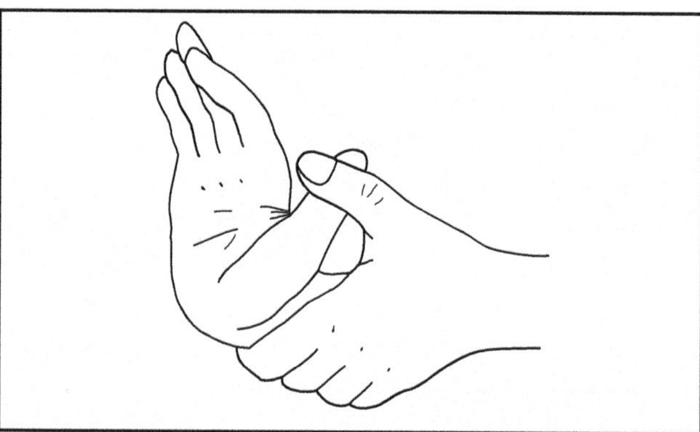

- Clench the fist. Release, forcefully fanning out the fingers. Do five times; repeat at least five times a day.
- With the fist clenched, palm up, resist an attempt of the other hand to hold the wrist down on the forearm.

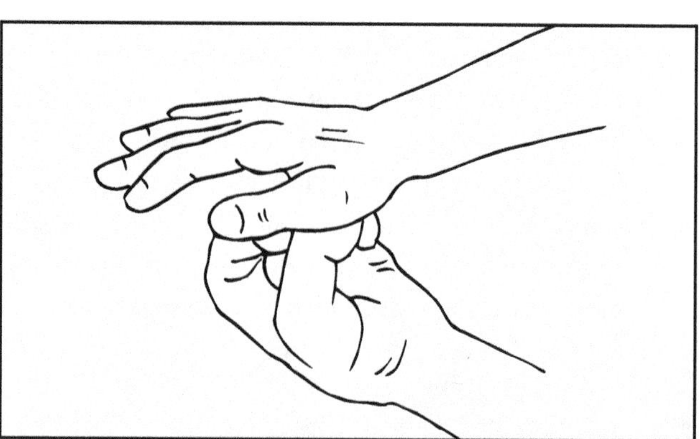

- With fist clenched, palm down, resist a similar attempt of the opposite hand to fold the wrist on the forearm.

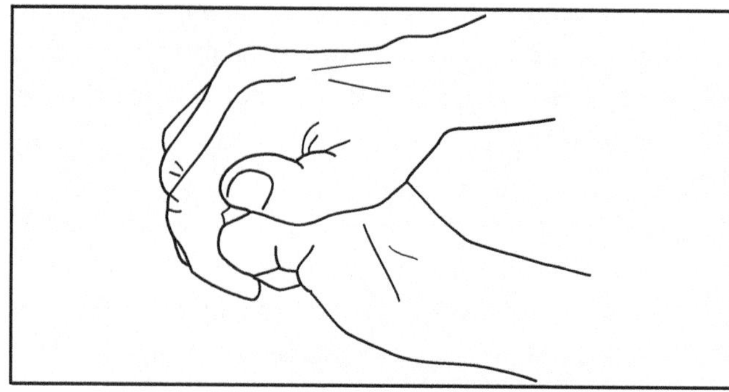

- Resist the same type of pressure with the thumb side of fist up.

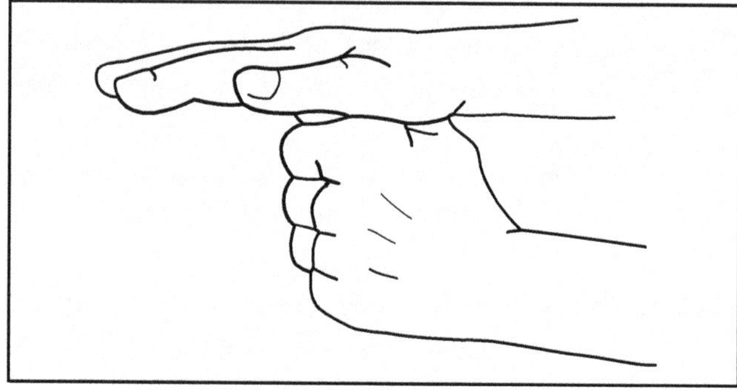

- Resist a similar attempt to fold the wrist up while the fist is palm down.

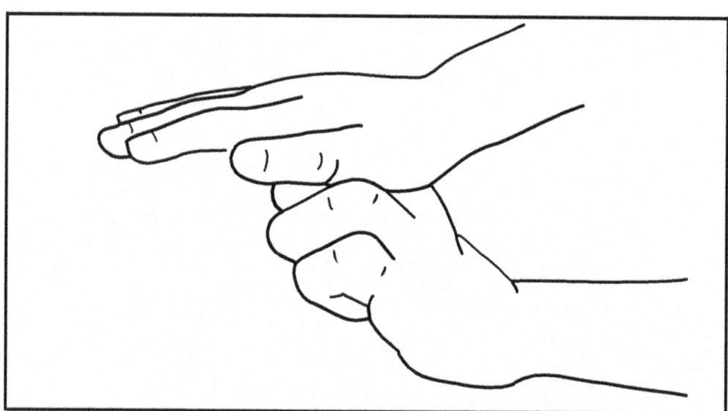

- With palm flat on a table, bend forearm onto hand.

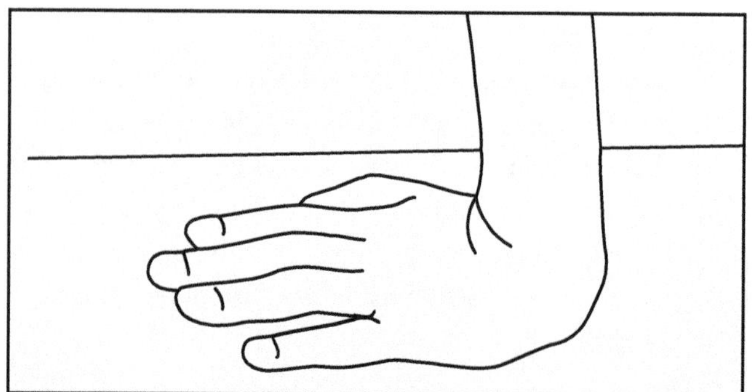

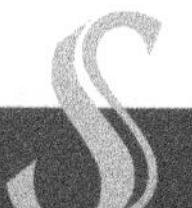

Ganglion Cysts

These cysts are lumps under the skin most commonly seen on the wrist, usually on the backside but sometimes on the palm surface as well. They can go away if the cyst is irritated such as by puncturing with a needle and pulling a thread through it which is allowed to hang free on the entry and exit path of the needle. A clean bandage is put over the cyst so that it can take up the fluid that will ooze from the cyst along the thread ends. A portion of thread should extend from each side of the wound approximately six inches, and each day about half an inch of thread is pulled through the cyst from one side or other.

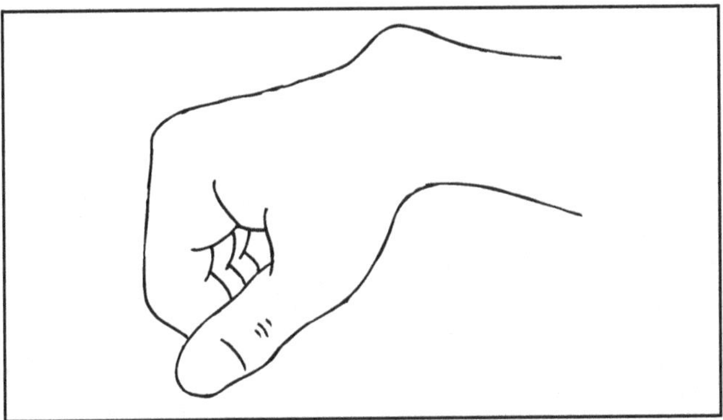

One week after the fluid has completely stopped flowing, the thread can be completely removed. The irritation that occurs from the thread will usually cause the cyst to disappear. Be very careful to keep everything clean so that an infection does not occur. Should it become infected (red, tender, with pus) the thread should be completely removed and hot and cold soaks can be instituted to encourage more rapid healing. At the same time take an antimicrobial herb. Usually it does not become infected, but if it does use the hydrotherapy and herbal antimicrobials. You can be encouraged that infection will also cause the ganglion to go away, usually permanently.

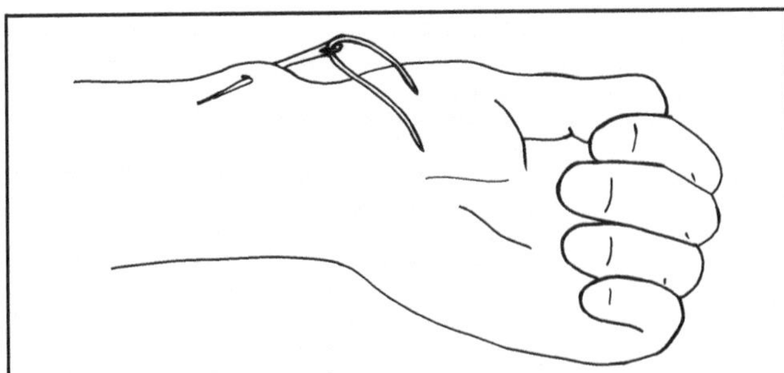

Some doctors used to hit a ganglion cyst with a large book, such as a large dictionary weighing about 5 to 10 pounds. The force used to hit the ganglion should be enough to rupture the cyst but not enough to break a bone. Support the wrist on a table with the cyst uppermost and give it a sharp blow with the large hardcover book.

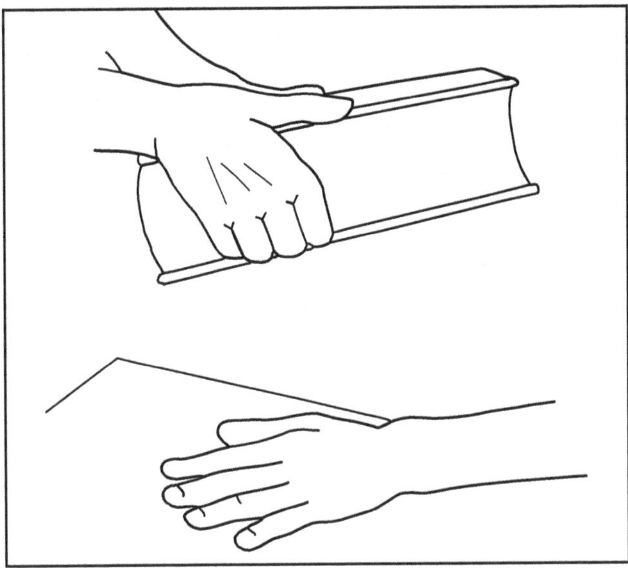

Sometimes tight binding around the wrist with a splint on the palm side, extending from the middle of the palm to halfway to the elbow, wrapped snugly with a bandage, can cause the cyst to disappear. If none of these measures are effective, the cyst may have to be removed surgically or you may simply decide to live with it.

Hammer Toes

Several foot conditions of older people, while minor in themselves, can be painful enough to cause lameness and varying degrees of disability. Hammer toe is a deformity of the toe in which the last joint of the toe is bent downward.

The simplest and most effective treatment is the application of adhesive-backed felt pads wherever the toes touch the interior of the shoe.

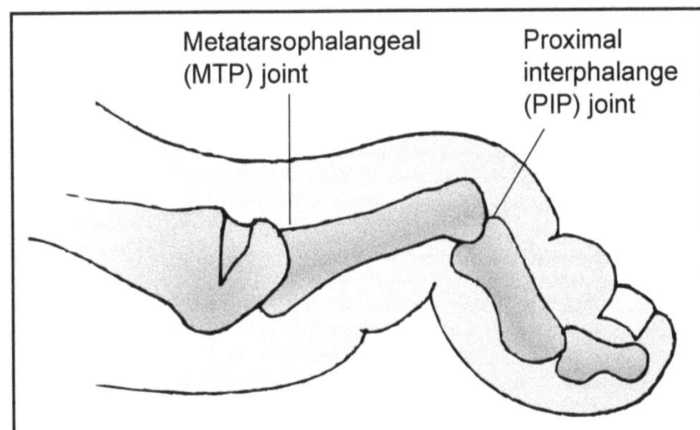

It is equally important to wear properly fitted shoes made of soft leather or other very resilient material that does not constrict toes. Often less expensive shoes will mold more

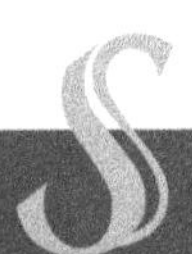

readily to the foot than more expensive quality leather that does not yield.

Running shoes are often made of synthetic materials that do not "give" as leather and some cloth ones do. Socks should be of cotton or other stretchy fabric to prevent restriction of extension of the toes.

Stretch your calf, which will stretch the tendons in your foot, as you would for leg cramps.

Walk on your tip-toes. This exercise will encourage your toes to bend and flex.

Use a hot foot bath for 30 minutes each night if you are not a diabetic.

If you are overweight, maintaining proper weight will help to relieve hammer toes.

Heel Spur

A heel spur is a thickening of a normal ridge on the principal bone of the heel, the calcaneus.

Repeated trauma to the heel from excessive weight or insufficient padding of proper shoes is the usual cause. Treatment includes weight loss, hot foot soaks (30 minutes each night), stretching the calf muscles, and strapping (see "Sprains" within this section).

Leg and foot exercises may seem to be a very small treatment for such a severe pain, but I can assure you that any exercising or stretching you do will make it better. A small investment of time and effort will pay large dividends.

- Follow the instructions for leg cramps standing two feet from a wall, bracing your hands against the wall at shoulder height, and while keeping the heels flat on the floor, lean the chest fully into the wall. Hold that position 10 seconds, push away from the wall for 5 seconds, and return into the wall another 10 seconds. Repeat this three times four times daily for two months.
- Walk on tiptoe on a carpeted surface for at least 10 seconds three times daily.
- Walk on the outsides of your heels, barefoot, on a carpeted surface for 10 seconds three to four times daily.
- Do a half squat, slowly bringing yourself back to the upright position four times, repeat four times daily. Walking up and down stairs is very good for this condition.
- Get some heel pads from a medical supply store. They have cut out pieces on the heel. Use those in your shoes.
- Every night, before going to bed, put your foot in hot water, as hot as can be tolerated, for 30 minutes. Then end in cold water, preferably about 30 seconds of nearly ice cold water. If you have insulin dependent diabetes, you should not put your feet in hot water.
- A firm massage for 30 minutes to the heels can be very helpful.
- If you have access to ultrasound treatment, a long treatment session, about 30 minutes in length, can be helpful for spurs.
- If you are overweight, correct the condition.

Knee Pain

The following tests will help you discover the source of your knee pain.

Valgus Stress

Have the patient lie down and bend the knee at a 20-degree flexion with the examiner's hands on the foot and the calf. The examiner should push the foot to the outside (laterally) while keeping the knee straight in front to force the knee medially, which will put stress on the medial collateral ligament. It will result in pain if the problem is there.

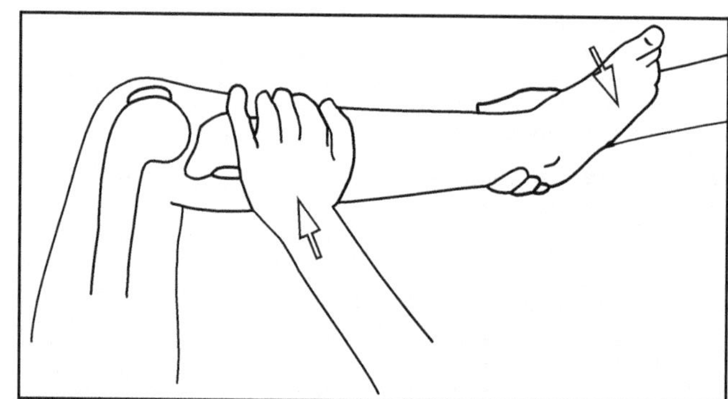

Varus Stress

This is done in the opposite way to the above test, and, if it elicits pain, indicates that cartilage is rubbing on the bone.

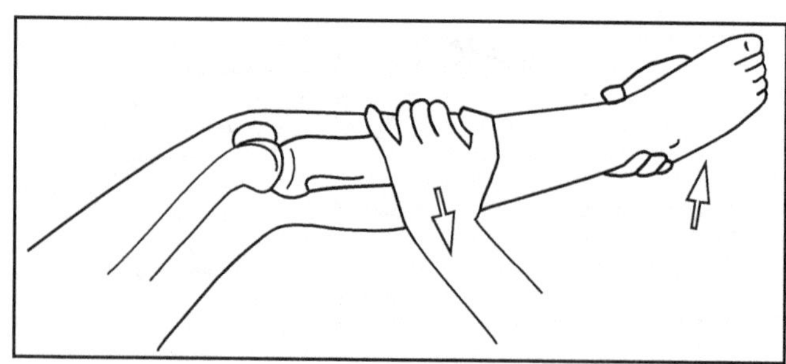

To treat this issue, protect from trauma for months or years to encourage the gradual replacement of cartilage. That means practicing all the suggestions below, especially the suggestions about weight. Figure 100 pounds for your first

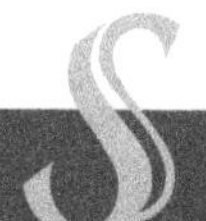

five feet in height, and five pounds per inch thereafter if you are a woman, and six or seven pounds per inch if you are a man, depending on how muscular you are.

Anterior Drawer Test

With the patient lying down, knee flexed to 60- or 70-degree angle, stabilize the foot with one hand. Put the other hand behind the knee. Stand at the patient's foot, and with the hand behind and under the knee, pull straight in front of the patient (toward examiner standing at the foot). If the deep ligament right under the knee has pain or extends out too much, the cruciate ligament has a tear or a bad sprain.

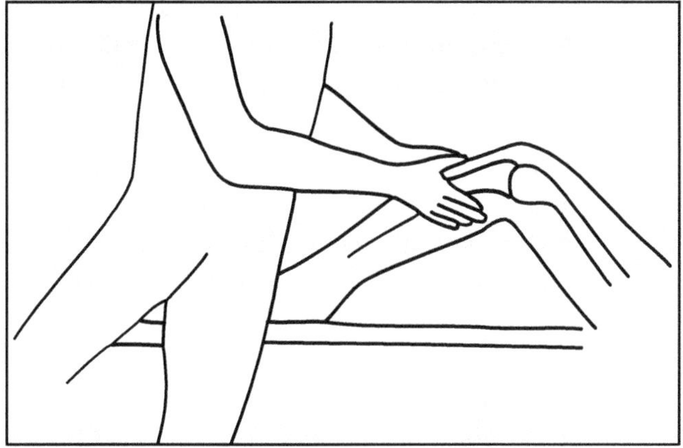

If this is the case, use crutches, stay off it as much as possible, be patient, and wait. Let time pass for it to heal. After a few days, hot and cold applications done simultaneously will give a reflex action that can help heal. If it is still painful after two to four weeks, see a physician about prolotherapy with natural ingredients, most usually glucose.

Posterior Drawer Test

This tests for laxity in the cruciate ligament. With the knee flexed 90 degrees, push on the tibia with your hand placed on the tibia just below the knee. It is the opposite movement to the one in the anterior drawer test.

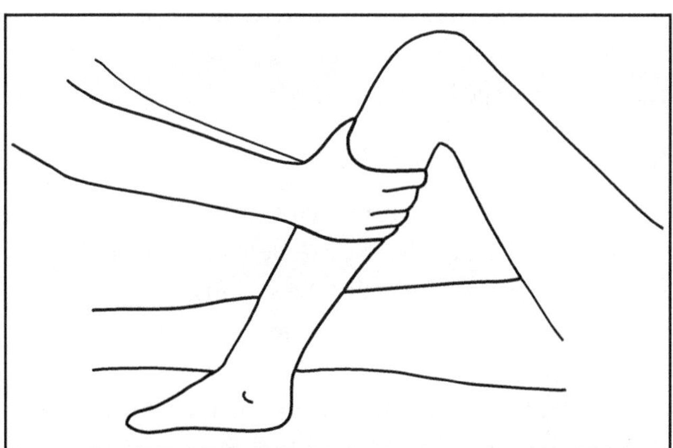

To treat a lax cruciate ligament, do a modified prolotherapy. It is done by deep pressure with the thumb in the area of the pain, frictioning the area to the point of pain for 10 minutes. Do this deep massage daily to encourage the ingrowth of fibrous tissue to strengthen the lax ligament.

Treatment of Knee Pain

Much knee pain begins with allowing the knees to drift outward. If a person stands with the toes pointed outward in a splayfoot position, a strain is placed on the internal structures of the knees. If, while sitting, the knees are allowed to fall widely apart, the twisting of the joint places a strain on the knees. Climbing steps or descending steps with the toes pointed outward strains the knees, especially if the step taken upward or downward is a long step.

Do not start normal physical activities too quickly, or without proper warm-up, as this can start a cycle of recurrent injury to the knee and chronic pain.

Apply ice packs in acute knee pain or recent injury to diminish swelling and stop the pain. These are effective for about 48 hours. Then the ice can be replaced by alternating hot and cold compresses. The swollen joint treatment can be summed up by the acronym RICE—rest, ice, compression, and elevation. The knee joint should not be compressed or wrapped as tightly as other joints. When elevating the knee, use pillows to prop the knee in a slightly flexed position to keep down swelling and pain.

Complete rest may require the use of crutches and perhaps even splints. One to five days of rest are important for an injured knee, as an injury to the knee can develop chronic pain for years if not properly treated.

Knee surgery recovery requires patients not to put full weight on the operated leg for one to four weeks depending on the type of surgery. Once the patients have the go-ahead for full weight bearing, then the process of restoring the knee begins. Recognize that, having rested the knee, it is now more vulnerable and susceptible to re-injury. Inactive muscles, tendons, ligaments, and bones lose their strength and suppleness. As a general rule, for every week of complete rest, a month of active restoration is required.

Hot compresses in the daytime and charcoal compresses at night can be very helpful. A liniment made of arnica is often surprisingly helpful. (See "Arnica Liniment" in the *Herbal Remedies* section.)

Stay slim. Even 10 pounds more than is normal for the person can increase the risk of sustaining and maintaining injury or re-injuring the knee after healing or surgery.

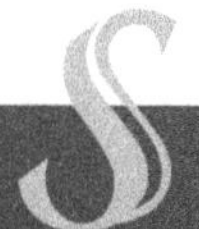

Deep knee bends may strain the knees. The person with knee pain should arise from the sitting position by assisting the rise with the hands, lifting the weight as much as possible with the hands until the weight is almost directly over the feet.

Take some herbal anti-inflammatory herbs such as white willow bark, licorice root, and hawthorn berry. One tablespoon of each of these in a quart of gently simmering water for 15 to 20 minutes will make a one-day supply. Make it up fresh daily.

Some cases of chronic knee pain have been almost miraculously cured by about four to five months of daily application of red pepper extract. Put one teaspoon of red pepper (hot pepper or cayenne) in one cup of rubbing alcohol. Allow the pepper to settle and apply some of the alcohol to the knee in all areas having pain. Apply six times a day for six days, and then drop down to two applications a day. If it is effective, you should experience pain relief in two weeks, but the applications should be continued twice daily for four or five months after the pain has stopped.

Do the following exercises to gradually increase the knee's range of motion, strength, and endurance. Strengthening the muscles surrounding the knee helps to stabilize and support the knee. Flexibility is best improved by self stretching.

- Endurance is increased by walking, climbing stairs, swimming, and aerobics that don't over-stress the joints. If exercises cause pain, stop. Swimming or other water workouts may be the best exercise for people with recurrent knee problems. Avoid jogging, basketball, tennis, and other twist and turn exercises. Bicycling can exacerbate knee pain if the person is not careful to keep the knees pointed straight in front, rather than drifting outward. Walking, cross country skiing, or low impact aerobics may be the best exercise.
- Rope training and fitness machines are good tools for increasing strength. Books can be obtained from the library or on the Internet on these exercises, or you can join a fitness club.
- While sitting in a chair extend your legs so that only your heels rest on the floor. Then tighten the muscles on the fronts of your thighs (quadriceps). Hold the tension for two seconds then release. Repeat five times. This exercise causes the secretion of synovial fluid, a nutrient rich fluid that cushions the knees and encourages healthy cartilage.
- From the starting position in the exercise above, lift your entire leg a few inches off the floor and back down. Repeat 10 times. The next day hold the leg up one second at the height of the lift. Each day increase the time by one second up to five seconds. When able to do this easily, increase the number of times each day you do the exercise until you can easily perform them four times a day.
- While standing supporting your hands on a chair or wall, lift first one leg then the other straight up behind you. This motion strengthens the hamstring muscles on the back of the thigh. Repeat 10 times.
- Glucosamine sulfate is very effective for knee pain. Take 1,000 milligrams three times a day until you get relief, then drop down to 500 milligrams three times a day. It is a synthetic nutrient supplement somewhat like the chemical components of cartilage. This has been helpful in some cases. Quite a lot of studies have been done on this substance, and it is apparently as safe as honey or salt. Take two of the vegetarian variety pills three times a day for two months.

Morton's Toe

Severe foot pain can result from a Morton's neuroma, a swelling of a nerve that goes to the toe. One method of treating it is to tread on the painful area for about 10 minutes. This measure can relieve pain, and in about two weeks it may stop it completely. Massage can also help, concentrating firm pressure on the painful area. Put a quarter-sized pad of moleskin under the end of the bone next to the toe having the neuroma. This measure can rotate the bones in such a fashion as to cause the nerve that has the neuroma to slip out of the way of pressure and heal. On top of the quarter-sized moleskin put a nickel size piece of moleskin in pyramid style. Then top it off with a dime size piece of moleskin.

Make certain that shoes fit correctly, as improperly fitted shoes are a common cause of rotation of the bones of the toes, which puts pressure on and causes the swelling of the nerves because of chronic irritation.

Muscle relaxants

Use the following herbs as muscle relaxants: catnip, chamomile (goes to the central nervous system to relax muscles), peppermint, passion flower, rosemary, black cohash wild cherry, and yarrow (related to thujone, which is in marijuana).

Massage, hot baths, heating pads, hot water bottles, and, for some, ice packs can all give muscle relaxation.

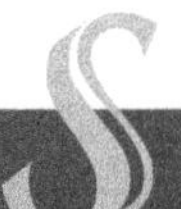

Osgood-Schlatter Disease

This is a disease of children characterized by tenderness, pain, and some swelling just below the knee that is self-limited and always disappears with time. The best treatment is rest, hot and cold applications to the knee, and sometimes elastic bandages. It may be worth a trial to see if the child has a food sensitivity. Hormone pills, hydrocortisone injections, and plaster casts add risks to this benign condition and should not be used.

Osteoporosis Pain

For the pain of osteoporosis or any skeletal pain, take two drops of food-grade hydrogen peroxide in a glass of water three to four times a day.

Plantar Fasciitis

Plantar fasciitis is recognized by low-grade pain in the beginning located on the sole of the foot just at the junction of the heel pad and arch and spreading to the arch of the foot. Pain may be felt immediately beneath the heel pad where the plantar fascia (a sheet of specialized fibrous connective tissue) inserts into the calcaneus bone, the principal bone of the heel. The inside of the heel may be more likely to cause pain than the outside. It is caused by microscopic tears and inflammation of the plantar fascia, which results from repeatedly bending the foot while walking. The injury may occur because the ankle is not as loose as it should be because of tightness in the calf. Swelling is not usually present, but tenderness is likely.

Treatment

- Ice massage 20 minutes several times a day
- A prolonged firm massage of the area
- Anti-inflammatory herbs
- Running shoes with soft heels. Some have found relief from wearing hiking boots.
- Each day stand two feet from a wall, support yourself with hands placed at shoulder height on the wall in front of you, lean into the wall while keeping the heels flat on the floor. Hold the stretch about 10 seconds, push away for five, and repeat three to six times at one session. Repeat approximately five sessions throughout the day.
- One of the best remedies we have found is red pepper extract. It can be purchased from a pharmacy or prepared from cayenne and rubbing alcohol. (See "Tincture, Extract" in the *Herbal Remedies* section.) Rub the extract on the heel six times a day for six days, then drop down to two times a day for about three to six months, or until the condition is healed.

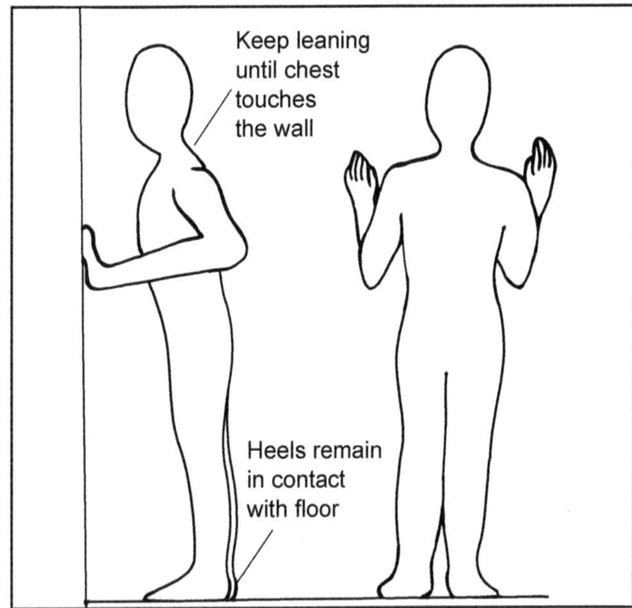

- A semi-rigid heel cup and a soft rubber pad in the shoe can help. There are over-the-counter pads for the shoes that sell for around $10 that have been found in a study to work better than the custom made shoe inserts that cost hundreds of dollars. Since heel pain is the most common reason people go to a foot doctor, it is important to know that you can get good relief without the more expensive methods.
- A specific remedy that we consider natural is prolotherapy or the injection of a concentrated glucose solution into the plantar fascia performed by a physician.

Sciatica and Slipped Disc

Sciatica is most commonly caused from rupture of the intervertebral disc. Usually the person has had some indication for years that there was something wrong in the back before the final herniation occurs. The typical pain from a herniated disc in the lumbar region is pain in the upper mid buttock. Typical sciatica occurs from this kind of slippage.

When the long and very large nerve named sciatic, which supplies the muscles of the thigh, leg, and foot, and the skin of the leg, running the entire length of the leg, becomes inflamed pain is felt in the areas associated with the sciatic nerve, buttocks, knee, leg, and even foot in severe cases. It may be caused by a slipped disk or inflammation in or around the vertebral bones. An abnormal condition in nearby blood vessels may starve the nerve or press on it. Hardening of the arteries can cause reduction of blood supply and pain in the nerve. Poor muscle tone or contracted ligaments may also cause a problem with sciatica.

Repeated activities that cause a resting of the elbows on the knees for long periods, which flexes the back, can increase the risk of developing a bulging disk in a place to cause sciatica. Sneezing while in this kind of position compounds the force on the disks, sometimes causing a weakened disk to rupture.

In order to determine if you have sciatica, evaluate your condition by answering these questions:

1. Is the pain sometimes better or is it constant? If the latter, it needs vigorous treatment to prevent its progressing to acute inflammation and disability.
2. Is it felt in the buttocks, knee, or foot? The greater the distance from the low back to the end of the pain, the more difficult to treat. The severity of the case is reflected by the proportion of the leg involved.
3. Do an exercise to determine if your leg pain is because of a knee problem or sciatica. Bring the knee on the painful side up to the waist while lying flat on the floor. Then cross the foot of that leg over the other leg at the level just above the knee and anchor the foot against the knee. Very gently, with your opposite hand, pull the knee toward the floor on the opposite side from the pain. If a muscle spasm causing sciatica is present, it will hurt when it is stretched. Gentle stretching loosens the muscle. A similar stretch can be done while sitting on the floor or in the bed. Again, with the knee bent, place the ankle of the affected side behind the opposite knee on the outside. Hold it there and gently pull the knee toward the opposite side from the pain. If it is sciatica, pain should occur in the middle of the buttocks and travel down the thigh toward the ankle.

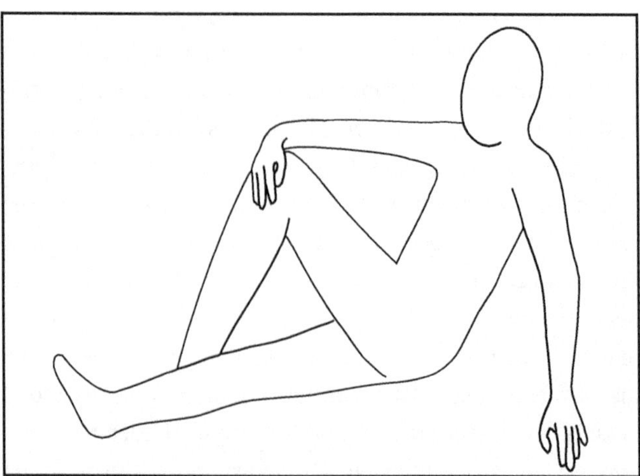

Treatment

The treatment for acute sciatica is broken down into several phases. The first phase is aimed at centralizing the pain (bringing it close or near to the back only, if possible, making it recede from the thigh, leg, or foot). The second phase is stretching and conditioning the nearby structures. The third phase is aimed at prevention of recurrence by promoting general health of the body and especially the nearby structures.

Phase A—*Used for acute and disabling sciatica.*

Lie on the abdomen with enough pillows under the chest for neck comfort, and a pillow under the ankles for toe comfort (or hang the feet off the end of the bed).

Then put the same number of pillows as you have under the chest, plus one more, under the abdomen so that the lumbar spine is in the neutral or slight flexion position.

While in this position, put heat on the back. The objective is to get pain out of the ankle area even if it is worse in the thigh. Patients often find that the pain moves up their leg. After about an hour you should be able to tell if the pain is less, or relieved in the thigh, leg, and foot, and has moved to the buttock, or even all the way up to the back. If it has moved farther down the leg or has become worse, then your sciatica is not caused by a bulging disk. It may be because of irritation on the sciatic nerve as it passes through the foramen ovale (a large opening for the nerve to pass from the interior to the exterior of the buttock).

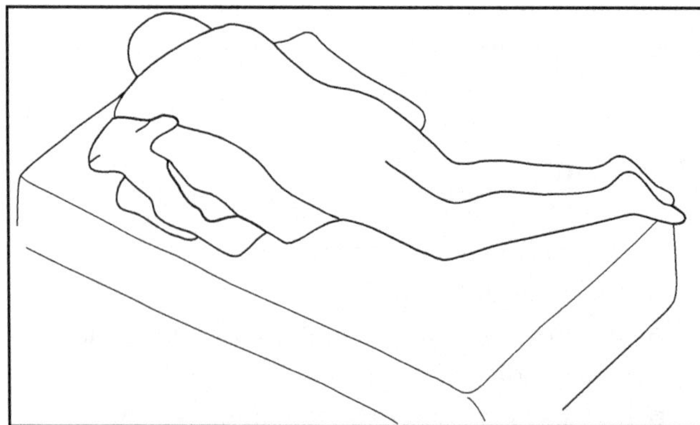

While still lying on the abdomen, move both legs toward the painful side so that the patient is in a sideways bend toward the painful side. Remain in this position for 15 to 60 minutes. Increase the degree of the bend toward the pain and hold for 15 minutes if possible, or decrease the bend if the patient complains severely, depending on whether the pain is less or more.

If the patient gets centralization of pain to above the knee or above the thigh, or even significant lessening of pain in the leg or foot, then you are ready to slowly reduce the flexion of the spine. Do so by reducing the number of pillows under the abdomen, or by putting another pillow under the chest. Do not move off the pillows! Simply do a pushup to get readjusted.

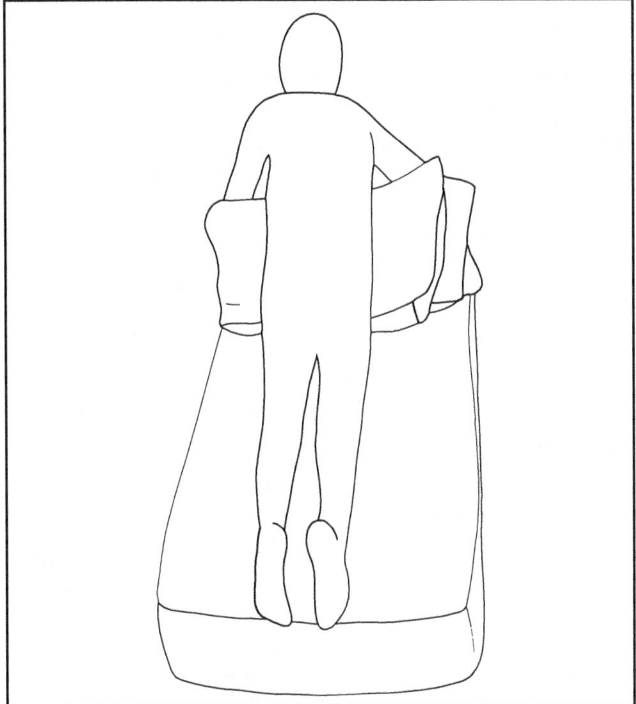

To ensure that you are ready to start removing pillows from under the abdomen, you should do a form of a pushup in which you put your hands to the sides of your shoulders and lift your head and shoulders and a portion of the upper back. Then slightly twist to the right and twist to the left, and then make a hump-back and then tilt your head far back. If any of these movements causes an increase in pain, rest again for a few minutes in the same position and then perform the pushup again. Bear in mind that when you first start doing this range of motion for your upper back, you may have some increase in pain at first. The pain should decrease or return to involving only the back after you continue to do a few twists and bends of the back.

After you have done one pushup and the twisting movement, again rest for about one minute, then do the pushup again with the twisting and bending movement, repeating the pushup about 10 times with resting in between. Do not try to push up too high or twist or bend too far in any direction. If the pain is less, then roll to the side without pain, keeping your arms held overhead while rolling and remove one of the pillows under the abdomen. Roll back onto the remaining pillows. Rest again for about 10 minutes. If the pain is still not increased and a subsequent pushup trial produces no pain, you are again ready to roll as a log and remove the remaining pillows. Rest in this position for one or two minutes, then again roll to the normal side and put a pillow under your chest. Keep the legs straight down.

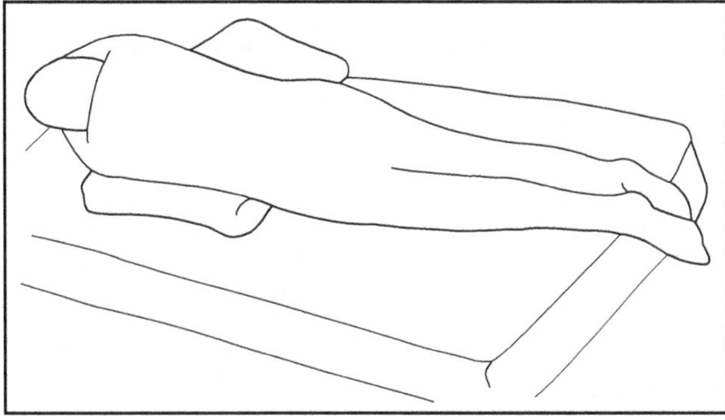

If the pillows under the abdomen do not lessen the pain, try gently bending the painful leg and then moving the non-painful leg over toward the painful side, moving only a small range at first. Hold this position several minutes to see if it succeeds in bringing the pain up from the foot and leg into the thigh, buttocks, or back. Then move the leg still further toward the painful side, always moving the painful leg first. As soon as the pain moves up to the thigh of the painful side, bring both legs back to the midline as the pain could move to the opposite side. Next do the pushup and twisting and bending exercise again.

Then gradually put the back in slight extension (head and shoulders lifted up to make a backward bend). Make no abrupt change to get in extension. You may need to go very slowly. This part of the treatment takes quite a lot of time in some people, an hour or more, so be prepared to be patient.

Phase B—*Used when pain is better and more tolerable.*

Stretching exercises such as given for leg cramps are helpful during this stage. Face a wall and stand two feet away from it. While keeping the heels flat on the floor, lean the chest into the wall for 10 seconds. Push away for five, and repeat three times. Then turn with your side to the wall and, from two feet away, lean the hip into the wall, 10 seconds in and five out, three times. Turn the opposite hip toward the wall and repeat. If this side movement causes pain, move closer to the wall to do the exercise. Gradually increase the distance day by day from the wall. Repeat the series four times a day for 60 days.

Winging and bridging exercises to strengthen the back. Lie on the back and support the body on heels and shoulders, keeping all other parts off the floor (bridging). Lie face down,

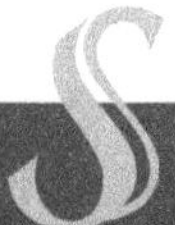

and support the body on the abdomen keeping all other parts off the floor (winging). Hold each of these three seconds on the first day. Build up to 30 seconds three times daily for 90 days.

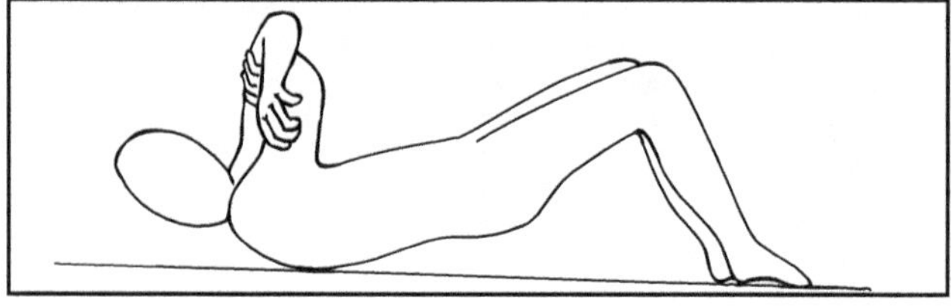

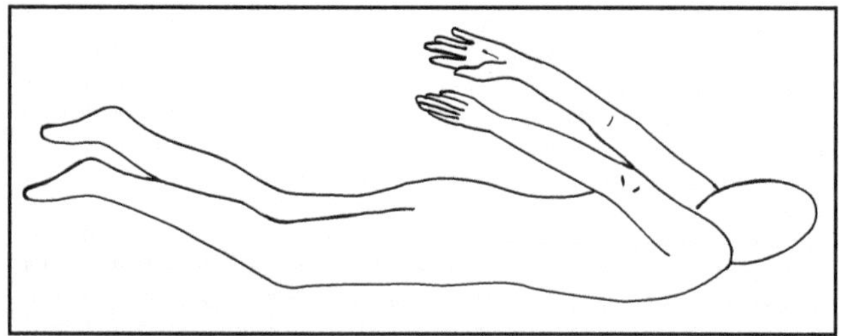

Place hot compresses over the buttocks, thigh, leg, and ankle. Leave the heat on for 20 to 30 minutes, interrupted every 3 to 5 minutes for 30 to 60 seconds of ice cold compresses.

Try using an ice pack to control pain. Crush ice and put it in a plastic bag within a second bag to guard against leaking. Use an ice massage in acute sciatica for the first 72 hours unless it makes the pain worse. Afterwards, heat treatments are the best choice.

If the muscles of the low back or buttocks are tender to the touch, an ice massage may be applied instead of heat. Block the area with towels and rub ice over the area, keeping the ice constantly moving. Freeze water in a seven to nine ounce styrofoam cup, and tear the bottom off so that the upper portion can be held while the bottom portion of the ice is exposed. This size is ideal. Ice cubes may be used if you are unable to make your own larger cube. Continue ice rubbing the painful area for 12 to 15 minutes.

An effective but gentle exercise is done by sitting away from the back of your chair with the knees separated slightly and the feet flat on the floor. While keeping the back straight, bend forward and place the right forearm on the right thigh. Extend the left arm up toward the ceiling and, while exhaling, turn and look up toward the left hand. Hold for three breaths, and repeat with the other side. To increase the stretch even more, bend forward and place the right hand along the outside of the left foot. Then continue as above.

A most effective remedy for sciatica in men is simply not carrying a wallet in the back pocket. Prolonged sitting puts pressure on the sciatic nerve and can cause a full blown case of sciatica.

Phase C—*Used at all stages.*

The most favorable diet for sciatica is a totally plant-based diet with no free-fats, free-sugars, or dairy products. If you have high blood cholesterol or triglycerides, your back may be weakened by hardening of the arteries in the low back area, which causes reduced nutrition of the bones and disks. These biochemical problems should be corrected immediately to prevent further injury to the back.

Experiment with omitting nightshade foods (tomatoes, potatoes, eggplant, and peppers) from your diet. An irritation from a food sensitivity may also be a part of the problem.

Scoliosis

Scoliosis is a sideways curvature of the spine that begins most often during the growth spurt just before puberty. Girls are affected more frequently than boys. Most cases are quite mild and hardly call anyone's attention. While scoliosis can be caused by conditions such as cerebral palsy and muscular dystrophy, the cause is usually unknown, but we have theorized that wearing constrictive clothing in childhood may cause asymmetrical development of the skeletal structures and blood vessels, resulting eventually in curvature as growth proceeds in an asymmetrical way.

From time to time during childhood, the parent should have the child bend over from the standing position, allowing the arms to dangle loosely perpendicular to the floor. The parent then looks down the spine with a light coming in from one side or the other, but not directly overhead. From this position an early spinal curvature can be easily seen, as well as the elevation of one shoulder blade, which is usually the most clearly visible abnormality when the disorder begins.

Treatment

The most favorable diet is a plant-based diet. Avoid high protein, high fat, and high sugar foods.

Begin correct posture at once, insisting that it be maintained. The head must be brought into a "neutral posture." That means the cheek bones must be perpendicular to the collar bones. A helper will be needed to guide the person into the correct posture. Then get the shoulders back and down. Do this by reaching overhead as far up as possible, then bringing the arms in an arch backward, reaching as far as possible. Then letting the arms rest at your sides with the shoulders relaxed downward, not held upward by the ears. Notice that you are now standing tall. Get the hips in a neutral position by tilting the hip bones backward a bit. Next relax the knees slightly forward to the neutral position. Stand slightly on the outsides of the feet to avoid pronation of the feet. You now

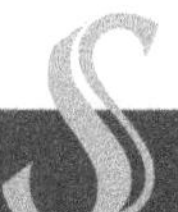

have perfect posture. You should be able to stand for an hour without any fatigue except of the feet.

Do not lift heavy objects more frequently with one hand than with the other, such as a backpack, books, bag, a lunch box, etc.

Most school children carry backpacks weighing about 30 percent of his or her body weight, with many school children carrying heavier packs. Adult workers in industry, etc., are not allowed to carry weights exceeding 25 to 30 percent of their body weight. If a child should have a tendency toward scoliosis, carrying such a heavy weight could make the child have a much more severe case, even requiring corrective surgery (*Journal of the American Medical Association* 282 [1999]: 1427, 1472).

Special exercises for the development of muscular strength should be instituted at once. These include household labor, making certain that both arms are used equally to ensure symmetrical development of the back muscles.

Do the following stretching exercises for the back for five minutes twice a day.

- Raise the hands and arms straight overhead, reaching as high as possible.
- Bend forward, touching the toes.
- Bend backward with hands stretched overhead.
- Hold each of these stretches for two to six seconds.

Tight waist bands must be avoided and make sure to keep the extremities warm.

If these measures are not successful, a physician skilled in the treatment of children with this disorder should be consulted.

Spinal Stenosis

The condition typically affects adults after age 50 and often results from arthritis, excessive use of the back, and aging. One vertebra may slip forward on another vertebra and cause pressure. Usually conservative measures such as stretches, heat, cold applications, compresses, massage, and exercise can be successful in controlling pain.

Lumbar stenosis sometimes causes back and leg pain. For this pain there is often relief by lying on the back with one leg bent and pulling the bent knee up to the chest about 10 times in a row. Then swap knees and pull the flexed knee up to the chest again about 10 times. If relief of pain from lumbar stenosis does not occur with these measures done four times daily for three months, it would be worth a try to do prolotherapy before drugs or surgery are considered. While the prolotherapy will not change stenosis, a fair proportion of spinal stenosis patients have their pain from more usual mechanical causes such as disc injury, ligament sprain, or strain. For these, prolotherapy can be very helpful. For some individuals with severe stenosis, it can be that they will not get relief from any measure, and decompression surgery is suggested, but even that is questionable as to whether it will bring relief.

For cervical stenosis, one can try chin tucks with the chin tucked well down as the head glides forward, but one must do this with care not to continue to push into positions that aggravate any numbness or tingling that has resulted from cervical stenosis.

Of course, the usual methods of pain control should be instituted. These include hydrotherapy, massage, and herbal remedies. (See "Pain Control" in the *Conditions and Diseases* section.)

Sprains

These are injuries in the area of a joint, usually the ankle, in which a sudden movement or fall stretches or overstrains the connective tissue fibers belonging to the ligaments, muscles, or tendons so that they are torn or ruptured. Blood or tissue fluid may accumulate around the joint in the soft tissues. If it is ascertained that no bone is broken, the treatment of the sprain should begin immediately.

Treatment

Stay off the foot from the time of injury. Walking on a fresh sprain makes the injury more extensive. Try to put pressure instantly on the ankle with your hands to try to minimize the bleeding into the tissues from torn fibers or blood vessels.

Extremes of temperature, extreme cold or extreme heat, will stop internal bleeding when applied promptly after the sprain. As soon as possible after the accident, seat the patient (if not a diabetic) in a chair in front of two deep pails of water—a very hot one maintained at 115°F to 118°F and the other with ice water. Plunge the injured foot into the hot water for exactly two minutes, then into the ice water for 30 seconds. (Note: If the person can only tolerate the very hot water for 20 seconds and takes it out of the hot water, you should immediately plunge it into the icy water for the same length of time.) Dry the injured part and wait 10 minutes. The objective for the first part of this treatment is to force a closure of any bleeding blood vessels, which will reduce the extent of the injury. This part of the treatment is done only once.

After the 10 minutes are up, elevate the foot and apply an ice bag to the ankle for 20 to 60 minutes. After that dry the

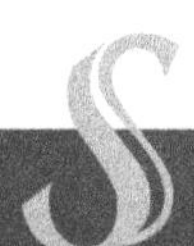

foot thoroughly but very gently, causing as little movement as possible, and strap the foot.

To strap the foot, place it in a neutral position. Then the big toe and its attaching bone in the foot are pressed down toward the sole while the little toe and its attaching bones in the foot are gently pressed upward toward the top of the foot. Two strips of one-inch tape are placed from the bump just behind the joint of the big toe (the one which usually gets bunions) extending around the back of the heel and ending at the same bump beside the little toe.

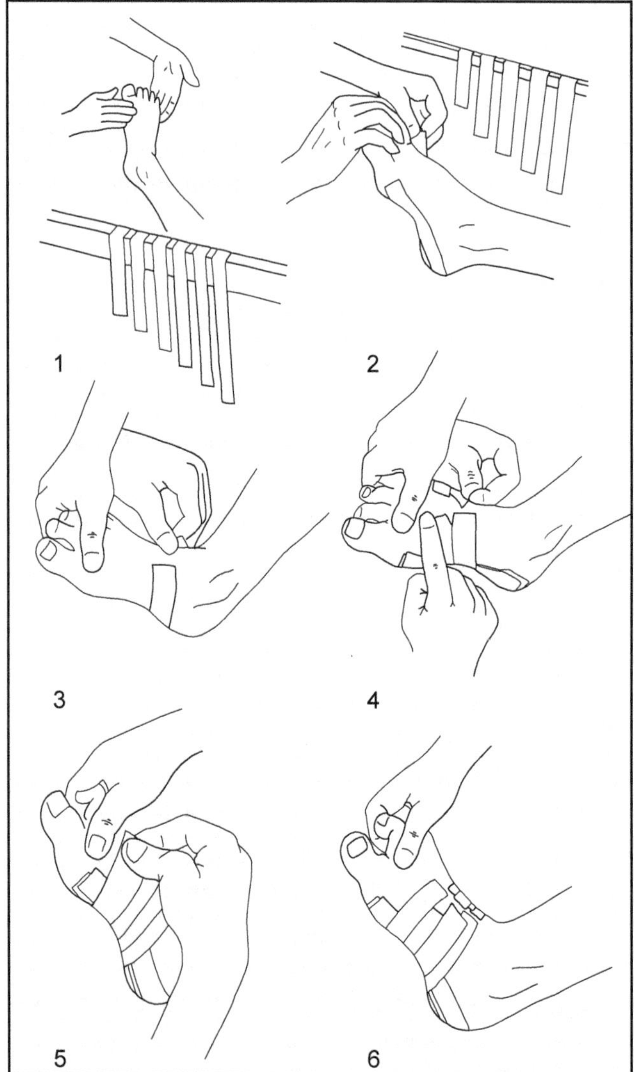

Then four to six strips of one-inch adhesive are put as stirrups under the sole of the foot, beginning the first one just in front of the place where the heel pad joins the arch, tilting the tape toward the toes and ending on the top of the foot with the tape pointing slightly toward the toes rather than straight up toward the leg. Place the second tape lapping over about halfway of the first tape in exactly the same manner as the first. The tape should overlap on top about one inch. Continue in this fashion until the fourth strip of tape ends about the base of the toe. Extra long feet may require a fifth or sixth one. During the placement of the strips of tape, which go under the sole of the foot, the foot should be held in the position described earlier.

A firm bandage such as an ace bandage can be applied over the strapping or in place of the strapping beginning at the base of the toes and extending well above the ankle, each round of the bandage covering one-third of the last wrap. Keep the patient's weight off the foot for about 24 hours. It is best not to walk on it until it is healed, so it is wise for the patient to use crutches.

Some have found a compress of vinegar most helpful, especially where strapping cannot be done immediately. The compress can be saturated with vinegar and put in the freezer for 5 to 10 minutes and applied to the injury. It warms up quite comfortably. Cover it with a plastic bag to retain moisture, and wear it overnight.

A compress of castor oil can also be used. Wet a piece of cotton cloth with castor oil, wrap it around the ankle, slip a plastic bag over the cloth, and fasten it in place with tape or hold in place with a large sock. Wear it overnight. The castor oil increases the T-cells in the tissue beneath it.

As soon as pain has diminished, gently move the ankle through the entire range of motion that can be done without pain, to regain full mobility. Contrast baths, first in very hot water for three minutes, then in cold for 30 seconds is an excellent healing modality. Make five exchanges. Do not use hot water for diabetics, but plunge in ice water for 10 minutes. When activity is resumed the person should have the ankle braced or strapped as described above, to prevent re-injury while the tissues are still tender.

Most ankle injuries are not associated with a significant fracture and do not need X-rays. In general, you need a doctor's opinion, and possibly an X-ray, only if:

- You heard a crack when you hurt your ankle. You can feel a snap when the ankle only suffers a simple sprain, but you do not hear it.
- The ankle is extremely swollen and otherwise misshapen.
- It hasn't improved in pain or swelling after five days.
- Pressing one particular spot on the ankle bone causes sharp pain.
- You feel numbness in the ankle or foot.

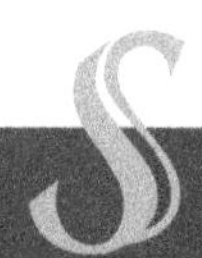

Tennis Elbow (Epicondylitis, Tendonitis)

A pain when moving or pressing on the outside eminence of the elbow is called tennis elbow. Once the pain gets started, it is difficult to get rid of it, as the inflammation continues because of continued movements that put a strain on that particular tendon. A movement that rotates the arm on itself is likely to cause tennis elbow. The diagnosis is made by a typical history, tenderness over the bone at the side of the elbow and the muscles between the two bones of the forearm, and weakness of the hand. The weakness may be so severe as to cause dropping of even lightweight objects. Doing a repetitive movement sufficient to put a strain on the tendons on the top of the elbow brings it on.

Treatment

The most important beginning treatment is modified rest for three or four days. Especially, restricting the rotational movement of the arm can be healing. This does not mean entire immobilization, as that will tend to make the disease worse and lead to muscle atrophy, but it does mean elimination of all movements that cause pain. When the pain is felt, however, it is already too late to avoid some degree of re-injury. Do not rest for a great length of time, as more than two to four days can result in muscle shrinking and stiffness.

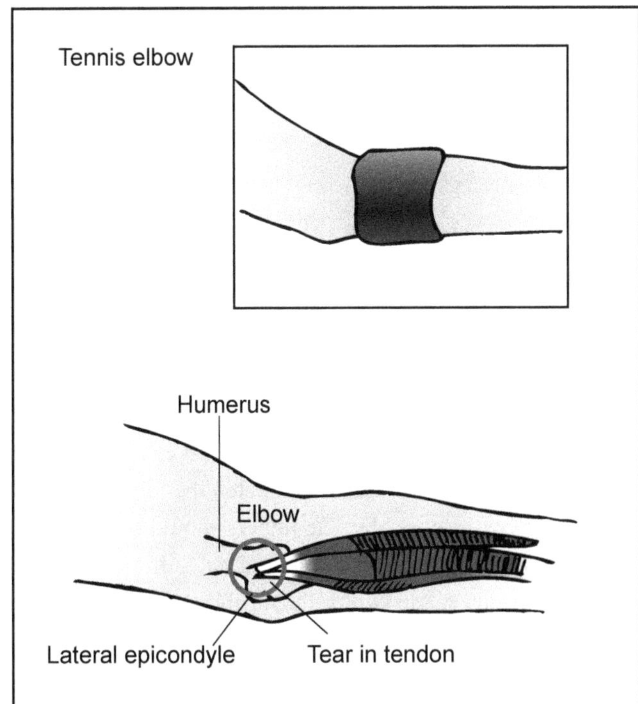

A 2.5 inch band held in place by velcro worn just beneath the elbow on the muscles of the forearm can be helpful. The gentle pressure on the muscles of the forearm actually pump soreness and swelling away while the wearer continues to work. It allows normal circulation and can be worn comfortably for hours. It should not be worn at night.

When the disease is in the early stages it should not be taken lightly, as it may get much worse quite quickly. Applying ice 30 to 90 minutes twice daily can relieve pain. Ice applied over the painful area is soothing and encourages healing. Some people will find heat more soothing than ice, which may be applied by a hot arm bath. In our experience the ice is usually more healing, although the heat may be as soothing.

A hand gripper, used 5 to 10 minutes four times a day, with the elbow straight and the wrist bent outward to one side to stretch the tendon, aids in healing and strengthens the muscles. This will prevent stiffness and contracture of the extensor tendons, making it difficult to close the fingers.

Locating trigger points in the painful muscles, both of the arm and forearm; applying firm pressure for 7 to 10 seconds; and moving in ever widening circles, taking point by point to relax the trigger points, although painful while the pressure is being applied, can exert a healing benefit. Vigorous and very firm rubbing should follow the trigger point pressure. The treatment requires an hour or more to adequately initiate the healing process. Expect great improvement in three days.

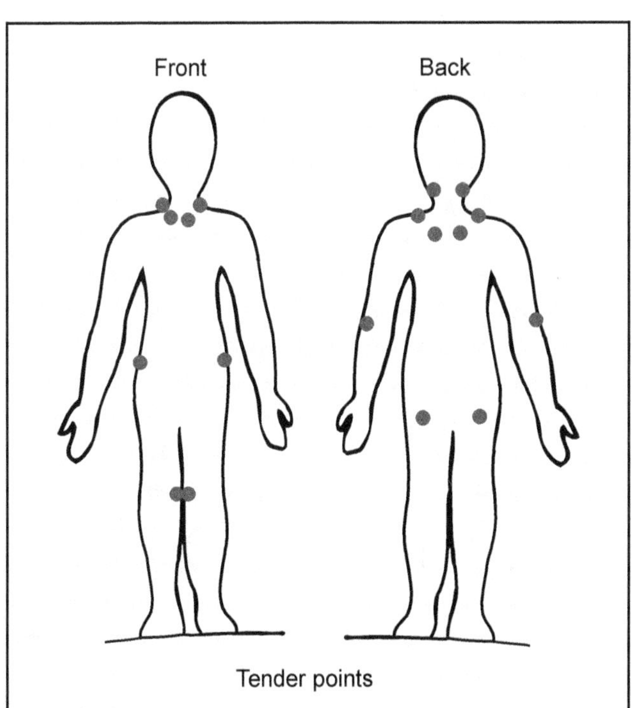

Tender points

Stretching exercises for all muscles having tenderness around the elbow can hasten healing. A tendon stretch, made by extending the arm so the hand is on the outside of the knee

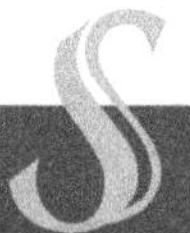

while sitting, then turning the closed fist to the extreme lateral (outside) direction, will exert a stretch on the muscles on top of the arm. The stretch can be increased by assistance from the opposite hand. Then repeat the stretch, turning the fist in the opposite direction. Move the extended arm from side to side, overhead, behind the back, etc., to repeat the stretch in as many planes as you can reach. Each plane stretches other muscle fibers not stretched in other positions. Repeating the stretch several times daily accelerates healing faster than most other self-induced treatments.

Another good exercise for healing is four to six weeks of daily use of a one-pound weight, with the palm down, arm on a table, lifting the wrist upward and rotating slightly outward, and holding for five seconds. Return to the palm down position, grip the weight again, lift and rotate as many repetitions as you can do. Continue daily until 15 repetitions can be done with ease. Then increase the weight one-half pound at a time, until 8 to 10 pounds can be lifted without pain.

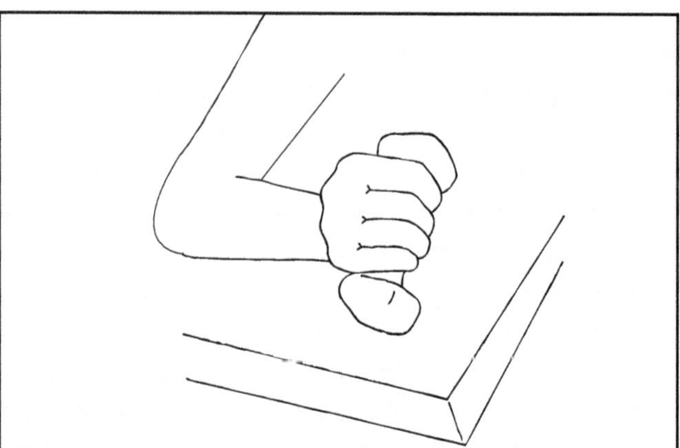

Another helpful exercise begins with the arm hanging downward, holding a dumbbell and rotating the forearm 180 degrees to bring the dumbbell into the horizontal position. Repeat 15 times.

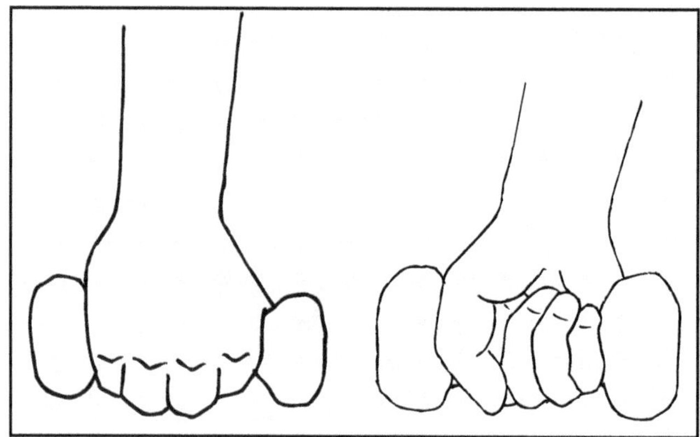

A very simple yet most effective method of treatment is working with a firm rubber band. While wearing a tennis elbow band on the forearm just beneath the elbow, place all five fingertips into the band. Then stretch the fingers to open them as widely as possible. The fingers should be separated at least an inch. If one rubber band is not sufficient to give a strong resistance, use two or three rubber bands. Do 15 to 20 repetitions every three to four hours throughout the day for one to two weeks. This same treatment is also useful for carpal tunnel syndrome in many patients (*The Physician and Sports Medicine* 22, no. 9 [September 1994]: 29).

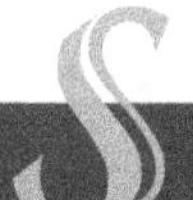

Vigorously rubbing the elbow and forearm with firm pressure on the deep structures in the painful areas can be very helpful. Rubbing with aloe vera gel or cream prior to the massage enhances the healing benefits. Or you may use liniments containing arnica or menthol as a massage oil. Aloe vera ointment is a good massage lubricant to aid healing of tennis elbow. Massage the aloe ointment until it is dried and reapply the second time, using about 15 minutes of firm but gentle rubbing of the area after the second application.

Try also omitting nightshades from your diet for about a month to see if that helps. It is sometimes a cure.

Trigger Finger

This is a common condition in middle-aged people and can be diagnosed by the fact that the finger "sticks" at a certain point, usually in flexion. A hard nodule can be detected in the line of the crease in the palm nearest the fingers. This hard nodule is because of a thickening of the tendon sheath, making it difficult for the two long tendons to glide in or out of the mouth of the sheath.

Treatment

Put pressure on the nodule for one minute six or more times daily while gently opening and closing the fingers, trying to do so in such a way that the finger will not lock in the 90-degree flexion position.

Soak the entire hand in ice water, with ice floating, for five minutes just prior to bedtime and increasing each night by one minute until 20 minutes have been achieved. Use a timer so that the full length of time is achieved. Continue for 40 days total.

If any kind of trauma is occurring such as carrying heavy loads in the hand, playing certain musical instruments such as the harp or guitar, using a hammer, shovel or heavy hoe, opening jars that are stuck, etc., discontinue the activity until one month after the treatment has finished.

Each night wear a castor oil compress in the palm made by pouring castor oil on a thin cloth until it is saturated, placing it in the palm, and covering the entire hand with a bread bag fastened at the wrist by taping or wrapping with an ace bandage. Continue the oil for at least two hours a day, or preferably overnight for about three months. The castor oil is said to raise the T-cell population in the area and assist healing of the problem.

The lump may completely disappear in the palm if the finger is immobilized for three weeks.

Heat may also be applied successfully to a trigger finger. Simply soak the hand in water at about 108°F to 112°F for 20 minutes each day for 30 days. We believe heat is not as effective as cold, but some patients prefer this treatment.

Tape a small neodymium magnet to the inside of the trigger finger to abolish pain and straighten the finger.

Take one to two glasses of celery juice or puree per day. About three or four large stalks blended will produce a glass of juice or puree. Also, one to two glasses of cucumber juice acts as a diuretic and assists in reducing swelling in the affected tendon.

A skilled chiropractor may be of help. The chiropractic work of adjusting the hand and finger may require about three weeks until the finger stops triggering. Some people heal quicker.

Take 100 milligrams of B6 three times daily. Some say that within the next six months the trigger finger will be completely healed (*Nutrition and Healing* 6, no. 3 [March 1999]: 7).

Skin Diseases

Acne

Acne occurs mainly on the face, chest, shoulders, and back. Acne is usually limited to the adolescent years when the oil glands of the skin go through a similar period of active development as the rest of the body, causing them to develop a sensitivity and an overgrowth in susceptible persons whose glands may go through the same kind of process as the interior of the nose goes through in hay fever. The cystic form of acne—large, painful lumps deep in the skin—can be chronic, widespread, and disfiguring. Pimples, red spots, blackheads, whiteheads, and swollen areas usually occur just at the time in life when social relationships are the most important. Most experienced dermatologists and acne sufferers will attest to the value of avoidance of chocolate, fats, and sweets.

It is also well to promote slow and steady growth in children. This is done by implementing a healthful diet and lifestyle. Slow down the growth of children if they are in the tallest, fattest, or biggest percentile of growth charts. This is done by eliminating all fast food and junk foods and between meal eating. Severely limit all concentrated foods such as sugar, margarine, mayonnaise, salad oils, cooking fats, nut butters, and fried foods.

To determine foods to which one is sensitive, perform an Elimination and Challenge diet and see if the pimples are reduced by the elimination of certain foods. (See "Elimination and Challenge Diet" in the *Dietary Information* section.) As soon as the acne clears up, begin adding foods, one every five

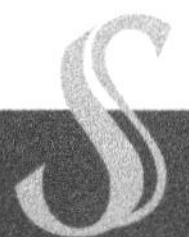

to seven days, which were formerly eliminated. When a food causes the pimples to return, make a list of those foods and omit them for at least one year to see if the body heals itself. Acne usually runs its course in 10 to 15 years.

It seems clear to us that in youngsters who have had early puberty the major cause is sensitivity to certain foods, particularly to the combination of sweets and fats, but many other food sensitivities are frequently involved. The value of avoidance of a high fat, high sugar diet is attested to by the fact that Eskimos who had eaten little or no sweets prior to 1950 and had had no acne whatsoever had a veritable explosion of acne after the Alaska-Canada Highway went through. In eight short years this population who had always had a high-fat diet from whale and seal blubber, and other animal fats, now began taking around 120 pounds of sugar per person per year, up from around 20 pounds per person per year. Overnight diseases they had never had before became as common as on the mainland—acne, diabetes, carious teeth, gallstones, and appendicitis.

Treatment

The most important matter is diet. Various food sensitivities such as milk, sugar, citrus, chocolate, fats (margarine, mayonnaise, fried foods, cooking fats, salad oils), nuts, peanuts, wheat, honey, yeast, legumes, and all animal products have been implicated. Animal fats from meat, milk, eggs, and cheese are an important cause of acne. A plant-based diet will be found to be most helpful. All chemicals, additives, conditioners, etc., should be removed from the diet as much as possible, along with coffee, tea, colas, and other soft drinks. Eat liberally of all fruits and vegetables, especially those that are green or yellow.

Avoid foods high in hormones—all animal products, wheat germ oil, peanut and corn oil, and vitamin E oil. Of course, all drugs containing hormones should be avoided if possible.

Avoid being overweight or overeating. Being overweight, even a small amount, stimulates the production of hormones that contribute to acne. Overeating encourages "leaky gut," which has become in recent years a suspect in a wide variety of disorders, including skin diseases.

Drink plenty of water daily, sufficient to keep the urine quite pale. This will make skin secretions thinner and more easily discharged. Good posture and deep breathing, along with daily exercise out of doors in the sunshine for an hour or more provides good circulation to the face and adds poise and a sense of well-being. These measures also relieve stress, which worsens acne. Do not get your exercise from competitive sports as they increase stress. Exercise neutralizes stress and is very important.

Salty foods as found in fast food, chips, pork, fries, dairy products, ketchup, mustard, and vending machine items should be reduced for all and eliminated for some. A salt-free diet is completely curative for an occasional case. The removal of salt must be absolute. Try it for three weeks to see if it helps. Use the same rule of thumb for eliminating salt as hypertensives. These rules of thumb include the following:

Oral zinc sulphate, about 135 milligrams, significantly improved acne in 64 patients in an experimental trial (*Clinical Pearls News* 9, no. 12 [1999]: 233). Zinc can become toxic if taken indefinitely; so I recommend discontinuing after about two to four months.

Iodine triggers acne and is present in approximately 30 times the daily requirement in the typical food served at fast food restaurants. It is especially high in beef from the additives in animal feed, from the salt in the fries, and in the buns. Avoid high iodine foods such as sea foods, seaweed, kelp, beef and pork, iodized salt, some swimming pools (the disinfectants), many soaps such as Betadine. Bromides are chemically related to iodides and may promote acne. They are found in some soft drinks, cooking oils, and many cough medicines.

Avoid tobacco, even secondhand, the use of drugs, alcoholic beverages, and any other toxic substance.

The use of antibiotics should be especially avoided, as several of them have been described as having severe long-term effects, even on the next generation!

Use 100 percent cotton clothing and bed linens rather than synthetic fabrics.

Many cosmetics and lotions contain chemicals that may aggravate acne. Dermatologist Nia K. Terezakis, M.D., states that some of the most popular commercial skin care products may be the greatest culprits in skin problems. Dr. Terezakis suggests compresses of cornstarch, baking soda, or a combination of the two.

Cleansing the skin every four to six hours will discourage bacterial growth. Washing may be done with or without a washcloth. Then rinse in lukewarm water. Repeat a second time. Some individuals have had good results from washing with lemon or lime juice and then rinsing, or by applying a small amount of lemon or lime to the wet skin after washing and rinsing as above. Lemons and limes have an acid pH in which human skin does well. The juice is also keratinolytic (softens or dissolves the scale on the skin) and antibacterial. Failure to cleanse the skin thoroughly and touching the skin often with the fingers makes acne worse. Do not prop your

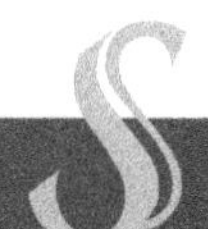

hands against your face. Touch the skin only with a clean tissue, even to scratch an itch.

Do not squeeze pimples or blackheads as this often pushes the blackhead down into the skin. Use a pimple extractor to remove blackheads and pustules rather than squeezing.

Shampoo nightly and keep hair off the face either by short haircuts or pinning up the hair.

A light coating with plain vinegar, red or white, can also encourage the increased peeling of the skin scales. A light brushing with a soft brush during washing the face also helps the peeling process.

Sunshine will help acne by increasing the peeling of the surface keratin and preventing blockage of the skin glands. Do not allow sunburning. The relaxation associated with sunbathing may also benefit acne.

Some individuals get pimples and a rash around the mouth from their own saliva, caused by licking around the lips or drooling on the pillow at night. A heavy application of petroleum jelly around the mouth at night and perfect restraint from licking will cure these cases in a few days.

Heat treatments are healing, with hot compresses 20 minutes three times a day using hot water, hot golden seal tea, hot baking soda water, or hot comfrey compresses. End each treatment with a splash of ice water or a 30-second ice-cold compress. Also, an ice massage over the face three minutes once daily can reduce inflammation. One young man felt his acne was helped by a 10-second application of ice every 30 minutes as often as he was able to do it during the day.

Pine tar soap should be lathered on at night very heavily, rubbing the face with the bar and leaving it to dry. It will "pull" all night. Rinse it off the next morning and lather up freshly and dry the face without rinsing. Any treatment that causes irritation should be discontinued, including the pine tar soap.

Be regular in all your activities, as the natural body rhythm will assist in clearing acne. The most healthful sleep pattern is early to bed and early to rise. Regularity can be very beneficial in both preventing and treating acne. Eat on time, sleep on time, study, exercise, and have devotions on a set schedule. Regularity promotes good circulation, which has a healing benefit.

Warm extremities, particularly the hands and feet, will be helpful to promote good circulation to the skin. The skin reacts as a single organ, and habitual chilling of the extremities can reflexively reduce the amount of blood flowing to parts of the skin.

Herbal tea compresses may be used such as witch hazel, ephedra, mullein, slippery elm, and white oak bark. Compresses may be applied hot or cold.

A tincture of cayenne can be enormously helpful in some cases. Make the tincture yourself by putting one-half teaspoon of red pepper (cayenne) in a jar with a screw cap. Add four ounces of ordinary rubbing alcohol. Swirl the solution. It may be used immediately but does not develop full strength until three weeks. Then the alcohol portion may be poured off the red pepper into a dark dropper bottle. Use the dropper to scatter drops over the face while gently spreading evenly with cotton-tipped applicators. Avoid introducing into the eyes, mouth, or nose.

(See also 'Rosacea, Acne Rosacea, Adult Onset Acne, Menopausal Acne' in the "Skin Diseases" entry.)

Aging Skin

Aging of the skin is revealed by many signs such as wrinkles, dry skin, and discoloration. We will examine a number of different conditions below.

Wrinkles

Skin loses its elasticity as it ages and, with the thinning of the skin and the loss of fat, it looks less plump and smooth. Gravity also pulls at the skin, causing it to sag. Wrinkles are much worse in the sun exposed areas since sun is a major cause of aging skin. Sun exposure causes skin cells to make enzymes that weaken connective tissue in the skin (*Science News* 149 [February 10, 1996]: 93). Avoid excessive sun exposure to the face during the middle of the day.

Cigarette smoking is also very contributory to wrinkles.

Dry skin

The skin becomes drier, more flaky, and itchy with aging.

Both wrinkles and dryness can be helped by a drop of castor oil mixed with about five or six drops of ordinary nongreasy hand lotion emulsified between the hands by vigorous rubbing, and spread gently over the wrinkled, dry or scaly areas. Petrolatum or lanolin are also very good for moisturizing the skin. Possibly the best is coconut oil.

You may use facial packs to help flatten wrinkles. The stinging nettle leaves, soaked for 20 minutes to get the astringent action activated, can be used to make a facial pack.

Cranesbill can be simmered for 20 minutes and applied to the skin as a facial pack.

To improve skin texture, harden nails, and strengthen hair growth, take a short cold bath daily. (See "Hydrotherapy" in the *Natural Remedies* section.)

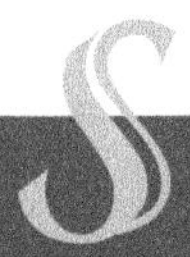

Skin lesions

Warts, age spots, liver spots, scaly spots, and cancers are more common as the skin ages. A basal cell carcinoma is the commonest form of cancer. The squamous cell carcinoma is also fairly common in the sun exposed areas; melanoma is a less common but more serious form of skin cancer, also more likely to occur in sun exposed areas. Severe childhood sunburns can result in melanomas; therefore, the most frequent areas melanomas occur are the upper back, the chest, and lower legs. Skin cancers are best treated by surgeon.

Cherry angiomas

There are harmless, small bright red domes created by dilated blood vessels that occur in most if not all middle-aged and elderly people. Cautery with an electric needle is the best treatment. But the only reason to treat them is for cosmetic concerns.

"Broken" capillaries, skin varicosities

These are dilated blood vessels often on the face but also on the thighs and ankles, and sometimes elsewhere. They are usually related to sun damage.

Bruising

Many seniors complain of black or blue marks on the arms and legs that are very superficial and caused by very little trauma. These become superficial because of the loss of fat and connective tissue that weakens the support around blood vessels. Bruising that occurs in areas always covered by clothing may represent something more serious such as the bruising caused by medications that interfere with blood clotting or some internal disease.

Flat and Polyplike Skin Growths

For flat rough skin growths on the hands and arms coming on with aging, take the yellow-blossomed bitter weed common in the south and southwest, also called sneeze weed, and crush the leaves, flowers, and stems together to produce juice. Rub the juice generously on the lesions daily, or more often as you can. Usually within one month the lesions disappear. Combine this remedy with vinegar spread on the growth every morning after showering and a brisk rubdown with a coarse towel to hasten the process. The elongated skin tags can be removed by strangulating with waxed dental floss.

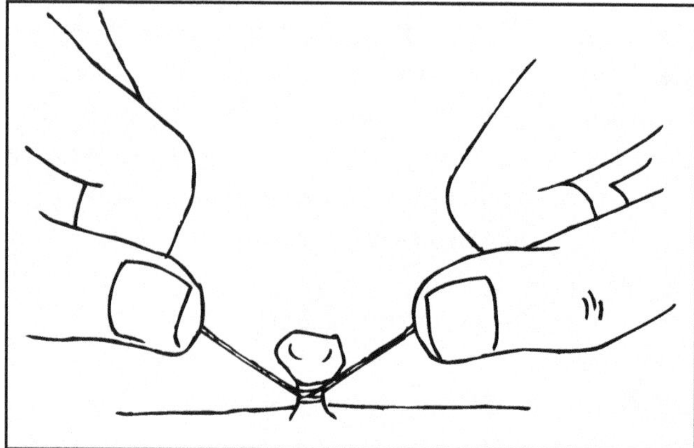

Freckles, Pigment Areas, Age Spots

To remove pigmented facial areas after pregnancy: Cut a green papaya and rub the milky sap from the skin of the papaya on your skin. Apply daily for one month. Onion juice and vinegar applied to these freckles, age spots, and pigmented areas, will help to fade them. Lemon juice spread on them daily, or a thin-slice of lemon applied as a poultice at night can help fade pigment in the skin. Hydrogen peroxide applied three to four times daily to pigmented spots will sometimes help.

Alopecia, Baldness, Hair Loss

There are three types of hair loss, general thinning, hereditary pattern baldness, and loss of hair in unexpected spots. Hair loss in both men and women is caused by a combination of factors—genes inherited from either parent, stress, unknown factors, and the effects of the hormone testosterone on hair follicles. In women only the adrenal glands produce testosterone. Estrogen counteracts most of its effect until menopause, after which time a woman may have thinning in the same pattern as the baldness of her father and her brothers.

In women, hair loss can also be caused by allergic reaction to hair dyes, and other hair cosmetics, physical and emotional stress, childbirth and lactation, the wearing of wigs or hair styles that pull tightly on the hair.

Many drugs, including beta blockers, certain anti-arthritis drugs, blood thinning drugs, and even aspirin can cause or promote hair loss. Large doses of supplemental vitamin A (over 25,000 IU per day) can cause hair loss.

Spot baldness can occur without any known association and at any age. Alopecia areata may be found in persons who are functioning entirely normally, but since alopecia areata has been found in persons who have low functioning of the immune system, it would seem advisable to use some of the immune system boosters and certain herbs known to have

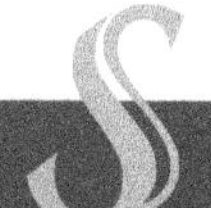

antioxidant and immune stimulant qualities. The principal immune system booster is echinacea. It is often used with a healing herb such as golden seal. Antioxidant herbs such as rosemary and licorice root can also be used. These may be taken as a tea or in pill form (*Southern Medical Journal* 88, no. 4 [April 1995]: 489–491).

It has been shown that the use of aromatherapy is effective in treating spot baldness in men and women. A study was reported in 1998 from the dermatology department of Aberdeen Royal Infirmary in Forest Hill, Scotland, of a trial with aromatherapy. The dermatologists took a group of 86 patients with alopecia areata and put them into two groups in a random fashion. One group was treated by massaging essential oils of thyme, rosemary, lavender, and cedarwood in a mixture of carrier oils (jojoba and grape seed) into their scalp daily. The control group used only carrier oils for their massage, which was also done daily. Measuring the results by photographs by two dermatologists, independently, showed that 44 percent of the patients in the aromatherapy group showed improvement compared with 15 percent of patients using only the carrier oils. The degree of improvement was significant. The researchers concluded that aromatherapy is safe and effective for the treatment of alopecia areata (*Archives of Dermatology* 134, no. 11 [November 1998]: 1349–52).

Rub a halved clove of garlic over bald or thinning areas of the scalp. Repeat at least three times daily. You may leave the garlic juice on the area, or it may be rinsed off if it smells too strong. However, allow the area to dry before rinsing it off. You should notice results in a few weeks if it is going to help (Jude C. Williams, *Jude's Herbal Home Remedies* [St. Paul, MN: Llewellyn Publications, 1996]).

Some have reported benefit from the use of aloe vera, both in spot baldness and falling hair. Rub it on the area of hair loss four to six times a day, and drink one to two ounces of the commercial liquid or gel two to three times daily, 10 minutes before meals.

For some people, nettles tea, four cups daily for two or three months, can make the hair grow thick. It should be used in the form of tea and not as pills.

Eating two tablespoons of flaxseed, freshly ground each day, at two meals can encourage healthy, normal hair growth. The ground flax can be sprinkled on cereal, a salad, or into juice.

Persons with celiac disease, sensitivity to gluten, have been observed to have more baldness in small areas of the scalp. For alopecia areata, one should try a period of abstinence from the gluten grains to see if the baldness is because of a gluten sensitivity (*Gastroenterology* 109, no. 4 [1995]: 1333).

Areas of baldness have been successfully treated by a gluten-free diet, not only in those who have celiac disease, but others who have alopecia can use a gluten-free diet and hopefully expect complete disappearance of the alopecia areata (*Clinical and Experimental Dermatology* 23 [1998]: 230).

Boils

Boils are red, tender, warm, and very painful lumps in the skin. A yellow or white point at the center of the lump develops when the boil is ready to drain or discharge pus. An abscess is also a collection of pus; however, it can occur anywhere in or on the body. A boil often involves a hair follicle.

In a severe infection, multiple boils may develop at one time along with fever and swollen lymph nodes. Those most likely to get boils are individuals who carry staph germs in the nostrils, have diabetes, are obese, are malnourished, or use certain immunosuppressive drugs. Boils are most often found on the back, stomach, underarms, shoulders, face, lips, eyes, nose, thighs, and buttocks, but they may also be found elsewhere.

The treatment for a boil is two-fold. One way is to reduce the boil and dissipate the inflammation. The other is to bring the boil to a head, which always brings tissue death. To dissipate or reduce inflammation, alternate hot and cold applications. To bring the boil to a head, use steady heat applications.

To prevent future boils and to help a present one, begin a plant-based diet, paying special attention to removing sugar and honey from the diet. Be sure and take a daily shower to get rid of germs on the skin. Getting plenty of sunshine will also help kill bacteria. Additionally, herb compresses of yellow dock, charcoal, and hops are helpful.

Contact Dermatitis

This skin rash is an inflammation caused by sensitivity to a substance with which the skin comes in contact. It may be manifested as rashes, hives, cracks, burning, sores, or irritations. A good example is poison ivy, but many plants, wood, fur, silk, wool, dye, resins, plastics, rubber, metal, and many other things can cause contact dermatitis. (See 'Poison Ivy' under "Skin Diseases" in the *Conditions and Diseases* section.)

Corns

Corns and calluses on the feet are thickened layers of skin caused by repeated pressure or friction from shoes. Favorite locations are the side of the fifth toe, top of the second toe, bottom of the foot just behind the toes, and anywhere else the shoes rub the foot.

Treatment can be as simple as filing the thickened area with an emery board or nail file. For calluses on the bottom of the foot, a small carpenter's electric file can be used to good advantage by one with a steady hand and good grip.

Crush a clove of garlic and the white part of a spring onion together. Apply a small amount to the corn, and tape it in place. Replace with a fresh application every day or so.

Dandruff and Seborrheic Dermatitis

Dandruff is often a part of a larger disease called seborrheic dermatitis, which is caused by excessive secretion of the sebaceous or oil producing glands. Symptoms may vary widely from nothing more than dandruff to a full fledged seborrhea in which the whole scalp, eyebrows, nose, crease beside the upper lip and mouth, chin and down the breast bone are covered by greasy crusting scales with red irritation underneath.

The cause is probably sensitivity to something being contacted or to foods. It is often seen in people who are heavy users of animal products, sweets, fats, fried foods, and nut butters. Soap sensitivity or shampoos may play a part in this disorder.

Some suspected causes are genetic predisposition, emotional stress, drugs or other factors that can block vitamin B6 function, including hormones used for replacement therapy, dry skin especially in cold weather, and irritants such as soaps, harsh scrubbing, and drying lotions that contain alcohol and nutrient deficiencies especially of B vitamins, choline, methylamine, inositol, and magnesium.

Treatment

Success depends largely on frequent shampooing, massaging the scalp, and close attention to the natural laws of health. Anxiety and emotional strain often make the condition worse.

Generally it is a good policy to avoid soap, but if soap needs to be used, a good soap to use on the skin is pine tar soap.

Avoid all shampoos containing soaps. Detergents, however, may not cause dandruff. Use a pure detergent concentrate such as Basic-H or L.O.C. (Shaklee or Amway products, respectively; however, do not use their shampoos because they contain soap and fragrance). Many people are cured of dandruff after one or two shampoos during the first week.

An aloe vera shampoo may be very helpful. Scoop out the inner part of the fresh aloe blades, blenderize, and use about one-fourth cup as a shampoo.

Some have found that dish detergent without fragrance, used as a shampoo, is effective in banishing dandruff.

A plain water shampoo used daily or several times weekly can cleanse the scalp adequately and keep the hair in good condition, thus avoiding soap altogether. A bit more water, rubbing, and time may be needed.

We have found it very helpful to use a vinegar rinse following shampooing. At one time this was a very common practice to keep the hair shiny and soft. Simply pour a little vinegar into a cup of water (one to four tablespoons of vinegar), and pour it through the scalp and hair after the shampoo. Towel dry. Pure vinegar may be used if the scalp is not tender.

Some persons have dandruff or seborrhea because of food sensitivity. The Elimination and Challenge diet may be necessary to find the cause of some types of dandruff.

Pour one pint of boiling water over one-half cup of fresh chopped parsley. Let it stand 30 minutes. Massage the tea into the scalp, wrap a towel around the head, and allow it to stay on 15 minutes. You may rinse again if you like, or simply towel dry. This may also be used as a final rinse after shampooing (Jude C. Williams, *Jude's Herbal Home Remedies* [St. Paul, MN: Llewellyn Publications, 1996]).

Taking supplements with omega-3 fatty acids, and a multi-vitamin and mineral supplement including 400 micrograms of folic acid and B12 each, and 50 to 100 milligrams of vitamin B6 may help. Zinc, magnesium, and flaxseed oil are also helpful.

Overweight persons tend to have seborrheic dermatitis more frequently than lean persons. Losing weight may be curative in many individuals.

Eczema

Three types of eczema deserve special mention—allergic dermatitis, infantile eczema, and sensitivity eczema such as dishpan hands.

Eczema is a non-contagious skin rash with a number of possible causes such as a change in the weather, temperature, the intensity of light, foods, clothing fabric, chemicals, animal dander, cosmetics, etc. There is a familial likelihood of

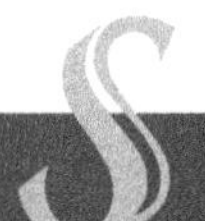

developing the disease, and some people are apparently born with sensitized skin. Any material that touches the skin could cause eczema. The appearance of skin lesions on the scalp may differ greatly from eczema on the face or groin.

Eczema may occur from the age of infancy to old age. Infantile eczema is a manifestation of allergy. Symptoms include redness of the skin, weeping, oozing, crusting, dryness, cracking fissures, scaling, thickening, and sometimes intense itching. Small blister-like bumps may occur at the edges or in the beginning stages.

Babies may develop a red, itching rash that may involve only the cheeks, or may spread to the entire body. This disorder begins about the age of two months, and usually lasts until the child is about two years of age. It is much more likely to occur in non-breast fed babies or in families having a history of allergies. These children are more likely to develop asthma or hay fever in the future.

Treatment

Begin any treatment routine for eczema with an Elimination and Challenge diet. Breastfed babies have much less eczema, but even they may become sensitive to the foods eaten by the mother. The most common problem foods are eggs, milk, and soybeans, but any foods may be involved. It may be difficult to identify the particular food that is responsible for the eczema, but a very careful Elimination and Challenge diet must be performed on the mother, watching for signs of clearing in the infant. (See "Elimination and Challenge Diet" in the *Dietary Information* section.)

Reducing the salt or sugar intake can be of great help to individuals with allergic dermatitis or atopic dermatitis. Some improvement in itching usually occurs after three to four days of salt restriction, but the major improvement occurs after about three or four weeks (*Lancet* 344 [November 26, 1994]: 1516).

Many drugs cause eczema, and even if they are not the cause, they may prolong or worsen eczema. Try to test all medications, nutrient supplements, and herbal remedies as some may be involved in the eczema.

Common inhalant allergens such as house dust, pollens, animal danders, smoke fumes, etc., can all cause a problem.

Avoid the use of chlorinated water for bathing, drinking, or cooking. Use bottled water, distilled water, purified water, or water to which a tablespoon of charcoal is added to a gallon of water and allowed to settle.

Do not use soaps, bubble bath, or bath oil for infants, bearing in mind that nothing is on the baby's skin that will not be removed by plain water.

The application of oils such as evening primrose oil, olive oil, or a mixture of olive oil and lime water shaken together may be used as lubricants or as healing agents. Plain castor oil has been used on eczematoid rashes (scaling, cracking, and reddening of skin) with good success by some patients. Apply two or three times a day in covered areas but after every hand washing for eczema on hands. Evening primrose oil applied to the inflamed skin after a soothing bath can be very effective. It may also be taken internally as it is a rich source of gamma-linolenic acid, an essential fatty acid, a precursor of certain prostaglandins.

The most effective treatment we have found for the hands is Vaseline milk. Vaseline milk has helped many to heal. While the hands are still wet from washing or from the bath, a lump of petroleum jelly is taken between the palms and rubbed vigorously to mix with water still on the hands. For a child also still wet from the bath, the milky fluid developed from rubbing petroleum jelly vigorously must then be gently smoothed over the skin of the child, the motion of the smoothing being in the same direction as the lines of the skin. If the direction is across the skin lines, it will tend to break open the eczema and make microscopic cracks that can be more easily irritated by a sensitizing agent. Only a thin coating is required.

A wonder formula for eczema consists of four parts soybean or similar oil, one part cocoa butter, one part strong comfrey root tea, and one part aloe vera gel (99 percent pure, bottled kind). Melt the cocoa butter and combine the ingredients. Unrefrigerated in warm climates it will keep about three days, in the refrigerator, about a week. It will separate and must be stirred or shaken. It is gooey, but it works well. Use in the evening before bed, and cover the area with a towel, cotton glove, or sock, or whatever is appropriate for the area, until the mixture is absorbed into the skin.

Aloe vera gel, red clover, golden seal tea, comfrey tea, or witch hazel tea may all be applied to inflamed areas to prevent itching or promote healing. Red clover and golden seal tea may be used as cold compresses for their astringent action.

For eczema that covers most of the body, take daily baths in hot water (about 110°F) for three minutes. The method is to submerge oneself for three minutes in the water, step out of the bath water and fan the skin for one minute, then re-submerge oneself and step out three additional times for a total of twelve minutes. If the eczema is located only on the hands, a similar treatment of hot and cold hand baths could be applied to the hands as a trial to see if it helps (*Journal of Medicine* 25 [1994]: 333).

Charcoal tub baths, putting one-half cup of powdered charcoal in a small tub of lukewarm water, and submerging oneself for 30 minutes twice daily may offer relief. Finish with a tepid rinse to remove much of the charcoal and pat dry. Some residue will remain on the skin. While this treatment is being used, clothing may be stained.

Various other baths are helpful, including sun baths (start with 20 minutes sun exposure each side per day, building up by five minutes daily) and oatmeal baths. (For information about these baths, see the *Natural Remedies* section.) An alkali such as baking soda can also be added to the bath water. If the climate permits, one can then dress without drying to allow the alkaline water to moisten the clothing a bit. For some, vinegar (acid) baths are best, for some the alkaline bath. A starch bath may be effective to relieve itching and weeping in the wet lesions and often also in dry.

It is important to prevent bacterial growth or yeast infections in the skin lesions. This may be done by frequent bathing in warm water to which one-half cup of vinegar has been added to a baby's bathtub of water, and equivalent quantities for adult eczema. If showers are preferred, pour a quart of water over the skin after the shower to which has been added four tablespoons of vinegar.

Avoid overexposure to water if the eczema is dry, but weeping eczema can be dried by the use of wet dressings or frequent warm baths, every one to three hours. The old motto "If it is dry, wet it; and if it is wet, dry it," applies very nicely to eczema. Oil should be applied to dry lesions.

Flare-ups can often be stopped by using a fever treatment.

Cotton or silk clothing should be worn next to the skin, and synthetic fabrics should be avoided. Wool or suede can be irritating. Dyed clothing may cause eczema, and all new clothing should be washed thoroughly and rinsed an additional cycle before touching the person struggling with eczema, particularly a child. Bed linens should be soft and laundered without detergents.

One of the most important things is to avoid scratching. While scratching does not cause the disease, it certainly keeps it going. For children, they must wear gloves covered by mittens or socks, especially at night to prevent scratching the lesions during sleep. Trim the fingernails right down to the quick to avoid daytime scratching. Rubbing across the skin lines must be avoided, and the application of any kind of medication must be done in the same direction as the skin lines to avoid opening them up and causing microscopic cracks.

Keep the skin temperature warm at all times, as chilled skin does not heal readily.

If all else fails to control itching, a brief hot bath or shower lasting two to four minutes will almost always control itching for several hours.

A diet high in omega-3 essential fatty acids such as flaxseed, walnuts, etc., is very helpful in treating eczema. Stress is a major factor in some promoting eczema. Ginkgo, licorice, dandelion root, and various local applications of soothing lotions containing camomile, witch hazel, or zinc oxide can reduce inflammation and itching.

Case Reports

We had a patient who came to Uchee Pines Institute with severe eczema, which he had had most of his life. He was a nineteen-year-old black man who had just graduated from high school, but because of his eczema, which caused an unsightly whitish flaking of the skin, he withdrew from social contact and remained indoors with the plan never to leave the house again. He was a heavy user of dairy products and was not very careful with his diet. He was also overweight. After coming to the institute, we modified his diet and prescribed warm charcoal baths by putting one-half to one cup of charcoal powder in a tub of lukewarm water. He soaked in this once or twice daily for an hour or two, finishing with a tepid shower (no soap!). Within three weeks, his eczema had cleared completely for the first time since he was two years old. He has remained symptom free since then. Both diet and the baths were healing for him.

We also had a young fourteen-year-old patient with a severe swollen, red, scaling eczema on her left nipple and the surrounding pigmented area measuring approximately three inches in diameter. She had had the eczema for more than two years and had gone to three different dermatologists and had faithfully taken every medicine that had been recommended. The eczema was as bad or worse than when she saw the first dermatologist. We prescribed for her bee propolis dissolved in Eucerin Creme; as much as she could dissolve and still have it creamy so that she could easily rub it on. This was to be applied two or three times daily. She was instructed never to scratch the area, not even through her clothing. Additionally she underwent an Elimination and Challenge diet that was salt restricted and fat restricted. She was prescribed a totally plant-based diet with an emphasis on fruits and vegetables except for those restricted in the Elimination and Challenge diet. Within a month her eczema was markedly improved, and by six weeks she had no rash left.

Acrodermatitis Enteropathica

This rare kind of eczema-like disorder has symptoms of dermatitis, diarrhea, and loss of hair. The symptoms do not appear in breastfed babies, but they generally appear within non-breastfed babies within the first 4 to 10 weeks of life or within a week or so of the introduction of cow's milk.

It has been discovered that impaired zinc absorption is probably the underlying problem. Aspirin, calcium supplements, soymilk protein, and cow's milk interfere with the absorption of zinc, and should be avoided. The mother should make a herculean effort to re-establish breastfeeding, even if it has been several weeks since the baby was weaned. Herbs to encourage breastfeeding are blessed thistle, milk thistle, and red raspberry leaf. They may be used singly or mixed. Use one heaping teaspoon of each of the herbs to one cup of boiling water. These should be used as teas rather than as capsules or tablets. Take three to four cups per day for six weeks or more. Exercise and sweating promote milk production.

A daily dose of zinc of around 15 milligrams can be given to infants. The zinc supplements dramatically reverses the symptoms. A behavioral change is usually the first sign of improvement. The infant is less irritable, less anxious to be held, and a better sleeper within one or two days. The skin clears and the appetite returns and diarrhea stops within a few days. The dosage can be reduced to 5 to 10 milligrams daily for about one month as soon as symptoms begin to improve. You may be able to get a zinc liquid from a drug store, but, if not, you can make up your own liquid using a 50 milligrams tablet or capsule dissolved in one tablespoon of warm water. Give the baby one teaspoon of the liquid each day, which will contain 15 milligrams per teaspoon.

The breastfeeding mother should follow a diet high in legumes and whole grain products, which are high in zinc. Many types of greens, popcorn, and pumpkin seeds also have large quantities of zinc. Dandelion tea and dandelion greens added to other greens, or to salads, can be very helpful in the mother's diet.

Feet, Cracked and Peeling

The heels often become cracked and peel excessively, usually because of a superficial fungus infection of the skin. Spread a thin layer of Murphy's Oil Soap, rubbing it in as a lotion. In a short time the skin usually becomes soft.

Use a vinegar, calendula, and myrrh solution (see "Lotion" in the *Herbal Remedies* section). Moisten the skin twice a day for about six months, and the skin will usually become smooth. For resistant cases, a year may be required to heal the condition.

Vitamin E oil can be used on thickened, cracked heels to soften and heal them.

Natural fibers, especially cotton, were once thought to be the best material for absorbing moisture, but now it is recognized that a mixture of synthetic and natural fibers for socks makes them much more absorbent and better at keeping the feet dry. If feet or hands are especially damp try soaking them in a pan of tannic acid solution for 30 to 45 minutes prepared by steeping four to six tea bags (grocery store type such as pekoe or green tea) in a quart of boiling water for 30 minutes (*Physician and Sports Medicine* 24, no. 8 [1996]: 91).

Fungus Diseases, Fungus Nails, Athlete's Foot, Ringworm, Tinea

Fungus Nails

If a dark streak on the nail that looks somewhat like a splinter under the nail develops, immediate action should be taken. If such a streak occurs, scrape the dark discoloration off the nail entirely with a sharp blade such as a knife or scissors. If you can scrape all the discolored area off, you will have gotten rid of the fungus, as it is in the discolored area. If allowed to spread, it permanently ruins the entire nail, causing it to become thickened, deformed, dead, and separated from the nail bed.

To prevent fungus nails, keep the nails trimmed short, do not wear tight stockings, socks, or shoes, or allow bed covers at night to fit tightly over the toes so that blood is pressed from the nail bed. Pressing out the blood weakens the resistance of the nail against fungus.

It is more difficult to eradicate fungus from the fingernail than from the toenail. You must be both diligent and persistent. Nail fungi are related to athlete's foot, and often caused by the same fungus. Avoid the use of oral medications for fungus nails, as they are all powerful and toxic, resulting in potential injury to the body. As soon as the medication is discontinued, there is a high recurrence rate for the fungus nail. Little is accomplished of permanent good, and a risk to the future health is taken by administering the medications.

Treatment for Fungus Nails and Athlete's Foot

Trim the nails as closely as possible, and scrape what is left as thin as possible. If a crumbly material collects under the nail, trim off all the nail, lift it up off the nail bed, and remove the corners, if possible, where they are embedded in the cuticles.

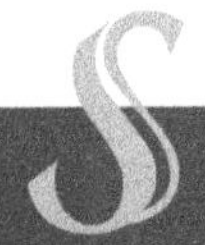

Do not allow pressure on the toenails from socks or shoes, as that presses the blood out of the nail and makes the nails more susceptible to fungus growth.

Make a vinegar extract of myrrh and calendula. (See "Lotion" in the *Herbal Remedies* section.) While it is being made, apply vinegar to the toenails four times a day for 21 days. Then start once or twice a day with the herb extract. For fingernail fungus, take a portion of the batch you make and add an equal quantity of DMSO (obtain from a feed store), and apply 6 to 20 times a day, after each hand washing, and while sitting around in meetings.

Black walnut tincture has been used by some to treat toenail fungus. Black walnut has one disadvantage in that it turns the skin purple or brown. We have not found it successful in all cases of toenail fungus, but it may be tried.

Tea tree oil has been successful in early cases of fungus nail. Apply it twice daily until the part infected with the fungus grows completely out and is no longer visible.

One part Citricidal (concentrated grapefruit seed extract), and one part DMSO (dimethyl sulfoxide) can be mixed together. Then apply a small drop to each affected nail four to eight times a day and after each hand washing. Be certain to moisten the cuticles as well. The medicine will discolor the nails, but they eventually grow out smooth, not cracked or chipped, and of normal color.

One patient reported that he got very good results for fungus fingernails by boiling down one cup of bottled concentrated lemon juice to four ounces, to which he added one teaspoon of myrrh gum. Dab the concentrate on the fungus fingernails six times a day, and after each hand washing. Avoid prolonged contact with water, especially with water to which soaps or detergents have been added. He reported several fingernails healed with this recipe.

Ringworm, Tinea

A ring-shaped infection, ringworm is the commonest of superficial fungus diseases, also found in dogs, cats, and other domestic animals, and spread by contact with infected sources. The skin generally carries several species of inactive fungi that can be aroused by conditions favorable to their growth, such as excessive perspiration, heat, moisture, lowered general resistance, or friction. The fungi may attack hair follicles of the scalp, beard, or elsewhere; nonhairy skin surfaces or nails. The infections are unsightly and uncomfortable. Ringworm usually starts with small red, slightly raised, round or oval sores that gradually enlarge and become redder. Blisters may follow, with some itching and burning, and healing toward the center. Some ringworm infections are highly contagious, such as ringworm of the scalp. The hair loses luster and becomes brittle and breaks. The scalp becomes covered with grayish scaly patches and short stumps of diseased hair. Temporary baldness may occur.

This superficial fungus infection can be treated in essentially the same way athlete's foot is treated, with vinegar or herbal treatments. Simply smear the affected area with vinegar four to six times a day or, if located on the back or groin, twice a day for 30 to 60 days. It will usually disappear in that time.

Since a variety of fungi may be involved, no one treatment can be said to be effective in all cases. Try one type of treatment and then another if the first is not effective.

Treatment

Wash the area or shampoo the hair daily with pine tar soap. Cut the hair short.

Rub a small amount of vinegar on the area four to six times daily, keeping the skin clean and dry between times. Usually only 30 to 60 days are required to clear up the fungus infection.

For very resistant cases use a vinegar extract tincture of calendula and myrrh. (See "Lotion" in the *Herbal Remedies* section.)

Garlic, freshly cut and applied in thin sections held on with tape, has healed the infection in as short a time as 10 days. The garlic may also be blenderized with a little water and applied as a soak, compress, or poultice.

Castor oil, strong golden seal tea, and borax have all brought healing in certain cases.

Ingrown Toenails

This is a painful condition in which the nail grows so that it cuts into one or both sides of the nail bed. While ingrown nails can occur in both the nails of the hand and feet, they occur most commonly with the toenails.

The condition can be brought on by injury or fungus infection of the nail or surrounding skin. It may be caused by the way people walk, by wearing tight shoes, or by improper trimming or neglect to trim the toenails. Sometimes after trimming the nails a sharp spicule of nail breaks off and is left behind that acts as a tiny sword stabbing through the skin and leading to infection.

To treat an ingrown toenail, thoroughly wash and dry the foot. Then put a little wisp of cotton up under the edge of the nail to lift the nail away from the skin. An even more effective alternative to the cotton is a tiny bit of folded un-waxed dental floss. It is more manageable than cotton and equally effective. It can be wedged under the nail with greater ease since the ends can be grasped easier with the two hands. Then trim the ends short to lessen the possibility of accidentally removing it.

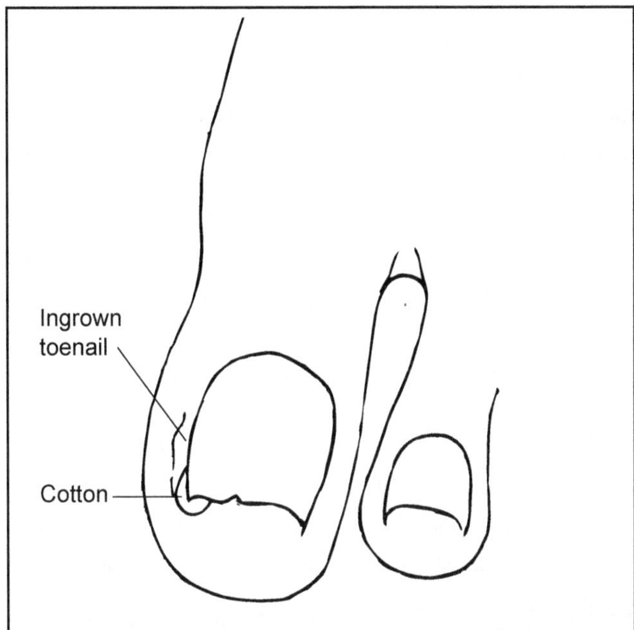

If the nail is surrounded by a swollen and oozing zone, you should soak it in hot water for 30 minutes twice a day. Wait until enough swelling has subsided so you can grasp the edge before putting the cotton or dental floss under the nail edge. Alternating hot and cold footbaths, or hot baths alone, can be used to heal an infected ingrown toenail. When the toe is swollen, red, and tender, the hot footbath can relieve pain and congestion.

A callous formed by an ingrown toenail can be treated by placing a tiny bit of salicylic acid on the area, blocking it from spreading to the normal skin by carefully applying some kind of waterproof tape before applying the acid. When the callous is soft enough, it can be carefully lifted off. This will relieve pressure and abolish the inflammation. When the ingrown toenail becomes infected, a portion of the nail that has become ingrown needs to be removed. Sometimes professional help is required to accomplish this removal.

Itching

Itching is caused by an irritation of the fine terminations of the sensory nerves in the skin. Itching is carried over the same nerve pathways as pain. It occurs in many different diseases and may erupt from sensitivity to certain foods, drugs, chemicals, fabric, dust, lice, scabies, sensitivity to animals, fungus infection, diabetes, gout, jaundice, and nervous disorders. Another cause is a lack of moisture in the skin from failure to drink enough water or the need to apply a lubricating lotion on the skin.

To control itching, the cause must be ascertained and eliminated if possible. Suggestions are applicable also for itchiness of the perineum of women.

Investigate whether chronic or recurring itching is caused by a food allergy (see "Elimination and Challenge Diet" in the *Dietary Information* section) or an environmental thing that may contact the skin.

Keep the skin as moist as possible by drinking lots of water.

Take a tepid starch bath for 10 to 90 minutes (30 minutes is the usual time) using a high starch substance such as oatmeal ground in a blender or cornstarch added to the water. One cup of dry rolled oats can be ground to a powder in the blender on low speed. Put this into a sock and tie the top of the sock. Wet the sock in the bath water by holding it under the faucet and rub or pat the itchy skin with the oatmeal-filled sock.

A hot bath for 20 minutes, keeping the head cool once sweating begins, can also be curative for itching, especially from chigger bites, giving as much as eight hours of relief. This is very good for itching that requires large parts of the body to be treated. Several tablespoons of cornstarch can be added to the bath water and dipped onto the skin. After finishing the bath with any of these high starch or baking soda substances, do not dry the skin but pat yourself dry with the hands and get dressed.

One patient reported instant relief of "bottom itch" from making a powder from rolled oats in a seed mill or blender. She mixed the powder with water to make a paste. She spread this on the anus and perineum for itchiness and erosions. The patient reported that relief came immediately with the application of the paste. It would certainly be worth a try. (See also "Pruritus Ani" in the *Conditions and Diseases* section.)

One cup of baking soda to about three inches of water in a bathtub can be very helpful. This is called an alkaline bath.

For unexplained itching of any type, try rubbing one of the following into the itching area: vitamin E cream, cocoa butter lotion, or safflower oil with vitamin E mixed in. You may also use a mixture made of equal parts of sesame oil and mineral oil into which has been stirred two ounces per pint of basil leaves from the kitchen. Heat these together in boiling water in a double boiler for one to two hours. Strain. Cool and store in a bottle.

Apply a light coat of baby oil, chamomile lotion, aloe vera gel, vitamin E or castor oil, almond, olive, coconut, lecithin, mineral oil, or petroleum jelly. These are all very good

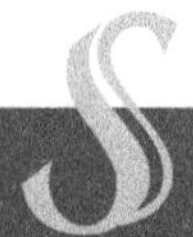

for itching associated with a dry rash. The use of lubricating ointments or lotions following showers or baths, particularly hot baths, will cure a large percentage of "winter itch."

Avoid soaps and any other practice that will dry the skin or cause skin sensitivity.

A brisk rubdown with a coarse dry towel after a cool shower on areas most likely to be dry such as arms, legs, and upper back will stimulate the skin to produce more oils. Do not use this rubbing for eczema as skin lines may open or crack.

Wet the fingers in water; then dip them in salt and rub the affected areas with the salt that clings to the fingers. After the skin dries, brush off the extra salt. There may be a bit of burning at first, but a cool sensation and relief of itching usually follows.

Ice also calms an itch. Rub the itching area with an ice cube. When the itching starts up again, rub with another ice cube. If ice is not available, wet a paper towel in cold water and lay it over the itching area. Ice rubbed over the itchy area or immersion of itching feet or legs into buckets of ice water can bring relief.

Wet dressings may be applied by using old sheets cut into appropriate sizes and squeezed from cool water and laid over the itchy area for 10 to 15 minutes, allowing the cloths to air dry. A mild unscented lotion may then be applied.

Some kind of acid solution such as lemon juice or vinegar diluted one to four with water may bring relief to itching areas.

Hot compresses laid over the itching skin will bring relief in seconds. Witch hazel and cool compresses may also be used to stop itching. Follow these compresses with some kind of moisturizing lotion or oil.

Keep the fingernails short. If you accidentally scratch, as during sleep, at least you will not scratch deeply. It may also become obvious that mittens need to be worn at night to minimize scratching while sleeping.

Mix or blend 10 drops of an essential oil such as Melaleuca, mint, lavender, or nard with three to four ounces of commercial aloe vera gel or the pulp from a blade of aloe vera. Put the mixture in a washed hair spray bottle and spray the involved skin. Shake well before each use.

For nonspecific itching or for itching from insect bites or poison ivy, try spreading toothpaste, not gel, on the itching area.

When jaundice produces itching it can be relieved by giving guar gum or charcoal by mouth. Use a heaping teaspoon four times a day (*European Journal of Clinical Investigation* 28, no. 5 [May 1998]: 359–63).

(See also 'Eczema' and 'Scabies' in the "Skin Diseases" entry and "Itching" in the *Conditions and Diseases* section.)

Keloids

Keloids are exaggerated scars, raised, shiny, and dome-shaped, colored from pink to red. Some keloids become quite large and unsightly. Aside from causing cosmetic problems, these scars tend to be itchy, tender, develop bleeding points, and become painful to the touch. They may start as the healing process begins or start some time after the injury and extend beyond the wound site. Their cause is unknown, but there is a greater tendency to develop keloids in persons who are not vegetarians and those who use a high fat, high sugar diet.

The most effective treatment is prevention, as the only definitive treatment once they occur is surgical excision, which may itself result in a second keloid. It is rare that a keloid will spontaneously regress, but it occasionally does, leaving a depressed scar. It is always well worth a trial to give echinacea, Pau d'Arco, blue violet, and chaparral tea by mouth, at the same time one applies hot compresses for a series of 30 daily sessions, 20 minutes each session. The tea is made by putting a heaping tablespoonful of echinacea, Pau d'Arco, and chaparral in one quart of water and boiling gently for 30 minutes. Set it off the fire and add two tablespoons of blue violet. Steep for 30 minutes. Strain and drink the quart over a one-day period. Make it fresh every morning.

Try to prevent keloids with the following routine. After surgery or an injury, the keloid-prone person should immediately switch to a plant-based diet, if not already on one, using no meat, milk, eggs, or cheese. All free fats such as margarine, mayonnaise, fried foods, cooking fats, salad oils, and nut butters should be removed entirely from the diet. Take no free sugars. Avoid ginger, cinnamon, nutmeg, cloves, black and red pepper, vinegar in any foods, including sauces and breads, all fermented foods such as the fermented type of soy sauce or sauerkraut, and alcohol, tobacco, and all prescription or other drugs. Use simple meals comprised of one type of grain such as rice or bread, and two simple dishes such as baked potatoes and green beans. With a simple salad, the meal is complete. These simple vegetarian meals should be maintained for a full month after surgery, and perhaps three months.

Do not overeat. Get plenty of outdoor exercise every day for a month.

You can try to prevent their coming by rubbing the juice of fresh aloe on the scar four times a day for two months.

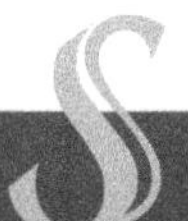

Hot and cold compresses—three minutes hot and 30 seconds cold—should begin on the fifth postoperative day and be maintained until 21 days after surgery.

Keratosis or Solar Keratosis

A keratosis is a roughened and thickened area of skin usually present on parts of the skin that have been exposed to the sun in the past. They are sometimes pigmented from tan to dark brown.

To treat these areas, omit free fats from the diet for a period of months.

You can also rub the area each night with coconut, olive, or tea tree oil to soften the lesions. This will often make them fall off.

Ice the keratosis nightly by rubbing it with an ice cube for five minutes for 28 days. This will sometimes remove a small keratosis. However, treatment by a dermatologist may be required to remove the lesions.

Use raw carrot and raw broccoli put through a heavy duty food processor, juicer, or blenderized with some water or vegetable juice, enough food to make one cup. Take this cupful with leaf lettuce five or six times or more each week as a salad at lunchtime. Some have reported that senile keratoses and spots suspicious of cancer can disappear within three months on this regimen. At the same time eliminate all free fats from the diet, and the skin can heal itself more efficiently.

Apply a cream to the skin every night made by mixing a bit of your hand lotion with 4 to 10 drops of castor oil and about a teaspoon of vinegar. Apply the vinegar first. Next, mix the lotion and the castor oil by rubbing vigorously between the palms, then smooth gently onto the skin. Every morning wash the area with warm water, rubbing the skin with the fingers. Once a week scrub the area gently with a luffa sponge or nylon scrubby from the kitchen. The vinegar softens the scales and allows the removal of the lesion.

Also in the morning, moisten all the scaly patches with vinegar and let it dry. Vinegar assists in the removal of scales.

Other applications that can be used include castor oil, tea tree oil, vitamin E oil, vinegar, or some of the commercial products available from drug stores for warts. Vinegar and any mild acid acts as a softening agent for keratin. After a few days of applying the acid, soak the keratosis in water and remove the crusts.

Avoid being in the sun without a large hat or other protection against the sun's rays.

Lichen Planus

Lichen planus is a recurring, itchy, and inflamed patch occurring most frequently on the arms below the elbows, but it may be on the legs and arms, trunk, or inside the mouth. The lesions often have a faint purplish color and sheen on cross-lighting. They tend to be symmetrical and are of unknown cause. If it gives no symptoms, no treatment is needed.

We recommend for lichen planus that you determine whether a food sensitivity is the cause of the problem. During a trial period of eliminating foods, the skin lesions should disappear if your lichen planus is related to a food sensitivity. When the skin lesions have disappeared, you should then begin adding back foods, one group every two weeks until each group has been added back that you wish to have. There are some groups it may be best to leave out permanently for the sake of your general health, even if they are not involved in lichen planus.

During the first six weeks, take a heaping tablespoon of activated charcoal in a large glass of water four times daily. Take a short cold bath daily four days a week, and a hot bath once a week, bringing the mouth temperature up to 101°F while keeping the head cool. Obey all health laws to the letter. Get to bed at least two hours before midnight, and preferably three.

Licorice root tea is also a good treatment. Use one rounded tablespoon of the powder to a quart of water, simmer gently for 15 minutes, without straining, drink one cup four times a day. Watch for sodium and water retention with some degree of swelling of fingers and feet to let you know you have taken enough and should discontinue the herb.

Melanoma

(See "Cancer" in the *Conditions and Diseases* section.)

Nails, Split fingernails

A principal cause of split fingernails is water, or more specifically alternating periods of wetness and excessive dryness. Persons whose nails split easily should wear cotton lined rubber gloves when washing dishes or cleaning with water. Immediately after exposure to water, apply a moisturizing lotion.

Keep the nails clipped short to prevent breakage. File in only one direction, not back and forth, which can also create splits. Don't overuse nail polish removers, especially the acetone ones as they leave the nails dry and brittle. Look for nail polish removers that contain acetate instead. Calcium, gelatin, or vitamins will not improve the nails.

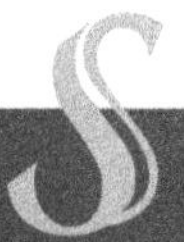

Another cause of splitting nails is a superficial fungus infection. For this, use the fungus fighter for nails given earlier in this section on skin disorders. (see 'Fungus Diseases, Fungus Nails' in the "Skin Diseases" entry.)

Poison Ivy, Poison Oak

Treatment is the same for these plants and all other poisonous plants causing a dermatitis.

If you are exposed to poison ivy or any other skin irritant from plants such as nettles, look around where the plant grows and you will find a plant growing such as mint, plantain, or any broad leaf or juicy plant (not grasses and not usually tree leaves). Crush the leaves and rub the skin where the ivy came in contact with your skin. Rub only the exposed area, as you must not spread the irritating oil from the poison ivy plant. Often within a few minutes the stinging will stop, and in the case of poison ivy a rash will not develop when the first contact is treated this way. Then, as soon as possible, wash any area exposed to poison ivy with soap and water to remove any residual irritating oil from the poison ivy plant, which is the cause of the rash.

Poison ivy and poison oak can be treated with Basic-H rubbed all over the exposed area. Some have felt they were protected from getting the contact dermatitis of poison ivy by spreading pure detergent concentrate such as Basic-H or L.O.C.over the skin before taking a walk in an area where poison ivy is known to grow. These detergent concentrates can be obtained from a marketing company in your area.

Mix powdered golden seal and honey to make a poultice. Others have used petroleum jelly and flowers of sulphur or petroleum jelly and golden seal powder, but these mixtures can stain clothing. Usually within a couple of days the rash will completely clear up with this treatment. Mix equal quantities of honey and golden seal powder, spread it on the rash, and cover it with a gauze bandage. Change the dressing daily.

A paste made from powdered golden seal root with water is both soothing and healing.

Burdock, a relative of the sunflower, has large leaves. These leaves provide one of the simplest poison ivy cures. Simply vigorously rub a leaf over the affected area and the itch will subside in minutes. Apply many times daily for rapid healing of the rash of any poisonous plant.

Comfrey root can be crushed and simmered in a little water (two tablespoons of the fresh root to one cup of water) for about five minutes. You can then use the water as a wet dressing or the lightly boiled roots as a soft poultice on poison ivy or bee stings. You may also crush jewelweed and rub it on poison ivy. Any part of the plant can be used. It is one of the best treatments for poison ivy.

Milkweed stems broken or crushed into cold water provides an excellent remedy for poison ivy. Strain off the cold water and spread some of the whitish water on the lesions.

Mint leaf tea, made by steeping a large handful of fresh mint leaves in a pint of water for 15 to 30 minutes, can be spread several times daily over the poison ivy affected skin.

Thistle root is good for poison ivy. Take a handful of fresh roots and place in about a pint of gently simmering water. Simmer for 25 minutes, strain the liquid, and then use the root directly on the poison ivy or insect stings.

Other remedies include acorn tea, chicory tea, hemlock bark, spicebush root, sweet fern tea, and yucca roots.

For the skin rash of poison ivy, take the thin membrane from between two onion layers and lay that on the skin rash. If the thin membrane cannot be obtained, take a very thin slice of onion and place it on the rash.

Hot compresses or a hot shower or bath can stop the itching. It also tends to promote healing. Although it may appear that it tends to spread the number of blisters in some people, it will minimize the length of time one must spend in treating the blisters. If itching becomes intense and intolerable, running hot water over the area will stop an itch for several hours after the first minute of intense burning.

Aloe vera is healing for poison ivy, as are charcoal compresses.

Wet dressings or cool water soaks are comforting and may prevent secondary infections. The wet compresses should be changed every 8 to 10 minutes for an hour, and repeated on alternating hours, an hour on and an hour off. This helps with intense itching.

Some have spread lemon juice over the rash several times daily, or wet salt, vinegar, or moistened baking soda. Good results come from any of these treatments.

Blended oatmeal mixed with a little water and spread over the rash as a paste can be soothing.

The white portion of a banana peel rubbed directly on the rash can bring relief for as long as four hours.

Commercial poison ivy preparations can easily be substituted by using these natural methods for relief.

Psoriasis

This is a chronic inflammatory skin condition, one of the 10 most frequent skin ailments. It affects both men and women, usually after the age of 15. It is non-infectious, of unknown cause, and tends to run in families. There may be difficulty in digesting fats. Fungus growth in the skin lesions

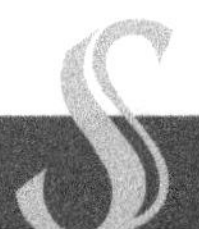

may produce a part of the symptoms. The first sign may be an eruption of pinhead size, bright red spots that group together to form larger ones becoming covered by silvery, white scales. If the scales are removed, tiny bleeding points are seen beneath. Itching is not a usual feature, and the general health is usually not affected. There is, however, an associated complication that occurs in some: psoriatic arthritis. This arthritis is of the rheumatoid type and can be disabling.

Most frequent sites for the lesions are elbows, knees, backs of the arms and legs, scalp, and sometimes the chest and abdomen. Fingernails, toenails, palms, and soles may be affected. Areas most likely to receive trauma or pressure will often be affected.

A plant-based diet is the most favorable diet for treating psoriasis. Free fats should be avoided—margarine, butter, mayonnaise, fried foods, cooking fats, salad oils, and nut butters. Use foods that are low in tryptophan. Plant-based foods high in tryptophan include baked potatoes, bananas, seeds, beans, peanuts, hummus, lentils, etc. Avoid free sugars, including honey.

A study on patients with psoriasis revealed that patients who consumed large amounts of fresh fruit, fresh tomatoes, and carrots were less likely to develop psoriasis. The study also revealed that overweight people are at increased risk of psoriasis (*British Journal of Dermatology* 134 [1996]: 101–06).

Prevention of skin dryness with high humidity environments and the application of skin lubricants following bathing promotes healing.

Avoid emotional stress and anxiety. Get daily out-of-doors exercise to control stress.

Olive oil massaged into the scalp, followed by a hot towel compress for 30 minutes, should be used before shampooing the hair. Do not rub the scalp vigorously during shampooing, and always avoid scratching the scalp. Trauma worsens psoriasis.

Avoid sun burning as this is trauma to the skin and can make psoriasis worse.

Petroleum jelly applied to dry scaly areas can keep the scales softened. Crush calcium tablets and mix with petroleum jelly and apply to the affected areas.

The use of grapefruit seed extract has been helpful on the skin lesions in some cases. Apply two to four times daily.

Arachidonic acid applications by a poultice with air excluded for 24 to 48 hours five to seven times brought complete clearing of psoriasis in some cases. The acid can be obtained through a drug store or health food store. Also, taking 12 grams (one tablespoon) of eicosapentaenoic acid for six weeks resulted in modest improvement of psoriasis in one reported case.

Spread Murphy's Oil Soap on the affected areas one or two times a day. It will often work well for several weeks or months, and then, as with other remedies for psoriasis, it might be necessary to switch to another remedy for a while. After a few weeks it may be helpful again.

Various baths such as seawater bathing, starch baths, and herbal tea baths (golden seal, echinacea, comfrey), and the addition of one cup of vinegar to any hot bath, can be very helpful. For extensive body involvement, add half a cup of 32 percent food-grade hydrogen peroxide to a tub of water and soak for 30 minutes daily. Be seated in the water before adding the peroxide.

We offered a young man some clay poultices for a very bad psoriasis flare-up on his arm. It disappeared almost overnight.

Celery seed, gotu kola, sarsaparilla or parsley may be used as a tea taken internally, or applied externally. Try making a tea of parsley, soaking a cloth in the tea and applying it to the area. Let the cloth dry. This should be done daily for 30 days.

Coleus forskohlii contains a nutrient compound called forskolin, which possesses a number of properties. It may be used in eczema, psoriasis, and angina (*The American Journal of Natural Medicine* 1 [1994]: 10).

Make a vinegar extract of calendula and myrrh, one ounce of each, in half a cup or more of vinegar. Also place two tablespoonfuls of golden seal powder in the vinegar. Swirl from time to time. You may use the vinegar as a lotion to wet each lesion four times daily.

Apply garlic oil during a flare-up, in addition to taking one teaspoon per day of raw sesame oil along with three cups of cranberry juice.

Hot pepper ointment may be very helpful for psoriasis. A cream may be purchased from the pharmacy, or you can make your own extract by putting a teaspoon of red pepper powder from the grocery store into a jar with one cup of rubbing alcohol. Put a label on the jar with tape, making a notation that this is a poison so that it will not be mistakenly placed in the kitchen. Rub the areas of psoriasis with the alcohol that has soaked with the red pepper. It should be applied two to four times daily with a cotton-tipped applicator.

Other topical treatments include vitamin A oil, aloe vera gel, or strong comfrey tea rubbed on the lesions every night.

Use Australian tea tree oil, 20 to 40 drops in an ounce of olive oil. Massage into lesions twice a day. If too strong, decrease the amount of tea tree oil.

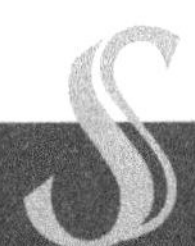

Use milk thistle by mouth to enhance the function of the liver and immune system to help fight the psoriasis.

Toxins derived from the bowel can be a factor in psoriasis. A three- or five-day intestinal cleanse may be helpful in treating psoriasis. The diet in psoriasis should be high in natural vitamins and minerals, and there should be a supplement of one tablespoon of flaxseed oil daily (*American Journal of Natural Medicine* 3 [1996]: 8).

Rosacea, Acne Rosacea, Adult Onset Acne, Menopausal Acne

(See also 'Acne' in the "Skin Diseases" entry.)

It is not normal to continue to have adolescent acne into the thirties; nevertheless, it does occasionally occur. For such a person it is usually a part of what is called "adult acne" or rosacea. The person is probably allergic to certain foods.

Check yourself for food sensitivity. This step is very important. Such foods as milk, sugar, citrus, chocolate, free fats (margarine, mayonnaise, fried foods, cooking fats, salad oils), nuts, peanuts, wheat, honey, yeast, legumes, and all animal products have been implicated as allergies for some people. Animal fats from meat, milk, eggs, and cheese are an important cause of acne. A totally plant-based diet will be found to be most helpful. All chemicals should be removed from the diet as much as possible, along with coffee, tea, colas, and other soft drinks. Eat liberally of all foods richly colored green or yellow. A careful attempt should be made to discover any other food sensitivities by doing an Elimination and Challenge dietary procedure. (See "Elimination and Challenge Diet" in the *Dietary Information* section.)

Become a total vegetarian. Do not use meat, milk products (read labels), eggs, or cheese. Do not use vinegar (read labels), nutmeg, ginger, cinnamon, cloves, black or red peppers. Chew your food to a cream before swallowing. Take small bites, chew thoroughly, and eat slowly. "Leaky gut" is now being implicated in this disease, and one of the causes of leaky gut is believed to be eating too much, too many varieties at a meal, and chewing too little. Never overeat.

Get plenty of exercise, water, and sleep. Bring all your health habits up to par. Drink 10 to 12 glasses of water daily between meals, and do not drink with your meals.

Do not use soaps of any kind, including liquid skin cleansers, hypoallergenic soaps, etc., the exception being the pine tar soap. Shaving should not be done with a shaving cream. Perhaps an electric razor requiring no creams would be best. Use pine tar soap. (Users should test themselves for sensitivity to it. One person broke out in a rash from head to toe when using it.) If not sensitive, lather up at night and leave a heavy lather on the face to dry overnight. Actually rub the bar on the moist face. It will "pull" during the night. Wash it off the next morning using more pine tar soap. Rinse, dry, and apply a thick layer of Bag Balm immediately after rinsing. Get this from a feed store and insist on this name. Similar products are not as effective. Wear the salve for at least an hour and preferably all morning, but even wearing it 10 minutes will help a bit. Then wipe it off. If you must wash the face, do so with either plain warm water or the pine tar soap.

We have one patient with rosacea who has kept her rosacea under control with Bag Balm alone for several years. If she leaves it off, however, she begins to get pimples and a rash again.

On-The-Spot made by Neutrogena is good for single spots or particularly resistant pimples. The best face cream for daytime use is Neutrogena Hand Crea. It comes in a tube. Only a small amount is needed, as it is very concentrated.

Try tincture of cayenne, which you can make by putting one-fourth tablespoon of red pepper into a jar with a lid. Pour about two ounces of rubbing alcohol onto the red pepper and swirl. The alcohol can be used immediately but does not develop its full strength until after three weeks with the red pepper. Pour out the alcohol when ready, and store it in a dark bottle. The alcoholic extract can be applied daily to the pimples using a cotton-tipped applicator. The same tincture is good for many other skin lesions such as fever blisters, shingles, and herpes genitalis. For these conditions it can be applied once an hour.

Black Chinese tea, two to three times the normal strength, can be used as a skin bath.

Rosacea may be caused by a skin mite that lives in hair follicles. Purchase all new face creams if there is any chance of a germ or skin parasite having been transferred to your lotions, creams, or makeup by your fingers. The mite named Demodex folliculorum has been implicated in this disease. The mites stimulate, and they themselves are made more active by food sensitivities. The mites can be treated by using compresses of garlic, grapefruit seed extract (diluted), golden seal powder, or other antibacterial, antifungal, or antiparasitic herbs. Bear in mind that Artemisia annua (wormwood) is one of the most effective antiparasite herbs known. A compress using this herb could be very helpful against the skin parasite.

Consider that a rash may be because of the sensitivity to the frames of glasses. If you wear glasses, you might consider changing the type of material of the frames you wear.

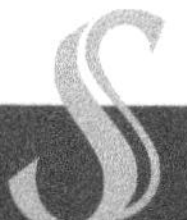

Use apple cider vinegar and natural sea salt in a solution of one-half teaspoon of salt to one ounce of vinegar. Use as a face wash for skin and glasses.

White iodine used three times daily for three to four days has been effective for some.

Drink two cups of fenugreek tea daily as a treatment for adult acne.

Case Report

A physician shared the following with us: "I would like to review for you the experience I had with rosacea personally since we have had several patients who responded similarly. I began having pimples on my face just under my eyes in the soft tissue. Gradually the pimples increased in number and in severity until they covered my cheeks. Through the next several months my cheeks and jaws became covered with pimples about down to the edge of my nasal flanges. It was about a year before it began to clear up above and started involving my upper lip and extending outward toward my ears almost in a line. As it moved downward, it seemed to clear above. I never had any pimples on my forehead. But after about another year it began to clear on my cheeks, still involved my upper lip and moved to my chin.

"For four years I continued to have pimples. During this time I suspected I had some kind of sensitivity, but everything I tried led to a dead end. Finally, a physician friend suggested perhaps I might be allergic to certain common foods, and upon her suggestion I did an elimination and challenge diet and discovered I was allergic to wheat, yeast, cucumbers, principally, but also to honey, certain other grains, and some beans. I had been a total plant-based eater (no meat, milk, eggs, or cheese) for about 20 years, and did not have to test myself on foods of animal origin.

"Within two weeks of leaving off wheat, I was clear of all pimples, but I still had a red rash, more prominent after eating. It was then that I eliminated all the gluten grains. Within two more weeks the rash had disappeared. For four years I avoided all the foods to which I was sensitive, except for rare small accidents. Then, one day I accidentally ate something with wheat and did not break out. Before that if I even took the small piece of unleavened bread at communion at our church, I would break out within an hour. I was very hopeful when I did not break out to the accidental ingestion of wheat, but dared not test myself again for an entire week. At that time I took a small bite of bread. No pimples. A week later I ate half a slice. Again, no pimples. For the last several years I have been able to eat wheat and other gluten grains (barley and rye) without getting either a rash or pimples, providing I do not eat a large quantity at one time. I am also able to eat yeast and cucumbers. I am very careful not to eat them frequently, but on the days I do eat wheat, I eat a fairly normal amount."

Scabies

Scabies is caused by an invasion of the skin by the microscopic itch mite that lives on the surface, but her eggs are laid under the skin. The female burrows under the skin and may remain a long time, traveling along a tunnel and laying eggs in the burrow. The skin reaction to her burrow may leave red, itchy lesions in a line more or less straight or slightly curved; one of the diagnostic clues. Most frequently involved are the fingers near the webs, the toes, ankles, knees, armpits, breasts, and external sex organs of boys and men.

To treat the itch, use cool soaks, starch baths, calamine lotion, and hot baths.

To eradicate the mite:

- Blend a clove of garlic in a small amount of cold water. Wet a cloth in the garlic water and apply to the affected area, or actually soak the hands or feet in the garlic water. If cotton cloths must be used, cover them with kitchen plastic to hold the compresses in place for two to eight hours. Test yourself for garlic sensitivity by starting out with only one hour. Wait for 8 to 12 hours to see if redness or irritation develops. Do not walk in shoes while the compresses are on the feet. They are very likely to blister with walking.
- Make a salve from anise seed by boiling two tablespoons of anise seed in one-half cup of water very gently for 20 minutes. Strain and pour the residual (should be at least two ounces or one-quarter cup) hot liquid into an equal quantity of vegetable shortening or coconut butter. Set the container with the hot liquid into a large bowl of ice and stir vigorously until it begins to set well enough it will not easily separate. Keep it refrigerated and apply to all affected areas four to eight times daily.
- Use an ointment made by stirring flowers of sulfur (from the pharmacy) into petroleum jelly or liquid soap. Use approximately two ounces (four tablespoons) of petroleum jelly or liquid soap and two teaspoons of flowers of sulfur (a powder). Mix them together, heating slightly if necessary, and store in a small, clean cosmetic jar. Take a warm soaking bath before application of the sulfur ointment. Apply each night to all affected areas three to five times. Do not

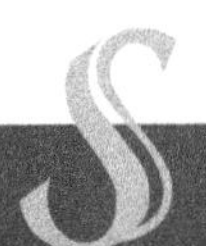

bathe during the treatment period. Remember that the ointment can stain clothing.

- Launder clothing daily in hot water (140°F) or iron with a hot iron to kill the parasite. The mite cannot survive 120°F for longer than five minutes.
- Keep fingernails short to discourage scratching, and treat all members of the household at the same time if there is any evidence of spreading to prevent cross- or re-infestation.

Sebaceous Cyst

This cyst is produced from an ingrown area of skin that somehow turns inward. It begins to accumulate shed skin and skin oils and becomes quite rancid over time. One of our patients called from Virginia and told us how she got rid of a sebaceous cyst. It was small, less than half an inch. Her treatment may not work for larger cysts, but she used this remedy: three minutes hot (moist towel) and one-minute ice rub. Repeat three to five times. Try to lift the cyst out by pressing at its base on both sides with two credit cards. Try to turn the cyst inside out. Our patient said hers came "out whole with an awful odor."

Skin Ulcers

For active, chronic skin ulcers apply a paste made of baker's yeast to clean up the ulcer and to encourage the healing process.

When a bedfast patient begins to get a reddened area of skin over a bone or other pressure point, start treatment immediately. With one patient we used an ice cube to massage from the outside toward the center of the red area, including the center also. It only took two or three applications of this to completely heal. We did not wait for the skin to break.

Honey poured on the ulcer, or confectioner's sugar (fructose) sprinkled generously on the ulcer, can stop infection in a few days and clean up an ulcer. Apply a bandage over the honey or sugar. Smelly ulcers can be deodorized by charcoal.

Fifty-nine patients with wounds and other ulcers, which had failed to heal with conventional treatment, were treated by pouring in unprocessed honey. Infected wounds became sterile within one week of the application of honey. The honey cleaned up the infection in the ulcers rapidly and promoted the growth of skin from the ulcer margins (*British Journal of Surgery* 75 [1988]: 679).

Sties

These painful lesions are inflammations of the glands at the base of the eyelashes. Sties are characterized by an acute onset, usually short in duration, 7 to 10 days, with or without treatment. I have found hot compresses adminstered while bending over a sink, using a folded washcloth held under the hot water, one after the other as hot as can be tolerated, for about 10 minutes two to four times daily, will often clear up a sty in a day or so. If they are more persistent, you can try one of the following treatments.

Steam fresh cabbage until limp; drain, apply as a compress for 15 minutes. Keep the compress covered to keep it warm.

Place the inside peeling of a raw potato on a paper towel. Fold and apply to the eyes as a poultice (Jude C. Williams, *Jude's Herbal Home Remedies* [St. Paul, MN: Llewellyn Publications, 1996]).

Wear a charcoal compress on the eye at night until the sty heals.

Hot and alternating cold compresses—the hot for three minutes, the cold for 30 seconds—can be healing in one or two days if applied four or more times a day.

Sun Sensitivity, Photosensitivity

There are many drugs capable of causing photosensitivity reactions. Some common ones are as follows: anticancer drugs, antidepressants, antihistamines, antihypertensives, antiparasitic drugs, antimicrobials, antifungals, antibiotics (tetracyclines, griseofulvin, sulfonamides, phenothiazine, piroxicam), naproxen, Tretinoin, diphenhydramine, birth control pills, and antivirals. Antipsychotic drugs, diuretics, hypoglycemics, NSAIDs (non-steroidal, anti-inflammatory drugs), sun screens such as para-aminobenzoic acid (PABA-405 solar cream), avobenzone, benzophenone, cinematize, homosalate, and others (Xanax, amantadine, Amiodarone, benzocaine, Tegretol, Librium, Atromid, oral contraceptives, Topicort, Norpace, Accutane, Phenergan, quinidine, Retin-A) can result in photosensitivity (*Sun and Skin News* 10, no. 1 [1993]: 1).

A few herbs may also cause sun sensitivity: bergamot oil, oil of citron, lavender, lime, sandalwood, cedar, citrus rind oils, musk, and St. John's wort.

A sensitivity to sun in which a person may break out in hives has been described as a part of other diseases such as lupus, herpes, and the group of blood disorders known as porphyria. Several drugs and other substances are also known to trigger sun sensitivities such as prescription drugs, the

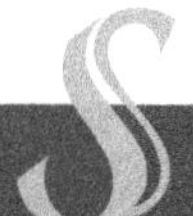

bergamot oil in certain perfumes, soaps, and the coal tars in medicated soaps and shampoos. Some common plants such as parsley, celery, limes, figs, etc. can cause sun sensitivity in some people.

Sunburn

The reddening of the skin because of sun exposure is a first-degree burn. This may be followed by blistering and peeling, which signals a second-degree burn. There are a variety of treatment options.

Cool compresses will help to relieve pain, as will cool or tepid baths. The use of baking soda or vinegar in the bath can be helpful, two to four tablespoons of either. Do not use soap.

Generously spreading a thick layer of petroleum jelly over the burned area and applying a light shirt or gauze dressing can relieve much of the discomfort.

Spreading aloe vera, oatmeal water, or baking soda and water paste over the burned area can be soothing and healing. Aloe vera is especially beneficial. Baking soda is slightly anesthetic. Drink lots of water as a burned area may lose much fluid. Avoid commercial sunburn products as they can cause damage and are no more helpful than home remedies.

Apply vinegar generously, and when dry, reapply. The vinegar is slightly anesthetic.

Varicose Ulcers, Stasis Ulcers, Stasis Dermatitis

Varicose veins in the legs can cause the feet to swell, and the blood flow to the heart to be slowed because of incompetent veins. Sometimes a rash begins to develop with itchiness and reddish or purplish discoloration. This stasis dermatitis may advance to the point of an ulcer, which is hard to heal. All manner of creams, antibiotics, and other medicines may be used to no avail. The ulcer continues to deepen and widen.

For varicose or stasis dermatitis and stasis ulcers, one of the most effective remedies ever devised is that of the Unna Boot. It is a rigid bandage that supports both the skin as well as the veins and clears a severe case of stasis dermatitis in an almost miraculous way. The formula for making the paste to be used with the Unna Boot is as follows:

- Two-thirds cup zinc oxide
- One and one-third cup glycerine
- One and one-half cups water

Fill a measuring cup to the 200-milliliter line with gelatin. The unflavored animal gelatin obtained from a grocery store gelatin can be used.

Pour the gelatin into the water stirring constantly. Allow the mixture to stand 10 minutes. Heat in a double boiler until the gelatin dissolves. Add the zinc oxide, which has previously been rubbed to a smooth paste with the glycerine, using a rubber spatula from the kitchen. Carefully stir the zinc oxide into the melted gelatin until a smooth jelly results. Set aside in a warm place.

Wrap the foot from the base of the toes around the ankle and up the leg two inches or more above the upper edge of stasis dermatitis and/or stasis ulcer. One or two layers only of roller gauze are required. The heel and the toes should be left free from gauze wrap. Using a small paintbrush, paint the warm (check to make certain it is not too hot) liquid over the layer of bandage until it is saturated. Then roll a second layer of gauze over the paste, again using one or two layers of gauze. The method of wrapping the roller gauze onto the leg is identical to that used for an elastic bandage. Do not pull the gauze tight, only snug. Allow the paste to harden at least 10 minutes before walking on it. Full hardening requires up to two hours, depending on the temperature of the room and the humidity.

If the ulcer is not infected, the Unna Boot can be left on up to two weeks if it is kept dry and cool. If it becomes ragged or soft or saturated with ooze, it can be replaced at any time. When the bandage is to be removed, cut it off with sturdy kitchen shears, or it can be soaked in warm water for a few minutes and cut off with ordinary household scissors. The leg and foot are then rinsed and wiped clean before the application of the next Unna Boot. You may use any left over paste from the previous boot.

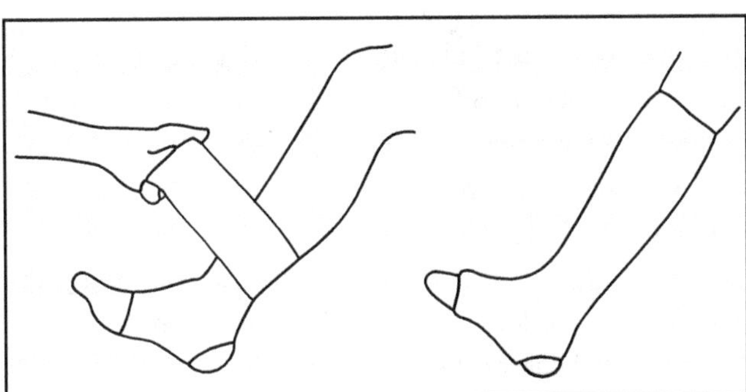

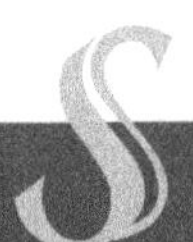

Vitiligo

Vitiligo is a disorder of pigment in which there is loss of melanin from the skin. It usually begins on the hands or around the mouth or eyes. Its significance is cosmetic and appears otherwise harmless. Treatment is slow and often unsatisfactory. The following suggestions may be helpful.

A product named Melagenina Plus was developed by Dr. Carlos Cao. It is made from an alcoholic extract of placenta and is used in combination with ultraviolet light. The area to be treated should be free of cosmetics, deodorants, etc. Cleanse the skin before the application of the product and wait at least one hour after application before bathing. Apply directly to the depigmented areas. Spraying is the best means of application and a cotton swab or cloth should never be used, as the active ingredient will remain on the swab and the alcohol will be the only thing reaching the skin. Apply every eight hours followed by 15 minutes of sunlight or an infrared lamp at a distance of about 15 inches. Success rate is reported by Cuban doctors to be close to 99 percent.

In about 40 percent of patients new areas of hypopigmentation begin to show up after the treatment begins. As they appear, they should simply be included in the treatment regimen. The more dark the skin, the quicker the results. The face usually requires four to six months of treatment. Baldness or hair loss associated with vitiligo is also benefited by the treatment. Psoriasis can also be cured with Melagenina, according to the Cuban doctors. Seventy-seven percent of psoriasis patients treated experienced a total cure after five years. You will use approximately one bottle per month.

One milligram of Vitamin B12 and 5 milligrams of folic acid, two times per day, along with sun exposure, significantly improved vitiligo in a majority of patients (*Actadermatoligica Venerial* (Stockh.) 77 [1997]: 460).

One doctor cured his vitiligo by taking moderately high doses of the vitamin B family. The B vitamins should be taken for several months.

Some physicians consider vitiligo and fibromyalgia to be expressions of low thyroid function, along with water retention, low body temperature, weight gain, cold sensitivity, dry skin, muscle weakness, arthritis, high blood pressure, slow heart rate, and constipation.

Slice a piece of fresh ginger or garlic clove. Rub the affected region until the juice is gone and hot sensations are generated in the skin. Repeat three to four times per day until the skin pigmentation returns to normal. Sun exposure after treatment hastens repigmentation.

PABA cream plus vitamin B6 spread on the area three or four times a day should be followed by sun exposure. One hundred or more sun exposures of 10 minutes each have been found effective.

Sometimes rubbing orange peel daily on the depigmented spots and then cautiously exposing the skin to the sun for 10 minutes can bring repigmentation. Do not allow burning, as that increases the risk of cancer of the skin.

Eight people got slow repigmentation over a period of many months with the following three vitamins: folic acid, 1 to 10 milligrams per day; vitamin B12, 1,000 micrograms every two weeks if taken by injection or 500 micrograms three times a week if taken by mouth; vitamin C, 1,000 milligrams every two weeks, intramuscularly, or 500 milligrams daily. Since vitamin C can deplete copper, we do not recommend it be taken longer than a year. A small supplement may be in order.

We have not used L-phenylalanine, which is an amino acid, but others have recommended it. Take 50 milligrams per kilogram of body weight per day (for the average 150-pound person that would figure out to be 3,500 milligrams per day) along with exposure to ultraviolet-A radiation therapy. It seems a bit hazardous for sunburning, which would then increase the risk of skin cancer, so if you try this remedy use extreme caution.

Some studies have shown patients with vitiligo to have a deficiency of hydrochloric acid in the stomach. Take a dilute solution of hydrochloric acid or betaine hydrochloride. Repigmentation with this treatment took a year or more. Take one dose four times daily.

St. John's wort makes one more sensitive to ultraviolet radiation and may assist in repigmentation. It may be worth a try, but guard against sunburning.

Since it has been shown that persons with compromised immune systems may get vitiligo, it may be of help even in those who have no demonstrable problem with the immune system to take echinacea, a known stimulant of the immune system. Other anti-inflammatory herbs are rosemary and licorice root.

Warts

These are usually hard growths on the skin producing few if any problems except when on the palms, soles of the feet, or in the perineal area around the genitals. They are caused by viruses and often precipitated by prolonged chilling of the skin. This accounts for the fact that children who play outdoors tend to get more warts than children who play indoors. These viruses have a narrow range of temperature,

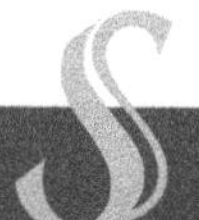

which they tolerate. Therefore, extreme heat or extreme cold will usually have a beneficial effect.

Warts are slightly contagious. About 7 percent of school children have warts. The peak incidence of warts is between 12 and 16 years, before it sharply declines. The average wart disappears within a year.

Treatment for Warts

Soak the wart for 30 minutes daily for 30 days in about 112°F to 115°F water to which has been added some blenderized garlic (optional). Nine out of 10 warts, even those that are very resistant, will disappear with this treatment.

An ice massage for 12 to 20 minutes daily for 21 days will often cure warts. An alternative to ice massage is an ice water soak for 20 minutes daily for 21 days. This treatment is most effective.

Applications of softening materials can be used, after which you should try to scrape off all the wart with the fingernail, or the edge of a credit card:

- A slice of fresh pineapple, garlic, aloe vera pulp, raw potato, papaya, or sour apple can be attached with a piece of adhesive.
- The milk of fresh figs or fig leaf sap may be curative. Apply a drop daily for several days or weeks.
- Wheat germ oil, castor oil, the juice of cabbage, or milkweed sap may all be helpful. Apply a drop daily, cover with a band-aid for several days, or even weeks.
- Crush marigold flowers, and apply to the wart using waterproof tape. Continue to refresh daily for three weeks or more.
- Apply several layers of waterproof adhesive tape to the wart, and leave covered constantly for six-and-a-half days. Remove the tape and scrape. If the wart is still present, reapply the tape after 12 hours and again leave on for six-and-a-half days. It may be necessary to repeat this procedure several weeks.

Comfrey compresses may be used. (See "Comfrey Compress, Poultice" in the *Herbal Remedies* section.)

One of the simplest treatments is to soak the wart in a concentrated saltwater solution. To obtain a 30 percent solution add one and one-half teaspoons of salt to one-half cup of water. Soak the wart for 20 minutes two or three times a day for three weeks.

Two patients have been reported to develop multiple flat warts while receiving tetracycline. When the tetracycline was discontinued, the warts disappeared. Other antibiotics may produce the same effects.

Sunlight has been shown helpful in the treatment of warts. Dr. W. E. Nelson, author of a prominent pediatrics textbook, suggests sunlight exposure sufficient to cause redness of the skin.

For genital warts acemannan, a derivative of aloe vera, is very effective. A good source of the acemannan is a compound called Carrington Wound Gel that is very beneficial for genital warts, although it is marketed for dermatologic conditions other than warts. The gel should be applied once nightly until the warts are gone, usually about two months.

For warts on the cervix use hot garlic douches daily for six weeks, along with echinacea and golden seal by mouth, and vitamin A suppositories inserted nightly for six weeks.

Treatment for Plantar Warts

These miserable warts occur on the soles and may cause much pain when walking. They may have the appearance of warts elsewhere, or may be smooth on top. Plantar warts often develop beneath pressure points on your feet, such as the heels or balls of your feet.

For plantar warts soak the foot daily for two weeks in water as hot as you can stand. (Diabetics should not use this treatment if their doctors have told them not to put their feet in hot water.) After three minutes in hot water, plunge into ice water for 20 seconds and then back into the hot footbath. Repeat the exchanges five times for a total of about 20 minutes of treatment time. Do this treatment nightly for 30 days. After 15 to 20 days, take scissors with very sharp points, clip around the edges through the dead skin, and try to dig the wart out with your fingernails, starting with the edge you have clipped.

If the hot baths fail to remove the warts, you should scrape the warts after soaking for 30 minutes in warm water that has dish detergent added to it to help soften the hard parts. If you can work your fingernail or a knife blade under one edge of the wart, try to lift it intact out of its bed. You can sometimes remove it with a little patient effort trying to avoid damaging the underlying tissue. Be careful attention to avoid infection. That means being very clean with all your instruments and materials. It is not necessary to try to sterilize the area or the instruments. Follow this treatment with the application of softening material described in the basic treatment of warts.

Make a paste of Comet cleanser as a scrub three to four times daily for as long as required to get rid of the warts. Apply the paste and let it stay on the wart for 5 to 15 minutes.

Then scratch the wart with your fingernail for three to five minutes, keeping the paste on the wart. Bear in mind that the surrounding skin should be scrubbed as little as possible.

Change socks twice a day to keep the feet very dry, as warts grow best in a moist environment. Apply talcum directly to the feet, and wear shoes that breathe. Nylon stockings must be worn with absorbent shoe liners. Wear white or light colored socks since dark ones retain more moisture.

Apply one or two drops of castor oil directly to the wart and cover with a bandage or tape. Apply the oil daily, and in time the wart can be removed effortlessly with your fingernail or a knife blade.

Rub garlic oil on daily or use a fresh garlic mini-poultice if you are not sensitive to fresh garlic.

Place the inner side of a fresh piece of banana skin over the wart and tape in place. This is changed daily after washing the affected area. Once a week the thickened outer horny layer is removed. The maximum time required for the complete disappearance of the warts is approximately six weeks.

Papain and bromelain (from papaya and pineapple, respectively) can also soften the skin of a wart. You can make a paste of the two enzymes and apply it to the wart. Cover it with a bandage only if needed. The sock may be adequate. When it is soft, after several days of applications, it is easy to remove with the fingernail or a dull blade.

Sleep

Insomnia

Does a poor night's sleep make you drowsy so that daily activities are difficult to perform? Is lack of sleep affecting your ability to concentrate either on the job or when you read? Do sleepless nights make you irritable with friends or family the next day? Does it take you longer than 30 minutes to fall asleep at night? Do you sleep less than six hours per night? Do you wake up frequently and have a hard time going back to sleep at night? If the answer to any of these questions is yes, you probably have a sleep problem that should be addressed promptly. In this way you can prevent an acute and temporary sleep loss from becoming chronic.

It is important to sleep from six to nine hours each night, as people with chronic insomnia are more likely than others to develop several kinds of emotional or mental problems. They are also more likely to have difficulty recovering from a physical illness. Insufficient sleep can impair memory, learning, and logical reasoning. Inadequate sleep can cause one to make improper decisions concerning moral matters. Inadequate sleep can rob you of your motivation to exercise, which brings in its train a list of serious health problems. Furthermore, inadequate sleep can be dangerous, leading to serious or even fatal accidents. More than 200,000 automobile accidents annually are estimated to be fatigue related.

Any degree of sleeplessness during the time when it is appropriate to sleep is termed insomnia. Almost 10 times more women report sleep difficulties than men, involving about a hundred million Americans at any one time.

Losing as little as one to two hours of sleep each night can leave people not only drowsy but also disturbed in hormone production, reaction times, psychomotor skills (enough to impair driving ability), certain essential functionings of the immune system, and an increase in an inflammatory molecule called TNF-alpha. (Remember that inflammatory substances in the blood increase risks of heart attacks, hardening of the arteries, cancer, and osteoporosis.)

Impaired quality and quantity of sleep is a common complaint particularly among older persons. Recent research indicates that too much sleep may be worse for you than too little sleep. The lowest mortality hazard ratios for men and women were with seven hours of sleep. The hazard ratio increased to 1.1 for five hours of sleep, and to 1.17 for nine hours of sleep. The use of sleeping pills was associated with an increase in mortality to 1.15 to 1.25. Insomnia was not related to any increase in mortality. An excess mortality in women of 83 percent and in men of 78 percent occurred with greater than eight hours of sleep per night. The mortality associated with short sleep duration accounted for only 17 percent of the excess in women and 22 percent of the excess in men. The conclusion was that insomnia and short sleep duration are not significant hazards to health. Sleep in excess of nine hours per night accounts for approximately 80 percent of the mortality associated with sleep. The use of sleeping pills is associated with increased mortality risk (*Archives of General Psychiatry* 59 [February 2002]: 131–36).

Causes of sleep loss include stress, school or job related pressures, marriage problems, depression, lifestyle stressors (for some that means alcohol, caffeine, exercising too little or too close to bedtime, a shower taken in the evening, eating close to bedtime), taking a nap in the afternoon, mental activity close to bedtime, smoking, shift work, jet lag, a distracting environment, a physical condition that causes pain or discomfort, medications such as steroids and asthma, blood pressure, depression medication, or sleep disorders such as sleep apnea or narcolepsy. It is estimated that 40 percent or more of women have trouble sleeping, whereas only 30 percent of men do. Early to bed, early to rise is still good advice.

Sleep deprivation lowers the percentage of natural killer cells in the blood. Working straight nights causes more sleep disturbance than daytime shifts or late afternoon and early evening shifts. Both quantity and quality of sleep are disturbed. Workers with rotating shifts over five days moving clockwise have fewer problems than counterclockwise rotations. Fixed evening shift workers were found in one study to have stronger immune systems than night shift or rotating shift workers based on a research report by the American Sleep Disorders Association. Findings were presented at a meeting in San Francisco on June 17, 1997.

Surgeons who stayed up all night the night before an operation made 20 percent more mistakes and took 14 percent longer to complete surgical tasks than surgeons who had had a good night of sleep. They also exhibited poorer dexterity and greater signs of stress, as much as with a blood alcohol level of 0.10 percent, which is enough to get a driver arrested in many states (*Lancet* 352 [1998]: 1191).

Remember that older people may feel very good on less sleep and may function quite well on six to seven hours of sleep nightly, but they still need rest, as much or more than in younger years. Naps in the daytime can be very helpful.

Unfortunately many people are treated with drugs for sleeplessness who should do without them. And many more are treated with widely advertised products that induce sleep quickly. The habit of taking these drugs is easy to form and is quite dangerous. Side effects from them include depression, skin rash, anxiety, irritability, poor coordination, loss of memory, loss of appetite, digestive disturbances, problems with the heart, lungs, and circulation, poor vision, high blood pressure, liver and kidney problems, damage to the central nervous system, dizziness, confusion, and even insomnia itself. Many drugs, including alcohol, coffee, tea, colas, chocolate, and aspirin suppress REM sleep, which means that sleep taken will be of less benefit.

Two proteins each regulated by a different gene appear to control circadian rhythm—the body clock that underlies the sleep-wake cycle—body temperature, mental alertness, and sensitivity to pain, according to research at Rockefeller University.

Treatment

Using polysomnograms temperature and movement studies, a group of volunteers who were given either warm baths or hot foot baths were compared with controls who received neither treatment. The hot foot bath seemed to give the best performance with stage three being greater, sleep onset quicker, and body movements less during sleep with the hot foot bath than with controls. The warm bath was similar to the hot foot bath except that REM sleep decreased (*Journal of Psychological Anthropology and Applied Human Science* 19, no. 1 [January 2000]: 21).

There are many foods taken late in the day that can increase one's likelihood of being sleepless that night. Of course, coffee, tea, colas, or chocolate are well known to interfere with sleep. Even if falling asleep is not a problem, sleep later in the night may be disturbed. Vitamin C taken late in the day can keep you awake; food sources high in vitamin C include citrus fruits and their juices, kiwi, honeydew, cantaloupe, and strawberries, broccoli, Brussels sprouts, bell peppers, dark leafy vegetables, and tomatoes. Irish potatoes may contain sufficient vitamin C to cause insomnia in some.

Some foods that contain high levels of certain amines known as pressor amines can elevate blood pressure or cause sleeplessness. These amines include serotonin, norepinephrine, thyronine, tryptamine, and dopamine. Fruits including pineapple, banana, plantain, and avocado are fairly high in various amines. While these amines have the potential to keep one awake, it would probably be difficult for the normal person to eat a sufficient quantity to cause sleeplessness. Nevertheless, individuals who have a problem sleeping should notice their reaction to them, as some people are very sensitive to certain nutrients.

Dietary factors are often instrumental in producing insomnia or encouraging sleep. Monosodium glutamate (MSG) may produce sleeplessness, as can coffee and its relatives, tobacco, overeating, fatty foods, refined carbohydrates, salt, chemical preservatives, additives, and foods to which one is allergic. Any natural food high in carbohydrates and low in fats and protein can be expected to be high in tryptophan an amino acid that encourages sleep. L-tryptophan deficiencies can result in a serotonin deficiency, which can have a broad array of emotional and behavioral problems, including depression, anxiety, sleep disturbances, obsessive-compulsive actions, fear, anger, over-arousal, violence, aggression, and the inclination to commit suicide.

There are some prescription medicines that can cause insomnia: blood pressure medicines, diuretics, decongestants, cortisone and other steroids, Tagamet, Zantac, asthma drugs, and even some contraceptives (*American Family Physician* 51, no. 1 [1995]: 191).

To promote sleepiness, exercise during the day, especially out of doors. A warm shower can relax and soothe the insomniac, encouraging sleep.

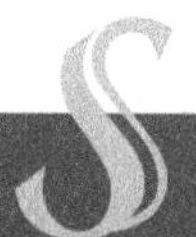

Massage is more soothing to newborn infants than rocking according to research done at the University of Miami and Duke University. Depressed adolescents often were distressed newborn infants who did not sleep well (*Infant Behavior and Development* 19 [1996]: 107–112). Adults given a five-minute foot rub have been shown to sleep better and to have lower blood pressure. A full body massage, but especially a back rub or a foot rub, can do wonders to relax the insomniac and encourage sleep. Massage the feet, squeeze the heels, and don't forget the ankles, especially the tissue around the anklebones on each side of the ankles. Also massage the scalp and eyebrows, forehead, and bridge of the nose. Massage the base of the skull and upper portion of the neck to induce sleep. These areas all tend to become tense during stress, fatigue, or burnout.

"White" noise of a fan, air conditioner, or recorded scriptures playing quietly can be an effective sleep producer.

The brain has ways to keep up with time so that sleep can be produced at the appropriate time. Until 1996 it was not known that there is a separate biologic clock in the retina of the eye; therefore, to set the biologic clock in the eye, go to bed at the same time every day, get up at the same time after six to nine hours sleep. If you must get up at night, use the most dim light possible and look at few objects while you are awake. Take a five to six ounce glass of water to rehydrate both the brain and the eye and go back to bed with the full expectation of returning promptly to sleep. Do not allow yourself to get in the habit of staying awake. Acute insomnia tends to become chronic and then generates anxiety. If you have insomnia, treat it promptly so as to avoid its becoming a chronic and more difficult to treat disorder (*Medical Tribune* 36 [1995]: 2).

Bear in mind that the hours before midnight are worth about two times the value of sleep after midnight. Therefore, if one expects to sleep four hours, try to go to bed at 8:00 o'clock. Those four hours of sleep will do you more good than all the remainder of the night if sleep begins after midnight. The reason for this may be in part because of the natural circadian rhythm of growth hormone, produced mainly in the early part of the evening and only during sleep.

Arrange your day so that the daily activities and room conditions are ideal to encourage relaxation and sleep—such things include social events, shower, exercise, stresses or challenges, temperature of your bedroom, fresh air, etc. Expect to sleep when you go to bed.

Be regular in all your habits, especially the hour of bedtime and arising time. Daytime naps may be taken before lunch. Pay attention to the air circulation in the room, the warmth of the room, the comfort of the bed clothes, and night clothes. Be sure the mattress is comfortable.

If you go to bed and tend to lie awake worrying, set aside 20 minutes early in the evening to use as "worry time." During this time you may meditate, write down actions you plan to take when you have time tomorrow, have prayer and Bible reading, and set your mind at ease for a good night's sleep.

Yawn yourself to sleep. Practice yawning, and before you know it you will be asleep (Jude C. Williams, *Jude's Herbal Home Remedies* [St. Paul, MN: Llewellyn Publications, 1996]).

Insomnia can be effectively treated with St. John's wort. Two capsules taken with a little water at bedtime are very effective.

A tea made from orange tree leaves has been found to be quite useful as a sedative and as a stomach tonic. It is quite effective, but is also quite mild, safe, and easily obtainable in areas where orange trees grow (*The Handbook of Pharmaceutical Practice*, reported in *Prevention*, September 1990, p. 135).

Lavender has been found to be an effective substitute for sleeping pills, which have serious side effects. Lavender oil is a gentle sedative with no side effects. A bit of the essence can be placed on a cotton or gauze sponge and pinned on the pillow or some other convenient place near the head to emit a nice fragrance in the room.

Herbal teas such as catnip, hops, mint, gotu kola, motherwort, valerian, passion flower, and chamomile are helpful.

A study done in a sleep laboratory showed that individuals given 600 milligrams of dry extract of valerian root one hour before bedtime fell asleep sooner, slept more efficiently, and entered into restorative slow-wave sleep. Older individuals could especially benefit from valerian root if they suffer from sleeplessness (*Pharmacopsychiatry.* 33 [2000]: 47).

An ancient Chinese remedy for insomnia uses fresh peanut plant shoots. Take one ounce of fresh peanut shoots, including leaves and stems, and pour one cup of boiling water over them. After steeping 30 minutes, the tea is drunk about 30 to 60 minutes before bedtime. Positive results are expected within the first three days, and a complete cure is reported in one to two weeks. Most patients according to the Chinese will not have a recurrence of insomnia. We suggest you get the peanut shoots by planting peanuts in flower boxes or in a garden.

If, after you have done everything to promote sleep, you still cannot sleep, do not spend your time doing unprofitable things, instead pray while you lie relaxed in bed, keep your

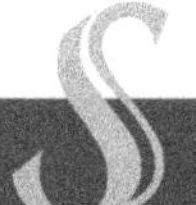

eyes closed, and think about the attributes of God, the spiritual growth you would like to have, and train the thoughts to dwell on heavenly themes—the home of the saved and the great sacrifice of our Savior to make eternal life within the reach of man.

Naps

We have an increasing body of evidence that human beings are natural nappers. The most favorable time for a nap is just prior to lunch. The second most favorable time is approximately two hours after lunch after digestion has gotten well underway and more than half finished. There is a slight midday drop in body temperature that encourages sleepiness. To nap increases mental function, reduces stress, and enhances the immune system. People differ in the length of time needed for the nap from a few minutes to half an hour. During the nap messenger molecules carry signals between the mind and the body to integrate many critical processes of healing and repair.

Persons who take a nap in the afternoon perform better, even though they get a good night of sleep. During a 30-minute nap a person may sleep more deeply than at night, particularly if the person is more than 60 years of age.

Sleep Apnea, Snoring, Daytime Sleepiness

Sleep apnea is a pause in breathing of 10 seconds or more. The cause of sleep apnea is unknown. Some feel that narrower airways than other snorers causes the apnea, which results from the tongue dropping back so far it gets sucked into the airway. Symptoms include excessive daytime sleepiness, fatigue, forgetfulness and irritability. It is estimated that between two and three thousand people die each year in their sleep because of sleep apnea. Since they sleep little during the night, they may have difficulty driving or operating machinery because of sudden uncontrollable drowsiness or brief naps. Complex problems may become more difficult for these persons to learn or grasp.

Sleep apnea often begins in mid-life and can be complicated by an increased incidence of accidents and heart attacks or strokes. It has been found that abdominal obesity, insulin resistance, and high levels of blood cytokine are all associated with sleep apnea and may contribute to the development of the problem (*Journal of Clinical Endocrinology and Metabolism* 85 [2000]: 1151). The pro-inflammatory cytokines can cause stiffness of blood vessels and lead to hardening of the arteries.

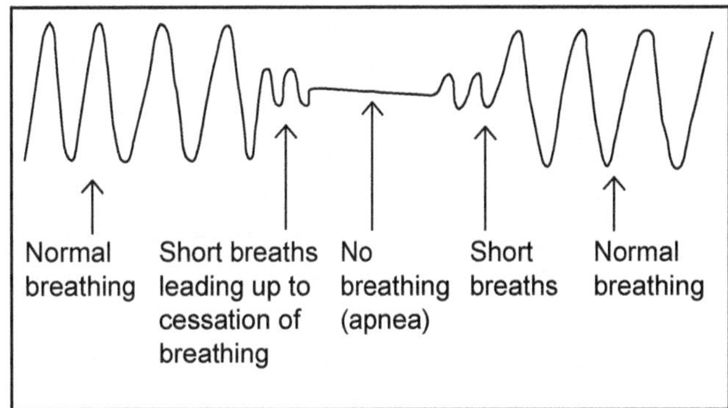

Night sweats often occur because of improper air exchange—breathing too shallow or too infrequently. To make this diagnosis, take an audio recorder to bed, placing the microphone in such a way that the sound of the breathing can be recorded, especially during the first part of the night. Record the breathing pattern for about an hour if possible. Notice if there are periods of very slow breathing or even absence of breathing. A period of absent breathing for 10 to 20 seconds or more repeated 20 or more times an hour is called sleep apnea. If you breathe less than 10 times a minute, it can be too little breathing, especially if your breathing is shallow.

Persons who have sleep apnea may need to use a machine to help them breathe deeply at night. If continuous positive airway pressure (CPAP) is used by individuals who have sleep apnea, there is an improvement in mental functioning, even if the user averages only three to four hours per night for use of the equipment. It improves mood and a sense of alertness as well (*Lancet* 343 [1994]: 572).

Because of oxygen depletion during breathing cessation, the heart has to beat faster to keep oxygen circulating, and it eventually becomes damaged or beats irregularly. They are also much more likely to suffer from hypertension. Those with sleep apnea are five times more likely to have high blood pressure than people who sleep normally. In another study of 50 men with high blood pressure, 26 percent had sleep apnea, a higher percentage than in the general population.

A remedy infrequently thought of is elevating the bed with two or three bricks under the bedposts at the head.

A tongue-retaining device can be obtained only through a sleep center, but it can be effective in eliminating apnea in 82 percent of cases.

Using a CPAP machine has a 90 percent success rate among snorers. Newer surgical procedures have an 80 percent success rate for snoring.

Not eating supper and taking a cup of mint tea can be helpful in both night sweats and sleep apnea. Being certain to get more than seven hours sleep, preferably a bit more than

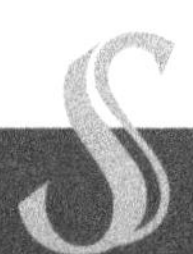

eight hours of sleep every night, can be helpful to combat sleep apnea and excessively slow breathing. One should be very careful to have fresh air in the bedroom at night, no restrictive clothing, and to avoid poor sleeping posture.

A number of heavy snorers were studied using nasal adhesive strips, which resulted in a statistically significant decrease in snoring and daytime sleepiness score. Another assistance for snoring is infrared coagulation of the inferior turbinates inside the nose. It consists of touching the infrared coagulator to the turbinates of the nose under a local or topical anesthetic. This opens up the airways in approximately 80 percent of patients. In some, not only do they stop snoring, but also their sleep apnea seems to go away as they again exhibit rapid eye movements during sleep.

The more snoring a person does during the night, the greater the daytime sleepiness. It has also been found that long durations of sleep were related to greater reported snoring. Individuals sleeping between seven and eight hours a night were considered normal, and those sleeping longer times or shorter times than seven to eight hours had greater measures of disease and lower psychosocial function according to a study done on 1,877 people aged 50–65 years (*Journal of Clinical Epidemiology* 47, no. 1 [1994]: 35). Women do not usually begin snoring until after about 50 years of age. Men often begin snoring at 18–20 years of age. Women often do not suspect that they snore.

Regularity in sleep habits, even if the number of hours spent sleeping is the same, greatly reduces sleepiness in the daytime. Those individuals also fall asleep more quickly after going to bed than those with an irregular sleep time, and sleep more soundly during the night. Poor concentration, a poor mood, and increased daytime sleepiness all result from irregularity in sleep time (*Sleep* 19 [1996]: 432).

Individuals who have sleepiness throughout the day, and especially afternoon drowsiness, should try extending their nighttime sleep by two hours for four successive days. This will help to relieve cumulative fatigue. The best way to do this is by going to bed earlier rather than staying in bed later in the morning, as early evening sleep is about twice as valuable as early morning sleep.

After about the age of 60–70, the body's biologic time clock sets the time for bedtime back to around 7 or 8 p.m. Then about eight hours later the morning alarm is set, waking individuals at 4 to 5 a.m. The problem is elderly people do not go to bed at 7 or 8 p.m. Therefore, they tend to have sleepiness and the ability to drift into sleep at almost any time they are still.

If you sleep only four or five hours per night, be certain to get to bed earlier rather than sleeping later in the morning. You will be more alert, and improve your overall performance the next day.

Treatment

Lose weight. Snoring will be aggravated by a thick neck. Even a few pounds of extra weight can mean the difference between snoring or no snoring. (See "Weight Control" in the *Conditions and Diseases* section.)

Alcohol and certain drugs cause snoring. Tranquilizers and depressant medications such as sedatives or allergy medications deepen sleep and lead to increased relaxation of the throat muscles and obstruction in the throat.

Make sure the bedroom is well-ventilated.

A supportive mattress with a low pillow to keep the neck straight and reduce airway obstruction is recommended. Do not sleep on the back.

A tennis or golf ball sewed into a pouch onto the back of a tight T-shirt that the snorer wears to bed can help the snorer no longer sleep on their backs after a few nights.

Dental devices can be obtained from a physician or dentist to realign the tongue or jaw.

Surgery on the uvula, tonsils, or soft palate will sometimes stop snoring.

The snorer should lie on one side or the other, and if one nasal airway is narrower and more easily blocked by congestion than the other, the wider side should be up.

Wear a snoring collar, something resembling the neck collars worn by persons suffering whiplash injuries.

Of course, one should eliminate smoking and any other cause of swelling of the nasal tissues—allergies, pollution, etc.

Hold the handle of a wooden spoon or a tongue depressor between your teeth for five minutes. Your jaw muscles are apt to feel tired, but you should keep bearing down.

Place your fingers against your chin, jaw slightly open, and press firmly for two or three minutes while you hold your jaw steady as you apply pressure. Your jaw involuntarily presses back, and you'll begin to feel an ache. This is the first step in making your muscles stronger.

With mouth closed, firmly press your tongue against your lower teeth until you feel an ache. Hold for three or four minutes.

Stick out your tongue and try to touch the tip of your nose. Repeat, holding 30 seconds each time.

Do these exercises morning, afternoon, and before bed. Don't expect immediate results as about four weeks are

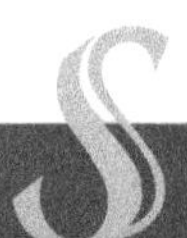

required to see an improvement. Continue the exercises for two months, and then drop down to only once a day.

Slipped Disc

(See "Skeletal Problems" and "Numbness" in the *Conditions and Diseases* section.)

Smell

Smell can be lost by trauma such as a blow to the head, nasal sinus disease such as chronic sinusitis, and, most commonly, viral infections.

Mumps, especially in adults, can cause loss of the sense of smell. Sometimes there will be a gradual return of smell in a few weeks, but often the condition is permanent.

Being very careful with general health is the first step in treatment. It is especially important to get plenty of water. Our most successful treatment has been the use of 50 milligrams of zinc daily for two to three months. If you have not had a return of smell in that time, you should stop the zinc, which has been implicated in the development of Alzheimer's disease. Do not continue for more than six months if you have not yet had a return of smell.

Snake Bite

(See the *Home Emergencies* section.)

Sore Throat

(See "Colds" in the *Conditions and Diseases* section.)

Spider Bite

(See the *Home Emergencies* section.)

Spinal Curvature, Scoliosis

(See "Skeletal Problems" in the *Conditions and Diseases* section.)

Sties, External

(See "Skin Diseases" in the *Conditions and Diseases* section.)

Stomachache

(See also "Abdominal Pain" in the *Supplemental Information* section.)

One important cause of stomachache, which people rarely consider, is tight belts. Some people wear the belts or bands of their pants or skirts as much as three inches too tight.

The first thing to consider is that all vinegar, aspirin, and alcohol must be absolutely stopped, as these are the commonest ingested cause of gastritis and peptic ulcer. You will be much better off without them as they also adversely affect the pancreas, the brain, bladder, bones, and the entire digestive tract. Also avoid hot spices such as chilies, ginger, cinnamon, nutmeg, cloves, and black and red pepper.

Eat your meals on a strict schedule until your stomach is entirely healed, choosing to skip a meal altogether than eat an hour or more off schedule. Unsweetened Swedish bitters can aid digestion and stop stomache.

Do not drink more than four ounces of liquids (juice, beverages, gravies, soups, and thin sauces) at a meal as these dilute the digestive juices and interfere with the protective faculties of the stomach.

Be very careful to drink plenty of water between meals. One of the recognized causes of gastritis and peptic ulcers is inadequate water drinking. Juices, soft drinks, and other beverages do not supply the place of water.

We also recommend that you take slippery elm tea, one teaspoonful per cup of warm water, four times a day. You must also avoid all antacids, other drugs, and any food you know that hurts you. You must eat only two meals a day—breakfast and lunch—skipping supper. This is most important in the healing of your stomach, as it needs to be resting several hours every day. If you are not better in several weeks or months, then you should get a diagnostic workup to determine the cause.

Take a full dose of charcoal, one heaping tablespoon of powder in water for an adult. May also take four capsules or up to eight tablets as one dose.

Lie down and rock your abdomen back and forth between your two hands in a churning action.

Lie facedown in bed. This is especially helpful for children with a tummy ache.

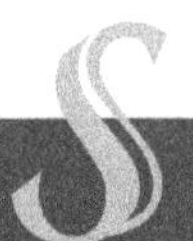

A lick from your moistened fingertip of mint oil can be helpful. Catnip tea can also settle the stomach and ease pain.

Take one small blade from an aloe vera plant. Peel the green off and eat one to three teaspoons of the inner pulp.

Use one teaspoon of honey to the juice of one lemon. Mix with water and drink.

A quarter teaspoon of fresh ginger root mashed in water or blended in a blender can aid digestion.

Stress

Early warning signs of stress include the signs of adrenal insufficiency. These may include chronically low blood pressure, fatigue, low stamina, sensitivity to cold, pale fingers, and addictions to either sweet or salty foods. Other symptoms are irritability, forgetfulness, temper flare-ups, reclusiveness, and loss or gain of weight and appetite.

Beginning in childhood the stresses of life can be minimized by simply reducing the noise level in the home. Chaotic homes produce children with less development of their intellectual skills. In addition they have delayed language skills, trouble mastering their environments, and increased anxiety. Establish a quiet place where children can spend some time by themselves. Read to your children in quiet places. Have a regular schedule. Have a place for everything and keep it in that place. Or if you are short on space, learn how your home can function smoothly without storage room to put away things.

Stress-giving foods such as caffeine, sugar, sodas, and all refined foods can increase one's stress. Certain minerals can be lost as a direct result of stress such as magnesium, calcium, zinc, potassium, sodium, and copper. Most richly colored fruits and vegetables have anti-stress properties. These include the richly colored greens, yellows, orange, reds, blue, etc. Foods that are high in B vitamins such as beans, nuts, brewers' yeast, and whole grains, especially popcorn, also reduce stress. Good sources of manganese, another stress-reducer, include bananas, whole grain cereals, and nuts.

Eyelid twitching, which is often a sign of stress, can be relieved by hot compresses for 20 minutes and by reducing stress.

If you have a troublesome matter causing you stress, try to give it the mildest name you can think of as well as your emotional reaction to it. Now ask your heavenly Father to help you control the emotion involved in this problem. Have faith that you will gain help from this method.

Effective communication is essential to maintaining good relationships. Learn to express yourself constructively, especially when facing conflict. If a close friend or family member seems to have a problem with you in some way, face the problem by simply asking, "Have I offended you or caused you trouble in any way? Is there some contention between us?"

Make a priority list of irons you have in the fire now with the most important things listed first. You should decide how to manage overload after a weekend or a vacation. Following is a suggested list to help you make plans:

- Schedule the first day very lightly.
- Assign workload in three categories:
  - Important and urgent
  - The 70 percent rule—who can do this task at least 70 percent as well as I can. Let that person do that task.
  - Non urgent work to be done as soon as possible
- Plan the next day's goals the afternoon before, as you will be better able to decide what needs to be done.
- Before sleeping make a to-do list of tasks for the next day, ranged in urgent and less urgent groups.
- Schedule tasks early in the day.
- Angle your desk away from windows to avoid distractions.
- Eliminate photos and all distracting, unrelated materials from your desk. Have a clear desktop. Only keep materials for one day on your desk. You will be surprised how much this single factor speeds up work performance.

Teach yourself how to sleep. If you must, use soft foam earplugs, and if distracting light such as streetlights disturb you, wear a silk sleep mask. Don't eat a heavy evening meal. If a supper is eaten at all, make it only fruit or fruit and bread. Avoid caffeine in any form from coffee, tea, colas, or chocolate.

Remove noise from your environment as much as possible.

It has also been shown that exercise and relaxation lower anger-hostility expressions, particularly concerning individuals who are likely to talk about their problems. Blood pressure was reduced, heart rate was reduced, and overall benefits were experienced (*Journal of Behavioral Medicine* 14, no. 5 [1991]: 453; *Research Quarterly for Exercise and Sport* 63, no. 1 [March 1992]: A-78). Further, talking about problems implants the problems deeper in the consciousness.

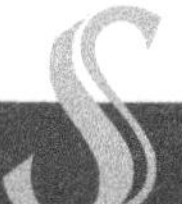

It is well known that serious personal problems can increase the likelihood of stress of severe enough proportions to cause the immune system to function poorly. Freudian psychology has for several decades advised that persons having problems "talk out their problems to prevent their being bottled up inside the mind." We do not agree with Freud's theory as verbal repetition of the problem is harmful and fixes the problem more firmly in the mind. Research provides evidence that Freud was wrong. If a person talks about problems they are experiencing, the immune system suffers. Natural killer cell activity shows evidence of cytotoxicity, the effect being greater the more hostility is generated by speaking of the troublesome problem. We can now be certain that talking about problems harms other systems—nervous, mental, gastrointestinal, even musculoskeletal—as well as the immune system. It is better to make it a habit to keep one's problems to oneself and to speak earnestly to the Lord in prayer concerning such matters. When praying about problems, begin the prayer by asking the Lord for control of any hostility (*Psychosomatic Medicine* 58 [1996]: 150–155). There are times when a troubling problem must be discussed with someone, but generally, speaking and complaining about problems multiplies difficulties. Choose your confidant carefully and make sure it is someone of your same gender.

Take a ten-minute break every day. Find a quiet spot, close your eyes, and allow the mind to dwell on heavenly themes. Pray out loud to our heavenly Father.

Stress can be treated by making something orderly in the life. This one thing may be an orderly household, schedule, checkbook, car, or children's schedules. A scrupulously clean and orderly kitchen goes far toward making a happy home.

Managing time becomes essential to managing stress. Following are helpful techniques to keep you organized:

- Always start the day with your own personal devotions, meditation, and prayer. That means going to bed early enough so that you can get up a full hour in advance of the time you must start dressing.
- Get everything in your life in order, including making a daily schedule.
- Make an accounting system for your money.
- Recognize a central priority. This may be your work or time with your children. That which is the central priority for that day should be written down so that you can organize all other things around it.
- Learn that you can save minutes here and there that count up to hours in a day, and days in a year. Most busy people add time to their lives by saving these few minutes here and there that most people squander. Five minutes saved in dressing, five minutes saved in eating breakfast, five minutes saved in a telephone call gives you one quarter of an hour to do something else.
- Do not start a two-hour job that requires an outlay of equipment when you have only five minutes.
- It is well to take a moment at the end of the day while you are meditating and praying to make plans for tomorrow. At this time the Holy Spirit has more access to your mind with connections with the day you have just spent than at any other time in your future life. Therefore, spend a few minutes writing out a list of what you must do tomorrow before retiring.
- Most people waste a lot of time after waking up, before getting up, and while dressing. Simplify your closet and your bathroom so that everything not needed day by day is put in a box and set on a shelf well out of the way; preferably on the back shelf of a closet where it is out of sight and will never need dusting. Then the two or three items that you need every day for dressing can be kept in prominent places, easily accessible without knocking something else over, and can be easily cleaned with a single swipe.
- Save time in cleaning your bathroom by using towels that are ready for the laundry. If this is done twice a week, it will not stain the towels and will save a major cleaning operation. Floorboards can be dusted in the same way, as can high shelves, windowsills, and commode bases.
- Choose what you plan to wear the night before, and set it out or hang it aside in your closet.
- Always put scarves, sweaters, coats, etc., in their places rather than dropping them on a chair. The extra second or so required to fold and put it away will not be missed now as much as the hours that must be used for a major clean-up job.
- Organize your desk. The major thing about organizing a desk is how to manage paper. A load of paper comes onto your desk daily from the mail, delivery services, and your own notes on telephone calls, etc. You must have a place to file these, or your desk will get swamped. Then every time you approach your desk you must thumb through 20 items to find the one item you need. This wastes a lot of time. Whereas, a file cabinet that has folders labeled 'Things to do,' 'Bills paid,' 'Bills to be paid,' 'Correspondence done,' 'Correspondence to be done,' 'Children's schooling,' 'Equipment

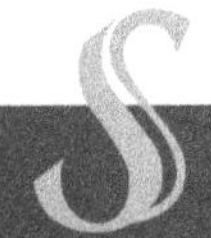

manuals,' 'Guarantee slips for equipment,' etc., saves time. Such a file is invaluable to keep a desk organized.

- An important thing about filing papers is to determine what needs to be kept. If the information is available in a library, your computer, or some book you already have, do not file it; throw it away. Have your calendar nearby when you open the mail so that anything with a deadline can be added to your calendar. Have a desktop box, or tray, labeled with your spouse's name, secretary's name, children's names, etc. Put information relating to something about them in each box as necessary. Then, the next time you see one of these persons take the items in the box to them.
- Almost everyone can get large amounts of things done early in the day, and very few things done from late afternoon till bedtime. Therefore, plan to go to bed early so that you can save an hour of time for getting things done in the morning, which may so increase your productivity that you will find you cherish the practice of going to bed early. Sleep taken before midnight is worth roughly twice what sleep after midnight is worth. All unpleasant or stressful tasks should be done in the morning. Anything requiring intense concentration should be done in the morning.
- Keep a yearly calendar. Some things must be done once a month, some things once a year, and others once a quarter. Window washing falls in the once a quarter, or once a year category, and should be written on the calendar in advance. Mailing birthday greetings, or writing to a shut-in who never writes back, should be put on the calendar so they will not be forgotten.
- Make apologies and correct irritations immediately. These unpleasant duties become more difficult with each passing day.

Each January set goals for yourself to accomplish that year. The list should be reviewed at the beginning of each month. Whatever it is, the goals should be written on your calendar so they can be accessed easily. You should make a progress sheet for each goal with the following information:

- Starting date
- How much must be finished by a certain time
- When the task is half done
- When a review should be made of the task by some independent or objective person
- The finish date

Correct Sabbath observance is essential to handling stress. Use the Bible method of observing the Sabbath, being careful in every item.

Keep the extremities warm as cold stress is an important factor in irritating the nervous system.

Do not overeat as biochemical stress arises from over indulgence of the appetite.

Avoid any foods to which you are sensitive, as food sensitivities are often the cause of an irritated nervous system. Use the "Elimination and Challenge Diet" in the *Dietary Information* section to discover food sensitivities.

If a skin rash is present, get rid of it, as skin afflictions are often the cause of an irritated nervous system. So is any physical affliction such as cystitis, chronic constipation, etc.

Warm or neutral baths at about 97°F to 99°F can be very soothing. Be sure to keep the mouth temperature below 100, and keep the head cool with cold compresses.

The use of sedative herbal teas can give enormous relief. These include catnip, hops, skullcap, St. John's wort, valerian root, and others. Boil one quart of water and then turn it to a very gentle simmer. Add one rounded teaspoon of licorice root powder to the simmering water for 20 minutes. Then set the pot off the fire and add one tablespoon each of catnip and chamomile. The mixture should steep for 30 minutes, then strain. Drink the resulting tea throughout the day, or you can use one cup four times a day. One cup at bedtime is helpful for sleep.

Stroke

If you have had any of the following conditions, you are at risk for a stroke:

- Heart attack
- Angina (chest pain during physical activity)
- Unstable angina or coronary insufficiency (the symptoms of a heart attack, but with no increase in the enzymes that signal heart muscle damage)
- Intermittent claudication (severe leg pain, usually upon exertion, that results from an inadequate blood supply)
- Congestive heart failure (symptoms like breathlessness and severely swollen ankles caused by the heart's failure to pump enough blood and oxygen)
- An electrocardiogram that shows you have left ventricular hypertrophy (an enlarged heart muscle)
- A systolic blood pressure (the higher of your two blood pressure numbers) higher than 170

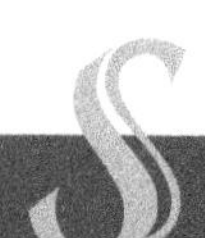

- Atrial fibrillation (irregular heart beats in the upper chambers of your heart)

Roller coaster rides and similar forms of amusement with rapid up and down and back and forth movements can rupture blood vessels in the brain and cause hemorrhage (*Neurology* 54 [2000]: 264).

Ischemic stroke from artery blockage is 89 percent more likely to occur between the hours of 6:00 a.m. and noon, and hemorrhagic stroke are 52 percent more likely between 6:00 a.m. and noon. TIAs are 80 percent more likely to occur in the morning. Strokes of all kinds were least common between midnight and 6:00 a.m. The new thrombolytic treatments such as tissue-plasminogen activator can significantly reduce the long-term effects if taken within three hours of symptom onset. Blood pressures rise by about 20 percent just after waking. A stroke is much more likely to occur in persons who are regularly exposed to passive smoke (*American Journal of Public Health* 89 [1999]: 572).

Atrial fibrillation causes 15 percent of all strokes in the United States. If you add congestive heart failure, disease of the heart valves, or a history of heart attacks, hypertension, smoking, or previous stroke, to atrial fibrillation it will increase the risk of stroke mortality by 40–60 percent (*OBGYN News*, March 1, 1996, p. 42).

The contraceptive pill increases the likelihood of having a stroke. A low-dose pill (50 milligrams of estrogen) can triple a woman's risk of thromboembolism (*British Medical Journal* 312 [1996]: 83; *Lancet* 346 [1995]: 1375). Hormone replacement therapy in menopausal women carries a similar risk. Low levels of testosterone may increase the risk of stroke in elderly men.

Blacks are twice as likely as whites to have dangerous strokes that are fatal (*USA Today*, March 13, 1992). Similarly, blacks have almost a 33 percent greater rate of high blood pressure than whites. We believe blacks should begin checking themselves every three to six months for high blood pressure, obtaining their own blood pressure cuff and stethoscope by age 25. Begin natural treatments for hypertension if there are two consecutive readings above 140/85.

Patients who spend more than 48 hours in intensive care in the hospital increase the risk of developing blood clots by 33 percent. The prolonged inactivity can lead to the formation of clots as well as to heart failure.

When a person over the age of 60, or one who has recently had anesthesia, takes a long plane trip, they are in danger of developing blood clots in the legs. If a blood clot forms, when the person gets up from a sitting position the blood clot dislodges and goes to the lungs, causing a life-threatening pulmonary embolism or the development into a pneumonia-like illness. To prevent these problems, walk around the plane cabin about once every two hours and, while seated, repeatedly tense and relax your leg muscles every 15 minutes or so. Yawning and stretching can also help blood flow. Drink plenty of fluids. Elasticized stockings also help during long plane trips. The stockings help prevent blood from pooling in the legs. Since intestinal gas expands at high altitudes, it can interfere with passage of blood from the legs back to the heart. Eat lightly and only of foods you know will not produce gas before taking a long jet flight. Wear very loose clothing and a loose belt as well as avoid gas-producing foods before and during the flight (*Lancet* 347 [1996]: 1697).

Fibrinogen levels can be measured. A relatively high white blood cell count can predict an increased risk of having a cerebral thrombosis. Men with a white blood cell count above 8,100 had a 39 percent increase in the risk of strokes compared with those having white cell counts below 6,600. The effects were increased in persons who smoked (*Journal of Chronic Disease* 35 [1982]: 703). Persons with the cleanest blood, such as those taking a plant-based diet and avoiding fumes and smoking, have the lowest white cell counts.

Walking 10 miles per week was associated with a significantly lower risk of stroke. The risk of stroke is lower in people who engage in moderate levels of exercise than at either low levels or excessively high levels of exercise (*Clinical Pearls News*, 9, no. 3).

A folic acid deficiency may increase the risk of strokes, perhaps being responsible for 15 to 20 percent of heart attacks and strokes (*N Engl J Med* 1995; 332:286-291).

Vitamin B6 and folic acid, which are found in legumes, greens, and grains, reduce the risk of both stroke and heart attack, regardless of homocysteine levels. At least seven milligrams of B6 and 400 micrograms of folic acid are minimal intakes to accomplish the best good (*Circulation.* 2004; 109: 2031-2041).

The risk of having a stroke is about 30 percent lower in men who remain physically active after the age of 40 compared with sedentary peers. Stroke is more than 90 percent higher in men who have poor lung function compared to men with high levels of lung function. Low intensity activities such as walking and swimming may offer the greatest benefits in preventing stroke (*Annals of Internal Medicine* 130 [1999]: 987).

Avoid overeating as a custom of life. Unusually large meals are reported in many elderly people just prior to having a stroke. A blood pressure change may occur just after eating

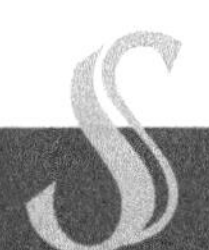

a heavy meal. Over-secretion of insulin, which occurs as the blood sugar from a heavy meal goes up, has an unfavorable effect on blood vessels (*Medical World News*, October 3, 1969, pp. 13, 14).

Good hydration cuts the risk of fatal strokes and coronary heart disease. A study done on 34,000 Seventh-day Adventists for six years showed that those drinking at least five glasses of water a day had a significantly decreased risk of heart disease, strokes, and complications of diabetes. If the blood is not well hydrated, strokes and heart attacks are more likely to occur. Those drinking five or more glasses of water a day had a 44 percent decreased risk of stroke compared to those who drank two or fewer glasses of water. It is of interest that drinking fluids other than water—juices, soft drinks, coffee, or tea—did not affect the incidence of fatal heart disease or stroke. From this study we can say that the best beverage for cleansing and diluting the blood is water (*Internal Medicine News* 31, no. 19 [October 1, 1998]: 6).

Two or three small glasses of purple grape juice a day reduced platelet aggregation by 40 percent in two studies of healthy subjects and Rhesus monkeys. This would make grape juice as protective as a daily aspirin. Unlike aspirin, however, the flavonoids in purple grape juice remain effective when adrenalin levels rise (*Medical Tribune,* May 1, 1997, p. 26). Also, unlike aspirin, grape juice has no mortality or morbidity rate associated with it.

Ginkgo biloba taken daily offers some protection against strokes.

Stroke Warning Signs

- Sudden weakness, numbness, or paralysis of the face, arm, or leg, especially on only one side.
- Blurred or decreased vision in one or both eyes; fleeting loss of vision in one eye.
- Difficulty or inability speaking or understanding simple statements; confusion.
- Dizziness, loss of balance, or loss of coordination, especially when combined with another symptom.
- Sudden very intense headache with no other obvious cause.
- Any one of the following: sudden nausea, fever and vomiting, brief loss of consciousness, fainting, confusion, convulsions, loss of taste or smell, and sudden onset of numbness, tingling, weakness, or clumsiness.

Ischemia means severe reduction in oxygen supply. A TIA (transient ischemic attack) is a tiny stroke that often warns of a more serious one to come. Thirty percent of people who have TIA's will have a major stroke days, weeks, or months later. Stroke is the third leading cause of death in the United States, causing 150,000 deaths per year. A TIA is a momentary lapse of power in an arm or leg, or the fleeting loss of vision in one eye, or inability to speak correctly for a few moments.

If one or more of these symptoms lasts only 5-30 minutes, it is probably a mini-stroke. The risk of full-fledged stroke is as much as 10 times greater than average after a mini-stroke.

It has been discovered that in persons who have a TIA the blood is often quite thick and has a slow-flow condition somewhat like honey on a cold morning. It is not known whether the TIA comes first and causes the thick blood, or whether the thick blood comes first and causes the TIA. We favor the latter position. We believe that too many red blood cells and plasma containing too many nutrients and wastes cause a TIA (L. Dintenfass and G. V. F. Seaman, eds., *Blood Viscosity in Heart Disease and Cancer* [Pergamen Press, 1981]).

Treatment for TIA's

As soon as the condition is recognized, the person's temperature should be adjusted. If they have been working in the hot sun, cool the face with cool cloths, not ice. If they are chilled, give a hot footbath while keeping the face cool with cold compresses to the face, forehead, and neck. A hot footbath will often drain the blood from a congested head. This can often be observed with draining of the flushed face, resulting in less agitation. The hot footbath can be placed in the bed while the patient is in a semi-reclining position. Keep the head cool, as described above.

A glassful of water every 10 minutes for an hour will often be beneficial, or taking the water in the form of herbal teas such as ginkgo, juniper berry, yarrow, or a sedative tea.

Treatment for Strokes

The sooner a stroke or an impending stroke is recognized, the smaller the probability of a massive stroke. If a person who has just had a stroke can be taken to a center for stroke treatment, and the proper treatment with minerals and intravenous fluids is begun immediately, the smaller the area of the brain suffering permanent damage, and the less extensive the disability resulting from the stroke. Treatment must begin within six hours to be most protective. If a stroke center is inaccessible, begin your own treatment at home as soon as possible. First, while they can still swallow, give a glass of water every 10 minutes for an hour. Give the first two

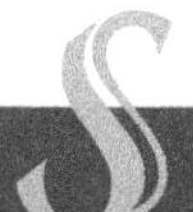

glasses of water as a solution of magnesium and potassium. If you can get capsules of these minerals from a pharmacy, open enough capsules to supply 400 milligrams of magnesium, and around 4 milligrams of potassium. Dissolve this in 16 ounces (one pint) of water. You may add lemon juice if that will make it more palatable. If the person can swallow (this is important as fluid or food must not be given to a person who cannot swallow because of the likelihood of getting it into the lungs) give the entire pint at once. If swallowing is impossible, give the mixture by rectum, not more than eight ounces at once or it may not be retained. Fluids by rectum must be at body temperature to encourage holding it in; but by mouth the temperature should be either pleasantly warm or cool, as the patient prefers, to prevent nausea.

Zinc supplements are shown to reduce brain injury after stroke. Start with 30 milligrams immediately or on the same day as the stroke if the patient can swallow. Next day give the same dose twice a day; and the third day begin on a routine of 15 milligrams three times daily. Continue for one to two months. Use this same routine for any form of head injury, such as after an automobile accident or fall.

Hot footbaths can reduce congestion in the head following a stroke. The hot footbath can be used promptly if the stroke is because of a hemorrhage or if high blood pressure is part of the case. It is important that the water temperature be comfortable at first, as very hot water can cause the blood pressure to go up for about three to five minutes. After the foot bath has been in progress a couple of minutes, hotter water can be added. Of course diabetics should not have foot baths hotter than about 102°F to 105°F.

Stroke Recovery

Cornflower tea is said to aid in returning the use of limbs after stroke, if used regularly, such as four cups a day (Jude C. Williams, *Jude's Herbal Home Remedies* [St. Paul, MN: Llewellyn Publications, 1996]).

Teas that are helpful for stroke recovery include bilberry, feverfew, garlic, ginger, ginkgo, quercetin, and white willow bark.

During the recovery phase, stroke victims can be helped by mirror therapy. Victims have regained their ability to move a paralyzed limb by watching themselves move the opposite extremity in a mirror. After four weeks of treatment in this way, improvement should be noticeable and sometimes dramatic (*Medical Tribune* 40, no. 2 [1999]: 6). Start with the undamaged side and stand in front of a mirror to make certain motions that the damaged side cannot yet do.

Recuperation in a Stroke Victim

- Let them do as much as they can, but don't put them in situations they cannot handle.
- Expect some unreasonable fear from the patient.
- Understand that anger may be a part of their recovery.
- Encourage survivors to help themselves. A survivor that helps design his/her own program is more likely to stick to it.
- Insist that a survivor return to normal activities, but very gradually. Stress aggravates a stroke, but so does inactivity. Do not become a recluse.
- Expect that some directions will be new, and some old dreams may need to be abandoned. Develop new dreams.
- Join a support group. You may get some very good ideas from them.
- Contact the American Stroke Association, the National Stroke Association, or The Agency for Healthcare Policy and Research.

It is often recommended that aspirin be taken, but there are many side effects to taking aspirin such as stomach upset, nausea, vomiting, and gastrointestinal hemorrhage—not only hemorrhage in the intestinal tract but also hemorrhage inside the brain is at greater risk of occurring, even in low doses of aspirin. Aspirin also depletes the body of certain essential vitamins and minerals, especially iron. Liver damage can occur as well as allergic reactions such as hives, wheezing, ringing in the ears, chronic nasal mucus, headache, confusion, and sometimes low blood pressure followed by collapse. Aspirin is also blamed as a factor in macular degeneration, now the most common cause of blindness in the Western World.

The use of Warfarin (coumadin) is also often prescribed, but this too has hazards of its own and may not be the best answer to the problem of strokes. Controlling the underlying disease may be much more feasible and productive. Atrial fibrillation carries a six-fold increase in risk of strokes. The other diseases carry two to three fold elevations in risk. Exercise daily, red or purple grape juice, garlic, and a plant-based diet eliminating free fats can give a risk rate lower than with either of these, and without the side effects. One or two fresh garlic cloves per meal seems to be as protective as other measures against the development of blood clots inside blood vessels (*Prostaglandins Leukotrienes and Essential Fatty Acids* 63 [1995]: 211, 212).

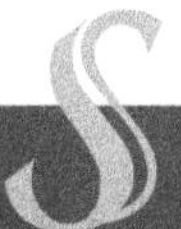

Sudden Infant Death Syndrome (SIDS)

Pregnant women who drink caffeinated beverages may put their babies at increased risk for sudden infant death syndrome (*Archives of Disease in Childhood* 78 [1998]: 9). Caffeine also has a link to infertility, spontaneous abortion, and birth defects. Our recommendation is that coffee, tea, colas, and chocolate be avoided by girls and women, especially during pregnancy and lactation.

Do not have a smoker in the house where there is a baby under one year of age.

Keep the child's extremities warm.

Do not put a baby on its tummy to sleep.

Swimmer's Ear

Swimmer's ear is an infection brought on by getting water in the ear, followed by the development of inflammation or infection in the ear canal.

The objective of treatment is keeping the ear clean and dry. Pour the ear full of plain rubbing alcohol, immediately drain it out, and dry the ear as well as possible with a tissue wrapped around the smallest finger—do not use Q-tips or any instrument inserted into the ear. The finger is quite adequate.

Soft sponge earplugs may be saturated with herbal tea to keep the application next to the infected area. Use astringent teas such as golden seal, comfrey root, mullein, slippery elm, witch hazel, or white oak bark.

Alcohol-vinegar drops may be put in the ear several times daily, or the entire ear canal may be filled with the mixture, immediately drained out, and the ear dried with a tissue wrapped around the smallest finger. This treatment is especially effective for fungus ear. Mix two ounces of rubbing alcohol with two ounces of vinegar, and keep on hand for use after swimming.

The application of heat in any form for 10-20 minutes will promote healing and relieve pain. Use a hot water bottle, desk lamp, heating pad, or hot compresses.

To relieve pain, ice water can be dropped into the ear from a melting ice cube. As soon as pain is relieved, dry the ear with the alcohol procedure discussed above.

Syphilis

Syphilis is a sexually transmitted disease caused by *Treponema pallidum*, a germ similar to the germ causing Lyme disease. It has three phases when untreated. Primary syphilis typically has a painless sore somewhere on the genital area, perhaps with swollen lymph nodes. Secondary syphilis comes on about two weeks or more later, characterized by a generalized rash, often with a rash on the palms and soles, one of the few diseases causing a rash on the palms. The tertiary phase of syphilis comes on years later with gumma or balls of necrotic tissue that can be destructive to bones, liver, brain, heart, etc.

Fever therapy will rapidly heal the primary chancre, but the fever baths must be prolonged in order to prevent secondary syphilis from occurring. To treat a syphilitic eye infection such as interstitial keratosis, iridocyclitis, or gonorrheal conjunctivitis, use fever treatments (*Medical Bulletin of the Veterans Administration* 7 [November 1931]: 1083–85). (See also "Gonorrhea" in the *Conditions and Diseases* section).

Fever treatments in three-hour sessions for syphilis were adopted in 1937 and were generally used until the early 1950s. Prior to that, five-hour sessions up to 105°F and 106°F rectally at weekly intervals for a total of up to 50 hours were the usual course, the average patient receiving 36 hours of fever treatments. After 1937 about 25 hours of fever were used on the average patient. The three-hour sessions can be given at weekly or semi-weekly intervals to ambulatory patients and three times weekly or even daily to those under constant surveillance. The first treatment is about one hour at 102°F to 103°F rectally, the next at 103°F to 104°F, the third at 104°F to 105°F, and the remainder 105°F to 106°F. The length of time is gradually increased until the patient is able to take three hours of fever at 105°F to 106°F rectally. If the temperature must be measured in the mouth rather than by an indwelling rectal probe, the numbers are one degree less for each reading, starting with 101°F to 102°F orally.

In treating syphilis it is well to be aware of an unusual, always puzzling occurrence, the Jarisch-Herxheimer reaction. It is generally a single episode of headache, flushing, sweating with fever that may go up to 104°F, starting some 2 to 12 hours after beginning any drug treatment for syphilis. It occurs in approximately 50 percent of cases of early syphilis after the first dose of penicillin. It was first observed after mercury treatments and was seen also after bismuth and arsenic. Most of the reactions last 24 hours or less (*British Journal of Venereal Disease* 47 [1971]: 293-4). We have no

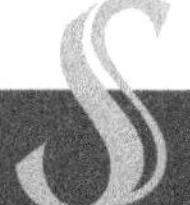

information that it occurs with hydrotherapy, but it is well to remember that the reaction has been reported in the course of treating syphilis with several other methods of treatment.

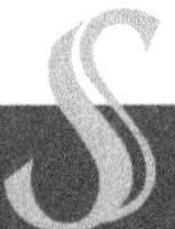

Tardive Dyskinesia

(See "Mental Disorders" in the *Conditions and Diseases* section.)

Taste

The surface of the tongue, the soft palate, and other areas of the mouth can detect four flavors: sweet, sour, salt, and bitter. Various combinations of these probably account for all the flavors we experience. Taste buds are replaced on the average of about every 10 days, and things that affect this replacement are poor nutrition, hormone levels, medications such as insulin, and aging.

According to one study, because of poor taste perception, salt and sugar intake in those past the age of 65 is increased by 42 percent! Here are some better alternatives to adding these potentially harmful substances to food.

- Alternate bites of one type of food with bites of another, as both smell and taste sensations fatigue quickly from a single type of odor or flavor repeatedly experienced.
- Chew your food thoroughly in order to experience to the fullest the taste and smell-bearing molecules in the food.
- Drink tiny sips of water occasionally to clear the palate so the taste buds are freer.
- Choose foods for each meal that give a variety of chewiness, crunchiness, smoothness, roughness, as well as each of the basic four taste sensations—salt, sweet, bitter, sour. Since bitter is unpleasant, the taste of bland food such as bread, rice, potatoes, etc., can be substituted.
- Use less liquid in soups or sauces to increase flavor intensity. Cook vegetables and fruits with waterless techniques where possible. Steaming and baking preserve flavors better than boiling.
- Use a great variety of herbs. Fresh herbs are more flavorful than dried herbs. Grow some of your own herbs in flower boxes. Onion, garlic, and lemon perk up vegetables and grains nicely.
- Check your medications. Many are capable of diminishing taste or smell.
- Do not smoke, use alcohol, or hot spices, all of which can diminish taste and smell.

Teeth, TMJ

(See "Dental Care" in the *Conditions and Diseases* section.)

Temporal Arteritis

(See "Polymyalgia Rheumatica, Temporal Arteritis" in the *Conditions and Diseases* section.)

Tendonitis

This condition is recognized from the pattern of pain and can be experienced in any tendon of the body. It is less common than arthritis or bursitis, and when the diagnosis is suspected, it should be considered along with these other two conditions. The common cause of tendonitis is some kind of strenuous movement.

The best treatment is an ice massage. You can use a block of ice made by freezing water in a styrofoam cup. The small end of the cup can be torn off to expose the ice. The large part is held to keep the hand from getting too cold. Place towels around the affected area to catch the runoff water. Rub the skin over the more painful areas with the ice for about 10 minutes twice daily. In addition to ice massage, appropriate stretches, rest, and pendulum types of exercises, if applicable, should be utilized. The pain usually decreases promptly with this treatment.

If the tendonitis is severe, a two-week rest of the tendon may be necessary. Cortisone or prednisone, its close relative, should not be used as these are among the most powerful and dangerous drugs in modern medicine and will very likely cause other problems.

Tennis Elbow, Epicondylitis

(See "Skeletal Problems" in the *Conditions and Diseases* section.)

Tetanus, Lockjaw

The important thing in considering tetanus is to prevent infection in very traumatic wounds and deep puncture wounds that could allow the anaerobic (without air) growth of the *clostridium* germ that causes tetanus. The treatment of penetrating wounds should begin at their occurrence, keeping them open to the air if possible, giving excellent wound cleansing, alternating hot and cold baths, total body massage, poultices, and the proper use of charcoal, both internally and externally. With this treatment for wounds, the growth of the *clostridium* germ is discouraged.

Penetrating wounds such as nail punctures, animal or human bites, etc., should be treated by soaking the part in a strong hot tea made from plantain or golden seal. Treat tetanus before it begins by preventing infection in the wound. The broadleaf plantain can cause blisters in some people and needs to be used carefully. Instead of plantain, other soaking solutions can be used. One cup of vinegar should be added to each quart of hot water when penetrating injuries are soaked.

Aloe vera significantly decreases wound healing time, both when applied topically and taken orally. Golden seal, echinacea, astragalus, and grapefruit seed extract should all be used for two weeks after a penetrating wound.

A cup of charcoal powder should be put in water used to soak the injuried body part. Use a two or three-gallon tub full of water for a foot or hand injury. Charcoal should also be taken by mouth for its detoxifying properties.

Fever therapy has been successfully used by others for chronic tetanus, a condition in which a mild infection smolders in a skin cancer, bowel infection such as in a fistula, etc., and there is long-term tightness of muscles, difficulty swallowing, and sudden inability to make words sound precise (*Munchener Medizinische Wochenschrift* 92 [May 12, 1950]: 224-28). We believe fever therapy would be effective in acute tetanus as well, but we have not worked with such a case. If you are in a situation where no professional help is available, by all means try fever baths.

Thrombophlebitis

Blood clots inside a vein caused by irritation of the vein may occur because of injury, a nearby infection, or stasis of blood as in a varicose vein, obesity, pregnancy, surgery, prolonged bed-rest, long automobile or airplane trips, and congestive heart failure. Blood may clot more quickly in some people because of cancer, abnormality in the blood, oral contraceptives, recently having anesthesia, lack of exercise, dehydration, and a high fat, high-protein, high-sugar diet.

Symptoms include aching, especially severe upon standing or having the part hanging down, or while walking or climbing; swelling; heat; tenderness; redness; distended veins; and a firm tender cord felt in the tissues. After childbirth or an operation, a thrombophlebitis may occur in the calves, and is associated often with discomfort in the calf on flexing the foot up toward the leg. Involvement of superficial veins, which constitute most cases of thrombophlebitis, are not dangerous. Deep vein thromboses are dangerous, as the veins are straighter and can result in higher speed of blood flow with breaking off of portions of the blood clot, which then lodge in the lungs to cause pulmonary embolism.

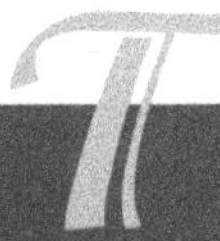

For persons prone to getting recurring thrombophlebitis, we recommend a low-fat, low-sugar, totally plant-based diet as the most favorable for this condition.

Food sensitivities are a cause of recurring thrombophlebitis in some individuals. If a case of recurring bouts of thrombophlebitis is unresponsive to other treatments, try the "Elimination and Challenge Diet," found in the *Dietary Information* section, for three to six months, then gradually add back a food group once a month until there is a return of thrombophlebitis. The treatment requires patience, but it can be very rewarding.

Donate blood to the Red Cross to keep the hemoglobin in the ideal range—10.5 to 12.5 grams for women, and 12 to 14 for men. The ideal hemoglobin range is lower than the range given in the laboratory, which is average for Americans, not ideal.

Avoid wearing constrictive clothing, particularly tight pants or constrictive leg gear such as pants, tights, or panty hose. Tight underwear, because of the elastic bands, can constrict both the abdomen and the groin regions, causing an increased risk of thrombosis in the legs. Chilling the extremities from inadequate clothing can also contribute to thrombophlebitis.

Exercises such as wading in water, swimming, bicycling, walking, gardening, and most other kinds of exercise are protective. It should be vigorous and kept up for 20-30 minutes daily.

Lose weight if you have any excess fat, as extra flesh promotes constriction of blood vessels.

Avoid extended periods of sitting while traveling, studying, or doing desk work. Avoid garters, girdles, and other restrictive clothing. Prop the feet on a small stool to relieve pressure on the thighs while sitting. Do not cross the legs or dangle the feet. Often take a deep breath, stretch the arms overhead, flex the legs, and yawn.

Practicing good posture and deep breathing are protective.

Do not sit long on the toilet, as that promotes slowed blood flow from the legs.

The herb horse chestnut is excellent for persons who have repeated cases of thrombophlebitis. One man we know could count on having thrombophlebitis in his legs about twice a year. For three years after he started taking horse chestnut he had no problem with thrombophlebitis.

Eat a fruit and bread diet for five days, avoiding fats, sugars, heavy protein foods, all animal products, vinegar, and irritating foods such as caffeinated and decaffeinated drinks, and spices.

Garlic, three cloves three times daily, minced finely and taken with meals, enclosed perhaps in a sandwich, will cause blood to be more normal in its clotting tendency. For deep vein thrombosis, the patient should be put to bed, given garlic and five ounces of red or purple grape juice every three hours and at meal times, and all unnecessary movement of that extremity avoided for five days.

The mainstay of treatment is elevation and heat. For deep vein thrombosis apply a folded hot towel on the extremity for 25 minutes, continuously, not alternating with cold, for the first three to five days. Then, apply hot and cold fomentations—five minutes hot and one minute cold repeated four times and performed four times daily.

For severe cases, continue with applications of moist heat 20-24 hours daily. That can be accomplished by wrapping the limb with a hot wet towel and keeping it hot with a group of hot water bottles or heating pads slipped into a large plastic bag and securely fastened to prevent any danger of electrical shock from moisture getting into a shorted area of the electrical heating pad. If the skin becomes waterlogged, allow it to dry for one hour, and then apply a thin layer of petroleum jelly to the skin before reapplying moist heat.

Keep the extremities warm as cool skin and tissue retard healing. Cold extremities also cause an increased risk of blood clotting inside other veins. (See also "Blood Clotting" in the *Conditions and Diseases* section.)

Thrush

Thrush is a fungal infection of the mouth in infants and occasionally in older persons with weakened immune systems. Thrush consists of white spots that may eventually develop shallow ulcers. Sometimes fever and gastrointestinal disturbances are present. The fungus may spread to the buttocks, groin, underarms, or other areas.

To treat thrush, make a saturated solution of baking soda in water by stirring as much baking soda as can be made to dissolve in a cup of hot water. When it has cooled, dip a cotton tip applicator in the solution and touch each lesion in the mouth. Garlic solution may also be used for swabbing. Blenderize two cloves in one cup of water, refrigerate the mixture, and swab in a similar manner as with the baking soda several times a day following the rinsing with water after every feeding. Another swabbing solution before the baby develops teeth is vinegar and water mixed one to one. After two or three days, switch to pure vinegar for swabbing if it does not cause an increase in pain. The vinegar acid can etch the teeth of older children or adults.

Rinse the mouth after each feeding with plain water. For babies, a bulb syringe can be used for this purpose. Rinsing helps prevent thrush.

Avoid antibiotics and steroids as these cause an overgrowth of the candida fungus that causes thrush.

Thyroid Disease

Hyperthyroidism (overactive thyroid)

There are many signs and symptoms associated with hyperthyroidism. It is not necessary to have all the symptoms to make the diagnosis. Following is a list of symptoms:

- nervousness and irritability
- palpitations and tachycardia
- heat intolerance and increased sweating
- tremors
- weight loss
- alterations in appetite
- frequent bowel movements, especially at night
- fatigue and muscle weakness
- thyroid enlargement (depending on cause)
- swelling of skin over shin bones (with Graves' disease)
- shortness of breath on exertion
- menstrual disturbance (decreased flow)
- impaired fertility
- mental or emotional disturbances
- sleep disturbances (including vivid or wild dreams, especially insomnia, but also sleepiness)
- changes in vision
- light sensitivity
- eye irritation
- seeing double
- prominent eyeballs
- lower extremity edema
- sudden paralysis
- lid lag when eyes look upward

The causes include:

- toxic diffuse goiter (Graves' disease)
- toxic adenoma (tumor)
- toxic nodular goiter
- thyroiditis
- iodine-induced hyperthyroidism
- excessive pituitary TSH (thyroid stimulating hormone)
- excessive ingestion of thyroid hormone

Treatment

Thiourea reduces the function of the thyroid. It is known to be present in large quantities in turnips, kale, cabbage, and rapeseed (*Endocrinology* 43 [August 1948]: 105). The use of cabbage juice may provide a convenient way to obtain the antithyroid component. Eat at least one serving daily of foods that contain goitrogens, which reduce the activity of the thyroid. Goitrin is slightly more active to suppress the thyroid hormone than the commercial drug propylthiouracil, which is widely used in hyperthyroidism. About 25 to 50 milligrams of goitrin is found in one to four pounds of fresh brassica, such as cabbage, rutabaga, cauliflower, broccoli, Brussels sprouts, collards, kohlrabi, or kale.

Avoid certain foods that contain pressor amines: sauerkraut (histamine), cheese (tyramine, tryptamine, and phenylethyl amine), bananas (dopamine, norepinephrine, and serotonin), and wine (histamine).

Use kelp quite heavily in your food. It is high in iodine and tends to normalize the thyroid function.

Butter and cheese increase the urinary excretion of iodine and should be avoided at this time.

The patient should take two to three pints of cabbage juice, at least one cup of tofu daily, at least four tablespoons of pine nuts daily, and at least one cup of millet daily until the condition subsides.

Use iodine in large doses, 1500 mcg per day. Iodine in this quantity inhibits the release of T3 and T4 (*Metabolism*. 1988 Feb;37(2):121-4). Use Lugol's solution or saturated solution of potassium or sodium iodide (SSKI).

Take 2,000 milligrams of quercetin per day. It comes in 1,000-milligram caps. Give one twice a day. It decreases inflammation in the thyroid and intestines. Onions are high in quercetin. Eat a whole onion, lightly steamed or baked, every day.

Digestive enzymes, pancreatic enzymes, trypsin, amylase, and lipase can be most important in hyperthyroidism.

Drink 8 to 12 glasses of water daily, sufficient to keep the urine pale and the bowels moving well.

Pay attention to bowel toxicity and function in hyperthyroidism. Bowel toxicity can lower the level of T lymphocytes, thus weakening your defense against thyroid inflammation.

Exercise will help to burn up extra hormones. It is best that the pulse rate does not go above 115-125 while exercising.

An ice pack should be worn over the thyroid area as you are able, up to five to seven hours a day. Apply the pack for at least 30 minutes at a time, and when the neck becomes quite uncomfortable, then the ice pack can be removed temporarily, only to be reapplied as soon as possible. With this treatment, cases of very acute hyperthyroidism have been helped, and the laboratory readings for T4 brought to within normal range in two to three months. Some cases may take more or less time.

To calm the nerves, give a neutral bath for 40-90 minutes, the water being neither hot nor cold.

If alternating hot and cold compresses cannot be used, a heating compress or a charcoal poultice to the thyroid area each night may be substituted. The heat treatment causes inflammation in the thyroid to subside.

Clay or charcoal in the maximum dosage is required to reduce the intensity of an inflammatory reaction in the thyroid gland. If inflammation is present, take one teaspoon four times a day in water, building up to two tablespoons of either, four times a day.

Concentrations in the blood of thyroid hormones, especially T4, fell during a study of bright and dim light treatments. It is believed that one of the reasons depressed patients improve is because of a reduction in the level of T4 with light therapy (*Biological Psychiatry* 40 [1996]: 899). (See "Mental Health" in the *Conditions and Diseases* section for information about light treatments.)

If the patient has not lost too much weight, a day or two of fasting per week is quite helpful. The following procedure may be useful:

- Three days of a water fast, or a juice fast if the water fast cannot be tolerated, will cleanse the bowel and reduce the total antigenic load. Antigens can be a cause of hyperactivity in some people. Fasting is sedating.
- Use GI stimulants as needed, such as flaxseed or psyllium seed (one to three tablespoons), or slippery elm tea. These may also tie up products from *yersinia*, various antigens, and some excess thyroid hormones.

Plant medicines that may help include the following:

- Bugleweed (*Lycopus virginicus*) inhibits iodine metabolism in the body and thyroxin production and other hormones.
- Use sedative herbs: valerian, passionflower, and skullcap. A good formula is one and a half quarts of water and two tablespoons each of valerian root and hawthorn berry; boil for 25 minutes. Add two tablespoons each of bugleweed, skullcap, nettles, yarrow, and passion flower. Cover, set off heat, and steep for half an hour.
- Milk thistle or silymarin is helpful as it encourages good function of the liver. The liver is needed now to help break down excess antigens.
- The following herbs are good for stabilizing or stimulating the thyroid: bladderwrack, bayberry, Irish moss, motherwort, oak bark, mandrake, and poke root.

Foods having red, yellow, and blue coloring in flowers and fruit can cause an inhibition of thyroid function. A form of millet commonly eaten by inhabitants of semi-arid regions called fonio (*Digitaria exilis*) has an inhibiting effect on the thyroid (*Nutrition* 12 [1996]: 100). Cooked millet six days old has a greater activity than freshly cooked millet by six times. The active principle increases with both long cooking and with aging. The action is because of flavonoids that can be extracted from the millet. The flavonoids are apigenin and luteo. These two flavonoids have potent antithyroid properties.

Give four drops (130 milligrams for a thyroid inhibiting dose) of SSKI (saturated solution of potassium iodide). This dose is sufficient to protect the thyroid after radio iodide exposure. Small children ages 3 to 12 need one to two drops; 12 to 18, two drops; newborns up to one month, one half a drop.

Essential fatty acids are critical to proper thyroid function because they are required for the integrity of every cell membrane. Essential fatty acids also improve the efficiency of hormones on the receptor sites, especially omega-3s. The only essential fatty acids are omega-3 and omega-6 fats. All others can be made in adequate quantities from foods that are consumed. In addition to ensuring plenty of essential fatty acids, the proper balance of zinc, vitamin C, and digestive enzymes will also help to stabilize thyroid function.

Also for the thyroid, alpha-lipoic acid and CoQ10 can be quite helpful. Foods that inhibit iodine utilization (goitrogens) include the *brassica* family foods, cassava root, soybeans, peanuts, pine nuts, and millet. Excessive quantities of iodine will also inhibit the conversion of T4 to T3. But inadequate intake of iodine causes the thyroid to be unable to manufacture T4. Iron or zinc deficiency, or high levels of heavy metals, including lead, mercury, and dental amalgams can cause impaired body response to T3 (the active form of thyroid hormone). Many prescription and over-the-counter drugs affect the thyroid. A few of the worst are lithium, amiodarone, phenytoin, and carbamazepine, but many others can also affect the thyroid function.

Case Report

One woman shares what worked for her: "Here is what I did for my high thyroid condition instead of Propylthiourea. I stopped eating dairy products, white flour products, textured vegetarian meat substitutes, all processed foods, and any junk foods. I also stopped eating out. I now use nut milks instead of commercial soy milk, drink eight glasses of water every day plus two to three glasses of carrot juice and cabbage juice, and make sure I have a good breakfast of grains with flaxseed sprinkled on top—also nut milk and fruits. I continue to take a multivitamin preparation and exercise daily in the open air and sunshine.

"The results are that:

1. My sleeping pattern has returned to normal, in fact I am catching up on my lost sleep.
2. The tremors in my hands and legs are gone.
3. My energy level has increased.
4. My heart palpitations have decreased, and my heart rate has slowed, but not normal as yet.
5. My weight has increased by 5 pounds up to 100 pounds, goal is 111 pounds as before.
6. I am not as hungry as before, so I take three meals daily.
7. Thyroid enlargement has decreased but not totally to normal.
8. Heat intolerance has disappeared and now I feel on the chilly side of normal.
9. Bowel movements have returned to normal.
10. Nervousness and irritability have disappeared.
11. Shortness of breath on exertion has decreased; I used to get winded just going upstairs to my bedroom, and my heart would pound. I don't notice this now.
12. Light sensitivity is improving, the sunshine is not so painful."

Hypothyroidism (low thyroid)

It may be that hypothyroidism is more undiagnosed than we have previously thought. These symptoms can be present for three or four decades, never being diagnosed. A small dose of thyroid hormone supplement may change the entire life. Symptoms of hypothyroidism may not all occur in any one person, but several of the following must be present to make a diagnosis:

- depression
- difficulty concentrating
- constipation
- cold extremities
- goiter
- poor resistance to infection
- delayed reflexes
- decreased concentration
- dry skin
- lack of energy, fatigue
- infertility
- cold intolerance
- slowed heart rate
- hair loss
- hoarseness
- anemia
- mental impairment
- fluid retention
- weight gain despite a loss of appetite
- increased cholesterol and triglycerides
- disrupted menstrual period (heavy or scant)
- weak muscles with stiffness and cramps

Treatment

Once the diagnosis is made, an attempt should be made to treat the hypothyroidism with natural means rather than with the hormone, using the supplement only as a last resort.

Omit margarine. Use a salt-free, oil-free, sugar-free diet until the thyroid is under control. Blood fats tend to be abnormally elevated. Fluid tends to accumulate, therefore, drink water abundantly to encourage the kidneys to throw off water.

Use oats, bananas, and plantain. Eat one serving of oats daily. A thyroid stimulatory nutrient is thought to be a component of oats.

Avoid corn, and some say to avoid soy products, but others say to use soy products therapeutically for low thyroid. In general, "vegetables" tend to suppress the thyroid, especially those listed for treatment of hyperthyroidism. Fruits can be more generally eaten. Avoid thyroid inhibiting foods as discussed in the hyperthyroid section.

Drink a cup of dulse tea daily, or sprinkle a little kelp on foods for flavoring daily instead of salt, for iodine. These foods tend to normalize the thyroid function.

Try to get sunshine on the skin every day the sun shines.

Exercise stimulates the sluggish thyroid. Increase exercise to three to five hours daily.

Take a hydrotherapy treatment to the adrenal area daily by either a cold compress from the shoulder blades and downward toward the waist on both sides under the shoulder blades or direct a cold shower to the same area. The reason to stimulate the adrenals is that they directly stimulate the thyroid.

Take a cool shower mornings and nights. The water temperature should be about 96°F or 97°F (skin temperature).

Direct a cold spray from the shower to the adrenal areas followed by tapotement (tapping with fingertips) over the area immediately beneath the shoulder blades to reflexively stimulate the adrenals, which will indirectly stimulate the thyroid. The tapping position is located by drawing a line between the lower angle of the shoulder blade and the waist at the side and estimating exactly halfway between those two points. Then, slide your finger from that point to the spine. You have now located the upper pole of the kidney. About three quarters of an inch above that point is the location of the adrenal. Forcefully tap your fingers, hand over hand, your wrists being like a hinge, to throw your fingertips onto the selected area. Follow the tapping with rubbing, as your fingertips should have caused a bit of smarting.

Hot compresses for six minutes followed by ice cold compresses 30 to 60 seconds can be stimulatory to the adrenals. Do three to five changes twice a day for seven days, then once a day for 30 days.

Use a charcoal compress over the thyroid every night during the entire night.

Do not use electric blankets or heating pads to warm up in bed, but force the body to put forth the energy to bring the body temperature up to a comfortable level. Regulation of body heat is a function partly of the thyroid. The brief period of coolness just after going to bed will stimulate the thyroid. An underactive or overactive thyroid gland affects every cell in the body, as the thyroid hormone affects the metabolism of all body tissues.

The following herbs may be useful: echinacea, chaste tree, dandelion, licorice root, milk thistle seed, hawthorn berry, bayberry, Irish moss, motherwort, oak bark, mandrake, poke root, false unicorn, astragalus, camomile, bladderwrack, *coleus forskohlii* and *commiphora mukul-guggul,* and Siberian ginseng. Use the same herbs as for PMS to stimulate or normalize hormone levels in women.

Check the temperature each morning before arising out of bed to get basal metabolic temperature. The measurement can be made in the mouth, the rectum, the vagina, or the armpit. If you are a mouth breather, select one of the other areas to measure temperature. If you keep your arms over your head when you sleep, select one of the other sites to measure. Armpit temperature is generally lower than oral temperature by 0.8°F, rectal and vaginal 0.8°F higher. You should use two thermometers at the same time, one in the mouth, and one in the armpit or other place you intend to use regularly, to check what your readings are. Thermometers should be shaken down the night before and left on the nightstand so that your muscular activity will not run your temperature up.

- For armpit temperature, if the temperature is consistently between 97.8°F and 98.2°F, you are normal.
- If above 98.2°F, then you may have an overactive thyroid.
- If you are below 97.8°F, you may be hypothyroid.

A number of factors can raise the temperature such as ovulation, pregnancy, infection, dreams, physical exertion before or after awakening. Some factors may lower the temperature such as heart failure, depression, asthma, lung diseases, emotional stress, or body position (arms away from body).

Thyroid supplementation

The use of a thyroid supplement may cause severe side effects. Doctors once said that while thyroid supplementation "may do you no good, it will do you no harm." We now know it can occasionally cause physical problems, sometimes severe, or even death.

Cardiac arrest is one of those rare things caused by excessive thyroid supplementation. In the person whose cardiac reserves are very low, the giving of thyroid supplementation may increase the metabolism more than the heart muscle is capable of supporting. A cardiac arrest may be the result.

Adrenal insufficiency can occur for very much the same reason as cardiac arrest. The adrenals will be functioning slowly because of the poor thyroid hormone, as every organ in the body is slowed in its metabolism because of thyroid insufficiency. To increase the need of tissues for metabolic support at a time when the adrenals have not yet recovered sufficiently from their having been low in thyroid, now makes the body recognize an adrenal insufficiency and will begin overproduction of adrenalin.

Diabetes mellitus or insipidus can be made worse by thyroid supplementation. Anticoagulants can be upset. The dosage in patients taking anticoagulants must be readjusted when thyroid supplementation is begun, and more Coumadin may be needed. In newborns, synostosis (closure of the ends of the growing bones before growth completion) can be caused by thyroid supplementation. For the skull bones to close early can mean the brain does not have enough room to develop as well as it should.

Thyroid supplementation also increases the need for insulin. Interestingly, estrogen supplementation increases the production of certain thyroid fractions, particularly thyroid binding globulin, and may act like giving thyroid hormone.

Thyroid supplementation will increase the need of antidepressants in many patients. It may turn a simple case of depression into a case of agitated depression. Cardiac arrhythmias may occur. Digitalis may become more toxic with thyroid supplementation.

For cretins, those who are born hypothyroid, after three years of supplementation, one should stop taking the thyroid medication. It may be that the thyroid will start up on its own after a bit of maturity occurs.

Angina and tachycardia may occur with thyroid supplementation, even without thyroid toxicity.

Hair loss occurs in some persons taking thyroid supplementation. Upon withdrawing the thyroid supplementation, the hair usually grows back within a year.

One complication may be osteoporosis. The longer a thyroid hormone is taken, and the higher the dose, the greater the likelihood of osteoporosis.

A few years ago some research was published relating thyroid supplementation with increased risk of breast cancer. Subsequent research has not supported this earlier finding. Nevertheless, some caution should be used when deciding to use any hormone supplementation. Certainly no woman should take thyroid supplement unless there are clear indications and the many natural remedies to stimulate thyroid function are not successful after an adequate trial.

Tic Douloureux, Trigeminal Neuralgia

This is a burst of pain, more frequent in women, consisting of an intense stabbing pain that strikes one or a combination of two or three of the facial branches supplied by the fifth cranial nerve. The attacks come in flashes without warning, violent, knifelike darts of pain. The face becomes twisted in spasms, and tears may flow freely, as well as saliva. The seizure lasts a few seconds and may clear up spontaneously with varying periods of relief. The forehead and eye may be involved, or the side of the face, lips, chin, or tongue. Usually the pain is on only one side.

Marginal mineral deficiencies in those with tic douloureux lead to a sensitive immune system, which can develop allergies. These individuals are also sensitive to stresses. In both adults and especially children, tics can develop more easily during these periods.

Treatment

Perform very carefully an Elimination and Challenge diet. (See "Elimination and Challenge Diet" in the *Dietary Information* section.)

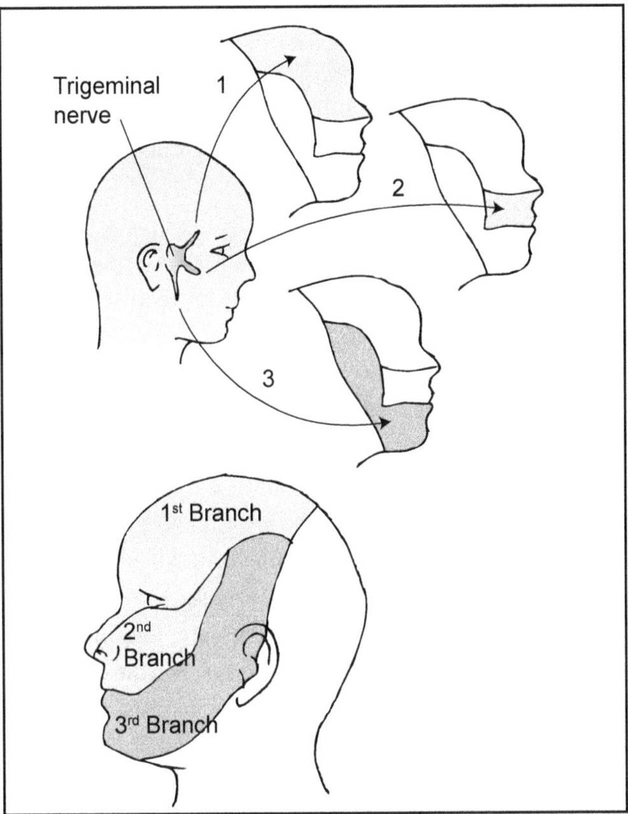

Administer vitamin B3. (See also "Food Nutrients–Food Chemicals for Disease" in the *Dietary Information* section.)

Try the same treatment as for cluster headaches.

Obey the natural laws of health.

A naturopath skilled in the use of bee venom says that trigeminal neuralgia can be successfully treated with bee venom. It is necessary to start with one sting per day; then to increase the number, one per day, until the fifth day; then five per day until the trigeminal neuralgia goes away. Usually only a few days are required, even for long-standing cases.

Tinnitus

Tinnitus is a ringing, roaring, or hissing in one or both ears, and may be caused by injury of the auditory nerve in childhood from an injury to the ears, various drugs, aspirin use, or to a brain disorder or various diseases in the head such as tumors. Occasionally wax in the ears is the cause of the noises.

Tinnitus was formerly thought to be only caused by a damaged ear; it has now recognized as originating in the brain itself. What happens is that an injury to the ears damages the auditory nerve. Then the brain rewires itself and may cause electrical signals that register as ringing. More than 10 percent of adults over the age of 70 are troubled by tinnitus.

White noise to mask the ringing has been the most important method of treatment up to the present time.

One patient took 8,000 IU of vitamin A once a day, and after a short period of time it cleared up her tinnitus.

Treatment

Use a low-salt, low-sugar, and low free-fat diet. Adopt a plant-based diet. Also, treat yourself for food sensitivities with an Elimination and Challenge diet. (See "Elimination and Challenge Diet" in the *Dietary Information* section.)

Avoid fatigue and stress. Avoid noisy environments, the use of alcohol, nicotine, caffeine (even if the beverages are decaffeinated), and marijuana. Aspirin is famous for producing head noises. A host of drugs have tinnitus as a side effect from Accutane and Achromycin to Zosyn and Zyloprim (*Alternative and Complementary Therapies,* May-June 1996, 145). Those drugs used for blood pressure, diuresis, arthritis, certain antibiotics, epilepsy medicines, and those given to control cholesterol are particularly likely to cause ringing in the ears. A person taking calcium channel blockers may develop ringing in the ears but will recover in 1 to 30 days after withdrawal of the drug (*Lancet* 343 [1994]: 1229).

Tinnitus is usually the most disturbing at night when all else is quiet. If the person will simply turn on an electric fan in the bedroom or put some other "white noise" in the bedroom, the tinnitus loses its annoyance. "White noise" may be the hum of an air conditioner or the gentle bubbling of running water, etc.

One patient reported that her ringing disappeared after her dentist corrected an uneven bite caused by a previous filling. Another patient told of a 60 percent clearing of her ringing in the ears the very day after she had a number (about 10) of silver fillings replaced by composite fillings.

Ginkgo biloba can be of benefit in reducing ringing in the ears. It increases blood flow to many internal structures. The dosage of 120 to 160 milligrams per day is therapeutic for tinnitus. While not every patient in a large study had a clearing of the ringing in the ears, many had a significant reduction (*Clin Otolaryngol.* 1999; 24:164).

Tonsillitis

Use the massage formula that follows to massage the throat and chest twice a day using gentle downward strokes for the throat and circular motions for the chest. The feet may also be massaged. Keep the feet warm at all times.

One ounce of base oil such as almond oil or jojoba oil (or olive oil in a pinch) to which has been added two drops of eucalyptus oil, one drop of tea tree oil, two drops of sandalwood oil, and one drop of thyme oil. The most important of these oils is the eucalyptus oil. Lavender oil or sage oil may be substituted for sandalwood or thyme oil. Dip your finger into the oil mixture and carefully insert it into the mouth and reach back as far as possible and rub the tonsillar area. The patient must breathe rapidly to minimize gagging while you massage the tonsils with the oil mixture. Do not dip the finger into the oil a second time, as viruses can live in the oils. Pour out into a smaller container enough to massage both tonsils.

Toothache

(See "Dental Care" in the *Conditions and Diseases* section.)

Tourette's Syndrome

Tourette's syndrome is characterized by involuntary or only slightly controllable outbursts of behavior that is out of context of the moment—facial grimaces or contortions, off color words or profanity, strange body movements, or strange sounds.

We have had two cases of Tourette's syndrome: one a 12-year-old boy in our patient program and the other an off-campus patient whom we advised but did not actually oversee his program. The following program should be instituted for two years without interruption. We found it to be helpful in both cases. The essential features of the program are as follows.

Country living is ideal for these children. The life should be as simple as it is possible to make it. The patient should go to bed early, and an easy but strict regularity in all things should characterize the life.

The patient should be given a non-stimulatory, plant-based diet, without free fat, caffeinated drinks (even if decaffeinated), sugar, honey, malt, rice syrup, dairy products, eggs, salty foods, gluten grains (wheat, barley, rye, oats), vinegar, or spices such as cinnamon, cloves, nutmeg, ginger, or black or red pepper. This diet should be carefully followed for three years. All "fast foods" and restaurant foods are likely to be stimulating to the nervous system and must be avoided.

No alcohol or tobacco should be ingested.

Fever baths three times a week should be performed.

No television, exciting reading, competitive games, or contact with children outside the home should be allowed. Home schooling is ideal for these children, and has been of the greatest help in controlling the problem.

There must be no overnight parties or parties of any kind. The child should lead a simple life.

Every night the child should go to bed in his own bed. At least three hours of sleep should be acquired before midnight each night, and four are better.

Train the child to recognize when an outburst is likely to occur and to pray for divine assistance to control the behavior fully. Each episode that has been controlled should be reinforced by a word of praise—"That was good," "You are making progress," "Let's take a walk and pick wild flowers for the dining table," etc. Ignore failures.

Pray with and for the child for complete control.

The mind should be occupied with purposeful labor, and time should be devoted to doing something for someone else.

One study showed that those with Tourette's syndrome had much better control of muscle tics and verbal outbursts if they wore nicotine patches (*Newsweek,* March 6, 2000, 53).

Magnesium supplementation may be helpful in controlling some of the symptoms of this tic. Several coexisting physical conditions with Tourette's include allergy, asthma, ADHD, obsessive compulsive disorder, anxiety, depression, restless leg syndrome, migraine, bruxism, heart arrhythmia, and heightened sensitivity to sensory stimuli including an exaggerated startle response (*Medical Hypothesis* 58, no. 1 [January 2002]: 47). These conditions are strongly related to food sensitivities, so we suggest performing the Elimination and Challenge diet. ("Elimination and Challenge Diet" in the *Dietary Information* section.)

Supplements such as catnip, skullcap, and valerian root teas, and magnesium sulfate (one-half teaspoon twice a day for a child) may be helpful.

Trigger Finger

(See "Skeletal Problems" in the *Conditions and Diseases* section.)

Tuberculosis

While TB is generally considered to be a pulmonary infection, it can actually infect many areas. It is caused by a very powerful germ that is not highly contagious, except with prolonged contact.

TB is still a big killer, killing more people (three million a year) than all other infectious diseases combined, the world over. About one-third of the world's population is infected with the TB germ, and eight million people get sick with it every year.

Between 1985 and 1991 the incidence of TB in the United States rose 13 percent overall, but in some U.S. cities the incidence of TB more than doubled. A new form is on the rise—multiple drug resistant TB (MDR TB). Antibiotics are failing more and more. If a hospital receives more than 200 TB patients in one year, from 1 to 10 percent of the hospital workers will come down with TB each year. Ventilation of rooms helps remarkably to reduce the incidence. For each complete exchange of indoor air for outdoor air, the concentration of infectious particles was reduced by 63 percent. Ultraviolet light can kill the germ, especially if the humidity is low (*Journal of Health and Healing* 18, no. 3 [1995]: 21).

In addition to the treatments listed in the case report, massage may be helpful. Get a full body massage one to three times a week to boost the immune system.

Use echinacea and golden seal for the immune system and for tissue healing. Use mullein and red clover for cough and as an antitubercular antimicrobial. Take one tablespoon each of echinacea and golden seal and boil gently for 25 minutes in one quart of water. Pour it all into a bowl containing one to two tablespoons each of red clover and mullein. Cover and steep for 30 minutes. Make fresh daily. One quart is one day's dosage.

Case Report

This is the story of a woman who had a long struggle with tuberculosis. In her late twenties she had her first attack of TB. She suffered 19 hemorrhages in 21 days, and it was feared she would not live.

She then spent 13 months in the TB sanatorium. No sugar was allowed as "it drew on the calcium which the lungs needed to enclose the germs in calcium capsules." She could have plenty of dried and fresh fruits and nuts. She learned that the most favorable diet should contain no meat, milk, eggs, or cheese. She took a cold shower every day. As soon as she was able to walk, she walked as far as she could without getting too tired. Working in the flowerbeds and vegetable gardens was also useful. She was given instruction on nutrition and general health, and it was emphasized that "contentment is the greatest thing in the cure." After 13 months she was pronounced "an arrested case" and allowed to return home.

She was well for seven years, but at age 36, after three years of a heavy program involving day and night work, she suddenly experienced a lung hemorrhage one night. This time, in a different sanatorium, she was given a very different program that consisted of absolute bed rest. However, she grew weaker and weaker and started coughing more and more. Her evening temperature gradually rose higher until it reached 102°F every evening. She coughed so much that her throat got raw. She suffered intense pain any time she tried to talk. Silence therapy was begun, as well as several drug therapies for her throat.

Her case deteriorated, and the doctors sent her home to die. She was not able to walk without assistance. Her outlook was so hopeless that she gave all her clothes away except something to be buried in. Yet, she lived 51 more years with no other breakdown with TB. Here is how she did it.

Her husband had taken nursing training and began an altogether different routine as soon as they got home. It was summer so he kept her out-of-doors all day, but not in direct sun, especially not during the middle of the day. He believed exercise for patients was a must. So with his help she walked from her chair 10 steps out and back, three times a day for one week; the next week 20 steps and the next 30, and so on until she could walk all by herself. Soon she was able to walk one-quarter mile three times a day. Then she began to take two baskets to pick up sticks for kindling the next winter. Finally, she was carrying tree limbs she picked up in the hollow. All this occurred within three months from the time she left the sanatorium.

In addition to exercise, she had heard that olives are good for tuberculosis, and that a TB patient should use plenty of high calcium greens (collards, turnip greens, broccoli, etc.), which are helpful to provide the extra calcium to wall off the TB germs. Within a year she was gardening, helping her husband some in his work, and doing her own housework. She began teaching again in two years.

She had only cold treatments—no hot ones. A tepid bath was for cleansing only. She had a cold mitten friction three times a day. Because there was no shower in her home, her husband gave her cold pail pours after he finished the mitten frictions.

A heating chest pack, which begins cold, was applied on retiring at night and removed in the morning. At the sanatorium she had been coughing almost all the time, day and night. The first night she was home her husband said, "Now for a heating chest pack."

She whispered, "Oh, that will kill me. I can't stand the shock of the cold cloths put on at first, and if they're too loose one can get pneumonia."

He said, "Don't worry, I'll fix it snug enough so no air can get to you." She coughed only three times that first night. The throat pain disappeared, and she was able to stop the silence therapy.

Not long after starting the hydrotherapy, her temperature became normal. She slept eight hours at night and took two naps during the day, one between 11 a.m. and noon, and another between at 5:00 and 6:00 p.m. She took a minimum of two glasses of water at 6:00 a.m., 11:00 a.m., and 5:00 p.m., with more in hot weather.

She died at age 87.

Typhoid

While the major diagnostic features of typhoid may be high fever with a slow pulse and diarrhea, the toxic effects of the germ fall mainly on the cardiovascular, nervous, and renal systems. Copious quantities of water and other fluids should be taken to dilute the toxins and reduce the likelihood of injury to the internal organs and assist the kidneys to keep the urine diluted. Small retention enemas may be useful for increasing the total fluids absorbed by the patient. If the patient has uncontrollable diarrhea or dysentery (bloody diarrhea), oral fluids, subcutaneous, or intravenous fluids may be the most favorable routes. When the disease is epidemic, in untreated cases the mortality of typhoid varies from 20 to 40 percent. With all forms of hydrotherapy, the mortality drops to 7.5 percent, and may be as low as 1 percent, about the same or better than with antibiotic therapy.

The treatments have three objectives: (1) elimination of the invading germs; (2) elimination of the toxins; (3) protection, maintenance, and comfort of the patient. As in all serious illnesses, treatments may need to involve all modalities of simple treatments—diet, massage, herbal remedies, active and passive exercise, charcoal, and water used internally and externally. To promote the most energetic phagocytic activity of white blood cells, food should be given on a regular schedule, two or three small meals daily, containing no free fats or sugars, and composed mainly of vegetables, fruits, and whole grains. The so-called antibacterial "herbals" such as garlic may be liberally used. Other herbs that must be used are goldenseal and echinacea, grapefruit seed extract, black elderberry, and any other antibacterial herb grown locally or available in health food stores.

A most useful adjunct to hydrotherapy, which must not be neglected in any serious illness, is massage, used for the relief of the discomforts of fever and prolonged bed rest, to stimulate the circulation, and to enhance immune mechanisms. Use copious quantities of charcoal for diarrhea control, adsorption of toxins from the intestinal tract, and encouragement of secretion of toxins from the blood into the bowel. Give one to three heaping tablespoons in a large glass of water after each loose stool, or at least four times a day.

The most useful remedy is water, given internally in abundance, and used externally as tub baths, hot and cold foot baths, cold or hot mitten frictions, cool showers or pail pours, etc. Select the treatment based on the major symptoms experienced. Keep the head cool at any time the fever is over 101°F by cool compresses squeezed from ice water.

Gentle cold baths reduce the rate of complications, especially in the respiratory and circulatory tracts. Hemorrhage from the gastrointestinal tract can be treated by brief (two to three minutes only) hot applications to the spine at 115°F to 120°F (*Journal of the American Medical Association* 34 [March 17, 1900]: 675).

Rather than hot saline bowel irrigations because of the danger of perforation, which is naturally greater in an infection of the bowel, it is safer to use the hot spine applications. Do not repeat the hot applications to the spine more frequently than once an hour.

Use external cold compresses and charcoal poultices to the abdomen.

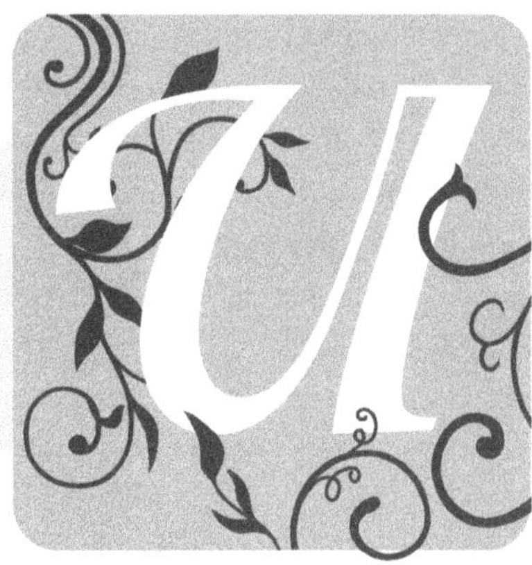

Ulcerative Colitis

(See "Colitis, Crohn's Disease, Ulcerative Colitis, Regional Enteritis" in the *Conditions and Diseases* section.)

Ulcers - Gastric, Peptic, Duodenal, Pyloric

An ulcer is a cavity in the lining and wall of the esophagus, stomach, pylorus, or duodenum. Gastric ulcers are peptic ulcers occurring in the stomach; duodenal ulcers are peptic ulcers occurring in the first 11 inches of the intestine. Duodenal ulcer is found in males about four times as often as in females, and is most frequent in 25 to 40-year-old men. Gastric ulcers occur in males two-and-one-half times as often as in females and is most frequently found in the 40 to 55 age group. Duodenal ulcers occur 10 times more frequently than gastric ulcers. In the United States 5 to 15 percent of the population have ulcers, but probably only about half of them are diagnosed. Many ulcers never produce symptoms severe enough to lead to diagnosis. Peptic ulcers apparently have somewhat of a tendency to run in families as they are two to two-and-a-half times more likely to occur in siblings of those who have ulcers. Ulcers tend to flare up during the spring and fall of the year.

Pain located just beneath the breastbone is a typical symptom of ulcers. Pain most frequently may radiate to the back in some cases. The pain is often considered to be heartburn or an empty stomach. The pain appears when the stomach is empty and is relieved by the intake of food. Some ulcers are not diagnosed until the person vomits blood. Severe ulcers cause pain at night and may awaken the patient at 2:00 or 3:00 a.m.

Causes

- Infection by *Helicobacter pylori* followed by increased acid secretion.
- Failure to drink sufficient water.
- Use of aspirin or other NSAIDs (non-steroidal anti-inflammatory drugs).
- Allergies or food sensitivities. Test yourself for allergies by omitting the 10 food groups known to cause most food sensitivities: (1) milk, (2) coffee, tea, colas, and chocolate, (3) citrus fruits and juices, (4) corn, wheat, rice, and yeast, (5) eggs, pork, beef, and fish, (6) tomatoes, potatoes, strawberries, and apples, (7) peanuts, soy products, and all beans, (8) cane sugar, cinnamon, and all spices, (9) lettuce, onion, and garlic (10) nuts and seeds. After two weeks begin adding back groups in the following order: #4, 7, 10, 3, 6, 9, 8, while permanently eliminating #1, 2, 5, putting at least three days between the reintroduction of food groups.
- White bread seems to act the same way tobacco does in the production of ulcers. Researchers felt that whole-grain bread might be of benefit to ulcer patients. Also the use of alcohol, and excessive dietary sugar, salt, and fat can causes ulcers.
- Insufficient intake of linolenic acid from nuts, seeds, whole grains, and beans may cause ulcers.

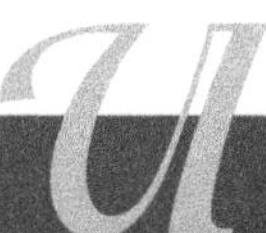

- Inadequate chewing, overeating, or under-eating. All food should be chewed to a cream before swallowing. Overeating and eating between meals slows gastric emptying, promotes excessive acid, and encourages ulcers.

Treatment

Ulcer treatment has changed drastically in the past few years. Frequent feedings, milk intake, and a bland diet are now discarded. It is now known that the calcium in milk stimulates acid production rather than decreasing it as was vigorously taught for many years. Milk does indeed initially neutralize stomach acid, but then the calcium promotes the secretion of gastrin, a hormone which triggers the release of more acid, giving a rebound effect.

Acid stimulation is not the only unfavorable result of alternating milk and cream and antacids on a regular basis during the waking hours. The incidence of myocardial infarcts (heart attacks) was more than twice as high in a group of ulcer patients treated with this regiment than in two other control groups. It is felt that the treatment caused the myocardial infarctions and deaths.

The bland diet has also been discarded. Bland diets do not relieve ulcer pain, nor do they speed healing of ulcers. Not only are they ineffective, but as a rule they are poor nutritionally.

You may very properly start your treatment routine with a fast for twenty-four hours. Drink plenty of water at room temperature, and do not fear that you will have severe pain. Most patients are surprised at the reduction of pain by fasting. Use licorice and hot applications to control pain. The presence of any food in the upper gastrointestinal tract is one of the chief stimulants to acid secretion, and reducing the frequency of food intake is far more important than the composition of the food. The six-feeding program can actually be harmful to the patient with an ulcer. The bedtime feeding is particularly dangerous. Gastric acid production is known to follow a circadian rhythm. We recommend a two-meal plan, with breakfast around 7 a.m. and dinner at about 1 p.m. with no between-meal snacks. Regularly scheduled meals allow one to take advantage of the rhythmic production of acid. If an evening meal is necessary, it should be light and eaten early.

Gastric ulcers may be caused by food stagnation in the stomach. Eating between meals slows gastric emptying and causes stagnation.

Chew food properly. Proper mastication mixes urogastrone from the salivary glands with food. Urogastrone protects the intestinal mucosa from erosion in animal tests.

Cabbage and several green leafy vegetables contain a factor known as "anti-gizzard erosion factor," later called vitamin U. It was observed that large amounts of fresh cabbage and lettuce protected guinea pigs from ulcers. The factor was found in the juice of cabbage, thus eliminating the need to eat huge quantities of cabbage. Sixty-two ulcer patients were given at least a quart of cabbage juice daily. The average healing time for seven patients with duodenal ulcers was 10.4 days, compared to 37 days for patients with standard therapy. Six patients with gastric ulcers healed in only 7.3 days, while six patients receiving conventional therapy required 42 days.

The cabbage must be freshly squeezed, and not boiled, as boiling destroys the factor. A mixture of 75 percent cabbage juice and 25 percent tomato or celery juice was used with patients who objected to the flavor of the cabbage juice. Raw celery has also been found to be high in the factor. Some patients develop gas, abdominal distress, bloating, and constipation during the first few days of therapy, but after the fifth day of treatment, digestive disturbances are rare. If symptoms become severe, the juice may be eliminated for a day.

Ordinarily it takes four to five pounds of cabbage to produce one quart of juice. Only fresh, green cabbage should be used. Wilted cabbage contains considerably less factor, and cabbage and cabbage juice held at room temperature for two or three days loses most anti-ulcer potency. Spring, summer, and late summer cabbages are suitable for use, but winter cabbages have very little juice.

Cabbage juice maintains its anti-ulcer activity for at least three weeks if frozen and preserved at approximately 0°C. The juice may be taken in four or five 6 to 8 ounce servings.

Aloe vera gel has been used in the treatment of peptic ulcers with good success. Two tablespoons of gel taken four times a day appears to be an effective dose. The author recommends that after healing of the ulcer, patients continue taking a single tablespoonful of aloe vera gel at bedtime. His group of patients had no ulcer recurrences after 18 months of follow-up. Apparently the gel inhibits the secretion of hydrochloric acid.

A diet high in sugar stimulates acid production. A high sugar diet for only two weeks drove stomach acid levels up by 20 percent in a group of healthy volunteers.

Dr. Maxwell Berry of Emory University reported to the 1956 meeting of the American College of Gastroenterology that 75 percent of peptic ulcer patients also have the

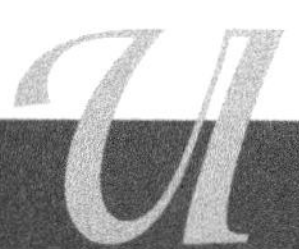

hypoglycemic syndrome. He stated that there was tremendous acid production in the stomachs of patients with low blood sugar. He feels that a very large percentage of people with the hypoglycemic syndrome will develop ulcers. Any problem with blood sugar should be treated.

Potatoes are often very helpful to peptic ulcer patients. Vitamin C has an important healing influence on wounds, and potatoes are high in vitamin C. Furthermore, potatoes have an alkaline reaction that assists in acid neutralization. Two or more potato feedings daily may be helpful. Potatoes may be baked, boiled, mashed, etc., but should not be fried, and milk should not be added.

Dried sweet almonds, well-chewed, raise the pH of the gastric juice, decrease hydrochloric acid production, and significantly inhibit peptic activity.

Ripe olives are known to be soothing to the stomach. Four to six olives may be taken with meals. Use only black or green ripe olives; avoid those canned in vinegar.

Millet is soothing to the gastrointestinal tract, and is usually well tolerated by peptic ulcer patients. Eat a low protein diet, as acid is formed most freely in response to the presence of protein in the stomach.

Peel, slice thinly, and spread plantains on a baking sheet and dry slowly in a barely warm oven. When thoroughly dry, pulverize in a blender. Take one tablespoon three times daily in water. This is a healing agent.

Caffeine and caffeine-containing beverages cause a prolonged increase in stomach acid output. Even decaffeinated coffee stimulates gastric secretion and should not be used as factors in coffee are harmful in addition to caffeine.

Do not smoke. Smokers have more gastric and duodenal ulcers, a higher death rate from ulcers, and slower healing of their ulcers. Smoking inhibits pancreatic bicarbonate secretion and promotes duodenogastric reflux.

For peptic ulcer pain apply an ice bag to the abdomen just above the navel or to the portion of the spine between the shoulder blades.

Remember that exercise neutralizes stress. Exercise daily outside in the fresh air.

Attention should be paid to dress. The extremities should be well clothed to balance the circulation and avoid congestion in the abdomen.

Avoid the use of any drugs. Aspirin has long been known to induce gastrointestinal bleeding. A single dose of aspirin tablets is sufficient to induce prolongation of bleeding time, and the effect may persist for up to two days. Alka-seltzer is irritating to the gastric mucosa. Steroids have potent adverse effects and may increase the incidence of complications. It is felt that many drugs (including aspirin) inhibit the synthesis of prostaglandins, and some feel that prostaglandins exert a protective influence of the mucosa.

Herbs for peptic ulcer include the following:

- Chew and swallow two tablets of deglycerized licorice tablets on arising, between meals, and at bedtime. Two more can be used at any time for pain, especially at night. This substance markedly increases upper bowel mucus production to give a protective coating.
- Take golden seal capsules four times a day just after eating and at bedtime.
- Echineacea can be taken in the same dosage as golden seal.
- Take grapefruit seed extract, which is antibacterial in nature, four drops in a glass of water three times a day. It is quite bitter, but if tolerated, increase after about a week to six drops in water three times a day.
- Myrrh or mastic gum is also good for peptic ulcer disease. Use the dosage given on the package four times a day.
- You may also use aloe vera, chamomile, licorice, slippery elm, catnip, and papaya.

Uremia

Uremia results from a failure of kidney function. It may be acute as from kidney injury or chronic as from chronic glomerulonephritis.

In acute cases give two treatments daily. Fluids may have to be severely restricted as the kidneys may not be able to put out much water, and the patient will become waterlogged and swollen. Gauge the intake by the amount of urine production, sweating, and the fluid content of the bowel movements.

Give a hot bath at water temperatures of about 106°F to 108°F for 15 to 20 minutes. The temperature level should be determined by the strength of the patient.

An alternative to the bath for very weak or sick patients is to put the patient in a lower-half body pack and cover the abdomen with a fomentation pack for 15 minutes. (See "Hydrotherapy" in the *Natural Remedies* section.)

Follow either treatment with a three-minute cold rub to the abdomen and the lower back, turning the patient on one side for the rub. Repeat four times. If necessary for the warmth and comfort of the patient, put a heating pad or several hot water bottles around the legs and over the thighs or

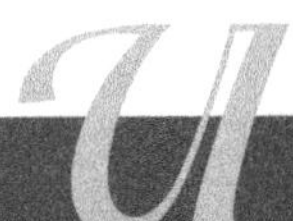

feet; or renew the hot pack underneath after the second cold rub. Finish with a brief cleansing shower or a sponge bath.

Several hours later put the patient into a very warm bath at 102°F or 103°F (or a full-body fomentation, add an abdominal pack, wrap the feet in a fomentation pack, and cover the patient well) to cause profuse sweating. Keep the face cool with an electric fan or cold cloths. Check the pulse periodically, and keep it well below 110 in a debilitated patient. Continue the bath or pack for 30 minutes. Finish with a cleansing shower to remove sweat, even from the head. Repeat daily until recovery, or the patient has entered a chronic failure stage. If the patient is in chronic failure he may become waterlogged and swollen. If so, this same treatment may be done to get rid of excessive body water. If shortness of breath occurs, you may put blood pressure cuffs on three extremities at a time, rotating the one not in a cuff (or tourniquet) every 15 minutes. At this stage dialysis should be arranged if possible.

Treat uremia, either acute or chronic, with large charcoal poultices over the abdomen or back each night, and give by mouth one heaping tablespoon of powdered charcoal in a glass of water. An alternative to powdered charcoal is four to eight charcoal tablets by mouth four times daily. Give enemas as needed to prevent constipation from the charcoal. A charcoal enema may be helpful in removing toxins. Chronic, progressive uremia indicates more than 90 percent loss of kidney function and will require renal dialysis for survival.

Urinary Tract Infection

(See "Cystitis" in the *Conditions and Diseases* section.)

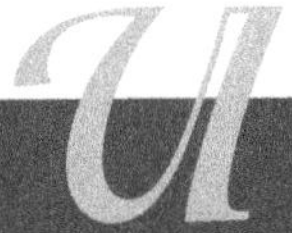

Varicose Veins

Varicose veins are swollen, sometimes tortuous, and sometimes painful vessels that have filled with a collection of blood. They are often without symptoms, but may look unsightly. Some women feel symptoms such as fullness, heaviness, aching, or pain in the legs, especially at about the time of the menstrual period, or after standing or sitting for a long time.

For pain in varicose veins, simmer a tablespoon of white oak bark in one quart of water for 30 minutes. The water may be strained, but that is not necessary. Store in a jar in the refrigerator. When the varicose veins give pain, rub the white oak bark tea over the varicose veins. A decoction of witch hazel can be made and used in the same way. Vinegar compresses as hot as can be tolerated may also help painful varicosities, whether they are on the legs or on the vulva. The compresses will relieve pain and reduce swelling and fluid retention. If this treatment is followed by putting on support pantyhose, the result is especially good. The hot vinegar or the herbal teas can be applied as often as five times a day. A tincture of witch hazel can also be rubbed onto painful varicose veins with good results. Bayberry or bilberry (berries or leaves) can also be used as the tincture or simmered in the fashion given above for white oak bark.

For bleeding varicose veins, especially after childbirth or even for cervical lacerations after childbirth, both shepherd's purse and cayenne in tincture form can be very helpful.

Valves in veins permit only one-way blood flow. In varicose veins the valves are damaged and stretched, so they no longer prevent backward flow. Thus, the veins dilate, becoming quite large in some cases.

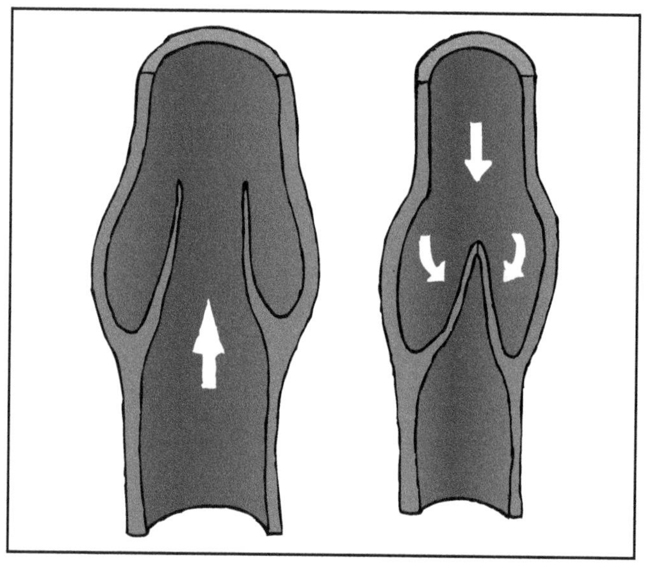

Hydrotherapy is very helpful for the pain of varicose veins or swelling, stasis dermatitis, or ulceration. Use the leg bath described in the "Hydrotherapy" entry in the *Natural Remedies* section.

Oxerutins from horse chestnut seeds given by mouth to patients with moderate swelling of the legs from varicose veins showed significant improvement with the horse chestnut extract (*Lancet* 347 [1996]: 292). The treatment period lasted eleven weeks and the dosage was 500 milligrams of oxerutins twice a day.

For varicose ulcers pick the fuzzy soft green leaves of mullein, steep them in hot water for five minutes, cool sufficiently to bear touching, and apply the leaves directly to the open sores, wrapping with a clean cloth. This relieves pain in sores and promotes healing. Apply daily for several weeks or until the leg ulcers are healed.

Vertigo

(See "Dizziness, Ménière's Disease, Vertigo" in the *Conditions and Diseases* section.)

Viral Diseases

There are several viral and metabolic conditions that may be helped by Coenzyme Q10 (CoQ10), in addition to the well-known use for nourishing and healing the heart muscle, these include AIDS, cancer, lung problems, pyorrhea, gastric ulceration, overweight, muscular dystrophy, and allergy (*Alternative Medicine Review* 1 [1996]: 11–17).

Vision Problems

For macular degeneration, one-half cup of spinach once a week will reduce your likelihood of coming down with this disease by one-third.

For diabetic cataracts, and glaucoma use one teaspoon of cascara sagrada in one quart of chia tea daily, along with one cup of nopales cactus daily. Additionally, wash the eyes once daily in eye bright tea. Drink one cup of eye bright tea daily.

Bilberry tea is specific as a strengthening and healing herb for the eyes. Take a cup of the tea four times a day.

Vitiligo

(See "Skin Diseases" in the *Conditions and Diseases* section.)

Vomiting

Treatment for Common Nausea and Vomiting

The treatment of choice in this kind of nausea is activated charcoal powder given in one to four tablespoon doses mixed with water and drunk with a straw. Every vomiting episode should be followed by taking the complete dose, the more intense the vomiting, the larger the dose. Even very severe nausea should receive the full dose, even if no vomiting is involved. If the dose is thrown up, take it again immediately.

Cold compresses to the head, or an ice bag to the stomach area, can often stop vomiting. A cold washcloth around the neck can stop nausea.

Some of the suggestions in the section below are also helpful for general nausea and vomiting.

Treatment for Morning Sickness, Nausea and Vomiting in Pregnancy

Use three small meals daily, allowing five hours from the end of one meal to the beginning of the next, the third meal should be only whole grains and fruit and taken several hours before retiring. Normally a person should not eat even a peanut between meals, but with nausea, some kind of dry cereal or crackers may settle the stomach. As soon as possible return to the pattern of nothing between meals, as continued eating between meals causes intestinal fermentation products to circulate to the baby.

Avoid all stomach irritants such as vinegar, spices, baking soda and powder, caffeinated drinks, sugar and its substitutes, free fats (such as margarine, mayonnaise, fried foods, salad oils, or cooking oils), drugs, TVP (textured vegetarian protein), and antacids.

Never allow any overeating. Don't eat sweet or greasy foods, especially no combinations of any two or more of the following: milk, sugar, eggs, or free fats. Free fats are digested slowly and can be eliminated from the diet, including margarine. Use only whole grains, not refined or polished.

Chew your food well. This may make the difference between good digestion and poor digestion. During pregnancy, digestion is normally slow. The slowing of the digestion can result in stomach irritation and nausea. Eat your food without beverages to ensure proper salivation.

Bananas and baked potatoes are usually tolerated well. Avoid dairy products, butter, cheese, and strong flavors or odors, as these are usually not tolerated well.

Oil-free popcorn, dry cereal, and breakfast in bed have been very beneficial for some. Meat, milk, dairy products, and eggs provoke nausea and vomiting in some.

A treatment that cured one woman's nausea was two tablespoons of freshly ground flaxseed sprinkled on cereal or stirred into juice or water, once or twice daily.

Eat plenty of fresh fruits and vegetables, or drink freshly made carrot juice or apple juice, one serving in the morning and one at noon. It is most favorable to the baby to be a total vegetarian during pregnancy, but if nausea occurs, it becomes even more important than previously to the mother as well, as the high nutrient content of a plant-based diet is most favorable for the baby's growth and development.

Berries of all kinds may help with morning sickness—strawberries, blueberries, raspberries, etc. Eat one-half to one cup or more at breakfast each morning.

Arise slowly from bed. Take several minutes to get from the recumbent to the standing position. Never lie down after eating as this slows digestion further and leads to irritation of the stomach or regurgitation into the esophagus to cause heartburn.

Allow no dehydration. Many glasses of water should be taken per day (eight to ten), along with additional herbal teas. Catnip or mint teas are helpful in nausea, one cupful as needed.

A glass of very warm water with a fresh lemon twist or lemon juice and honey can eliminate nausea for many women.

A tablespoon of carob powder made into a paste with water and nibbled will stop nausea in many.

As a preventive treatment, place an ice bag over the stomach 30 minutes before arising, or before meals, or whenever the nausea can be expected. It may prevent or sometimes cure a bout of nausea. Very warm water bottles, or a heating pad, placed over the stomach can also be helpful.

The *British Medical Journal* reported the location of a pressure point in the mid forearm, two inches above the prominence of the wrist bones, that is said to help post-anesthetic nausea and might help the nausea of pregnancy. The pressure should be sustained for several minutes, applied by opposing the thumb and forefinger at the two-inch area in the soft tissues between the two bones of the forearm.

Engage in outdoor exercise daily. Gradually increase the length and pace of the exercise until the exercise reaches that of the equivalent of about three to four miles of walking daily. Never engage in vigorous physical or mental labor immediately after eating.

Fresh air is helpful for most with nausea. Even sleeping out of doors has been found helpful.

Sunbathing out-of-doors has been found very beneficial. Use care to avoid sunburning, as sunburning can intensify morning sickness.

Life during pregnancy should be a study in regularity. Put all major functions concerned with health maintenance on a set schedule, such as bowel elimination, drinking water, exercise, meals, and sleep.

The clothing must be adequate to protect the extremities from chilling, as the internal organs will become congested. The stomach, if it becomes congested, has a tendency to malfunction and give the sensation of nausea. If the extremities are chilled, the blood vessels become contracted and blood leaves them but congests another area, perhaps the stomach or the placenta, causing it to function sluggishly. Use no bands, girdles, belts, or elastic that leaves a mark on the skin.

One of the best teas we have found is available only in summer. Take a double handful of green peach tree leaves and boil for half an hour in one-half gallon of water. Cool, strain, refrigerate, and use one tablespoon as needed for nausea. Do not drink excessively with your meals.

Sweet basil tea, catnip tea, and raspberry leaf tea have all been helpful, as well as diluted golden seal tea, mint, and sage tea. Sip the teas hot or cold as desired and as often as necessary.

Tea made from two teaspoons of ginger root powder to one quart of water, boiled gently for 5 to 10 minutes, can cure most cases of nausea. Take a tablespoonful of this tea any time you feel the need. One to two capsules of ginger root powder may also be taken one to four times daily for morning sickness.

Powdered red raspberry leaves or alfalfa herbs may be put in capsules and taken four times daily.

Wild yam, catnip, cinnamon, and mint oil are also good. Mint oil may be taken in small quantities by simply wetting a small portion of a finger from a mint oil bottle. Lick the oil off the finger. Mint oil relaxes the smooth muscle of the stomach and intestine and calms nausea, usually in about 10 minutes.

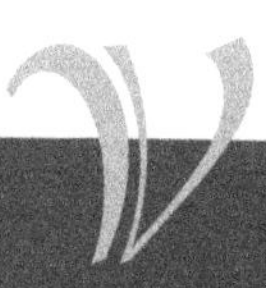

Warts

(See "Skin Diseases" in the *Conditions and Diseases* section.)

Weight Control

(See "Weight Control" in the *Supplemental Information* section for additional information.)

Sixty-four percent of American adults were judged in 1990 and 1991 to be at least some degree overweight. Since then the percentage has gone up. Obesity is the number one public health problem in the United States, almost neck and neck with smoking and drugs.

Being very strict with oneself until habits are established has been effective in changing the lifestyle for many persons who have had a problem with controlling appetite. One woman gave this as her testimony. "For example, not eating anything after dinner under any circumstances has effectively extinguished what was my lifelong night craving for food. I was known as a night grazer. This has been extremely liberating to me."

Obesity is primarily a result of lifestyle, helped along with a national preoccupation with eating. It is impossible to calculate the enormous amount of mental energy that goes into thinking about food, actually eating, and the drowsiness caused by overeating.

Once a person becomes overweight, he is likely to become highly, sometimes uncontrollably responsive to food stimuli. This is because of the stimulating quality of insulin. Overweight persons often have high blood insulin levels. We should regard being overweight as a controllable, and not a curable disorder. Being overweight is essentially an obsessive compulsive phenomenon. The compulsive overeater does not understand that the compulsion is controllable even though not curable.

Ghrelin, produced by the stomach to stimulate appetite, stops being produced when the appetite is sated. In response to the food eaten, insulin is produced by the pancreas. Insulin signals fat cells when the sugar and insulin balance are optimum. The fat cells then produce leptin, which signals the brain to turn off the appetite. If one takes in too much fat, or too much sugar, the system is altered and the appetite is not sated. Fructose is an especially crucial link to causing a sugar/insulin imbalance, insulin resistance of cells, and obesity in some people. A number of fast-foods and junk foods contain fructose such as beverages, commercial cookies, cakes, candy, and hot dogs. Another cog in the appetite wheel is the number and timing of meals throughout the day. The greater the number of eating occasions, and the later in the day these occasions occur, the greater the likelihood a person may become obese (*European Journal of Clinical Nutrition* 56 [2002]: 740).

The composition of the blood influences the absorption and secretion of the small intestine. An increase in salty and fatty foods causes an increase in glucose absorption. An increase in amino acids in blood causes a decrease in absorption of glucose and an increase in the secretion into the small intestine. Therefore, good advice for someone who is obese is "salty and fatty meals are a hazard to a weight reduction program."

Most people apparently eat about 18 percent more food than they think they are eating. According to a study

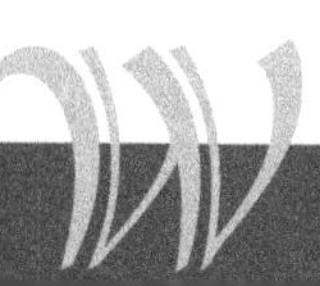

performed by the U.S. Department of Agriculture with 266 trained volunteers keeping a record of what they ate while their weight remained constant, the logs showed 18 percent less estimated than was actually eaten.

The vast majority of Americans could control their weight and cholesterol by following seven simple steps. These steps will lower the set point for weight in the body. A set point for any feature of our bodies is that point which the body recognizes as being "normal." It has to do with such things as the water level of the blood, the hemoglobin level, cholesterol level, sodium level, potassium level, and all other blood chemistry levels. These "set points" tend to creep upward with age. Is it a necessary factor of aging, or is it a problem with lifestyle, making it misinterpret excessive levels as being normal? So far as weight is concerned, it is a form of learning that recognizes a new steady state or a steady climb as being normal. It protects that position, or will climb to a higher weight by increasing appetite and reducing metabolism to maintain the higher level. To lower the body's recognized set point for weight as well as for cholesterol, the following seven steps need to be followed:

Seven Simple Steps to Weight and Cholesterol Control

1. Eliminate free fats and all dairy products. Totally and absolutely cut out all butter, margarine, mayonnaise, fried foods, cooking fats, salad oils, peanut butter, and all other nut or seed butters for the period of time required to reset the set point. It is not difficult to learn to enjoy foods without added fat. Almost all natural foods have some natural fat in them, even such fruits as apples, bananas, etc. Free fats make food more desirable but are not essential for health. You may eat the whole nuts, however, as fats from them are handled differently in the digestive process than free fats, which have been removed from their links with carbohydrates, proteins, and vitamin and mineral complexes.
2. Exercise immediately after meals for 10 to 30 minutes. Begin with a gentle stretching of the body for two to three minutes, then a slow increase in pace. Your exercise should be brisk or vigorous. Walking, yard work, vigorous house work, etc., will all suffice. Strive for one to two hours of exercise and/or useful labor per day.
3. Don't eat after 3:00 p.m.; only eat two meals a day. If you need to be sociable at dinnertime, pour yourself a cup of herbal tea and sip away. Carry tea bags with you for emergency use. Never eat a morsel, even a stalk of celery, or anything, between meals. Do not even cast a glance at other people's food. It will make you want some of it. Train yourself to look at their faces not their plates during a meal. If questioned regarding your practice, simply smile and say, "Doctor's orders." (That would be mine.)
4. The more raw foods eaten, the better it will be for your weight. If you find it particularly difficult to lose weight, try going a period of thirty days in which you eat nothing but raw foods. Breakfast could be fruits in any form (dried, canned without sugar, frozen, or fresh, but limit varieties of fruit to only three), with uncooked nuts or seeds. Lunch could be vegetables of any kind or quantity you desire along with corn on the cob or whole kernel corn; limit the varieties, however, to no more than four vegetables.
5. You should become a total vegetarian, at least until you have reached ideal weight, and probably permanently. And always bear in mind that the program that made you overweight in the first place will do it again. No animal product—meat, milk, eggs or cheese—is essential for good nutrition, or even desirable in this age of escalating disease in animals.
6. The greater variety of food you eat at one meal, the higher the set point. Have no more than four separate, simple items at a meal. A fruit salad could be apples and oranges with a generous quantity of sunflower seeds sprinkled all over it (perhaps one to two tablespoons). You may eat whatever quantity you would like of everything except nuts and seeds, which should be kept to one to four tablespoons, depending on the kind, using the following graduated scale from most fatty to least fatty: cashew, pecan, macadamia, sesame, walnut, almond, coconut, pistachio, sunflower, flax, pumpkin, and chestnut.
7. Minimize concentrated foods to lower the set points.

The motto must be "appetite under the control of reason." If you follow these seven guidelines, you will reduce your set point for weight control and cholesterol, which will help you to get a handle on these problems.

Do not eat stomach irritants as the irritation sets up motion in the stomach that sends messages to the brain indicating the stomach is hungry. These include vinegar, most drugs, hot spices such as cloves, and peppers both black and red.

All foods having high fiber content tend to have lower calories and exert a suppressive influence on the appetite. This includes beans, whole grains, fruits, and vegetables.

Outlast your cravings. Often a person suddenly has cravings for some specific food. If you force yourself to wait twenty minutes, you can reevaluate the situation, ask yourself why you think you need that food, and the craving is often much less intense. Cravings tend to build up a crescendo, peak out, and then decline. Choosing some kind of outdoor physical exercise such as a bike ride or a walk will suppress the appetite in most instances. Fats and sweets together tend to trigger the appetite and encourage cravings. Each by themselves tends to encourage appetite, but the combination is far worse.

A low-fat diet does less good if it is not accompanied by the removal of simple carbohydrates such as sugar, honey, malt, and alcohol from the diet. These simple carbohydrates can turn into saturated fats in the body and just as effectively damage the heart and blood vessels (*Journal of Clinical Investigation* 97, no. 9 [May 1996]: 2081–91).

Most people can achieve weight control very easily by making those changes in the lifestyle that will reset the set points for weight control. Some persons will need a support group. This can be most effectively achieved by organizing your own neighborhood weight control club. It may have as few as two or three people, or as many as fifteen or twenty.

Whooping Cough, Pertussis

This disease is characterized by a convulsive coughing leaving the patient out of breath and often being forceful enough to induce vomiting. A coughing or vomiting episode may be followed by a deep vocal inhalation through the mouth making a whooping sound. While children usually recover easily, whooping cough should not be treated as a trivial disease. It should be treated very carefully. If neglected, pneumonia can follow and may be fatal in young infants and the elderly. The commonest age for fatalities is under six months. With excellent family care, and attention to details of health laws, the disease can be handled better at home than in a hospital.

Symptoms during the first 10 days resemble an ordinary cold. The cough does not improve, however, and the second stage begins with the onset of the whooping sound. Isolation is desirable to prevent an infection from someone else spreading germs to the child, or exposing other children who may contract the disease. In adults who have a cold with a persistent cough for weeks, the culprit may be the whooping cough germ.

Treatment

The child should not eat large meals, as they are more prone to be vomited. The food should be nutritious, vegetarian, and free from concentrated foods such as free-fats and free-sugars. Fresh fruits and juices and plenty of water are most helpful. Each whooping episode should be followed by drinking a full glass of water to keep the secretions loose and the throat soothed.

Very young (under six months) or feeble children may require suctioning of the nose and throat to prevent aspirating secretions into the lungs and encouraging pneumonia. Water is the best cough syrup, and commercial medications for whooping cough should be avoided as a general rule as they dry secretions and promote retention of secretions, encouraging pneumonia. Sipping fenugreek or yarrow tea that has been steeped in freshly boiled water will soothe a cough.

A tepid water bath at 99°F for 10 to 15 minutes, the face and head being kept cool, will help whooping cough.

A hot bath, one minute for each year of a child's age, followed by a cool water pour and a brisk rubdown with a coarse dry towel, will usually be followed by sleep in a child who is having a hard time sleeping because of whooping cough.

Use a humidifier or steam kettle, keeping the bedroom well ventilated, but free from drafts. Tobacco smoke, cold air, and any kind of air pollutant should be strictly forbidden.

Always rinse the mouth after vomiting to prevent erosion of the enamel.

Sometimes an irritation of the skin develops from nasal discharges or vomiting. Petroleum jelly can be applied in these areas to keep the discharges off the skin.

Sunbathing will soothe a coughing spree. If it is chilly weather, a protected place should be found. Protect the eyes from the glare of the sun, particularly in small children as eye damage can result from sun exposure.

A danger in whooping cough is exhaustion from violent coughing. Besides the usual measures of good elimination, steam inhalation, light diet, and quiet, the patient will benefit by a daily or twice daily spinal steam pack. It loosens the mucus in the bronchial tubes, allays the irritating cough, intensifies the germ-killing activity of the white blood cells, and relaxes and soothes the patient. A small sip of honey-eucalyptus cough syrup may be given as often as needed. Stir a drop of eucalyptus oil into a tablespoon of honey and let the child nibble the solution.

If ever good hydration is needed, it is in whooping cough. Use every means to increase water intake, but do not give juices between meals if possible. Various types of hot or cool tea, mint, red clover, lemon grass, or catnip with a twist of lemon, a sprig of rose leaves or petals or geranium petals can all make water more appetizing. Mullein and slippery elm teas are soothing and have some expectorant effect.

Garlic is very good in whooping cough, as the active ingredient is excreted through the breath. Stir one-half teaspoon of kitchen garlic powder for each 20 pounds of the child's weight into half a glass of water, and give the solution to the child to drink.

Wilson's Disease, Copper Overload

Wilson's disease is a genetic disorder that results in excessive accumulation of copper in many parts of the body, particularly the liver. This condition is readily treatable, but if Wilson's disease is left untreated, it can be fatal.

Reliable and relatively consistent scientific data show a substantial health benefit from zinc supplementation as it blocks the excessive absorption of copper. Do not take more than 15 to 30 milligrams by pill. Zinc high foods are the safest way to increase the mineral in the body. Too much zinc by supplement has been suggested as one cause of Alzheimer's disease.

Wilson's disease is initially silent and may first be noticed as fatigue, absent menstrual periods in premenopausal women, or repeated and unexplained spontaneous abortions. In more advanced stages, there may be headaches, tremors, uncoordinated limb movements, unsteady gait, drooling, difficulty swallowing, and joint pain. There also may be strange thought patterns with unusual behaviors.

Most foods contain at least some copper, so it is not possible to avoid the metal completely. Foods high in copper, such as organ meats and oysters, should be eliminated from the diet. Sufficient copper may be obtained from such nutritious sources as nuts and legumes. Even these foods should be eaten in moderation by people with Wilson's disease. Grains contain significant amounts of copper but are important components of a healthful diet, and dietary restriction may be neither wise nor necessary, particularly if zinc is supplemented.

Zinc is known for its ability to reduce copper absorption and has been used successfully in patients with Wilson's disease, with some trials lasting for years. Researchers have called zinc a "remarkably effective and nontoxic therapy for Wilson's disease." The United States Food and Drug Administration has approved the use of zinc to treat Wilson's disease for maintenance therapy following drug therapy, although some scientists recommend that it be considered for initial therapy as well.

Zinc has also been used to keep normal copper levels from rising in people with Wilson's disease who had previously been treated successfully with prescription drugs. Zinc (50 milligrams taken three times per day) has been used for such maintenance therapy, although some researchers have used the same amount of zinc to successfully treat people with Wilson's disease who had not received drug therapy.

Zinc is so effective in lessening the body's burden of copper that a copper deficiency was reported in someone with Wilson's disease who took too much zinc (480 milligrams per day). Nonetheless, zinc may not help everyone with Wilson's disease. Sometimes increased copper levels can occur in the liver after zinc supplementation; however, leading researchers believe this increase is temporary and may not be harmful.

Zinc supplementation (25 or 50 milligrams three times daily) has also been used to successfully treat pregnant women with Wilson's disease. Management of Wilson's disease with zinc should only be undertaken with the close supervision of a doctor.

Copper is present in several dietary supplements, especially multimineral and multivitamin-mineral preparations. Supplements containing even small amounts of copper should be avoided by virtually all Wilson's disease patients.

Women's Conditions and Diseases

There are many conditions that are unique to women, and some that are much more common in women than in men, such as thyroid disease. In this section we will discuss some of these unique problems.

The Women's Health Initiative (WHI) presents evidence that hormone therapy does not prevent heart disease (*Annals of Internal Medicine* 137 [2002]: 273). In fact, the women in the treatment group had an increase of heart attacks by 29 percent. The WHI also found that combination hormone treatment significantly raised a woman's risk of invasive breast cancer, stroke, heart disease, and blood clots in the legs and lungs (*JAMA*, July 17, 2002).

Breast Cancer

(See "Breast Conditions" in the *Conditions and Diseases* section.)

Cervical Cancer

(See "Cancer" in the *Conditions and Diseases* section.)

Cervicitis

Cervicitis is an inflammation of the cervix, either acute or chronic. The most common symptom is a discharge that may cause irritation, itching, or a rash. Marital relations, careless douching, or swimming often causes it. There is a form of cervicitis called "virginal cervicitis," which is most frequently seen in unmarried girls but can be occasionally found in older women. There is redness but no erosion. The cause is not known. The discharge may have an odor or be odorless and may range in color from clear to tannish, yellowish, or brownish.

Treatment

Hot footbaths or hot half baths are very good for cervicitis. Many women get cervicitis because of habitually chilled extremities. The clothing of the lower extremities must be sufficient to keep the feet warm. That means the thighs must be warmly clothed, perhaps with several layers, to prevent losing heat.

The most important single treatment is the douche. For ordinary bacterial infections, we recommend hot garlic douches. For yeast infections use hot soda water douches, and for trichomonas infections use hot vinegar douches. If you do not know what kind of infection you have, start with the garlic, proceed to the vinegar, and end with the hot soda water, using each one for three days to test its effectiveness before switching to another one. If you get no benefit from the use of one solution, simply switch to another. Select a douche solution from our list of douche solutions described below and pour into a douche bag. The bag can be suspended from a position not more than about two feet above the hips. It may be hung on a chair-back, towel rack, shower rod, or it may be laid on the edge of the bathtub.

Sit in the tub in a semi-reclining position at about a 45-degree angle. Insert the nozzle, release the clasp, and allow the solution to flow into the vagina. Fold the lips of the vulva around the nozzle with the thumb and forefinger until sufficient solution has distended the vagina and a sense of fullness or pressure is experienced over the bladder. Shut off the clasp and hold the solution for as long as required to count slowly to 15. Let the fluid gush out. Repeat this procedure until all of the solution is used. Hang up the bag with the clasp open to encourage drainage and drying of the interior of the tube and bag. Continue douching for one month only. If discharge continues unabated after treatment, a Pap smear should be obtained.

Start a treatment series using three hot douches daily for three days for most ordinary infections, and then dropping to two douches daily for three days, then once daily for thirty days. Use all-cotton panties, and take showers rather than baths. Use no soap of any kind. Do not swim in public places or where there is any contamination of water.

Some cases of cervicitis will respond to a "perineal pour" as the only treatment. It is done simply by pouring one quart of water, to which has been added one quarter cup of vinegar, over the perineum, starting the stream into the pubic hair and allowing it to wash over the entire perineum, opening the folds with the opposite hand, even around the anus. The pour is done with each use of the bathroom, for bladder or bowel movements, and at least six times a day if possible. Keep up the pours for 30 days.

It is possible to become overly zealous and to over douche, aggravating or producing irritation. When the treatment course is over, stop.

Following are a variety of douche solutions:

- Hot water – The universally useful solution for vaginal douche is merely hot water, two to four quarts at 105°F to 110°F.
- Vinegar – For a vinegar douche, use one to four tablespoons of any kind of vinegar to each quart of hot water. For one treatment use two quarts of solution. This is the standard douche solution and should be selected for all ordinary infections and special cleansing. However, regular douching merely because you thought all women did is not recommended as it has been found that some who regularly douche have a greater tendency to develop cervical cancer.
- Baking soda – For the baking soda douche, use one teaspoon of baking soda to each quart of hot water. For one treatment use two quarts of solution. This solution is most applicable for monilia or yeast infections and should always be tried when vinegar is not successful within a reasonable treatment period, 5 to 10 days.
- Garlic – One clove of garlic may be blended in one quart of boiling water, cooled, and strained if desired. It is best to put the clove of garlic in the blender with only one cup of boiling water to blend. Put a kitchen

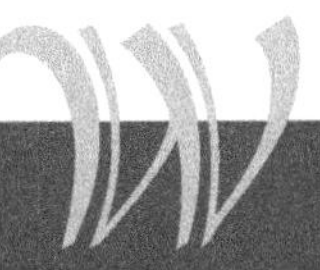

towel over the top and hold it securely as the hot water will pop the lid off if not held. Then pour in the other three cups. Use one quart of solution for a treatment. Use the garlic solution raw, or simmered for one to five minutes if the tissues are very tender and sensitive. Use it for infections that are resistant to the usual treatments or when you are uncertain which solution might be best.

- Styptic – For a styptic douche use comfrey, two heaping tablespoons of powdered tea leaves to one quart of boiling water. Mix and let it set for 15 minutes, strain, and use. For golden seal, use one tablespoon of root powder in one quart of water. Boil gently for 10 minutes. Use this douche for bleeding surfaces such as cervicitis or vaginitis.
- Charcoal – One tablespoon of charcoal may be added to a quart of water to make a charcoal douche solution for infections, ulcers, and viral diseases. It is very effective as a deodorant douche. Used hot it has more benefit.
- Lysol – Lysol is a 2.7 percent solution of phenol, water, and soap, a good antiseptic. Use one-half to one teaspoon of Lysol to one quart of water at 100°F to 105°F. Mix the solution well. Lysol occasionally causes a rash or burning. If that occurs, stop the use of Lysol, rinse off all surfaces with water (skin, vagina, and douche bag), and it should clear up promptly. May be used for ordinary antiseptic perineal care and for deodorizing the perineum, underarms, feet, or skin lesions that develop odor.
- Herbal – For trichomonas douching, thuja and bayberry tea is very helpful. Use one tablespoon of each steeped in a quart of just-boiled water for 30 minutes.

Childbirth Trauma

Any vaginal itch, cuts, burns, traumatized body parts, or perineal rash immediately after childbirth can be treated with astringent herbal compresses.

Take thin sanitary pads and cut them in half crosswise. Make strong comfrey tea by putting three tablespoons of comfrey leaves in a cup with boiling water. After half an hour, strain and pour the tea over the pads until they are saturated. Do not wring out. Put the pads on a cookie sheet or casserole dish and freeze. Remove individually and place in a labeled plastic bag. Return to the freezer. After birth of the placenta, before checking for tears, place the pads against the mother's perineum. It is soothing, healing, and slightly numbing to traumatized tissues. May be changed every hour for the first 24 hours.

Another herbal remedy that may be used for eczema, psoriasis, hives, poison ivy, or childbirth is as follows. Steep the following herbs in two quarts of boiling water: one to two ounces comfrey, two ounces shepherd's purse, one whole bulb of fresh garlic, one ounce uva ursi, one-quarter cup sea salt, and one ounce golden seal. If you are missing one or two herbs, go with what you have. After it has steeped for half an hour, strain it into a freshly scrubbed bathtub containing four to six inches of warm water. Continue the bath for 30 to 90 minutes, dipping the water onto the area involved, or onto the entire body.

Cystocele

(See "Cystitis" in the *Conditions and Diseases* section.)

Dysplasia, Cervical

The word dysplasia comes from two root words. *Dys* means abnormal and *plasia* means growth. In the cervix, dysplasia is one step short of being pre-malignant. Thus, the pathologist's reading of a tissue having the report of dysplasia, adequate follow-up and treatment must be done. The natural remedies are often curative within a few months.

Eating salads and drinking fruit juices may reduce a woman's risk of developing cervical cancer, so will avoidance of becoming overweight, breathing in tobacco in all forms, even secondhand smoke, and using coffee, tea, colas, and chocolate.

To treat dysplasia, chaparral tea can be used both orally and as a vaginal douche.

Use aloe vera gel or fresh crushed aloe pulp (the interior of the blades of aloe vera) under a contraceptive diaphragm worn overnight. The next morning remove the diaphragm and use a hot garlic douche. Repeat every day for 30 days.

Endometriosis

This condition results from the transplantation of the tissue that lines the interior of the uterus to other places such as ovaries, fallopian tubes, bowel, appendix, bladder, umbilicus, and internal abdominal wall. The cause for this transplantation is still not known for sure, but the most commonly accepted theory is that products of menstruation shed fragments of the inside of the uterus that are milked up in the fallopian tubes or the lymphatics by muscular contractions and are transplanted in other places while still living and take root. It is our belief that sexual excitation or marital relations during the menstrual period lead to uterine contractions that could

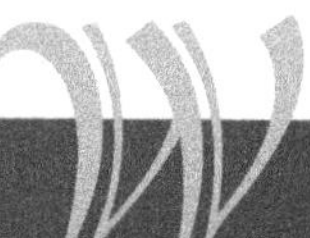

cause this backflow of living endometrial tissue. The old Levitical laws of the Bible prohibited sexual relations during or immediately following the menstrual period. It may be that prevention of endometrial implants was one objective of this law.

Internal fetal monitoring has been linked with subsequent development of endometriosis. The mechanism is still not clear.

Birth control pills stimulate endometriosis by preparing a fertile site for the transplants to grow.

Pain with the menstrual period, infertility, and abnormal bleeding represent the commonest symptoms. Other symptoms are low back pain and pain in the lower extremities; sometimes the back pain radiates down the legs. While it is rare in black women, up to 30 percent of white women suffer from this condition at one time or other. Pregnancy improves the symptoms, although it is a common cause of infertility.

Even sexual stimulation or thoughts can result in muscular contractions of the uterus, tubes, or vaginal structures and encourage endometrial transplantation (*Journal of Reproductive Medicine* 34, no. 11 [November 1989]: 887–890).

Endometriosis seems more likely to occur in women who have their periods beginning at twelve years or younger, menstrate for greater than eight days, have more painful menstruation, are more energetic in physical activity during menstruation, or have allergic reactions. Women are less likely to have endometriosis as the number of pregnancies goes up (*Chinese Medical Sciences Journal* 9, no. 2 [June 1994]: 114-118).

This very troublesome disorder has been found to be connected with the use of dairy products. In certain patients the connection is very obvious, since as soon as the person eliminates dairy products they cease having difficulties. It is certainly well worth a trial. Perhaps not all patients would be cured, but if a patient is helped by this simple measure, it is one of the easiest to institute. Other food sensitivities may intensify pain with the period. Follow the "Elimination and Challenge Diet" in the *Dietary Information* section.

Treatment

A diet high in plant sterols is quite helpful in endometriosis, including apples, cherries, olives, plums, wheat germ, coconut, carrots, legumes, sweet potatoes, all of the nightshades (tomatoes, potatoes, eggplant, and peppers), and all nuts. Garlic has a good level of plant sterols, such as ergosterol, sitosterol, and phytosterol, and may be taken in as large quantity as the patient finds practicable. Herbal remedies high in plant sterols include alfalfa, red raspberry leaf, black cohosh, licorice root, sage, food yeast, parsley, red clover, and anise seed ground and in food and simmered as tea. Evening primrose oil and flaxseed oil should be tried.

Many women may prefer to tough it out until the transplants burn themselves out and await the onset of menopause when endometriosis is automatically cured by the cessation of stimulation of growth by hormones. A very good way to treat the disease process in a younger woman is to wait it out, treating the pain with the suggested remedies until the implants have burned themselves out. This may take from one to five years, but pain tends to be worse at first and then better as time goes by.

The wall-stretch exercise is excellent for this condition. Draw a line parallel on the floor two feet from a wall. Facing the wall, stand with the tips of the toes on the line, and while keeping the heels flat on the floor, lean the whole body toward the wall, hands on the wall at about shoulder height. When the chest touches the wall, hold the position for 10 seconds, push back into the upright position for five seconds, then repeat the exercise three times. Turn to the side, putting the right outer edge of the foot on the line, and lean sideways toward the wall, attempting to touch the hip to the wall. Hold for 10 seconds and repeat. Do the same procedure with the left hip. Do the exercises three times a day for three days, then once a day for ninety days, then periodically for several years, until the symptoms no longer return.

A hot water bottle or electric heating pad over the low back for one hour at the very onset of the menstrual period can relieve pain for some people.

The application of heat by any method—hot sitz bath, fomentations, and hot foot baths—have all been reported to clear symptoms. One treatment routine includes a series of three fomentations over the low abdomen taken each of the first three days of the menstrual period for 12 months. For some this has resulted in complete clearing of symptoms.

Use the hot sitz bath alternating with the cold sitz bath, or hot and cold applications to the sacrum, feet, or legs, accompanied by much friction. A cold mitten friction should form a part of the regimen for these cases.

A large charcoal poultice covering the lower abdomen and pelvis at night is useful in pain relief.

Fibroids, Leiomyomata

Growth factors are responsible for the growth promotion effects on the smooth muscle of the uterus by estrogen and progesterone. Avoid being overweight as the increased estrogen can stimulate fibroid growth. The growth factors increase the number of receptors for estrogen and progesterone and provide the basis of the growth of the fibroid. The growth factors include epidermal growth factor, platelet-derived growth factor, keratinocyte growth factor, and both insulin-like growth factor and insulin. Since some of these growth factors are responsive to diet, in families having a history of early fibroids, the diet should be regulated so that insulin resistance and insulin over production will not be a feature of the woman's lifestyle (See factors on insulin resistance in the "Diabetes" entry in the *Conditions and Diseases* section.) (*Infertility and Reproductive Clinics of North America* 7, no. 1 [1996]: 5–18).

Uterine Fibroids

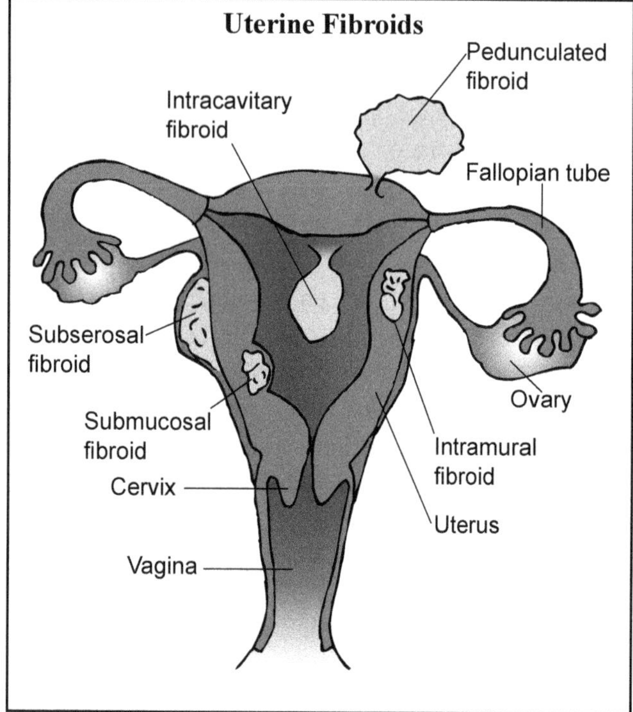

Most fibroids require no treatment other than providing relief for any kind of symptom the patient may have. Surgery to prevent the development of symptoms is seldom if ever warranted (*Obstetrics and Gynecology Clinics of North America* 22, no. 4 [1995]: 659). Wait until symptoms are intolerable before considering surgery.

It is believed by some naturopaths and chiropractors that these disorders are all because of a reduced quantity of tissue iodine in the uterus. Do not bother to take iodine by mouth as the iodine is taken up by the thyroid too quickly to get any into the uterus. The following treatment has also been used for fibrocystic breast disease.

Use two tablespoons of liquid chlorophyll, unflavored (which contains iodine). Use one teaspoon of liquid dulse. The woman should lie in the knee-chest position or on one side with hips elevated on a pillow, and inject the liquid with a bulb syringe as a retention douche. Wear a pad to catch any leakage. The next night the woman should lie on the other side and have the retention douche. Do the douches every night and stay in the same position as long as possible before moving. In two to three weeks the fibrocystic breast disease or fibroids will shrink if they respond to the treatment.

Fibroids are very common. In fact, 20 percent of women between the ages of 30 and 45 have these non-cancerous growths of the uterus consisting of a blend of muscle and fibrous (supporting) tissue, giving them the name fibroids. They are benign tumors of the same significance as moles on the skin. They tend to grow to a certain size determined by unknown factors, and just like moles, they tend to maintain that size with only minor, if any, additional growth for many years. Then, when menopause starts, they begin to shrink and eventually get to a fraction of their original size.

The most troublesome problem from uterine fibroids is bleeding, and the next is the cosmetic enlargement of the abdomen. I recommend that even with these problems simple remedies be applied and that the woman delay more invasive measures unless her symptoms force her to have an operation. Since the uterus shrinks as well as the fibroids after menopause, the bleeding usually stops promptly after menopause and the size of the abdomen reduces.

Fibroids, if large enough, can press on the bladder in front of the uterus or on the rectum behind the uterus, causing either scanty, frequent urination or constipation. Fibroids may interfere with the ability to become pregnant if they bulge into the interior of the uterus, and they may also be responsible for miscarriages. The vast majority of fibroids give little evidence of their presence, and a woman may have fibroids for years without knowing they are there. Multiple pregnancies can occur even with large tumors. An OB/GYN may feel large fibroids during a pelvic exam. But just because they are present, does not mean the uterus or the fibroids must be removed.

If you do not have any symptoms, you certainly should not have an operation. Uterine fibroids are benign tumors, and chances are good that you will not have any difficulty from them. The risk of anything serious happening if you keep them is far less than the risks of a complication or even death from the surgery.

The cause of fibroids is unknown. Although there are no natural treatments that will remove the fibroids, there are several things that can be done to shrink fibroids, but it is unlikely, if not impossible, that they will go away completely. The earlier in life they begin, the greater the likelihood they will grow to a fairly large size (large orange or grapefruit-size).

Most authorities say fibroids do not become malignant. Since fibroids are not malignant, my experience as a hospital pathologist evaluating hysterectomies led me to put very strict criteria on deciding a case for surgery: Her hemoglobin must be below 9.0 g, hematocrit below 27, pain quite incapacitating, and pressure on bladder or bowel quite severe.

Since hysterectomies are usually recommended for women with fibroids, it may come as a surprise to some women that if their fibroids are positioned just right and are present in an accessible area, the fibroid itself may be removed without removing the entire uterus. The procedure of myomectomy—removal of the fibroids alone—is in many ways, however, the more difficult procedure, often with more blood loss than a hysterectomy; and then, fibroids recur in one out of three women after myomectomy, particularly when the women are younger than 35.

Successful treatment consists not in the fibroids disappearing but in the control of bleeding or other symptoms and in avoiding an operation. It may take several months to a year of treatments for improvement to occur. Do not be discouraged if improvement is slow. The objective is to tide you over until menopause causes the natural shrinkage in size. The following are some suggested natural therapies for this problem.

Treatment

Eliminate coffee, tea, and other sources of caffeine as well as animal products from the diet, as these substances all promote the growth of fibroids. Avoid supplements that contain PABA or large amounts of folic acid. Alcohol and all toxic chemical exposure should be strictly avoided.

One woman had shrinkage of an orange-sized fibroid within about six months with the following treatment regiment:

- Become a total vegetarian—no meat, milk, eggs, or cheese. All free fats (margarine, butter, mayonnaise, fried foods, cooking fats, salad oils, and even peanut butter) should be removed from your diet. You may have some nuts, seeds, olives, and avocados, but no oil made from any of these foods, as free fats are metabolized differently than combined fats as they occur naturally.
- Prepare nightly castor oil packs, which should be worn all night. To make the castor oil packs, take about four layers of cotton flannel, saturate them with castor oil, and place directly against the skin over the low abdomen. Cover with a piece of plastic and tape in place. Then cover the plastic with a heating pad that has been protected by slipping it into a plastic bag. Keep the castor oil pack quite warm for one hour. Then the heating pad can be laid aside for the remainder of the night.

Another method of making a castor oil pack is as follows:

- Cut a piece of cotton flannel large enough to cover the torso from just below the breasts to the groin. The flannel should be wide enough to wrap all the way around the back as well.
- Cut a piece of plastic, such as a shower curtain, large enough to extend past the flannel two inches on all sides.
- Get a long, thin towel large enough to completely cover the plastic. Lay it on the bed first, and then lay the plastic on the towel.
- Then wet the flannel in castor oil. Spread the flannel on the top of the plastic.
- Lie down on the flannel and wrap the flannel around yourself first, then the plastic, then the towel.
- Pin it snugly in place with safety pins.
- Wear it all night (at least 8 hours) on a daily basis for six weeks.
- Take a two-week break and resume for six more weeks, and so on for a year.

An herbal suppository can be made from powdered herbs mixed with cocoa butter. Use red raspberry and equal quantities of wild yam pulverized and mixed with melted cocoa butter until you have a thin paste. Cool the mixture in the refrigerator until softly congealed. Scoop out tablespoon-size portions and roll each into suppository-size bars. Flatten slightly and cool in the refrigerator before inserting high into the vagina. Use one nightly.

Soy foods can be helpful for fibroids. The most helpful form of soybeans is the whole dry bean, soaked and cooked as ordinary beans. Eat about one-quarter cup of the cooked beans each day.

Hot sitz baths have been used by some OB-GYN physicians in an attempt to control uterine fibroids without surgery. The procedure for giving this treatment is as follows:

- Put about five inches of hot water in the bathtub and five inches of cold water in a smaller tub.
- Sit for three minutes in the bathtub in hot water with the knees drawn up out of the water. Have the water as hot as can be tolerated.

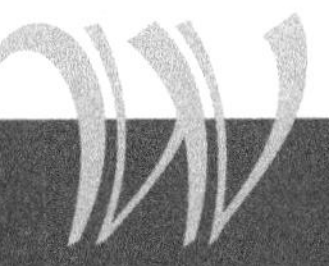

- Then, with the feet remaining in the hot water, transfer your seat into the smaller tub, having the cold water come up over all the area where hot water touched the skin. Keep the feet in the hot water.
- Sit three minutes in the hot water and 30 seconds to one minute in the cold water.
- Continue to add both hot water and cold water, keeping the hot water as hot as can be tolerated, and the cold water as cold as you can get it from the cold water tap, as well as adding ice from time to time to keep the water temperature around 45°F. If you positively cannot tolerate temperatures that low, raise the temperature to 65°F, or shorten the time in the cold tub to 30 seconds.
- The entire treatment should last about 45 minutes, alternating between the hot water sitz and the cold water sitz.
- When the time is finished, end with the cold water application, then stand in the cold water tub approximately 20 seconds. Step out of the tub and begin to briskly dry the body with a coarse, dry towel, vigorously rubbing the skin.
- Put on a bathrobe or wrap up in a sheet and quickly transfer to the bed and rest at least 20 to 60 minutes.
- Perform the treatment five days a week for six weeks.
- Note: If the cold-water tub cannot be managed easily in the bathtub, you can apply the cold part of the treatment by wrapping a slightly dripping, ice-cold towel folded into a triangle around the waist and hips, bringing it up between the legs like a diaper while standing in the hot water. You will need two large, wet, and dripping cold towels, one for the first 30 seconds of the one-minute cold phase, and the second for the last 30 seconds. Make your changes quickly. Then sit again in the hot water.

Take four capsules daily for six weeks of evening primrose oil, or 400 IU of vitamin E per day, or 20,000 IU per day of vitamin A. One or all taken each day can be helpful in some cases.

A foot rub will often help if there is pain or congestion of the fibroids.

A homemade medicinal tampon may help with fibroids:

- Cut well-washed and rinsed cotton fabric (old undershirts will be fine) in pieces about one inch by four inches.
- Lay one on top of the other until you have a small pile about one-quarter inch high.
- Tie a string tightly around the middle, and leave the ends of the string about eight inches long.
- Mix a teaspoonful of slippery elm powder and a teaspoonful of white oak bark powder with enough water and a teaspoon or more of French clay or powdered charcoal to make a thin consistency, about like mustard or ketchup.
- Spread this mixture on the cotton fabric layers, being generous and soaking the cotton thoroughly.
- Using the eraser end of a long but very sturdy pencil or similar sturdy instrument, insert the tampon into the vagina up to the cervix, leaving the long end of the string hanging out. The best way to insert the tampon is to lie in a dry bathtub. Drape the prepared cotton strips over the blunt end of the pencil and push the mid-section as far into the vagina as possible.
- Wear a protective pad to prevent any leakage from soiling your clothing.
- Follow these instructions five nights weekly for six weeks, immediately before bed, removing the tampon next morning by pulling firmly on the string.
- If for some reason the herbs are not used, Ichthammol Black Salve from a pharmacy or health food store may be used on the cotton fabric layers, being generous. Mix it half and half with vegetable glycerine, and follow the same procedure.

We suggest you take chaste tree berries, angelica root, squaw vine, licorice root, and raspberry leaf. Use one tablespoon of each of the herbs with one quart of water. All herbs that are not leaves should be put in the water and set to simmer for 25 minutes. The gentlest boil you can obtain is preferable, as too vigorous boiling can damage the active ingredients. When the herbs you are boiling have finished, add a tablespoon of any leaf herb and let them all steep together for 30 minutes. This is a day's supply. If it is slightly nauseating, you can eliminate that by adding a bit of nut milk with each cup of the tea. That should eliminate any nauseating effect from the herbs.

You may also take one of the following mixtures as an herbal tea: one part licorice root powder, two parts chaparral, one part cramp bark, one part false unicorn, and three parts red clover. Powder the mixed herbs in a blender. Put one teaspoon in a cup and pour boiling water over it. Cover, cool, and then drink both the liquid and the powder. Use one cup four times a day. Continue the herbs four 6 to 10 weeks.

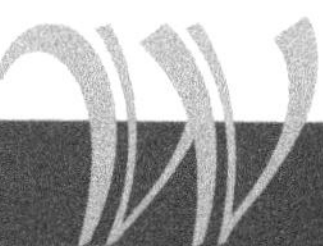

This mixture is reported also to shrink ovarian cysts, and endometriosis, as well as uterine fibroids. It will often abolish chronic vaginitis and other vaginal and uterine infections.

Another mixture you might find helpful for fibroids is chaste tree and milk thistle. Gently simmer one tablespoon of chaste tree for 5 to 10 minutes in one quart of water. Remove from the heat and add one heaping tablespoon of milk thistle. Steep for half an hour. Take one cup four times a day for three to six months. This mixture can be taken with the previous recipe. You may also find benefit from wild yam gel.

A patient told one of our doctors at Uchee Pines Institute about a treatment she used for fibroids that was very successful in helping her to control bleeding. She took two garlic capsules two times a day for six weeks; then once a day for six months; one-quarter teaspoon of cayenne pepper mixed in water with one teaspoon of golden seal powder two times a day; and one cup of echinacea tea twice daily for six weeks. While we do not usually recommend the long-term use of cayenne pepper, internally, in this case, if other remedies are not effective, it should be tried to see if surgery can be avoided.

If you are overweight, you are more likely to develop fibroids and to have complications from them. Learn to control your weight. One thing that can help is to avoid eating anything between meals or after 3:00 p.m. as food eaten then is more likely to be put on as fat than food taken at mealtimes. Be regular in mealtimes.

Fasting will temporarily shrink a fibroid. Start your fasting program with a three-day fast. Then, a day or two each week of fasting will be very helpful if the nutrient reserves are adequate—that is, you are not severely thin or very run down. (See "Fasting" in the *Dietary Information* section.)

In recent years we have had good success using an infrared dome. Even grapefruit-sized fibroids have shrunk to walnut size. She should use the dome one to five hours daily for six weeks or more.

Case Report

A 39-year-old white woman suddenly began bleeding at 2:00 a.m. one morning. She felt full in the abdomen. When she got up to go to the bathroom, she passed a number of large blood clots and some liquid blood. She recognized that this was not a menstrual period, but she had cramps with the bleeding. She saw her doctor the next day, and he found a grapefruit-sized fibroid. He told her the fibroid was doubtless the cause of the heavy bleeding. Her periods had been prolonged and more frequent and, at times, her hemoglobin level would drop down to around 10 grams, while usually running around 12.3 grams.

At this point, she had a D and C, and the surgeon recognized the presence of small fibroids just under the lining of the uterus, in addition to the grapefruit-sized one. He suggested a hysterectomy.

The patient postponed the surgery and began trying several types of home remedies. Her treatment was successful.

She took large garlic capsules for six weeks followed by odorless garlic in a concentrate. She started taking two of the large capsules twice a day, but switched to four tablets twice a day and later cut back down to two tablets a day. She found a preparation of cayenne pepper mixed with golden seal in a health food store. She took two capsules of that mixture four times a day.

Rose hip tea, two cups per day; echinacea tea, one cup two times a day; and burdock tea, one cup two times a day, were also taken. She borrowed an infared dome and began spending one hour under it in the morning, and one hour in the afternoon, and two or more hours after going to bed.

She emphasizes that she prayed to the Lord for assistance in successfully treating her fibroids. Within six weeks, the grapefruit-size fibroid had shrunk to a barely detectable size by the gynecologist. Her bleeding had greatly diminished, and within a year, she was back to the level of bleeding she had had before her trouble began.

Fissures and Fistulae

Anal fissures cause much pain, even to the point of being disabling for some people. Fistulae are tunnels that have eroded abnormally from the anus or vagina to the skin, or from the anus or rectum to the vagina or skin.

To treat fissures and fistulae, make your own suppositories.Use four ounces of coconut oil and two tablespoons of the following powdered mixture: one-third part golden seal powder, one-third part witch hazel powdered in a blender if not already in powder form, and one-third part comfrey root powder. Place the herbs in the coconut oil in a double boiler and boil for four hours. Refrigerate briefly, and when it begins to gel, dig it out by one teaspoon size lumps and roll into pencil-sized suppositories of the length needed to insert.

Insert one suppository in the fistula tract one to six times daily depending on the seriousness and acuteness of the condition. If you cannot penetrate the fistula, then put the suppository in the vagina, rectum, or elsewhere as close to the fistula opening as possible, even if a bandage must be used to hold it in place. If the suppository does not melt in two hours, put the unused suppositories back in the double boiler, melt and add one tablespoon of olive oil. When well mixed, follow the procedure above to make new suppositories. Powdered cranesbill or powdered garlic may be used instead of comfrey root in this formula. Continue for one month or more.

Hot sitz baths in herbal tea are also helpful and may be curative for fissures after a month or so. Sit in the herb tea in a shallow pan for 20 minutes, four times a day. The tea may be used for four treatments before discarding.

Labor

To encourage labor to begin around a woman's due date, take 10 drops of tincture of black cohosh and blue cohosh every hour until labor begins.

Menstruation Difficulties

Bleeding Abnormally

(See also "Hemorrhage" in the *Conditions and Diseases* section.)

The causes of menorrhagia, a loss of a larger amount of blood during menstruation than is customary, and metrorrhagia, a flow of blood between menstrual periods, are because of hormones, poor blood clotting, habitually chilled extremities—including when the young lady is growing up—or some emotional or psychological factor. The same herbs as used for prolonged and excessive menstrual bleeding should be used here.

Irregular Menstrual Cycles

Short-term fasting, from two to five days, suppresses certain hormones from the pituitary. This may be one of the reasons making dietary changes, such as becoming a vegetarian, may cause a loss of menstrual periods for several months. It is regarded as favorable for the overall health of the woman to have this hormone response to fasting (*Journal of Clinical Endocrinological Metabolism* 85 [2000]: 207).

Menstrual irregularity may occur from the use of meat and milk. There have been large studies showing that elimination of these food products from the diet can cause an improvement in regularity of the periods (*Tohoku Journal of Experimental Medicine* 169 [1993]: 245–52).

Blue cohosh root can be used as a regulator for the menstrual cycle. Simmer one heaping tablespoon in one quart of water for 20 to 30 minutes. Strain and drink one cup four times daily.

Chaste tree or vitex is amphoteric, meaning that if the function of the ovaries is too low, it tends to bring it up. If it is too high, it tends to subdue it. Chaste tree may be taken for excessive menstrual bleeding or for irregular periods.

Nettles and red clover are also helpful. Steep in hot water for four hours and use four cups per day. Mix the herbs equally, using one tablespoon per cup. Nettles is a wonderful herb. It is also used as a diuretic, galactagogue, and for general debility and convalescence.

Painful Menstruation

Causes of painful menstruation include lack of exercise, poor posture, poor hygiene, nervousness, tight bands around the waist, anemia, constipation, and habitually chilled extremities, particularly during childhood while growing up. Endometriosis, malpositioning of the uterus, inflammation of the pelvic organs, and tumors are more rare causes of painful menstruation. These must be corrected before any treatment can be successful.

Gynecologists have discovered that even a small amount of chilling of the lower extremities in girls during childhood results in a reduction in blood flow to the pelvic organs. It is believed by some that much of the pelvic distress young women experience is brought on by failure to properly clothe the lower extremities during childhood. Chilling of any part of the body results in a reduction in immune functioning. White blood cells become more sluggish and less interested in eating germs or taking up waste materials.

Exposure to cigarette smoke either by smoking or from secondhand smoke increases the likelihood of painful menstruation.

New research is showing that dysmenorrhea, painful periods, and menstrual irregularities may be tied closely with abnormal production of certain prostaglandins. Prostaglandins are extremely potent hormone-like substances produced in many organs of the body. The raw materials for their production are primarily fatty acids. When there is an overabundance of the wrong kinds of fatty acids, prostaglandin causes blood vessel constriction, contraction and spasm of smooth muscles, as in the uterus or arteries, which increases blood pressure, abnormal tendencies to clot the blood, etc. Saturated animal fats, partially hydrogenated vegetable fats, rancid fats, and the partially hydrogenated fats found in margarine tend to produce the bad hormones. Highly refined vegetable oils, though polyunsaturated, may be bad since protective antioxidants have been removed in processing. The oils as found in natural plant products—legumes, grains, fruits, and vegetables—tend to promote production of the good prostaglandins; these are the foods that should be used.

Some unfortunate people lack some of the enzymes necessary to produce the good prostaglandins despite a sufficient amount of the raw materials; it is rare to have a complete deficiency, but varying degrees of enzyme deficiency are common. For these women, it is essential to be on a diet with no free oils or shortening and use the natural plant foods in abundance. In addition, the use of evening primrose oil, with its abundance of gamma linolenic acid may be a great help. Use a dose of four capsules four times a day; or use cold-pressed flaxseed oil, kept tightly closed and refrigerated, in a dose of one tablespoonful twice daily. This amount will supply plenty of the beneficial omega-3 fatty acids. We advise the use of both of these substances if simpler dietary and physical methods do not give sufficient relief. Try the flaxseed oil first as it is much cheaper.

A number of authorities recognize an allergic factor in dysmenorrhea, menstrual pain. One study of 12 cases of dysmenorrhea revealed that eight patients became free of all symptoms when the foods to which they were sensitive were eliminated from their diet. The other four patients received partial relief, and the author felt that he had not been successful in identifying all of their food sensitivities. Wheat, eggs, milk, beef, chocolate, nuts, fish, beans, peppers, cauliflower, and cabbage were the foods listed as the most common causes of dysmenorrhea. We suggest the elimination of all of the most common allergens to test for allergy-induced dysmenorrhea. (See "Elimination and Challenge Diet" in the Dietary Information section.)

Forty-two young women were given omega-3 fatty acids and had a noticeable improvement in cramps and other menstrual symptoms, including headache and nausea (*American Journal of Obstetrics and Gynecology* 174, no. 4 [1996]: 1335).

Take three cloves of garlic with each meal the day before and the day of the expected menstrual period. Garlic all through the month is also very helpful, one clove with each meal.

Overeating, excessive salt intake, and being overweight all increase the probability of painful menstruation. Bring the weight to the ideal level. (See "Weight Control" in the *Conditions and Diseases* section.)

More benefit will be realized than you think possible from avoiding tea, coffee, colas, chocolate, tobacco, and alcohol.

A regular schedule helps the ovaries to keep things well regulated, thus diminishing pain.

Regular exercise can produce body chemicals that counteract painful periods. These chemicals are in the family of the endorphins that decrease pain.

Wear loose enough clothing to encourage deep diaphragm breathing in which the abdomen moves rather than the chest with each breath. The movement of the diaphragm massages the pelvic organs and prevents the congestion that causes a large part of menstrual pain. Singing or speaking lessons are helpful as it teaches good posture and diaphragmatic breathing.

To encourage diaphragm breathing, one may try this exercise. The woman should remove all clothing and lie on her back on a flat surface. She should flex the knees and place the arms at the sides to assist in the relaxation of the abdominal muscles. One hand is placed on the abdomen. The woman attempts to raise the hand as high as possible by lifting the abdominal wall and then seeing how far she can lower the abdominal hand. The exercise should be repeated 10 times each morning and night in a well-ventilated room. Initially this deep breathing may induce some dizziness, but with repetitions she will be able to complete the exercise.

Practice good posture at all times. Dr. L. J. Golub reported success with a twisting and bending exercise. The patient stands with the feet parallel and about 15 inches apart. The arms are outstretched to each side at shoulder height. Keeping the knees straight, the patient twists the trunk to the left and bends down to touch the floor with the right hand in front of the left foot. Return to the starting position and repeat the exercise with the right foot. The first week the exercise should be done four times daily. During successive weeks the exercises should be increased by two each week until a total of 10 repetitions per side are performed daily. Sometimes patients reported relief with the next period, but most people required three to four months before relief occurred. The exercises should not be started during a period as they may worsen the pain (*Journal of the Association for Physical and Mental Rehabilitation* 18 [July–August 1964]: 97–109).

A very good stretching exercise to loosen the pelvic ligaments is done as follows: The patient stands about 18 inches from a wall with heels and toes together with her side toward the wall. The elbow is put against the wall at shoulder height, the forearm and hand pointed downward and resting against the wall. Keeping the shoulders perpendicular to the wall and the knees straight, contract the abdominal and hip muscles and shift the hips toward the wall, attempting to touch the wall. The exercise should be done three times on each side three times a day, a total of nine stretching exercises per day. The study reported that mild cases got relief after about

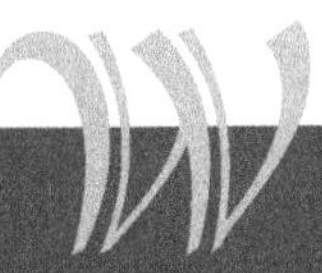

one month of exercises, moderately severe cases after about two months, and severe cases after three or more months (*Archives of Surgery* 46 [May 1943]: 611–13).

A hot water bottle or electric heating pad can relieve pain entirely in some women if applied to the back from the waist to the bottom of the seat at the very first sign of the onset of the period and maintained very hot for one hour.

Two hot tub baths per day will draw blood from the overly congested uterus to the outside of the body. A hot sitz bath 105°F to 115°F with a hot foot bath at 110°F to 115°F for 3 to 10 minutes can be curative in some women. A cold sitz bath from 55°F to 75°F for 2 to 10 minutes, with friction, using a washcloth or a brush and a hot foot bath, is preferred to a hot bath by some women.

Avoid constipation. (See "Constipation" in the *Conditions and Diseases* section.) A daily hot enema, hot vaginal irrigation (douche), hot tub bath, or hot foot bath, beginning four to seven days before the menstrual period is expected, are all beneficial. Then sit in a hot tub bath two times a day at the onset of the period (*Journal of the American Medical Association* 62 [April 25, 1914]: 1297–1301).

With the young lady lying face down, her head to the left, a person stands over her with the arms extended straight down toward her back and the heel of the hand placed just to the right of the spine and the opposite hand placed over the fist to increase the pressure. Using as much pressure on the extended arms as your body weight can give, or as much as she can tolerate, lean your weight into her back with the heel of one hand placed just to the right of the waist, and rotate. After a few seconds of pressure, inch downward, again repeating the firm pressure and rotation for several seconds, and continuing to inch down until pressure and rotation have been put on each inch of the spine all the way down to its end at the coccyx. Then begin working your way back up toward the waist, still only on the right. Spend at least five minutes doing this massage. Each time the heel of the hand is pressed into the back, a slight rotary movement is made to massage the large nerve trunks that come out principally on the right of the spine below the waist that affect the pelvic organs.

Sexual stimulation during the period should be avoided as it can lead to endometriosis and more pain.

Take a heaping tablespoonful of powdered charcoal stirred in a glass of water at the very first sign of the menstrual period and discomfort, and every half an hour until the pain is relieved. You may need four or five doses.

Put an ounce of mugwort in a glass container, and pour two cups of boiling water over it. Let it steep until cool. Drink both cups. It is an excellent remedy.

Another herbal treatment might include any five to seven of the following: blackberry, black cohosh, wild yam, cramp bark, chaste tree, black haw, caraway, catnip, chamomile, ginger, marjoram, meadowsweet, passion flower, bilberry, thyme, white willow bark, or yarrow.

Marjoram, the common kitchen herb, can stop menstrual cramps in some women. Mix one teaspoon of the herb with water. Drink the entire mixture, herb and all.

Catnip tea each morning and evening during the period may be helpful. Chamomile is said to relieve menstrual spasms. Peppermint tea may relax muscles and ease the pain.

An anticoagulant from soybeans, nattokinase, will help remarkably with dysmenorrhea. Take 200 milligrams per day.

A tea can be made by gently boiling the herbs for half an hour in one quart of water and taking as needed.

- 1 teaspoon black cohosh
- 1 teaspoon pleurisy root
- 1½ teaspoon false unicorn root
- 1½ teaspoon true unicorn root
- 2 teaspoons fenugreek seed
- 1 teaspoon licorice root powder

Miscarriages

A deficiency of the mineral selenium was found in 40 women who had recently miscarried. It may be that habitual aborters would be well advised to take selenium to prevent miscarriage (*British Journal of Obstetrics and Gynecology* 103 [1996]: 130–32). The long-term use of selenium supplements may not be advised, as there is evidence that large quantities of selenium increases risk for melanoma. A good dietary source of selenium is Brazil nuts. One nut per day will supply almost the entire recommended daily allowance. As a treatment, we recommend three nuts twice daily. The nuts carry no risk to one's health.

Wilson's disease may cause repeated and unexplained spontaneous abortions. (See "Wilson's Disease, Copper Overload" in the *Conditions and Diseases* section for treatment.)

The following herbs may also help to prevent a miscarriage: black haw, ginger, passion flower, red raspberry, and red clover. To stop bleeding after a miscarriage, use shepherd's purse.

When a miscarriage occurs, bleeding will most likely be similar to a heavy period. If the bleeding stops after one to three weeks, and menstrual periods start within about three months, there is no need for a D&C (dilation and curettage), the surgical procedure that removes the fetus.

To help the uterus to completely empty and cleanse itself, take the following herbs:

- Bayberry bark (or oak bark for difficult cases)
- Cayenne (a uterine and vascular stimulant)
- Golden seal (a healing herb and antibacterial)
- Red raspberry leaves (plant steroids)
- Eyebright (an astringent)

Alternating hot and cold compresses should also be used. Make the compresses of short duration and very intense. The hot compresses should be placed on the abdomen at 115°F to 117°F for one and a half to three minutes *only*. Follow the hot application by rubbing the abdomen for 30 seconds with large blocks of ice. It is best to have two persons applying the ice massage to keep it as cold as possible. If the bleeding has stopped, do not apply more. If bleeding continues to be heavy, this treatment can be repeated every four hours or at least twice a day.

If bleeding continues for more than four or five weeks, the uterus may require emptying by a D&C. Keep a close watch to be certain anemia does not develop.

Ovarian Cancer

(See "Cancer" in the *Conditions and Diseases* section.)

Ovarian Cysts

A cyst is a sac filled with fluid; ovarian cysts can be on or in the ovary. Unless it is larger than a small lemon, it should not be alarming. The proper course of action is to get an imaging study, probably an ultrasound, to establish its present size, and if no bigger in three months, leave it alone for another six months, at which time it can be re-evaluated. A stable cyst, causing no trouble, should not be disturbed.

Usually ovarian cysts do not require surgical intervention. The surgical hazards and the long-term complications are serious enough that it is not appropriate to operate for established benign conditions.

To treat an ovarian cyst, soak in a tub of water as hot as is necessary to raise the mouth temperature to 101.5°F, or thereabouts. If the patient is in excellent health apart from the ovarian cyst, she will have no difficulty raising her mouth temperature that high. She can bathe her face constantly with ice water while in the hot tub. The hot bath increases pelvic blood flow and encourages the body to heal the ovarian cyst.

After about 20 to 30 minutes of sitting in the tub, she should stand up, turn on the shower as cold as she can bear it, and rub herself vigorously while turning round and round in the shower for about 20 to 50 seconds. Then she should step out of the shower, rub herself briskly with a coarse dry towel, and then lie down for about an hour. Repeat the treatment five days a week for 15 treatments.

Repeat ultrasound examinations will usually show that there has been no progression of the cyst, or at most only a millimeter or so in a month, and probably even a regression in size. Ovarian cysts that have been known to be present for years need not be operated as they are clearly benign.

Postpartum Hemorrhage

(See "Miscarriages" or "Hemorrhage" in the *Conditions and Diseases* section.)

Premenstrual Syndrome (PMS)

Herbs helpful in the treatment of PMS include echinacea, chaste tree, dandelion, milk thistle seed, hawthorn berry, false unicorn, astragalus, camomile, Siberian ginseng, buchu, celery seed, nettle, parsley, sarsaparilla, and uva-ursi. Women with PMS who take an extract of chaste tree berry have less irritability, mood alteration, anger, headache, and breast fullness than women who do not (*British Medical Journal* 322, no. 7279 [2001]: 134).

The following herbal recipe may be used for PMS:

- 1 tablespoon chaste tree (Use 2 tablespoons for severe cases to stimulate the corpus luteum. That much may cause foul smelling gas, but it may be worth it.)
- 1 tablespoon of dandelion root (This is the most useful diuretic for PMS. Use buchu, another diuretic, for cystitis as a soother and antiseptic if needed.)
- 1 tablespoon of false unicorn
- 3 tablespoons of echinacea
- 1 quart water

Simmer all of the above ingredients for 25 minutes and pour over 2 tablespoons of skullcap. Steep 20 minutes. Take a little throughout the day, not all at once. At first take it throughout the month, but when symptoms seem to be cleared and well, try to stop taking the herbs. If symptoms return, begin again with the herbs only while the symptoms last.

Selenium contributes to progesterone production of the corpus luteum. It may be helpful in mild to moderate cases of PMS. One Brazil nut contains almost the entire recommended daily allowance. As a treatment for PMS, take three of the nuts twice a day with meals.

Calcium supplementation enabled 466 women to significantly lower the level of their premenstrual stresses as compared to 497 women who were not treated with calcium supplementation. The calcium-treated group had a 48 percent reduction in total symptom scores as compared to a 30 percent reduction in the placebo group (*American Journal of Obstetrics and Gynecology* 179 [1988]: 444).

Do not use black cohosh or licorice for PMS, only for dysmenorrhea, as they have plant estrogens in them that may worsen PMS.

Vaginal Itch

For itching around the vagina, use a perineal pour of one to four tablespoons of vinegar to one quart of water. Pour the mixture over the perineum through the pubic hair, opening all the tissues of the perineal area with the fingers of the other hand to make certain the vinegar water touches all portions of the perineal structures—this treatment can be very good for itching if done every time one uses the restroom. The water should be either hot or cold and not body temperature, as it is more effective in an extreme temperature.

Itching can also be helped by rubbing vitamin E oil on the vulva.

Vaginal itching and dryness may be helped by mixing angelica and alfalfa (if not already a powder, pulverize in a seed mill or blender) in glycerin from a pharmacy and using topically.

Vaginitis

Vaginitis is the name of an inflammation of the vagina associated with itching, irritation, and a discharge that may or may not have an unpleasant odor. Several causes include candida or yeast infections, trichomonas, or bacteria of several kinds. Frequently, the vaginitis can be successfully treated by paying attention to the outside only, using the perineal pour described under vaginal itch. Vinegar water is best for candida, and a saturated solution of baking soda in water is usually best for trichomonas. A garlic douch solution is usually best for bacteria. Use all solutions hot or cold as the extreme temperature will help aid circulation to the area.

The treatment time for all of the following treatments is one month in length.

- Use a low-fat, low-sugar, low-protein vegetarian diet.
- Use a hot soda water douche (one to three teaspoons of soda to a quart of hot water) once daily for 30 days. After one week if there is no improvement, switch to a hot vinegar douche (four tablespoons of vinegar to a quart of hot water). If no improvement after a week, switch to a hot garlic douche made by blenderizing one clove of garlic in one cup of boiling water until smooth, then add boiling water to make up one quart, and allow it to stand until the temperature falls sufficiently to allow douching. Generally, the soda water is used for trichomonas, vinegar for yeast infections, and garlic for any kind of vaginitis, especially bacterial.
- Use a hot or cold perineal pour after each bathroom visit, using one to four tablespoons of vinegar per quart and making sure the water flows into all folds.
- Another good treatment is a very hot sitz bath (just enough water in a large plastic basin to adequately cover the perineum) into which two cups of strong witch hazel tea and two cups of strong golden seal tea have been poured. Sit 30 minutes in the hot sitz bath two or three times daily until it shows signs of healing. The plastic basin can be braced in a bottomless chair for greater convenience.
- Avoid the use of pantyhose and tight clothing that encourages moisture retention, promoting the growth of germs. If pantyhose must be worn, cut with scissors to open the crotch seam at least six inches to allow moisture to evaporate.
- Keep the hair on the vulva clipped short.
- Avoid the use of antibiotics, cortisone-type medications (Prednisone, Ilosone, etc.), tampons, colored toilet tissue, and bubble bath or soap used in the perineal area, all of which may aggravate the skin.
- Avoid marital relations during infections. When the wife is receiving treatments, the husband should sit in a hot sitz bath once daily with one cup of vinegar added. All the folds and crevices of the foreskin should be retracted to allow the hot vinegar water access to all areas. The husband can reinfect the wife if he is not treated also.

Another form of treatment is the use of suppositories. Make suppositories as follows: Take enough slippery elm powder to make a ball about three inches long and the size of the patient's middle finger (two tablespoons more or less) and add sufficient water to make the slippery elm powder hold together. Knead the powder until it is quite stiff. Cut into three pieces, each one about an inch long, and set aside. Take a new sponge such as a sea sponge, and cut a portion of the sponge the size to fit into the vagina and completely fill the opening. Sew a piece of sturdy thread firmly to the sponge, leaving three to four inches of the thread to hang out. Smear the sponge with lubricant jelly and set aside.

Dip one piece of the slippery elm ball into boiling water and insert as far as possible into the vagina. Follow with the second and third pieces. Next insert the smeared sponge into the opening to hold the ball in place. Leave the sponge in for one to two days. Remove the sponge by pulling down on the thread. Irrigate the vagina thoroughly with a douche, using a cleansing agent such as yellow dock tea. Wait about six hours before repeating the pack.

Instead of slippery elm herb alone, some other herb may be mixed with it, such as goldenseal powder for infections, licorice root powder for hormonal problems, etc.

The suppository is very helpful in these conditions.

- Trichomonas vaginitis – This condition has a white to green colored vaginal discharge, more noticeable several days after a menstrual period, with vaginal itching, burning, irritation, pain, painful urination, and a foul or fishy smell. Risk increases with the use of oral contraceptives or HRT, the number of sexual partners, use of antibiotics, wearing tight jeans or nylon underwear, and depression or anxiety.
- Candida vaginitis – This condition has as its hallmark vaginal itching with a thick, curdy, almost cottage cheesy discharge.
- Chlamydia vaginitis – This affects 5 to 10 percent of sexually active women, but it usually has no symptoms until other infections develop such as of the cervix, fallopian tubes, or urethra, when the symptoms of pelvic inflammatory disease develops.

Vulvodynia, Vestibulitis

The diagnosis is made on the basis of chronic vulvovaginal pain made worse by marital relations or attempted vaginal entry that has no explanation and a biopsy that gives no specific grounds for pain.

The patient should be checked for dermatographism as it is sometimes present and helps to confirm the diagnosis. The patient should also be checked for a contact dermatitis such as a sensitivity to hand soap, laundry soap, talcum, hand lotions, etc.

To treat vulvodynia, switch to a plant-based diet, and use foods that are high in myoinositol—cantaloupe, citrus (especially grapefruit), beans such as pintos, and peanuts.

Oxalic acid has been implicated in the cause of pain in the vagina and vulva. Take no high-oxalate foods such as parsley, kale, leeks, escarole, dandelion, Swiss chard, beets, celery, parsnips, winter squash, yams, wheat, wheat bran, oats, popcorn, spelt, soy, sesame seeds, peanut butter, and green beans until the condition clears.

Calcium citrate can be helpful. Use the recommended daily dose on the package.

Daily douche using one tablespoon of a mixture of vinegar, calendula, and myrrh (make up the formula for fungus toenail medicine) diluted in one cup of hot water. Do the douche daily for six weeks. This may be alternated every other day with a slippery elm pack (See "Vaginitis.") Make plans to treat the vestibulitis for one year, but you may be significantly better in three months.

Licorice root powder tea may also be helpful.

Worms

(See "Parasites" in the *Conditions and Diseases* section.)

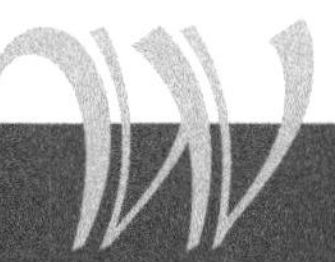

Xanthoma, Xanthelasma

These are flat, yellow plaques that may develop on the surface of the skin. The tumor is caused by cholesterol being deposited in the skin. The preferred location is the inner part of the lower eyelids, but it may also involve the upper eyelids or any other part of the skin, including the palms. The important matter in healing these cases is control of cholesterol. Do not take medications to bring cholesterol down. (See "Cholesterol" and "Weight Control" in the *Conditions and Diseases* section.)

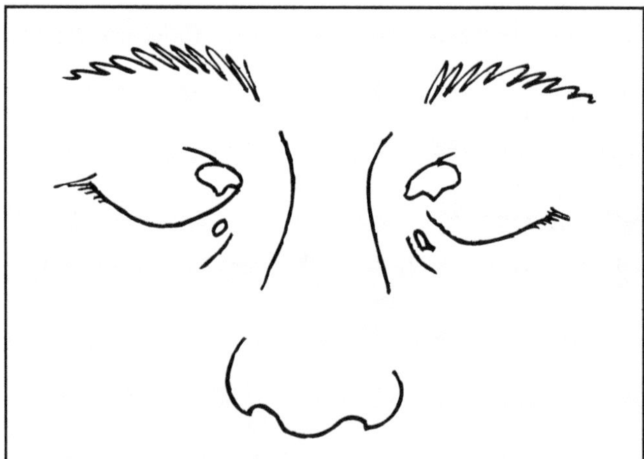

Case Reports

A young man in his thirties suffered a back injury that led him to stay at home and become sedentary. He watched TV all the time and ate junk food. When he came to Uchee Pines, his cholesterol was 2400 and his triglycerides were 1800! He had xanthelasmas on both upper eyelids. He also had mild angina.

After two weeks he became recommitted to Christian ideals and took a greater interest in working for improved health. Within five weeks his cholesterol was 350 and triglycerides 475. He was joyous. Gradually through the years his weight has continued to come down, as have his blood fats. He is now in good health, his back injury is completely healed, and he works on a daily basis.

Several years ago a woman came to Uchee Pines with xanthomas all over her body, including her palms and soles. Her triglycerides were 2450 and cholesterol was 425. She had mild diabetes, but was not taking insulin. Within two weeks she could tell that the skin lesions were "flattening out," but the doctor could not discern it. Her blood fats had fallen—triglycerides to 625 and cholesterol to 290. Within six weeks her triglycerides were 185 and cholesterol 180. The xanthomas also disappeared.

In both cases the treatment consisted of exercise, a totally vegetarian diet, two tablespoons of powdered charcoal in water by mouth four times daily, and wheat bran along with restrictions on free fats, free sugars, and textured vegetarian proteins.

Home Emergencies

Introduction

Of the millions of serious accidents that occur in the home every day, almost half are because of falls. We will discuss some of the commonest accidents within this portion of the book. Some accidents may require prompt treatment at the emergency room, but there are simple measures that can be done immediately that may save the life of your loved one.

This section is listed in alphabetical order as to the home emergencies that may arise, but the following applies to all emergencies. Every home should be equipped with a first aid kit, which should contain the following items:

- laxative herbs and aids
- medicine dropper
- bandages, various sizes
- gauze pads
- splints, wooden, 18 inches long
- water purification materials
- activated charcoal powder
- safety pins, large and medium
- adhesive tape
- other strong tape
- elastic bandages (such as Ace)
- scissors
- needles, sewing, large
- ear syringe
- tweezers
- magnifying glass
- thermometer
- blood pressure cuff
- stethoscope
- basin, 2-3 gallon size
- heating pad
- hot water bottle
- massage oil
- arnica oil
- alcohol
- iodine solution for cleansing
- herbs: hot pepper, catnip

Abdominal Pain

(See also "Abdominal Pain" in the *Supplemental Information* section.)

For acute abdominal pain consider saving urine, stool, vaginal discharge, and vomitus for future reference and for consultation by a physician, if needed. Specimens should be put in moisture proof containers, double bagged, and put in a refrigerator. Freezing is not usually necessary.

If pain is sharp, limited to one area, aggravated by movement such as coughing or sneezing, and lasts for more than three hours, there is probably an inflammation of the peritoneum (lining of the abdominal cavity) such as from an inflamed appendix, gallbladder, or fallopian tube.

If pain originates from an abdominal organ, the pain is often poorly localized and may or may not be colicky (worse and then better) in character. Usually tenderness is on direct pressure, but not on sudden release of pressure from the abdomen (rebound pain). Acute pain usually means acute dilation, distention, congestion, or pulling on an abdominal organ. The pain is generally felt above solid organs, in the center of the abdomen for small bowel involvement, and on the sides for large bowel involvement.

Very often pain originating in the abdomen refers to another part: irritation of the diaphragm gives referred pain to the area over the shoulder blade; distention of the bile ducts or gallbladder refers pain to the right sub-shoulder blade area; acute pancreatitis refers pain straight through to the back; an acute heart attack or pleurisy may refer pain to the abdomen or to either arm; pain in the rectum or uterus is referred to the low back; pain in the ureter radiates all the way down from the flank to the same side external genitalia; pneumonia often refers pain to the lower abdomen.

If the bowel is involved, there may be loss of appetite, nausea, diarrhea. If the urinary system is involved, the patient may have pain on voiding, blood in the urine, or pain in the flank. Consider also that abdominal pain may be because of hardening of the arteries, sickle cell anemia, diabetes, kidney failure, intestinal parasites, allergies, ulcerative colitis, peptic ulcer, or diverticulosis. Drugs may also be a cause of acute abdominal pain, as may alcohol and cortisone-like drugs.

You may simply wait and watch the patient with abdominal pain overnight if the person has a good appetite and normal bowel movements. However, be sure to eliminate appendicitis as a possible cause. (See "Appendicitis" in the *Conditions and Diseases* section.) A blood test to determine the white blood cell count may be needed to determine if the pain is from appendicitis or salpingitis or another serious problem.

Treatment

Check yourself for food sensitivities. Caffeinated beverages, spices, and the nightshades (solanine is the offending chemical in these foods and is found in tomatoes, potatoes, eggplant, and peppers) can cause abdominal pain.

Twenty cherries contain between 12 and 25 milligrams of anthocyanins, a dose which can be 10 times more effective than aspirin in relieving pain (*Nutrition Week* 29 [March 12, 1999]: 7).

Never overeat, as overeating intensifies pain.

Water has good pain-relieving properties. Drink 8 to 12 glasses each day.

Walk if you are able. Exercise is good for pain because it releases natural pain-relieving endorphins. If you cannot walk out of doors, lie out of doors in an area protected from the wind and where the sun is not too hot. Sunshine, even penetrating through your clothing, can bring relief.

Use a charcoal compress, laying it over the entire abdomen and sides. Pain relief will often come in a short while by the use of a charcoal compress.

Add one cup of cold water and one heaping tablespoon of charcoal powder to a pint or quart size jar. Tightly screw on a lid and shake it over a sink in case the lid leaks. When the charcoal powder is completely dispersed in the water, carefully unscrew the lid over a sink to catch any spills and pour the charcoal slurry into a cup for the patient. This is one adult dose. Drink the mixture three to four times daily to relieve abdominal pain caused by gas.

To control pain, use alternating applications of heat and cold, applied in a variety of methods—heating pad, hot water bottle, ice cap, or a jar filled with ice or hot water and wrapped in a towel. Other methods include a hot tub bath, a hot shower, a "short cold bath" (30 to 120 seconds in cold bath water of 50°F to 65°F). Hot water applied directly is usually the most effective—the temperature of the water being from 105°F to 110°F, but the easiest method should be tried first. Generally, the hot applications should be as hot as can be tolerated and the cold applications should be as cold as you can get them. Alternating hot and cold packs may be applied to the abdomen for aches and pains. Wring a towel from hot water and place it on the abdomen for three to six minutes. Replace the hot compress with an ice-cold compress for 30 to 60 seconds. Alternate in this fashion for three to five changes.

Use slippery elm tea for stomach or bowel pain, one teaspoon per one cup of water.

Anesthesia, Natural Methods

From time to time a situation arises in the home making it desirable to deaden pain. Removing a thorn or splinter from a sensitive area, or pulling a "baby tooth" from a young child are two examples. Of course, there are many others. Ice is one of the most effective at-home anesthetics. Among herbs, clove oil is one of the most effective. In addition, prolonged pressure or intense and repeated tapping are quite effective to produce anesthesia.

To use ice, simply freeze a styrofoam cup full of water. When it is ready for use, tear away the bottom. This prevents the ice from slipping out of the cup as it melts. Rub the place to be anesthetized. For example, let us say you intend to put a stitch in a small skin wound. Rub the ice over the wound and about an inch on all sides, keeping the ice moving. The ice causes pain at first, and then burning after about one minute, but then anesthesia sets in after about three minutes and continues for about three minutes. If you have clean hands, a clean needle, and clean thread ready, you have just enough time to set one stitch before the anesthesia fades and the skin must be re-iced. Then two to three minutes of icing will produce three more minutes of anesthesia, plenty of time to place a stitch, remove the splinter, or snip off a skin tag.

Clove oil is quite effective for giving pain relief for teeth. For centuries it has been used for this effect. If the clove oil is not available, a single clove bud can be put against the gum and held there for its anesthetic property. Clove oil (one part), mixed with hand lotion (ten parts) in a one to ten dilution, can stop itching or pain in the skin. If the clove oil stings the skin, dilute it more with the lotion.

Massage strokes may also be used to produce anesthesia. Repeated firm stroking will bring anesthesia, or at least greatly reduce painful sensations. The area should be repeatedly and rapidly rubbed for three to five minutes until anesthesia occurs. A second massage maneuver is firm pressure over the area for three to five minutes. If the pressure is firm enough, anesthesia or low sensation will follow the pressure. Repeatedly tapping the skin can cause loss of sensation for a short while, and is the most effective massage stroke for bringing anesthesia.

Allspice, the mints, and tarragon all have mild anesthetic properties. Oil of wintergreen is similar to clove oil but not as strong to produce anesthesia. The extract of any willow tree bark has some anesthetic qualities. These oils are for external use only.

Magnesium salicylate can be made into a paste with water or olive oil and used as an anesthetic on the skin or mucous membrane. Allow about 30–45 minutes for the best effect.

Automobile Accidents

The most important thing to do at an accident site is to have common sense and sound judgment, good observation skills, and a willingness to use your hands and eyes to help. Any intelligent person can perform a quick, systematic, head-to-toe examination of an accident victim.

The two most important things to ensure is that the victim's airway is open and any active bleeding is stopped. First, in an unconscious person, tilt the head back by putting your hand on the forehead of the person and gently depressing it downward while lifting gently on the chin, so that the head is tilted backward as far as possible to make a straight line from the nose and mouth to the lungs. This will keep the airway from becoming blocked by a relaxed tongue and palate. The second thing is to take a clean cloth and apply direct pressure with the palm of the hand on any cuts or gashes to stop the flow of blood.

No heroic measures are more likely to save a life than these two simple things.

Bite Wounds

If death results from an allergic reaction to an insect bite, it usually comes within 15 to 30 minutes after the sting. Other reactions are hives, itching all over, sweating, headache, tightness in the chest or throat, wheezing, shock, and dizziness. A little bit of swelling, about an inch or less, is a normal reaction to an insect sting. If the swelling extends beyond two joints of the extremity stung, or if the swelling is intense and quite extensive, you have an allergic reaction, which is usually not dangerous. But if sweating, shortness of breath, headache, nausea, chest or abdominal pain or faintness occur immediately, you may be dealing with a serious anaphylactic reaction, and the patient may need a respirator in the next 5 to 10 minutes unless you can stop the reaction with charcoal or an injection from a venomous bite kit.

Following are specific instructions for a variety of different bites and stings.

Animal Bites

Human bite wounds are the most likely of all bites to become seriously infected, and they should be washed as thoroughly as possible, irrigated with water and cleansed with hydrogen peroxide and any kind of good antiseptic available in the home, such as iodine or mercurochrome. Following the irrigation with the antiseptic, irrigation with water should again be done thoroughly. Dog or cat bites may be similarly treated, but the animal should be impounded and tested for rabies.

If infection should occur, soak the part every two to three hours in hot water or hot charcoal water, or apply hot compresses to areas that cannot be immersed, such as the face or trunk. Apply the wet heat for 30 minutes, 4 to 10 times a day, dressing the wound with comfrey compresses, or tea tree oil compresses, or other healing oils, ointments, or salves.

Snake Bites, Bee Stings, Spiders, Insects and Their Relatives

While snakes are more feared, more Americans actually die each year from allergic reactions to insect stings than from snake bites. Bees, wasps, yellow jackets, hornets, and ants are the principal offenders. Only two varieties of spiders, the black widow and the brown recluse, are dangerous to persons living in the United States. Most insect bites are not usually dangerous, but some people are intensely sensitive, and a sting or bite can be life threatening. For these persons venomous bites represent a serious emergency.

Bees and Wasps

The venom injected by the bee is composed of strongly acid or alkaline materials, a substance much like histamine, the chemical released into the bloodstream when one is having an allergic reaction. Some people have such sensitivity to the venom that the symptoms are quite dangerous.

After any sting, wash the spot and apply a cold compress. Use ice if it is available. Washing is important because some of the stinging insects such as yellow jackets and fire ants are scavengers and can carry infection. A charcoal bath applied immediately can assist in detoxifying some of the venom that has been injected. Take two to four tablespoons of charcoal slurry immediately by mouth.

The stinger should be removed by scraping it off with a knife or edge of a stiff credit card to prevent more venom being squeezed into the skin. Use care not to press on the fleshy part of the stinger, only on the hard sticker part that penetrates the skin.

Work fast to make a charcoal compress. Stir a few drops of water into a tablespoon or more of powdered charcoal to make a paste about the consistency of mayonnaise, and spread it on a folded paper towel about one-quarter inch thick. The charcoal may be placed directly on the skin, or one layer of the paper towel can be folded over it to keep from spreading the charcoal too widely. We have found charcoal compresses to be the treatment of choice, especially in very sensitive persons for whom the bee sting may represent a hazard to the life. In extremely sensitive cases, the charcoal should be applied with all haste, as minutes may count.

Vinegar is beneficial in the stings of wasps, hornets, and yellow jackets, followed by charcoal compresses, or used alone. Apply vinegar liberally on a cloth or paper towel to prevent itching, pain, and swelling. After about 20 minutes of vinegar application, make a charcoal compress, which should be kept on for 48 hours, changing it every four to eight hours.

Apply a paste of baking soda after carefully removing the stinger. Baking soda is as effective as vinegar to control itching and pain.

Insect bites should never be scratched when they are fresh. Scratching will spread the venom, which might have serious results in very sensitive persons.

If one has ever had a serious reaction to insect stings or bites, such as fainting, sweating, headache, chest pain with breathing, wheezing, severe weakness, and nausea, he should obtain an emergency kit containing injectable adrenalin and keep it near at all times. The next sting could be fatal if not treated immediately.

A remedy can be made by crushing several papaya enzyme tablets with enough water to make a thick paste. Apply the paste to the sting to break down the protein molecules of the venom.

Another very effective method to be used while in the woods when nothing else is available is to mix a bit of clay or fine soil with water. The soil can be obtained by digging into the ground several inches. This will also draw out toxins as it dries.

Comfrey root crushed and simmered in a little water (two tablespoons of the fresh root to one cup of water) for about five minutes may be used to diminish itching. You may use the water as a wet dressing, or the lightly boiled roots as a soft poultice.

Black Widow

The female black widow has a shiny black body and a scarlet hourglass figure on her belly. She is about half an inch long. The first evidence of penetration by her fangs is a sharp pain and a swelling and redness in the area. The black widow venom causes extremely severe abdominal pain and muscular tenseness, sometimes accompanied by pain in the extremities. Other symptoms may include inability to void, slowing of the heartbeat, a feeble pulse, and difficulty breathing or speaking. Delirium may also occur. In rare cases the black widow spider venom causes breakdown of red blood cells and some degree of kidney blockage. Deaths are rare from black widow spider bites.

Since the treatment for all venomous bites is about the same, we will describe the black widow bite as an example. The first treatment for black widow spider bites is to put the patient or the effected extremity in a tub of very hot water. If the pain recedes, it is confirmation of a black widow spider bite. The hot water will keep the pain away. Remember to keep the face and neck cool with ice-cold compresses and a small electric fan directed on the face. The pain can be quite severe. Watch the patient for 48 hours after the pain diminishes.

The bite is not usually very dangerous, but there could be some degree of circulatory collapse in a small child or in an aged person with blood vessel disease. The victim should drink plenty of water. From the beginning of the treatment with the hot water, have the victim drink a charcoal slurry made by stirring one or two heaping tablespoons of charcoal powder (depending on the size of the victim) into a glass of water and administering this every two hours until four doses have been taken. Remember that a small child cannot drink a lot of water. Put the dose of charcoal in a small glass for their slurry. Then drop down to a dose every four hours. You may discontinue the charcoal slurry when the pain is gone.

As soon as possible, apply a large, very moist charcoal compress. Change the compress every 10 minutes for the first hour, then every 30 minutes for the next two hours, then every hour until bedtime. Arise every two hours during the night to change compresses. If symptoms do not progress, or if they seem to be abating, nothing further needs to be done.

If a blister forms over the area of the bite, trim it off with scissors or scrub it off with a stiff bristle brush, if necessary being somewhat vigorous in the scrubbing motion before applying the next charcoal compress.

Keep up charcoal compress changes until the swelling ceases, making a schedule of four times daily after the first 24 hours.

There are immune serums that may be administered in an emergency room if the symptoms progress.

Brown Recluse

The bite of the brown recluse spider needs the above treatment for black widow spiders with charcoal compresses changed every 30 minutes for the first six hours, every hour for the next six hours, twice during the night, and three times during the second day. If symptoms do not progress, or seem to be abating, nothing further needs to be done. Keep up the four daily compress changes until swelling and redness cease.

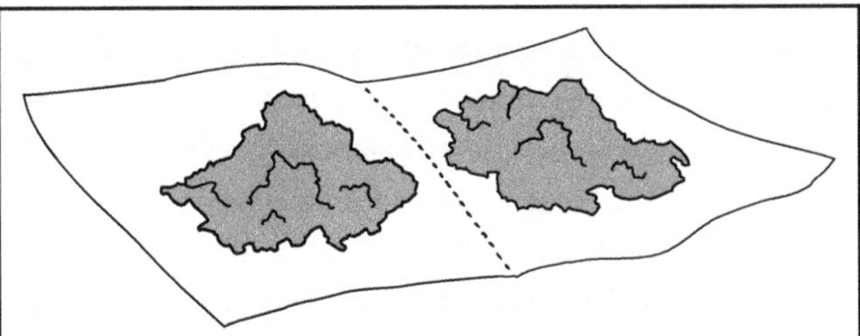

Chiggers, Mites

Chiggers are prevalent in the South for about three months each year. Chiggers are an almost microscopic wood mite that climb on people walking in the woods and migrate to the body creases and areas where the clothing fits snugly. A chigger bite shows up as a red pinpoint that severly itches for a few days.

Since it takes about two hours for the chigger to find its place and become embedded, one can prevent many bites by taking a bath within a few minutes of returning from the woods or grassy fields.

The following suggestions can prevent chiggers and/or help to alleviate the itch:

- Rubbing Basic-H or L.O.C. (commercial detergent concentrates) on the skin before going into the woods will prevent most infestations.
- A coating of any kind of kitchen oil will also prevent infestation. The oil suffocates the mites as they begin to bite.
- Once they imbed they turn bright red and may be easily scratched off with the fingernail, but itching will continue.
- Itching can be controlled by a 5 to 20 minute hot bath, which will usually give one about eight hours of relief. You may need three such baths per day.
- The inside of banana skins may be rubbed on the chigger bites, which helps in healing and itch control.
- Aloe vera leaves can be opened and the liquid rubbed on the bite to promote healing and relieve itching.
- Charcoal added to the hot bath water described above or applied as compresses encourages healing and can relieve itching at night.
- A dot of clove oil on an itchy lesion can stop the itch.
- Vinegar or baking soda paste may be used for itching.

Mosquito, Ant, and Other Insect Bites

Before entering an infested area, liberally rub all your skin that might get crawling or jumping insects such as chiggers, lice, ticks, or fleas with a pure detergent concentrate. This discourages their attaching to your skin.

As a mosquito repellant, rub lemon rind on all exposed areas. For a general insect repellant, you may use Skin So Soft, which leaves a residue on the skin that repels insects. Also, flowers of sulfur powder taken by mouth is excreted in the skin, leaving a residue that repels insects. A tablespoon of the yellow powder mixed with water, or honey or syrup, should be sufficient for one day. Dusting a bit of the sulfur powder in your socks repels chiggers and perhaps also ticks. However, it may leave your clothing yellow.

Onion and garlic, sliced and rubbed on an insect bite, can ease swelling and itching.

Ordinary black or pekoe tea leaves from the grocery store, moistened in a bit of hot water and placed on the bite, can be very helpful.

Crushed fresh dandelion leaves are sometimes helpful.

For chiggers, mosquitoes, and other insect bites use tea tree oil. The itching can be stopped by soaking in a hot tub for 5 to 10 minutes, or longer if necessary. The hot tub soak will provide several itch-free hours.

For relief of itching and stinging, spread vinegar, household ammonia, or a paste of baking soda or charcoal on the bite.

Scorpions

For scorpion bites, the prompt application of activated charcoal powder, directly on the skin within the first minute or so of the sting or bite if possible, may save a life. If you work or live in an area that is known for scorpions, it would be wise to mix up charcoal and honey and carry it in a small jar, such as an empty pill or cosmetic bottle, for immediate use. You may also moisten a charcoal tablet in a little water and smear it directly on the bite, while someone prepares enough charcoal to make a paste to spread one-quarter inch thick over the involved area and three inches on all sides. Apply a new compress every ten minutes for two hours if you are known to have a life-threatening sensitivity.

Meanwhile, or as soon as possible, prepare a large and very moist charcoal compress to extend two to four inches on all sides of the bite or sting, using four to six tablespoons of activated charcoal powder and sufficient water.

A charcoal bath, using half a cup of powder to a gallon of cool water in a foot tub, plastic trash can, or bucket is used to immerse the part to be treated. If there are stings on the trunk, a charcoal bath can be prepared by mixing one cup of powdered charcoal to a bathtub of slightly warm water. The person can lie in the tub, dipping the black water onto any affected part using a cup. The charcoal bath can help control general allergic symptoms such as hives or swelling. Charcoal powder, one tablespoon stirred in a glass of water, taken by mouth can also help control generalized symptoms.

Some kinds of meat tenderizer, such as Adolph's brand, will sometimes denature the protein portions of the venom, and should be kept on hand in high-risk areas. In addition, enzymes such as papain, bromelain, or slices of fresh papaya or fresh pineapple can be helpful in venomous bites when applied immediately. Simply moisten the skin over the bite and sprinkle the tenderizer on the area or slice the fruit and lay a slice on the bite. Change the application every 10 minutes.

For venomous bites there are devices somewhat like a miniature stun gun that claim to render a bite harmless by eliminating the protein in the venom. Search for "bug bite detox mini-zapper" on the Internet.

Snake Bites

The pit vipers such as rattlesnake, moccasin, and copperhead are the most dangerous snakes in the United States. Most bites occur below the knees; therefore, a person wearing boots in the woods is rarely envenomated even though struck or bitten by a snake. About 300 bites occur in Florida each year. Less than 10 people die each year in the United States from snake bites because of the availability of medical attention. Be prepared with powdered charcoal if you hike in the woods.

Venomous insect and snake bites should be treated quickly with charcoal compresses or baths. The part may be submerged in a tub of charcoal water large enough to completely submerge the part at least two inches. Or a large, soupy charcoal compress may be applied. A charcoal compress will assist in extracting the venom while medical attention is sought.

Bleeding, Nosebleeds, and Coughing Blood

(See "Hemorrhage" in the *Conditions and Diseases* section.)

Broken Bones

A broken bone is often recognized by failure of the limb to function properly. A homemade splint of a large magazine wrapped lengthwise around the extremity, or even a folded heavy blanket tied in place with handkerchiefs or strips of fabric, will serve to immobilize the part, reduce pain, and protect while being transported to an emergency room. Never attempt to put the broken ends of a bone back in place if they project into a dirt-filled wound. All dirt must be meticulously cleaned out or trimmed off before replacing bones or closing the wound.

In a field situation it might be necessary to attempt to set the bone yourself. This may be done by putting traction

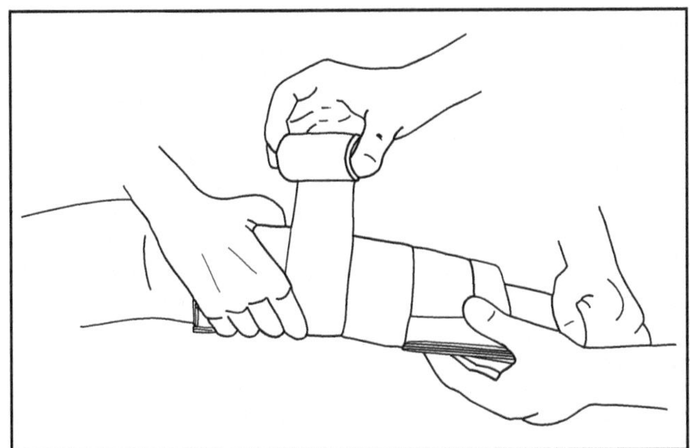

on the extremity sufficient to pull the broken ends back in perfect alignment. Expect quite a lot of pain. Get a helper to assist in stabilizing the end next to the patient if possible. After the bone is set, wrap it with some padding material and then fashion a splint securely enough to immobilize the part. This may be strips of wood or metal.

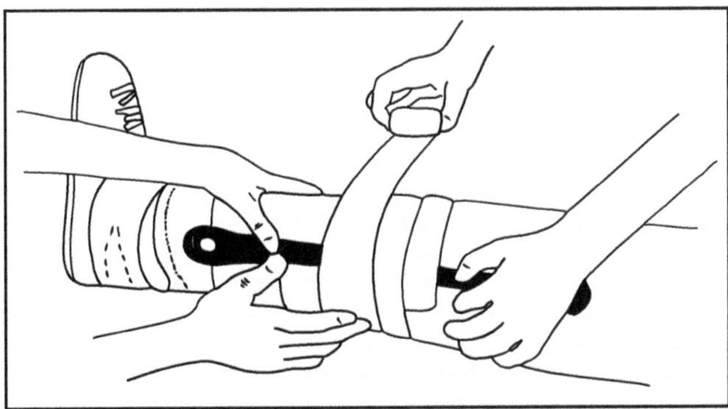

Knitting of the bones may require four to six weeks, during which time mild exercises may prevent some of the atrophy of muscles and promote circulation to the fractured part. Pain can be controlled by ice packs applied directly to the limb, or to the opposite extremity. If the extremity cannot be moved, exercise of the opposite extremity will help significantly to prevent atrophy of the affected part.

Bruises

An injury caused by impact in which neither laceration nor external bleeding occurs is called a bruise. Pain is sometimes followed by redness and swelling. Since blood oozes from broken blood vessels into the skin or deeper tissues, the skin may become dark blue before turning brown or yellow in a few days.

Ice packs can lessen the pain. An injury to the face can often be prevented from developing into a black eye by immediately putting pressure on the injured area to prevent bleeding into the tissue. After about 10 minutes of pressure, an ice compress can be applied. If the black eye develops, alternating hot and cold compresses will reduce the discoloration quicker than either cold alone or heat alone.

For treating bruises and preventing sprains and strains, keep some arnica oil on hand to rub on the area as soon as possible after the bruise or strain. A comfrey compress may also help clear the blood out of the tissue.

Burns

A burn may result from various agents ranging from steam, chemicals, grease, hot water, electricity, and the sun's rays. Burns are classified into three groups:

- First-degree burns involve only reddening of the skin, and usually only require treatment from cold water compresses, the juice of aloe vera leaves, or some soothing ointment, such as petroleum jelly. A mild sunburn is a first-degree burn.
- Second-degree burns include blistering of the skin as well as superficial reddening.
- Third-degree burns cause destruction of the tissue. Promptly covering the burn with cold, wet compresses, or soaking in cold water or saline to relieve pain is the best treatment for second- and third-degree burns. Aloe vera gel, or the juice from aloe vera leaves, may be used to keep the area clean and free from infection, as well as to prevent excessive loss of fluid. Cover the area with petroleum jelly and place gauze over the burn after the aloe vera juice has dried. To counteract shock, which in severe burns may be fatal, keep the victim lying flat with clothing loosened. Give as much water, or saline, as possible either by mouth or by rectum until arrangements can be made to transfer the victim to a burn center.

Other herbs useful for burns include chamomile, echinacea, gotu kola, and St. John's wort.

Burns with acid or alkali should be washed thoroughly at once with plenty of plain water. If this is done immediately, the burn will often only be superficial. If the chemical is not immediately removed, second- or third-degree burns may result. A solution of baking soda water can be used for acid burns once plain water has been generously used. Vinegar water may be used for alkaline burns.

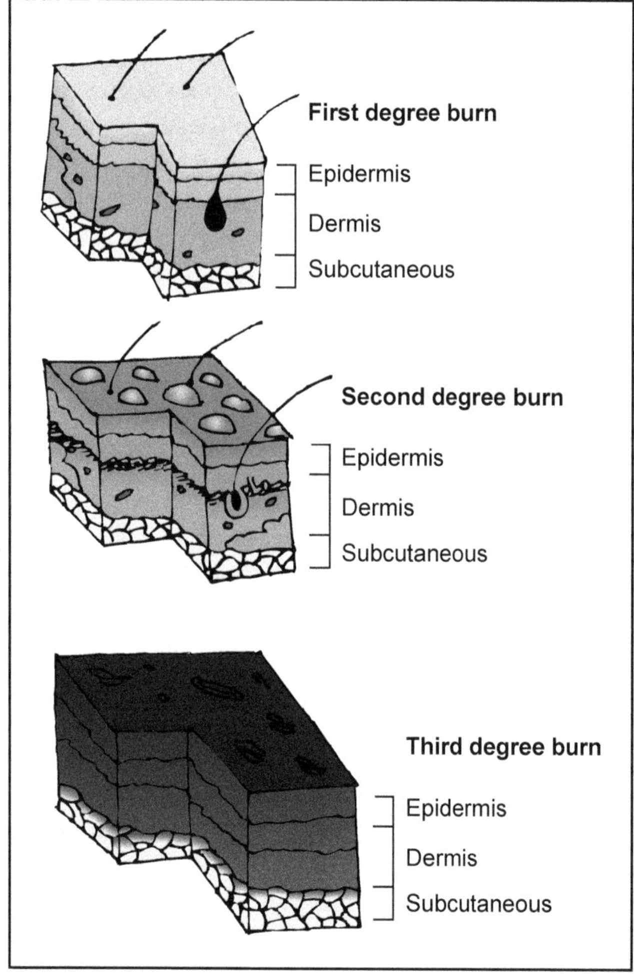

If the person has swallowed acid or alkali, give sips of water at once and then administer large amounts of charcoal powder stirred into water to adsorb some of the alkali or acid. DO NOT attempt to make the person vomit! The strong alkali or acid will burn the esophagus both going and coming. Do not try to neutralize the acid or alkali until you consult with a Poison Control Center, as some alkalis and acids almost explode in the stomach with household neutralizing substances such as baking soda. However, you may very safely use charcoal.

For flash burns of the eyes, take the clear gel from freshly broken or cut aloe vera blades and put it directly into the eyes. It brings rapid and total relief of symptoms and speeds up healing (*New England Journal of Medicine,* August 9, 1984).

For acute burns with pain, apply apple cider vinegar on the burned area. If it is on a large area such as the back, as in the case of a sunburn, it can be poured over the skin. Often the pain relief is immediate and scars are reduced or prevented. Also, for large burned areas, aloe vera blades can be sliced thinly and laid over the burn.

Choking and Other Foreign Objects

If an infant aspirates a foreign object into the windpipe, placing him face down and head down, but not upside down, may encourage coughing or spitting up of the object. If the object in the nose is a bean or other dried seed, it may swell if left a long time in the nose. Act quickly in those cases.

If a person stops eating, quits talking, and motions that they are choking stand the person up and perform the Heimlich manuever by using the following steps: get behind the person, press your clenched fist just above the waist and below the rib cage, thumb side toward the patient, and with your other hand rapidly and forcefully (as forcefully as you can) press your fist with the thumb pointed upward toward the back of the patient's neck. The air in the lungs should quickly expel the food by a coughing action.

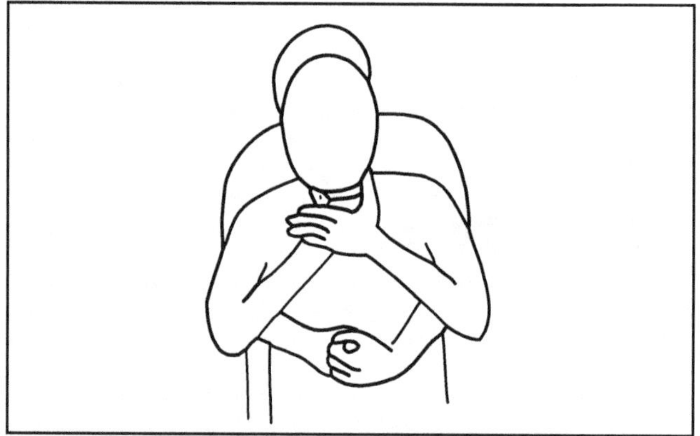

If the person cannot stand up and is sitting in a chair, have someone support the head and do the same maneuver, wrapping your arms around the chair back and the patient. Do the maneuver essentially as you did for the standing patient.

If the patient is lying down, put the patient on the back with the head turned to the side. Put the heel of your strongest hand above the waist under the rib cage in the center and give the same kind of very forceful, quick upward thrust. Repeat until the object is dislodged.

Foreign bodies in the ear, or insects, may often be removed by filling the ear with warm olive oil. The insect dies in the oil and can then be irrigated out with warm water. If it is an object, the oil will lubricate it so that it will hopefully fall out when the ear is drained. The water should be body temperature or dizziness may ensue.

A fish hook caught in the skin should not be pulled, but should be pushed. Cut the loop off the end with wire cutters and grasp the hook part and pull it all the way through.

Electrical Injuries

In the home there are two major sources of electrical injury, accidental contact with an electric current and lightning strikes. Most fatal electrical accidents actually occur in industry. In the home such accidents may result from faulty electric wire insulation or careless handling of lighting, heating, or refrigeration equipment.

When struck by lightning, the person falls to the ground as if a stunning blow to the head had been received. Blindness or deafness may ensue, along with paralysis, pain in the limbs, and sometimes hemorrhaging.

Dry skin offers a high resistance to electricity. Surface burns following an electric shock are greater and internal damage less if the victim has dry skin. Moist skin reduces resistance and permits the current to have greater access to the interior of the body with greater chance of death, although surface burns may be less severe.

A person suffering from an electric shock must be immediately removed from contact with the source of the current. If a live wire must be cut, an axe with a wooden handle is an ideal instrument. If one is not available, something made of rope, leather, or wood may be used to detach the victim from the electric current. Under all circumstances, the rescuer must protect himself from touching the victim as the current may be transmitted to the rescuer from the victim's body, or even from water in which the victim may be lying. The rescuer must be very careful not to step on wet ground, or especially on a wet floor on which the victim is lying. Throw a board or a piece of plastic on the wet ground or cover it with a blanket or coat. A leather belt, a dry rope, a wooden stick, or a hoe may be just the tool necessary to pull the wire off the person.

If the victim is unconscious or breathing has ceased, artificial respiration should be given at once and continued until medical help arrives. When the patient has resumed breathing on his own, the clothing should be loosened.

Once respiration and heartbeat are established, surface burns and injuries sustained in falling may be evaluated. Do not unduly disturb the resting person to attend to external wounds for the first hour unless there are life-threatening injuries on the surface.

Electrical burns may be treated as any other burn. Expect them to heal more slowly and show greater injury than thermal burns for the apparent extent of the burn.

Eye Care

Chemical Burns of the Eye

Immediately flood the eye (seconds count) with large quantities of water. The person can bend over a sink and rinse the eyes by water in the cupped hands. While the person is washing the eyes repeatedly for 10 to 15 minutes, someone else can prepare a saline solution using one teaspoon of salt to one pint of water, to which has been added one tablespoon of kitchen vinegar (not vinegar from pickles which contain spices, etc.) to be used for alkali burns, or one teaspoon of baking soda to the pint of saline for acids.

Eyelid Burns

For first-degree burns of the eyelids, the treatment of choice is gauze or cotton cloth strips onto which petroleum jelly has been smeared. Second- or third-degree eyelid burns are usually associated with extensive body burns as well and may need professional help.

Eyelid Lacerations

Lacerations of the lids do not need to be repaired provided the laceration edges fall together in a smooth line with no gaping opening and if the tiny opening at the inner corner of the eyelid is not involved in the laceration or the firm rim of the lid. If the inner corner is involved, the opening must be repaired in an operating room in order to prevent scarring of the tube that drains off tears, thus causing the patient to be constantly wiping tears.

If the lacerations are deep, particularly if the upper lid is lacerated, the muscle may be severed. This kind of laceration must also be repaired by a surgeon or the patient will be left with a permanent drooping of the eyelid. If the laceration is deep enough to involve the muscle of the upper lid, it may also be deep enough to involve the eye. If the laceration is vertical, the laceration must be repaired by a surgeon or the wound edges will notch in a staggered fashion, causing permanent unsightly scarring.

Foreign Objects

A tiny particle in the eye may be removed with a facial tissue. If it is caught under the eyelid, the lid may be turned up over a match stick or wooden toothpick. The eyelid can then be rubbed to remove the speck. If a speck appears on the eyeball itself, a facial tissue, cotton-tipped applicator, or clean handkerchief may be used to get it off. Touch the cotton against the eyeball, and the object will become attached to the cotton. If it fails to move, it must be removed by a medical professional. In this case, place a wet gauze or handkerchief over the entire eye and transport the patient to an emergency room.

Fainting

If a person has fainted, lay the person on the floor, apply cold water to the face, put the head on a small pillow, and fan the person to get plenty of fresh air to the face. The person may be lifted to a bed or chair as soon as consciousness is recovered. Offer cool water as soon as the person is revived, as fainting is often caused by acute or chronic dehydration. In addition, most kinds of medication can cause fainting.

Heat Stroke

If not caught early and wisely dealt with, heat stroke can be fatal. Heat stroke is a condition in which the body temperature continues to rise out of control, even up to 112°F, at which point protein breakdown occurs, followed rapidly by death. Body heat accumulates when the total heat production exceeds heat dissipation. If the situation is progressive, heat stroke will result. It is caused by a high work rate in very hot and humid conditions. If the ability of the body to lose heat is compromised for any reason, such as drugs or pulmonary disease, heat stroke develops in less extreme conditions. Dehydration predisposes to heat stroke by decreasing the efficiency of evaporation of sweat, which results in reduction of cooling of the skin surface. Also, the circulation is not as brisk if a person is dehydrated.

Circumstances that can increase the likelihood of heat stroke are obesity, cardiovascular disease, being unaccustomed to heat and humidity, advanced age, and alcoholism. The absence of sweating is regarded as an essential feature to distinguish between heat exhaustion and heat stroke. Heat stroke mortality is about 80 percent or more. Heat exhaustion acts somewhat like heat stroke, but sweating is always present in heat exhaustion. It is not as dangerous as heat stroke.

In very hot weather, particularly in closed rooms, persons may experience a rising temperature with dizziness, drowsiness, and fast breathing. Such a person should be taken to a cool place, immersed in cool water up to the neck, and ice should be added to the bath water until the mouth temperature drops to 101°F. If the person is sweating profusely, you do not have as much to worry about as if the person is not sweating at all. That represents the greatest danger signal! Quick action is necessary to save the person's life.

Give the person sips of ice water if conscious and not nauseated or vomiting.

Everything you do for the person must be done while the person is in the ice water, including artificial respiration if it should become necessary. If breathing should stop, administer artificial respiration by closing the nostrils, opening the mouth, and breathing your exhaled breath into their mouth, making certain that there is no obstruction to the airway. To tilt the head backward will ensure a free airway in most people.

Massaging the skin while the person is in the cold water helps accelerate heat loss and carries cool blood to the overheated brain and internal organs.

Poisoning

When a poison is taken internally or a drug overdose is expected, you should immediately call your regional poison control center.

If the package label says "Danger-Poison," then a taste (seven drops) up to one teaspoon is toxic. If the label says "Warning," a teaspoon to an ounce will be toxic. If the label says "Caution," an ounce to a pint is required before it is toxic. No warning label probably means that over a pint must be ingested in order to induce toxicity. Liquids or pelleted materials are more likely to be ingested in larger quantities than powders and solids or semi-solids.

A general guide is that you can expect pesticides, lye and other corrosives, petroleum products, and waxes and furniture polishes to give a moderate to severe poisoning. Soaps, cleaners, bleaches, and disinfectants will cause mild to moderate poisoning. Cosmetics may be either non-toxic or cause mild poisoning.

The most important first aid for poisoning is charcoal powder. We recommend that you administer about a tablespoon up to half a cup of activated charcoal powder stirred into water and sipped through a straw the minute poisoning is suspected. Then call your regional poison control center. Seconds may count in an instance of poisoning, so administer the charcoal while someone else calls poison control. It is quite likely you will already have administered the treatment of choice since charcoal is the universal antidote for poisoning. Every household should have powdered charcoal in the medicine cabinet.

Try to estimate an equal quantity of charcoal, or more, for the volume of the poison. Since one cannot overdose with charcoal, a sufficient amount should be given to take up all the poison. If the poison is in capsule or tablet form, use one teaspoon to one tablespoon of charcoal for each pill taken. Food poisoning can also be handled in this way. As much as half a cup of the powder may be needed in severe cases. Vomiting may be induced after taking the charcoal in any kind of poisoning except alkali and acid poisoning, kerosene and gasoline ingestion, or other hydrocarbons.

In addition to the charcoal, one may put on wet socks, cold wet pajamas, and cold socks on the hands, get into a large plastic bag, or between two plastic sheets in bed, and cover up snugly. This represents a heating compress to the entire body, or "wet sheet pack" modification. This will pull many toxins from the body.

Cadmium poisoning can be helped by chlorella, which is said to bind strongly to cadmium. If it binds to cadmium, it is possible that it will bind to other heavy metals. In cases of lead, mercury, aluminum, pesticides, copper, gold, nickel, or PCB intoxication or exposure, chlorella should probably be taken along with other methods to assist in the excretion of these toxic substances. Incidentally, in addition to protein, fats, and celluloses, chlorella has 3.3 percent glucosamine, which may be helpful in the leaky gut syndrome.

Garlic in moderately high doses (8 to 12 cloves daily, lightly steamed or baked) can help excrete lead, mercury, and other heavy metals. Large quantities of water should be taken for heavy metal poisonings for the purposes of encouraging excretion, diluting the toxic effect, and protecting the intestinal tract and kidneys. Do not force fluids in poisonings with overdoses of non-metallic poisons as the rate of absorption may be increased by drinking a lot of water or juices.

A general cleansing program is helpful immediately after any kind of poisoning. Intake of food should be small, or a juice fast should be done. (See "Cleansing Program" in the *Supplemental Information* section.)

Splinters, Thorns, Etc.

To remove splinters, fiberglass particles, prickly pear cactus hairs, or sand spurs that are sticking up above the skin, smear white liquid glue over the splinter and allow the glue to dry completely. Peel the dried sheet so that all the imbedded particles, or the splinter, will be lifted out. Spines from cactus and other small thorns will be removed easily following this method.

Natural Remedies

Introduction

The main objective of natural remedies is to stimulate the physiologic processes in the body in such a manner that they cooperate with the mechanisms of healing that were designed by a loving Creator to enable us to fight disease. The mechanisms built into the body include the immune system; blood cells; the skin barriers; stomach acids and digestants; the structure and chemical environment of natural body openings such as the eyes, nose, mouth, trachea, nipples, urethra, vagina, and anus; the natural resistance of certain organs such as the spleen, lymph nodes, stomach, thyroid, breasts, bladder, and rectum; and the responses from the blood vessels, lymph vessels, and nerves.

The variety of natural treatment modalities follows:

Therapeutic Diets

- Plant-based diet, without animal products
- Potassium broth or soup
- Low-cholesterol (see "Cholesterol" in the *Conditions and Diseases* section)
- Salt-free diet
- Sugar-free diet
- Fat-free diet
- All raw diet
- Juice therapy
- Allergy diet
- Elimination and challenge diet

Hydrotherapy

- Hot water, cold water, ice, steam
- Clay bath, mud bath, charcoal bath
- Herbal bath, mineral bath
- Foot bath, leg bath, arm bath
- Half bath

Irrigations

- Douches
- Pours
- Sprays
- Splashes

Compresses

- Wet dressings
- Hot and cold compresses
- Heating compresses
- Poultices: mud, herbal, charcoal, clay, vegetable

Massage

- Full body
- Diagnostic
- Specialized therapy, cross fiber, trigger point, etc.
- Foot, Neck, and Back rubs

Exercise

- Walking
- Stretches
- Jogging, running, jog-walk-jog
- Outdoor strolling or sitting
- Yard work or gardening

Sunning

- Sitting still to let the skin heat up
- Sunning clothed or unclothed
- Sunning while exercising
- Sunning while sitting or lying down

Herbal Remedies

- Teas, infusions, decoctions, tinctures
- Packs
- Suppositories

Fasting

- Total fast with water only
- Fruit fast
- Raw foods fast — fruits, vegetables, juices
- Grape, carrots, or greens fast

Supplements

- Plant hormone supplements
- Nutrient supplements
- Water supplements
- Non-nutritive elements such as silver

Special Devices

- TENS units
- Heating pads
- Compression devices
- Vacuum devices
- Hyperbaric chambers
- Massaging devices (chairs, bed)
- Cauterizing devices
- Depilatories
- Braces

In addition to this simple listing of natural modalities, this section of the book provides specific information about certain modalities. But before looking at specifics, we've included a section on the basic laws of health.

Eight (Natural) Laws of Health

Nutrition

Our bodies are built up by the food we eat; therefore, foods should be chosen that will best supply the elements needed for building up the body. The old saying "You are what you eat" has much truth. Eat whole grains, fruits, nuts (one to two tablespoons per meal), beans, and vegetables in as simple a manner as possible. Avoid all animal products, white sugar, and free oils. Unless the meal is all liquid, omit liquids at mealtime. Eat only what is sufficient—breakfast like a king, lunch like a prince, and supper like a pauper (if at all). Two meals are better than three. Take two meals about six hours apart. Have a set time for meals. Eat slowly and chew well.

Exercise

Make it a habit to exercise daily. Twenty minutes per day is minimal. One hour daily is better, but on certain days three to five hours may be needed. Do gentle exercise after meals.

Water

Drink 6 to 10 cups of water, as pure as possible, each day. Water is the best liquid to cleanse the tissues, inside and out. Take a daily bath.

Sunlight

Get 20 to 60 minutes of daily sun exposure. Sunlight destroys harmful bacteria, strengthens white blood cells, lowers blood pressure, allows blood to carry more oxygen, and causes cholesterol under the skin to change to vitamin D.

Temperance

Be moderate and mild in conversation, diet, work, study, recreation, and sleep. True temperance teaches us to dispense entirely with everything hurtful and to use judiciously that which is healthful. Avoid overeating, snacking between meals, caffeine, nicotine, alcohol, purging, prescription or nonprescription drugs, late bedtimes, tight bands and restrictive garments, and harmful and stimulating food.

Air

Breathe fresh, outdoor air as much as possible. Avoid smog, motor exhaust, and tobacco smoke. Take 20 deep breaths outdoors or near an open window two to four times per day. Spend more time out of doors and out of the cities. Hike and walk when possible. Keep correct posture with shoulders back to open lungs. Keep sleeping rooms well ventilated, being careful not to sleep in a draft.

Rest

Six to nine hours of sleep are needed for optimal performance. One hour of sleep before midnight is worth two after. Eating before bedtime disturbs the quality and restfulness of sleep.

Trust in Divine Power

Begin each day or end each day with a quiet hour or so alone with God in prayer and Bible reading, establishing a close relationship with Him. Talk to God and believe His promises. Be thankful, cheerful, and prayerful. These attributes produce endorphins, the hormones which fight disease and promote a sense of well-being. Churchgoers live longer. God is enabled to bless the health of those who trust Him.

Charcoal

Activated charcoal is a black powder of pure carbon. It can be manufactured from wood or bone. The medicinal use of charcoal is ageless, being used for poisonings, blood purification, odor control, and intestinal complaints. In recent decades, many other uses have been found for charcoal.

Charcoal may be used externally on wounds and bites, but it may also be mixed and swallowed to help with cholesterol, gastric issues, and poisonings.

To take charcoal by mouth, put one cup of cold water and one heaping tablespoon of charcoal powder in a pint or quart size jar with a secure lid. Replace the lid and shake over a sink in case there is a leak from the lid. When the charcoal powder is completely dispersed in the water, carefully open the jar over a sink to catch any spills. Pour the charcoal slurry into a cup for the patient. This is one adult dose, but it may be used for a child who has been poisoned. It is difficult to overdose on charcoal.

This treatment may also be used for poisoning with acetaminophen, amphetamine, arsenic, aspirin, barbiturates, camphor, cocaine, cyanide, digitalis, ergotamine, hemlock, Iodine, Ipecac, muscarine, narcotics, nicotine, opium, parathion, pesticides, phenol, primaquine, quinidine, quinine, salicylates, selenium, silver, stramonium, strychnine, etc,.

Charcoal by mouth is also the treatment of choice for nausea and vomiting, especially the travelers variety. It is also useful for sore throat, mouth and gum disorders, gastritis, and food poisonings.

Cholesterol

Activated charcoal has been found to lower the concentration of total lipids, cholesterol, and triglycerides in the blood serum, liver, heart, and brain. A study reported by the British journal *Lancet* found that patients with high blood cholesterol levels were able to reduce total cholesterol 25 percent with charcoal. About the best hoped for with drugs is 15 percent. Not only that, but while LDL was lowered as much as 41 percent, HDL/LDL cholesterol ratio was doubled! The patients took the equivalent of roughly one quarter ounce (approximately one tablespoon) of activated charcoal three or four times daily for six to eight months. Charcoal should not be taken near mealtime as food interferes with its best action. It should be taken upon arising, mid-morning, mid-afternoon, and at bedtime. It often takes quite a while before laboratory tests will show results as the lower levels of blood cholesterol tend to draw cholesterol out of the tissues that keep the blood cholesterol higher than it would otherwise be. Another study conducted by the National Institute of Public Health in Finland suggested that activated charcoal was as effective in reducing high cholesterol levels as the drug lovastatin.

Charcoal will take up most kinds of pharmaceutical medications as it treats medications as being poisonous. Since it will adhere to most poisons and inactivate them, it is necessary to take charcoal at least two hours from the time medication is taken, and even longer is desirable. For example, if you take blood pressure or epilepsy medication in the morning, take the charcoal in the evening. Charcoal therapy is certainly considerably less expensive, while possessing none of the dangerous side effects of cholesterol lowering drugs. Our own experience has been that charcoal is a valuable part of a total cholesterol reducing program, but that long-term lifestyle changes must be maintained to permanently reduce high cholesterol.

A group of 60 patients ranging in ages from 60 to 74 were divided into two groups. Forty were given activated charcoal for their high cholesterol, and 20 patients were treated with placebo. The course of treatment lasted four weeks. There was a 20 percent reduction in total cholesterol, 27 percent reduction in triglycerides, 20 percent reduction of apolipoprotein A, and Apo B dropped by 32 percent in the group that took the charcoal. There were also positive changes in the circulation and in the clinical status of patients in 60 percent of cases. In addition, exercise tolerance improved in 12 percent of the patients. At the same time, the control patients did not present any noticeable changes (*Klin-Med (Mosk)* 69, no. 6 [June 1991]: 51-3).

Poisoning

Most common poisons will be readily absorbed by charcoal. Nutrients, proteins, alcohol, and hydrocarbons like gasoline are not taken up. Whether a substance will be taken up by activated charcoal depends both on its natural ability to bind with charcoal, and whether the substance becomes bound to protein inside the body. As an example, valproic acid binds to protein and thus is not easily absorbed by activated charcoal (*Annals of Emergency Medicine* 25 [March 1995]: 356).

Wounds and Bites

Put one to two tablespoons of charcoal powder in a tall glass. Add water a few drops at a time until a paste about the consistency of warm peanut butter is obtained. Spread it onto one half of a folded paper towel. Fold over the other half of the paper towel to cover the charcoal paste. Lay the compress on the affected area, wettest side against the skin. Cover the compress with kitchen plastic wrap. Hold it in place with a bandage or strip of old cotton sheet or similar fabric. The compress may be left in place for up to eight hours, or changed every few minutes for recent venomous bites such as spider bites.

For larger wounds or areas of pain, a charcoal compress for the abdomen or a knee joint can be made by grinding three tablespoons of flaxseed in a blender or seed mill and mixing with one to three tablespoons of pulverized charcoal. Stir this mixture into one cup of water. Let it set for 10 to 20 minutes, or heat slightly to thicken. Spread over a square paper towel of the proper size, using enough to make the paste a quarter inch deep on the paper towel. Cover with another paper towel. The edge of the poultice should not have paste spread on it for about half to one inch all around to minimize leakage. Place the poultice on the skin, cover with a piece of kitchen plastic wrap that extends one inch over all edges and cover the entire plastic with an old towel to catch leaks that may develop. Use a binder or roller bandage to hold in place, pinning securely. A snug fitting garment, such as a knitted cap, can be used over a charcoal compress to hold it on the eye, ear or over the sinuses. A sweat shirt can help hold a charcoal compress snugly against the chest. Leave it on for 6 to 10 hours. Rub the area briskly with a cold washcloth after removing the compress.

It may be necessary to treat the patient with a charcoal bath. To do so, stir a cupful or more of powdered charcoal

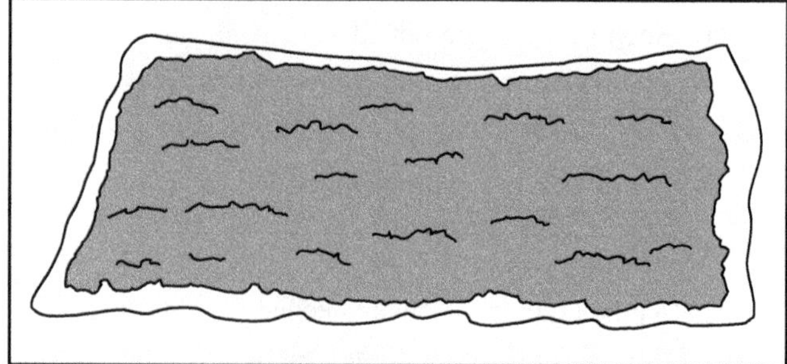

into the bathtub and let dissolve. The patient sits in the tub of black water for 30 to 90 minutes or more. The treatment is good for hives, ant bites, multiple bee stings, kidney failure, perineal rashes, etc. The charcoal will not damage plumbing or a septic tank, but it may permanently stain grout in a bathroom. To prevent staining, cover surfaces with plastic, and use care with the black water to avoid splashing. Shower off before using towels, as fabric can become indelibly stained with charcoal.

Clay Bath, Mud Bath

Clay may be dug from the ground. Recognize clay by the fact that it has no sand or humus but only finely compacted clay. Obtain enough that when water is mixed with the clay it should make a paste about the consistency of sesame tahini or a fruit smoothie. The mixture can be made in an outdoor children's swimming pool or other container. Warm the mud to about 95°F to 102°F, depending upon the need, with hot water or the sun. Have the patient sit in the tub until covered entirely with the mud. If the patient is comfortable, the mud bath may be continued for a half an hour to three or more hours.

In Europe mud baths have been found to be a more effective therapeutic measure in the treatment of soft tissue rheumatism, giving better relief from physical pain, than standard physical therapy (*Phys Rehab Kur Med II* [1992]: 92-97). In these studies the mud used for full body baths contained potassium polysulfide, sulphur, and huminic acids. The patients treated had osteoarthritis and nonarticular rheumatism.

A former student wrote us of the experiences they had with clay and mud baths in Guatemala. "Over the past 12 years we have used clay compresses in many different kinds of situations to very good advantage. At the Health Institute in Guatemala we had few ways to help patients. We were constantly experimenting with one remedy after another. Here are some ways we successfully used clay.

"We applied clay compresses routinely on almost every kind of patient. It was as routine as the quart of herbal tea they received daily ... the teas would be chosen according to their ailments just as the site for placing the clay poultice would be. If patients had arthritis, but the major organ affecting their health was their kidneys, we would put a clay poultice over their kidneys. If they had hepatitis it would go over their liver, etc. Almost invariably we found some site for a clay poultice.

"One woman I remember well had come to us with one breast already removed [because of breast cancer]. Clay compresses were the treatments she felt gave her the most comfort. She went home on a very different diet, and in much better health than when she arrived. She was back two years later for the same treatments. We sent her home again with the cancer apparently in remission as she had no signs or symptoms.

"We treated a number of diabetic leg ulcers with clay compresses successfully, in addition to a number of other ulcers on the extremities, such as the one on a young man's leg caused by leishmaniasis.

"We treated a man while we were there who had gangrene caused by a snakebite. A tourniquet had been put on his arm and left too long, and the surgeons were going to amputate but decided to try the clay just for experimental purposes. The clay, which usually takes all night to dry, if even then, took only a short time to dry on this man's arm. They kept reapplying it after each drying and noticed that the arm was beginning to revive. The blessing of the Lord saved the man's arm.

"We had an experience with a young man who had psoriasis. We offered him some clay poultices for a very bad flare-up on his arm. It disappeared almost overnight.

"An older woman who had a case of pleurisy while in Guatemala asked me to treat her with hydrotherapy and clay poultices every day in our treatment center. It was at this time that we first decided to add garlic oil to her clay packs. She told me that the clay compress with the garlic oil was the thing that relieved her congestion most and advanced her healing.

"Encouraged by our success with pleurisy, we decided to treat everyone with hepatitis with not just clay but garlic oil or chopped garlic in clay. The clay poultices were relieving in themselves and garlic may or may not have helped much. We found that the garlic could cause an irritation on the skin if we left it on longer than a few hours.

"Since I have come to Canada, I have experimented with clay on mothers who have blocked milk ducts. Again, it is one of the more effective treatments. And ... some like the addition of the garlic oil. One woman told me that it irritated her skin but the irritation on the skin seemed to relieve the internal pressure.

"Pink eye, a very common occurrence in Latin America, a kind of conjunctivitis especially aggravated by the little black gnats that hover especially around babies' eyes, is treated well with clay. We remember one girl at the Institute who had resorted to antibiotics for it. The antibiotics did not cure it. Then she tried the clay compresses at night and said they were immediately effective.

"Generally speaking we have found clay compresses very effective for any kind of pain. Clay holds its temperature better than charcoal compresses."

Deep Breathing Exercise

At the first evidence a cold may be coming, take a deep breath, hold for a slow count of 20, exhale through the nose, and hold breath out for a count of 10. Repeat 30 to 50 times. This procedure takes about 20 minutes and refreshes the blood to the tissues of the upper respiratory passages and carries away wastes and encourages healing. The deep breathing exercise may be done every two hours or at any time.

For hypertension, stress, appetite surges, and general health recovery, breathe in to the count of 4, hold it to the count of 7, and breathe out to the count of 9. Immediately breathe in again to the count of four, etc. and continue this pattern for 15 minutes twice a day or more until health is improved.

Epsom Salts Bath

Put one to two tablespoons of Epsom salts to each gallon of water in a bathtub. Sit in this mineral water at least 20 minutes. Use for any tub soak, muscle strains, sprains, colds, dermatitis, boils, etc.

Herbal Baths

The golden seal bath is done by simmering one-quarter cup of golden seal powder in a quart of water for 15 minutes, and pouring it into a bathtub of slightly warm water. Use this bath for infected skin lesions.

Comfrey, onion extract, garlic extract, etc. can be made similarly to the golden seal bath. Use comfrey leaves, a chopped onion, or chopped garlic with water that has been freshly boiled. Steep the herbs for 30 minutes before adding to the bathtub. Use for skin lesions, for disinfecting, healing, or soothing.

For a witch hazel bath, make it in the same way as for a comfrey bath, using one-quarter cup of the herb steeped for 30 minutes in boiling water. Add the witch hazel tea to a bathtub of water.

Hydrotherapy

Cold Applications

Cold Compress

Cold compresses are useful for rashes, sprains, swellings, inflamations, hot joints, etc. You will need cloths or cotton fabric pieces—wash cloths work well—and cold ice water or another desired solution. To administer the compress:

- Wring the cold water or solution from the cloth and lay it on the skin, molding it around body parts and folding it to fit the area.
- Renew frequently. Occasionally wipe the whole area with the cold cloth. Continue for 20 to 90 minutes.
- Dry thoroughly at the conclusion.

Cold Enema, Small

Use a bulb syringe that will hold about one-half cup of water. Use cold water and only one bulb full. Use after each meal. Gradually the colon will be trained to empty itself after meals if the exercise is continued for many weeks on a very regular schedule. Then the procedure can be discontinued.

Cold Mitten Friction

Procedure

1. Expose the right arm. Place one towel folded in half under the right shoulder, and a second one under the arm. Dip the mitts or washcloth into a basin of cold water between 50°F to 60°F or less. Squeeze out the excess water. Arrange the mitts on your hands. Use only one hand if washcloth is used. Catch one corner of the washcloth in the palm, wrap the hand with the washcloth, and catch the other corner in the palm, making a fist covered with the washcloth.

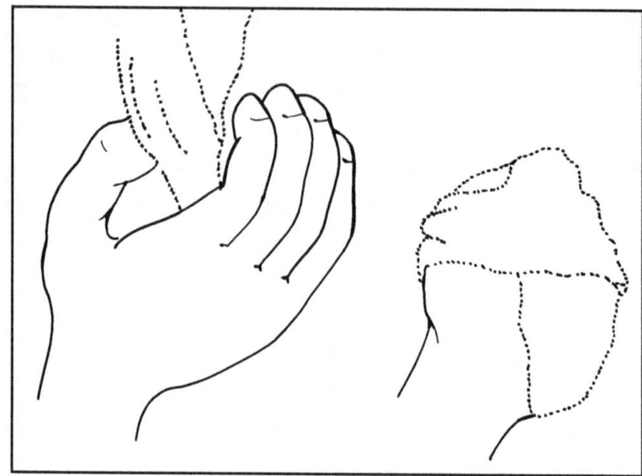

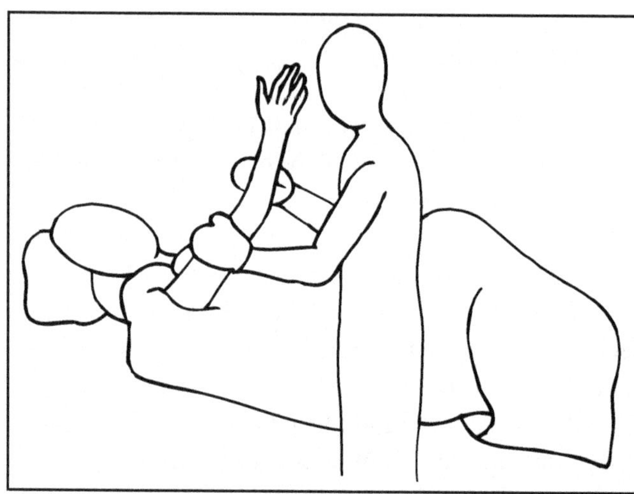

2. Begin at the fingers and work up the arm with a vigorous to-and-fro friction. You may dip the mitts again and repeat the process. If the skin is not yet pink, give a third rubbing.
3. Quickly remove mitts. Cover the arm with a towel, having the patient grasp the end of the towel in the hand. Vigorously rub over the towel, then wrap the towel around your hand and give a few long quick friction strokes to the whole arm. Rub the part with your bare hand to be sure it is thoroughly dry.

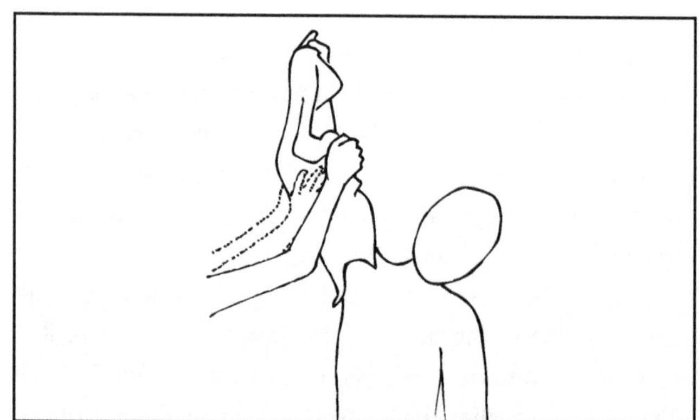

4. Replace the right arm under the sheet, and treat the left arm in the same manner.
5. Expose the chest and abdomen, placing a towel over each arm, tucking it well under the shoulders and sides to prevent chilling of the arms.
6. While standing at the bedside facing the patient, with the mitts on your hands, ask the patient to take a deep breath. Give a short to-and-fro friction, first to the chest up the midline, out over the shoulders, down the sides to the bedline, then back to the midline. Go over the surface twice, then quickly dip the mitts in the cold water and repeat. Dry briskly in the same way as for the arms. Cover the chest and abdomen with a towel or sheet and blanket. Avoid injuring the breasts or nipples, or getting the bedclothing wet.
7. Expose the right leg and foot. Bend the knee, place one towel under the thigh and heel lengthwise, another across the upper thigh. Proceed as with the arm. Dry, and friction the lower extremity. Cover. Repeat procedure for the left leg and foot.
8. Turn the patient to the prone position, pillow under the lower chest if needed for comfort, arms raised to the level of the head. Expose the back, including hips, and place towels at the front of the body. Give a to-and-fro friction with up and down movements; crosswise movements may also be used over the lower back and hips. Dip the mitts and repeat.
9. To vary the tonic effect, change the intensity and temperature of the water. More water left in the mitts and more friction will give a more vigorous reaction. Coarser mitts or a luffa sponge may be used for greater friction.

Effect

- Restores tone to blood vessels and muscles—called a "vascular gymnastic"
- Increases heat production
- Increases muscular, glandular, and metabolic activities of internal organs
- Increases phagocytosis and antibacterial activities
- Increases oxidation and elimination of bacterial toxins
- Produces a general tonic for prevention or treatment of cold, low energy and endurance, poor resistance to infections, tobacco and drug withdrawal, alcoholism, poor circulation, anemia, and low thyroid activity

Precautions

- The room should be at the proper temperature (75°F to 80°F), and the patient must be warm before beginning
- Give the friction vigorously with rapid movements
- Dry each part thoroughly with or without rubbing, leaving no dampness
- Be sure that the bed is not damp after a treatment
- If the patient does not have a good reaction, or dislikes the procedure, discontinue it promptly
- Avoid frictioning skin lesions or painful areas

Cold Sitz Bath, Short Cold Bath

Indications for the application of short cold baths are:

- Chronic diseases in which metabolism is below normal
- Low blood vessel tone as in congestive heart failure
- Low thyroid
- Diabetes (helps to clear excess blood sugar)
- Overweight
- Various skin diseases
- Infections: malaria, prostatitis, salpingitis, abscesses, and carbuncles
- Any disorder for which a fever treatment is indicated but for some reason the patient or the circumstances make it impossible for a hot bath

On the other hand, you would not want to use a short cold bath if the patient:

- Is cold
- Is excessively tired or debilitated
- Has poor kidney function
- Has high blood pressure (the systolic blood pressure rises with cold applications)
- Has an over functioning thyroid.

Procedure

1. Be certain the patient is quite warm.
2. Give the patient a vigorous cold mitten friction for five minutes while he is sitting in six inches of water in a bathtub, with the water at 70°F to 80°F. If absolutely necessary, the first few of these daily treatments may be for two to four minutes and at 85°F to 90°F. Gradually lengthen the time and cool the water, filling the tub higher until the hips are covered.
3. If the patient is debilitated, the cold mitten friction can be given with the patient lying down in bed. After the five-minute bath with the extremities being

vigorously rubbed with the cold mittens, the patient should rest in bed for one to one-and-a-half hours.

The cold mitten friction and the short cold bath are both very powerful treatments, and for the vigorous patient, these treatment methods should not be forgotten.

Ice Collar

Wrap an ice collar around the neck and keep on for 20 minutes or so for throat pain. Ice collars are c-shaped ice packs that can be purchased on the Internet. It is also quite acceptable to use sealable plastic bags that are filled with ice cubes or crushed ice. Double the bag to ensure no leaking.

Wet Sheet Pack and Friction Rub (Cold)

1. Tie a cold compress around the forehead at the beginning of the treatment.
2. Have the patient stand in a hot foot bath.
3. Soak a sheet in cold water at 60°F to 70°F and then wring it out.
4. Wind the wet sheet around the patient. Beginning under one arm, carry the sheet around the back, under the opposite arm, and across the abdomen. As the wrapping is continued, cover the first shoulder and arm, and tuck it in at the legs and neck. Fasten with clothespins or safety pins.
5. For the wet sheet rub, percuss and friction over the sheet quickly until the sheet becomes warm from the action of the friction and the body heat. At the end of the treatment, which should cover the entire skin surface, pour a pail of water at 70°F over the patient. A second pail at 65°F and a third pail at 60°F should be used. Two operators are best for this treatment. A cool, forceful shower gradually getting cooler can be substituted for the pail pouring if more convenient. However, the temperature cannot be as easily controlled.
6. Friction the skin dry with a coarse towel.

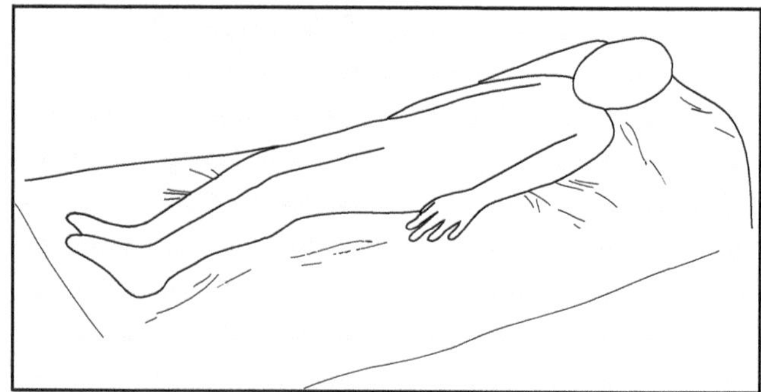

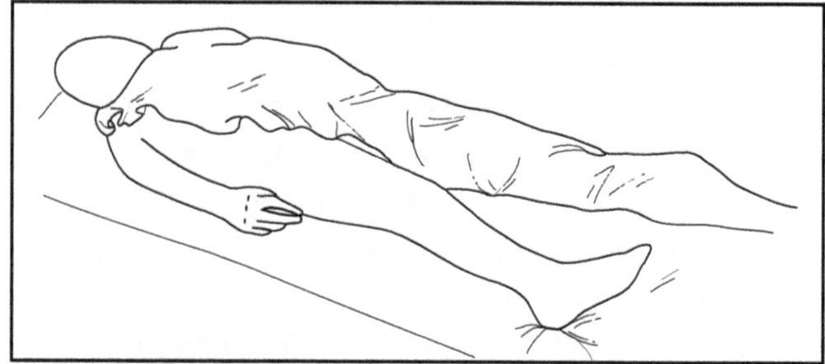

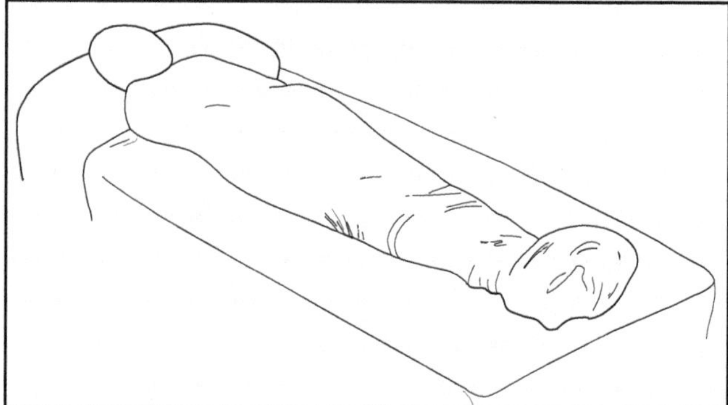

Neutral Applications

Neutral Bath

The neutral bath is given in the same way as the hot half bath, except that the temperature of the bath is around 94°F to 98°F. Except in mental or neurological diseases there is no need to sponge the face or forehead with cold water, as sweating is minimal or absent. It may be maintained from 10 minutes to several hours, even all day for a disturbed person or for intractable itching. If sweating begins, put a cold cloth on the forehead to keep it cool.

The benefits of the neutral bath result from the use of water so employed as to be absolutely non-stimulating, without mechanical friction or percussion and of such a temperature as to shield the body from the continued excitation resulting from contact of the skin with the clothing and constantly changing temperatures. The nerve centers, as a result of a total lack of excitation, are afforded an opportunity to accumulate a store of energy so that a recuperation, sedation, and energizing may occur.

If the person is going to work after a neutral bath, use a cold mitten friction and brisk rubdown. If one is going to bed, blot the skin dry, dress in soft clothing, and move slowly so as not to excite or stimulate the nerves. It may be used for insomnia, agitation, itching, depression, any mental illness, and lowering of blood pressure in acute hypertension.

Saline Purge, Saline Preparation

We do not use oral saline purges for several reasons. One is that the taking of salt water, even diluted, can overload the systems of some people who are very sensitive to salt. Unfortunately, people who use these saline purges usually do not distinguish between those who may have a familial sensitivity to salt and those who could accept additional salt. Generally, even salt added generously in our food is more than most people can tolerate even for one very salty meal and certainly not repeated doses or for long periods without injury to the kidneys or blood vessels.

Another reason we do not use the saline purges is that it is not in our philosophy to work in a way that causes a heavy taxation on the body, either by chemical or physical means.

Wet Dressing, Moist Soaks

The wet dressing is given with neutral water temperature. The evaporation of water from the skin surface results in vasoconstriction, relief of itching and congestion, and the removal of crusts. An infected dermatitis is effectively treated with wet dressings. Another purpose of a wet dressing is to keep an area of skin moist that would otherwise crack or dry and prevent healing. Squeeze a small linen towel from the proper solution, leaving it very moist but not actually dripping. Cotton pajamas, leotards, long-sleeved shirts, or cotton gauze can serve on large areas as wet dressings. After the pajamas are wrung out until damp and placed on the skin, cover them with dry pajamas. Never place plastic over a wet dressing as it prevents the necessary evaporation. Allow the moisture to evaporate slowly over a four- to six-hour period. The dressings are then completely removed and fresh dressings replaced. Boil all cloths used and sun dry if possible before reusing. Maximum benefit occurs at 48 to 72 hours, after which continued application of wet dressings is of little benefit.

The commonest wetting agent for wet dressings is plain water. Saline may be used over the eyes or elsewhere. Golden seal tea may be used for its astringent and antimicrobial action.

Hot Applications

Douches

Douching is not necessary for women with normal vaginal health. It has actually been found that some who regularly douche have a greater tendency to get cancer of the cervix Pregnant women should never douche. For most ordinary vaginal or cervical infections, start a treatment series using three hot douches daily for three days then dropping to two douches daily for three days, then once daily for thirty days.

Obtain a douche kit from a pharmacy. Select an appropriate douche solution from the list below. Fill the douche bag and attach the plastic tubing with the clasp closed. Attach the hook in the hole at the other end and suspend it from a position not more than 2 feet above the hips. It may be hung on a chair back, towel rack, or bathtub soap holder.

Assume a convenient position for the douche, lying or sitting in the tub at about a 45-degree angle. Sitting upright prevents a proper flow of the douche solution into all the crevices and folds of the vagina. Alternate positions are sitting in a shower stall or on the commode leaning back as far as possible. A low stool may be used to raise the feet off the floor a few inches. To get the air out of the tubing, release the clasp until the solution begins to flow out the end of the tubing and quickly close the clasp. Insert into the vagina and release the clasp, allowing the solution to flow into the vagina. To cleanse the many folds and creases, fill the vagina with fluid by folding the lips of the vulva around the nozzle with the thumb and forefinger until sufficient solution has distended the vagina and a sense of fullness or pressure is experienced over the bladder. Shut off the clasp and hold the solution for as long as required to count slowly to 15. Let the fluid gush out. Repeat this procedure until all the solution is used. Do not rush the procedure; allow 5 to 10 minutes to finish the solution.

Clean the equipment by washing with soap and water. Rinse well and hang it up with the clasp open to encourage drainage and drying of the interior of the tube.

- Hot water – The universal solution for vaginal douche is merely hot water, two to four quarts at 105°F to 110°F.
- Vinegar – For a vinegar douche, use one to four tablespoons of any kind of vinegar to each quart of hot water. For one treatment use two quarts of solution. This is the standard douche solution and should be selected for all ordinary infections and special cleansing.

- Baking soda – For a baking soda douche, use one teaspoon of baking soda to each quart of hot water. For one treatment use two quarts of solution. This solution is most applicable for monilia or yeast infections and should be used when vinegar is not successful within a reasonable treatment period, 5 to 10 days.
- Garlic – One clove of garlic may be blended in one quart of boiling water, cooled, and strained. Use one quart of solution for a treatment. Use the garlic solution raw, or simmered for one to five minutes if the tissues are very tender and sensitive. Use it for infections that are resistant to the usual treatments, or when you are uncertain which solution might be best. It often brings remarkable results in vaginitis.
- Styptic – For a styptic douche (one to stop surface bleeding of the vagina or cervix) use comfrey, two heaping tablespoons of powdered tea leaves to one quart of boiling water. Mix and let it set for 15 minutes, strain and use.
- Golden Seal – Use one tablespoon of root powder in one quart of water. Boil gently for 10 minutes. Use this douche for bleeding surfaces such as cervicitis or vaginitis. It is useful for both styptic and antimicrobial functions.
- Charcoal – One tablespoon of charcoal may be added to a quart of water to make a charcoal douche solution for infections, ulcers, and viral diseases. It is very effective as a deodorant douche.
- Lysol – Lysol is a 2.7 percent solution of phenol, water and soap—a good antiseptic. Use one-half to one teaspoon of Lysol to one quart of water at 100°F to 105°F. Mix the solution well. Lysol occasionally causes a rash or burning. If this occurs, stop using the Lysol, rinse off all surfaces with water (skin, vagina, and douche bag), and it should clear up promptly. This solution may be used for ordinary antiseptic perineal care, and for deodorizing the perineum, underarms, feet, or skin lesions that develop odor.

Enemas

The first rule is that a child under the age of 15 is never given but one child-sized enema in one day. An adult can usually take one enema after the other until the fluid comes back clear or nearly so. Many different fluids have been used for enemas including hot garlic, soapy water, plain water, charcoal slurry, Epsom Salts water, castor oil, or plain saline.

Have the person lie in a bathtub, on a plastic sheet in bed with a bedpan, or sitting on a commode or toilet seat. Select the enema fluid and pour it into the enema bag. Fill the tubing with the fluid, expelling all air. Shut the stopcock. Lubricate the nozzle tip with petroleum jelly, hand lotion, or a drop of liquid soap, and insert it into the rectum. Release the stopcock to allow the fluid to run into the rectum. You may need to elevate the enema bag high over your head to get the fluid to run in. The person should begin to feel full and will have the urge to expel the fluid, especially if the fluid is quite hot. Do not use fluid so hot you cannot hold your hand in it. The person can massage his abdomen to get the fluid to fill as much of the colon as possible. Once the patient cannot hold anymore fluid, the liquid should be expelled.

If a patient is unable to take fluids by mouth, a retention enema will in most instances be able to supply the entire water needs of the person. Simply place 8 to 16 ounces (1 to 2 cups) of lukewarm water or saline (1 teaspoon of salt to 2 cups water) in an enema bag and allow it to run slowly into the rectum. A specially prepared mineral replacement solution may also be used as follows: Simmer two tablespoons of wheat bran in two cups of water for 5 to 10 minutes. Strain and add two teaspoons of salt. Add sufficient water to the mixture to make two quarts (8 cups). If the patient has not eaten for a day or two, it may be desirable to add two to three tablespoons of white table sugar to the mixture for its protein-sparing effect. Lubricate the nozzle well, since repeated insertions, if not done gently, can be quite irritating to the anus and produce painful fissures. Repeat the fluid injection every two to four hours for a person not taking fluids in any other way until two quarts per day have been absorbed. More can be used in a sweating or dehydrated person.

The following enema solutions may be used:

- Water – Use plain hot water at 104°F to 110°F.
- Charcoal – Dissolve one to five tablespoons of charcoal in two quarts of water. For a retention enema use one tablespoon of charcoal powder to 8 ounces of lukewarm water, pushed in gently with an infant syringe. If a reflex elimination urge develops, the buttocks can be pinched together until the urge to eliminate passes. Use the charcoal retention enema for any toxic state such as snakebite, kidney failure, or drug ingestion or for inflammations and infections as ulcerative colitis, inflamed fissures or hemorrhoids.
- Golden Seal – Prepare golden seal solution as directed above under douche solutions. Most herb teas can be used double-strength as a cleansing enema, or regular strength as a retention enema.

- Oil – Use one to four tablespoons of olive oil in four to six ounces of warm water as a retention enema or to soften and lubricate impacted feces.
- Starch – First give a cleansing enema of 2 quarts of plain hot water. Then prepare a thin paste of starch (use kitchen cornstarch) in one to two ounces of cool water. Pour the paste into one pint of hot water. Allow to cool and inject into the rectum with a bag or bulb syringe. The starch enema is used to stop diarrhea or to relieve irritation.
- Epsom Salt – Use one teaspoon of Epsom salt per pint of water.
- Hot Garlic Irrigation Fluid – Follow the garlic douche solution formula.
- Castor Oil Enema – Use two tablespoons of the oil in a quart of water.
- Plain Saline – Use one teaspoon of table salt per pint of water.
- Unscented Castile Soap – Mix two tablespoons in a quart of water.

Fomentations

The fomentation itself can be referred to as a fomentation, a pack, or a compress. We will refer to it as a fomentation to simplify this procedure. The fomentation can be bought or made easily from many types of materials. One way is to fold a 30 x 36 inch piece of thick, brushed cotton laundry flannel into thirds and fasten with quilting thread, string, or colored yarn in six places throughout the middle of it.

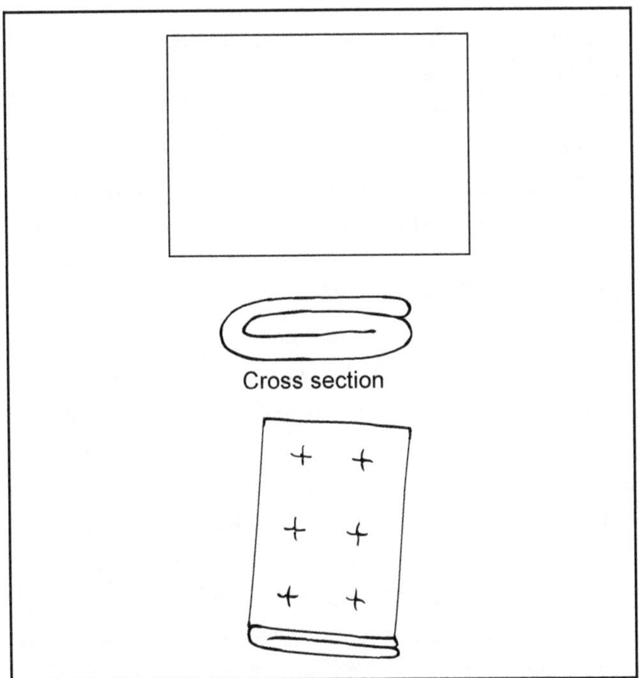

You will need the following items for the fomentation:

1. Three or four fomentations, as hot as can be tolerated
2. Two to four fomentation covers
3. Four large towels or more
4. Two to four wash cloths for cold compresses and cold mitten friction
5. One or two patient sheets (Extra sheet and blanket may be needed)
6. One foot tub with water approximately 105°F to 110°F
7. One basin with cold or ice water
8. One glass and straw
9. A canner or other large kettle rigged with a false bottom or rack

Once all of these items are assembled, go through the following steps for the procedure:

1. Protect the bed with a doubled blanket or a plastic sheet such as a shower curtain.
2. Have the person undress or only be wearing underwear or a light gown with a sheet draped over the patient.
3. Place one or two fomentations for the spine on the bed and cover well with towels to prevent burning.
4. Have the person lie on the compress and place the feet in a hot foot bath, if possible. If not, wrap the feet well in a fomentation or surround them with hot water bottles.
5. Arrange necessary towels (one to four depending on thickness) over the area to be treated.
6. Place the fomentation neatly in position and cover it with a towel, sheet, and blanket if necessary.
7. Remove the fomentation after the desired length of time, usually three to six minutes, and replace it promptly with a cold compress for 30 to 60 seconds; dry the skin after the cold application.
8. Use a cold compress to the head or throat after three to five minutes, or when sweating begins.
9. Have the person drink water, room temperature or hotter.
10. Repeat steps 5, 6, and 7 two or three times or more depending on the case, spending as little time during changes as possible.
11. Rub the thighs with a dry towel to remove perspiration.

12. Keep the foot bath hot by frequent additions of hot water, using care to avoid discomfort. (See "Hot Foot Bath" in this section for precautions.)
13. If desired, give a cold mitten friction, soothing back rub, or shower to finish. Otherwise pat or rub briskly to dry. Before removing the hot foot tub, pour cold water over the feet and dry well.

Avoid chilling or burning with compresses and observe for comfort and safety. If diabetic, do not apply heat to the feet.

Heating Compress

The heating compress is applied cold and covered, but it quickly heats up through the reaction of the body against the cold. The captured heat increases circulation of the covered area of tissue. Heating compresses can be applied to most parts of the body, including the feet, eyes, joints, abdomen, chest, throat, etc. The basic principle is the same for any part: a cold wet cloth applied to cause brief backward flow of blood, a layer to cover the wet one to prevent evaporation, and a final layer to prevent slippage of the compress while it is being worn.

We shall describe a heating compress for the throat. Get a strip of cotton cloth about 2 x 20 inches or long enough to wrap completely around the neck. Place the strip of cloth in ice cold water and then squeeze it out. Smooth it around the neck, avoiding dripping water on clothing or skin. Wrap a piece of plastic cut from a bread bag or similar material about 3 x 20 inches around the wet cloth, completely covering it so that no small bit is allowed out from under the plastic to cause wicking of the moisture and cooling of the compress. The objective is to cause a buildup of heat under the plastic. Cover the entire compress with a wool or synthetic fabric and pin in place with safety pins. Apply the compress snugly, but not so tight as to cut off the circulation or limit motion. The person can go to sleep with the compress. After about eight hours, remove the compress and friction the skin of the entire neck with a cold, wet, coarse wash cloth until dry and reddened—about 10 or 12 seconds. Immediately cover with a scarf or a turtleneck sweatshirt to keep the neck warm.

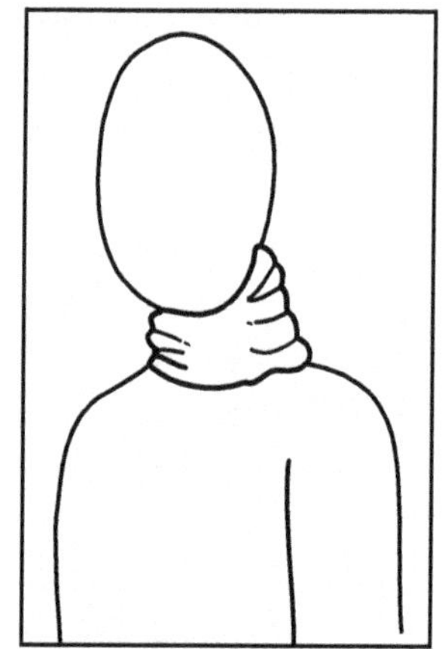

If the person does not warm up the wet compress, use a heat lamp, fomentation, heating pad, or hot water bottle to warm it up. Elderly, thin, or debilitated persons may have difficulty warming up the compress, especially if it is large. Avoid chilling.

If worn continuously day and night, the wet compress should be changed every eight hours, and the skin should be allowed to dry for at least one hour to avoid dermatitis from continuous moisture on the skin.

Hot and Cold Showers

For strengthening the immune system, take hot and cold showers, two to five minutes hot, 10 to 30 seconds cold, back and forth, alternating. The force of the water should be set as high as possible. Finish with a quick brisk rubbing with a coarse towel. Do this treatment twice a day.

Hot Bath, Fever Bath

The patient should get into the tub with the water at 102°F. After the patient is settled, raise the temperature of the water to about 108°F to 112°F and hold it there throughout the treatment. Keep the face generously sponged with cold water and an ice-cold compress kept to the forehead, one to the neck, and a third across the mouth and chin. Raise the mouth temperature to 101°F to 104°F, depending on the condition being treated. Keep it at that temperature for 20 minutes for the flu, but 45 minutes or more for Lyme disease or cancer. For children use one minute in the water for each year of their age. Record the mouth temperature on a notepad about every 2 to 10 minutes. Count the pulse at the same time, and do not allow the pulse to exceed 150 if the patient is 65 or older or debilitated. Discontinue the treatment if it approaches that level.

Finish the treatment with a cold shower or cold mitten friction. A cold shower for 10 to 20 seconds followed by a brisk rubdown with a coarse dry towel or a cold mitten friction with the patient lying down.

Hot Hip and Leg Pack

A single blanket is placed crosswise on the bed so that the upper edge will reach the waist and the lower edge will encircle the right hip, thigh, leg, and foot. A single or double thickness sheeting is next wrung from cold water and laid on the crosswise blanket. It should not extend beyond the edges of the blanket. The patient lies on the wet sheet, arms raised, and the wet sheet is wrapped around the abdomen and right leg and tucked in at the waist on the left. Place a hot water bottle, fomentation pack, or heating pad covered with a large plastic bag on the first layer of the wet sheet, which now covers the right abdomen. Subsequently the left side of the wet sheet is wrapped over the left thigh, leg, and foot and tucked in on the other side. Then the blanket is wrapped snugly around the patient and fastened with large safety pins or clothes pins or simply tucked in. The patient's arms are now brought down and a shirt is put on backward or a sheet and blanket used to cover the patient. General sweating should be produced.

Hot Foot Bath

For a hot foot bath, you will need the following equipment:

- Foot tub or large basin (in a pinch, use a trash can) about half filled with hot water (100°F to 110°F) preferably three to eight inches above the ankles
- Pitcher of very hot water
- Sheets or treatment blankets, according to the climate and patient's condition
- Two large towels
- Wash cloths for head compress
- Basin of ice water
- Bath thermometer, if available

To administer the procedures, drape one or two blankets over a straight chair and cover the blanket entirely with a sheet. Then place a large towel on the floor for protection with a tub of hot water on it.

Have the patient undress or only wear shorts, underwear, or a light gown and then sit on the chair with the feet in the tub. Wrap the person snugly, first in the sheet and then in the blankets, draping covers well about the tub and the patient's knees so as to avoid the circulation of air. A towel can be wrapped around the neck to hold the blankets snugly in place, and to catch the sweat from the face and head.

Apply cold compresses to the forehead. Change every two to three minutes during the height of the reaction.

Add hot water frequently during the treatment to keep the temperature up to the person's tolerance. Continue treatment for 20 to 30 minutes or even an hour or more if needed. Give water to drink when sweating begins.

To finish the treatment, have the patient hold the feet up and pour cold water over them. Place the feet on a towel on the floor. Dry the skin thoroughly. Have the person lie down for 30 to 60 minutes after the procedure.

While giving a foot bath, follow these precautions:

1. When adding hot water to the foot bath, push the feet to one side, and place your hand between the feet and the hot water. Pour the hot water against the tub and swirl it with your hand.
2. If the person perspires, dry the limbs thoroughly. The thighs are especially likely to perspire.
3. Do not end with cold water if the foot bath is given preceding a foot massage or during menstruation.

Hot Mitten Friction

Procedure

1. Have the patient lie on his or her back. Expose the right arm. Place one towel folded in half under the right shoulder to elevate the entire body quadrant and a second one under the arm. Dip mitts or washcloth into a basin of hot water (about 104°F). Squeeze out the excess water. Arrange the mitts on your hands. Use only one hand if a washcloth is used. Catch one corner of the washcloth in the palm, wrap the hand with the washcloth, and catch the other corner in the palm, making a fist covered with the washcloth.
2. Begin at the fingers of the right hand and work up the arm with a vigorous to-and-fro friction. You may dip the mitts again and repeat the process.
3. Quickly remove mitts. Cover the patient's arm with a towel. Rub vigorously over the towel, then wrap the towel around your hand and give a few long quick friction strokes to the whole arm. Rub the part with your bare hand to be sure it is thoroughly dry.
4. Replace the right arm under the sheet, and treat the left arm in the same manner.
5. Next expose the chest and abdomen, placing a towel over each arm and tucking it well under the shoulders and sides to prevent chilling the arms.
6. Give a short to-and-fro friction, first to the chest up the midline, out over the shoulders, down the sides to the bedline, then back to the midline. Go over the surface twice, and then quickly dip the mitts in the hot water and repeat. Dry briskly in the same way as for the arms. Cover the chest and abdomen with a towel or sheet and blanket. Avoid injuring the breasts or nipples, or getting the bedclothing wet.
7. Expose the right leg and foot. Bend the knee, place one towel under the thigh and heel lengthwise, another across the upper thigh. Proceed as with the arm. Dry, and friction the lower extremity and cover. Repeat procedure for the left leg and foot.

8. Turn the patient to the prone position, pillow under the lower chest if needed for comfort, arms raised to the level of the head. Expose the back, including hips, and place towels under the front of the body. Give a to-and-fro friction with up and down movements; crosswise movements may also be used over the lower back and hips. Dip the mitts and repeat.

Work quickly throughout the treatment. Once completed, cover the patient and have him or her rest for 30 to 60 minutes.

Hot Spine Applications

Alternate hot and cold packs in a narrow strip down the spine about three to six inches wide. Otherwise this treatment is the same as hot and cold alternating fomentations. A fomentation may be wrapped around the feet if the patient is not diabetic. Keep the patient well hydrated and the head cool.

Sinus Pack

For a sinus pack, you will need two trays of ice cubes, five small dry towels, hot compress for the spine, set of three compresses, alternating with cold to the chest, and a hot foot bath. Put one end of the treatment table or bed against the wall to secure the ice pack and pillow.

- Place the hot compress for the spine under the back. Put the feet in a hot foot bath on the table or bed with the knees bent as the first part of the hot compress procedure. (See the "Fomentations" entry in this section). Proceed with a set of three compresses to the chest, three minutes hot and 30 seconds cold. Leave the third hot compress on the chest throughout the remainder of the treatment.
- Put one tray of ice cubes in a small dry towel. Fold it over to make a pack 5 x 10 inches. Make a second pack. Put one ice pack covered by a towel under the back of the neck, centered on the edge of the cranium. Wet the top of the head slightly with water and place the second ice pack on the top of the head. Hold the pack in place with a pillow.
- Take two small towels and lay one on each side of the face, leaving the nose exposed.
- Dip two small towels in hot water and squeeze as a compress. Place it over the towels on the face. Cover with dry towels to preserve heat. Leave it on exactly three minutes! This is a stimulating treatment. Remove the compress and towels.

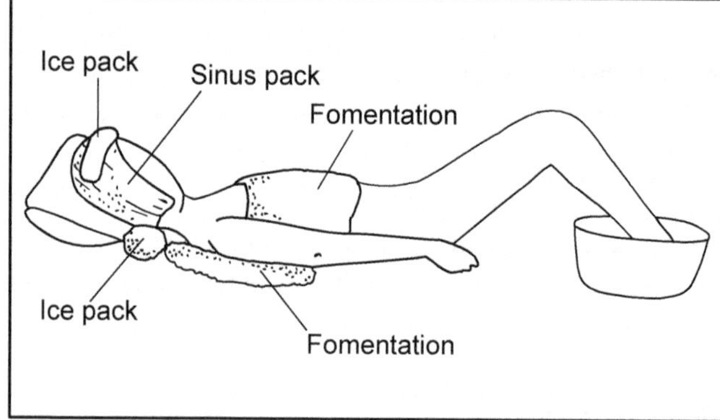

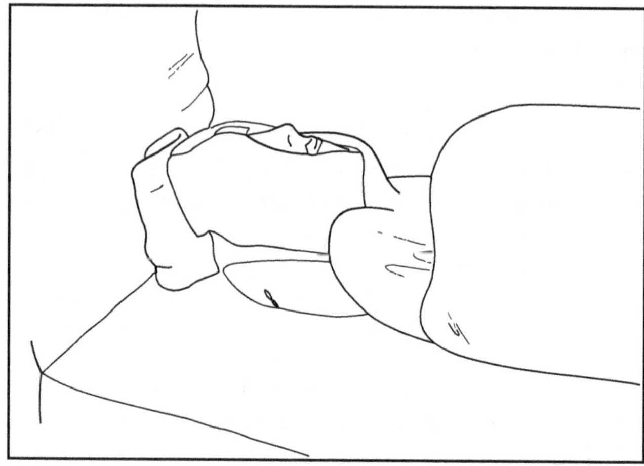

- Wring another small towel from the ice water and drape it on the face, molding it to the skin over the red area. There should be no delay between removal of the hot fomentation and replacement by the cold compress. Leave it on for 30 seconds. After drying briskly with another towel, repeat the procedure again three to six times. Finish off with a cold mitten friction or use a contrast shower.

Infrared Sauna

Infrared can be of great help in many conditions and should be used for either the whole body as a whole body sauna, or a limited area as in the use of an infrared dome.

Irrigations

Irrigations are excellent for cleansing surfaces, for delivering heat, and for giving a massaging or friction treatment. It can substitute for a gargle or the usual mouthwash if the area is too tender for other treatments. Following are two different irrigation fluid recipes:

1. Hot Garlic – Boil one quart of water. Blend one or two cloves of fresh garlic in about one cup of the boiling water until no particles remain. Add the remainder of the boiling water to the blender and allow the fluid to cool in the blender. This process should "cook" the garlic barely enough that it will not burn the tissues. In acute cases of quinsy, sore throats, acute vaginitis, etc., this can be a very excellent remedy to inhibit bacterial growth, and encourage circulation simultaneously. Obviously, do not use if the person is sensitive to garlic.
2. Hot Saline – Into one pint (two cups) of water put one teaspoon of table salt. The solution can be heated and used as an irrigation fluid for the nose, eyes, mouth, rectum, etc. Use care not to burn the patient with the hot fluid.

For streptococcal infections, use one quart of water into which one clove of garlic has been blended. If a Water Pik is used, the tip of the irrigator can be cut off to give a larger stream under less pressure. Use one of the lowest pressure settings. Strain the solution through a nylon stocking or gauze if particles clog the tubing. The solution may be used hot or cold. Charcoal is also useful for bacterial sore throats such as streptococcal or diphtherial. Mix one to four tablespoons per quart of warm or hot water. The bacteria adhere to charcoal. Garlic inhibits growth of bacteria, fungi, and viruses.

Hot garlic irrigation fluid is good for hay fever, colds, aphthous ulcers of the mouth or pharynx, acute tonsillitis or peritonsillar abscess (quinsy), streptococcal or diphtherial sore throats, or asthma.

Irrigation fluid may be self-administered. Fill the syringe with hot water or saline, expelling all air and completely filling the syringe. Bend over a sink and allow the run-off to escape into the sink. If the patient is treated in bed, administer with a basin held to catch the run-off water. .

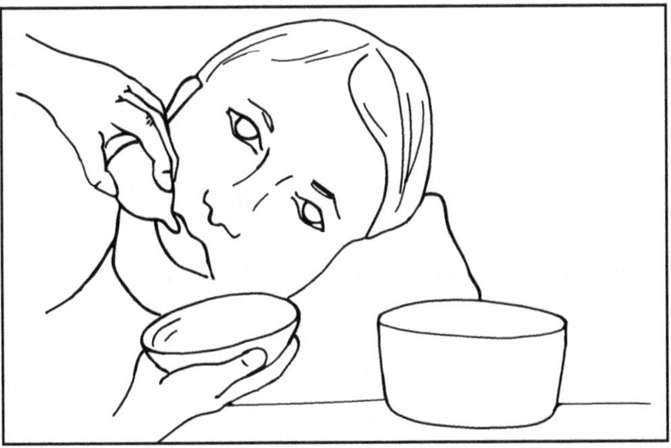

For a peritonsillar abscess, direct the spray toward the back of the throat, using as much heat as can be tolerated to gently massage the tissues and encourage dissipation of the infection. Use one quart or more of hot water or irrigation solution.

Irrigation is an excellent treatment for a beginning cold when used at 108°F to 110°F for about 20 to 30 minutes. It is said by some never to fail to prevent the cold from developing if it is used within the first two hours of symptoms. A peritonsillar abscess, acute pharyngitis, or tonsillitis will respond miraculously to this simple remedy if begun early. Be persistent in treatment of the more serious sore throats for a few days after symptoms subside. Do not stop the treatments too soon after rapid healing.

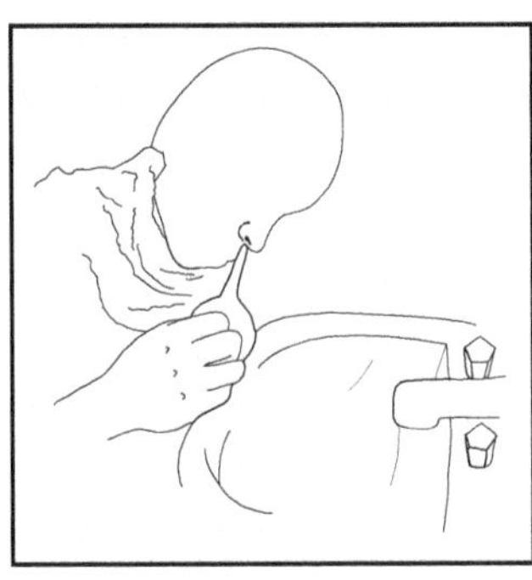

For a nasal irrigation, use plain water or the hot saline irrigation fluid above and insert the syringe nozzle into the nose and hold the nostril closed around the nozzle with a finger. The nostril can be completely occluded by wrapping the end of the nozzle with a large rubber band just bulky enough that it wedges snugly inside the nose upon insertion. Squeeze the bulb of the syringe with a steady stream, allowing the run-off to escape through the opposite nostril into the sink.

For an ear irrigation, the person should pull the ear upward and backward to straighten the canal and direct the stream of water forward and downward. An ear syringe should be pressed steadily to deliver water at a constant rate under very gentle pressure. If the water is hot the patient may experience some currents of fluid movement in the nearby semi-circular canals, causing sensations of faintness, dizziness, or nausea.

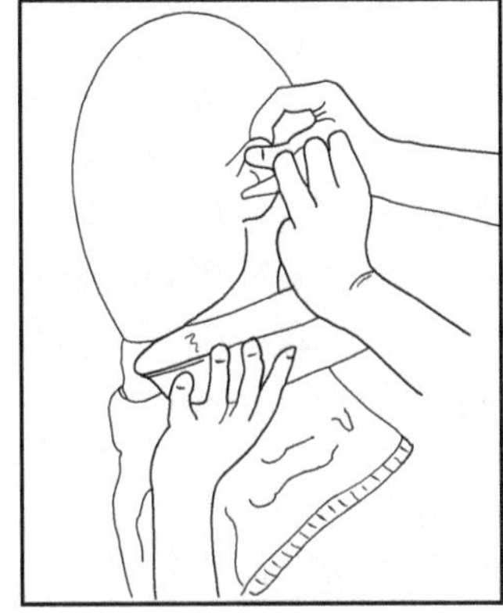

Irrigation of the ear is used in acute inflammation of the ear, to remove hardened wax, to remove insects or foreign bodies, and eczema of the ear canal. Ear wax may be softened by dropping a few drops of plain water or a little warm olive oil in the canal. Allow the fluid or oil to remain at least 30 minutes before tipping the head upright again. Repeat three or four times a day, and then irrigate the ear.

Kidney Stone Pack

To treat a kidney stone, a very large, hot fomentation (compress, hot pack) is required. It is necessary that the fomentation stay hot for a length of time. This is accomplished by keeping the fomentation hot with an electric device such as heating pads or with hot water bottles.

A series of layers will be required for this treatment. Spread a half-sheet across the middle of the bed, on it place a heating pad turned up to high, then a sturdy plastic square or garbage bag to ensure against electrical shorts, then the hot fomentation, next a towel or two, depending on how much heat the patient can stand from the fomentation. (Do not blister the skin.) Position the patient so that the area of pain is centered over this pack. Bring up the sheet on each side and pin it snugly around the body so as to hold the pack in place. Keep it hot for hours with the heating pad until the stone passes or the patient gets relief from pain. Keep the head cool by cold compresses. (For more information about fomentations, see the entry in this section.)

In addition to the fomentations, a person with a kidney stone may make the following recipe to help pass the stone:

- Black or Daikon radish, shredded
- Salt (Himalayan or sea salt) as for eating

Combine the radish and salt and let sit overnight, covered, in the refrigerator. Fast for 12 hours (overnight), and then drink 12 ounces of the squeezed or centrifuged (in a salad spinner) juice. Then wait two hours before taking anything else, even supplements.

Leg Bath

Use this treatment for varicose veins, phlebitis, arthritis, injury of an extremity, etc. You will need:

- A tall trash can filled with hot water (100°F to 110°F) preferably to the knee
- A similar tall trash can filled with cold water
- Two large towels
- Wash cloths for head compress
- Bath thermometer, if available

To begin the treatment, place a large towel on the floor with the can of hot water on it. Seat the person on a chair and place the affected leg in the can.

If sweating begins apply cold compresses to the forehead. Change every two to three minutes during the height of the reaction. Add hot water frequently during the treatment to keep the temperature up to the person's tolerance.

After three minutes remove the extremity from the can and put it in the cold water can up to the knee for 30 seconds. Then back into the hot can for three minutes. Alternate this pattern for 20 minutes. Give water to drink when sweating begins. Finish the treatment with 30 seconds in the cold bath.

Dry the skin thoroughly. Have the person lie down for 30 to 60 minutes.

Massage

The psychologic effects of a massage set up interactions that affect cell function. This can result in increased length of life for people who have had heart attacks, strokes, acquired immune deficiency syndrome, or cancer.

After one month of daily massage there was an increase in natural killer cell number and cytotoxicity as well as several subsets of immune cells. There was also an increase in overall cytotoxic capacity. Furthermore, there was a decrease in 24-hour urinary cortisol and catecholamines (stress hormones). There were significant decreases in anxiety and increases in relaxation. These findings were compared with the same patient, one month with daily massage, and one month without massage (*International Journal of Neuroscience* 84 [1996]: 205).

Patients who get massages enjoy the following physiologic benefits:

- An increase in circulation—skin, muscles, joints—with a reduction in congestion
- An increase in lymphatic drainage, reflexively, removing wastes
- Connective tissue increases in firmness and density
- Muscular tension is relaxed; headaches are relieved; blood pressure reduced
- Gastrointestinal motility is increased, which eliminates wastes
- Central nervous system is stimulated
- Swelling is reduced
- The pH of tissues is increased, which encourages healing
- The white blood cell count is increased

Abdominal Massage

- Take a full breath and hold for 20 counts, exhale fully and hold to the count of ten. Repeat 20 to 40 times. Do the exercise three times daily while driving or working. Take a "catch up" breath as needed.
- Lie on the back on a massage table or on a pad on the floor. Three positions are assumed one after another. Protrude the abdomen as high above plane as possible and hold for several seconds. Relax the abdominal muscles and assume an "on plane" position. Contract abdominal muscles to "hold in" the abdomen for several seconds. Relax and return to the "on plane" position. Repeat for about three minutes.
- A direct mechanical movement of solid contents of the colon or small intestine is seldom possible by massage, although gas is usually moved readily. It is the reflex action that achieves the benefit. Lie on the back and gently massage the colon. Begin with the fingers of the left hand over the cecum in the right lower abdominal quadrant. Make circular massaging movements, and then proceed up the colon a bit for the second series of circular movements. Follow the outline of the colon up and around the hepatic flexure. Change hands smoothly, and continue around the splenic flexure, descending colon, sigmoid, and rectum. Repeat 8 to 10 times.

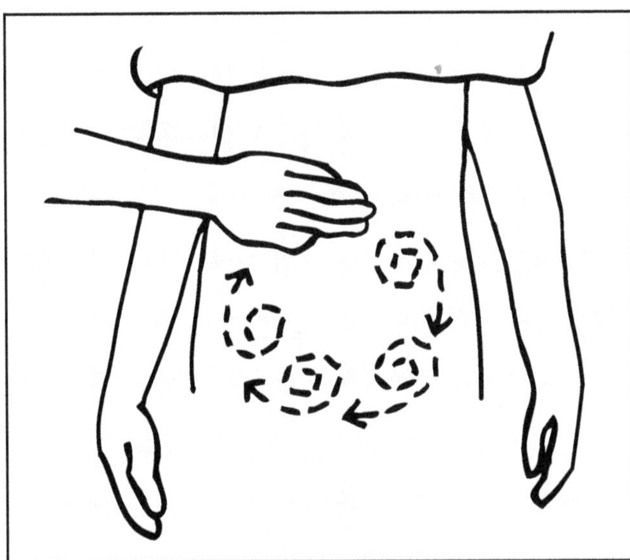

- Give a gentle percussion to the colon by tapping, spatting, and slapping.
- Gently knead the colon, four times as a minimum and up to 10 to 20 minutes.
- Deep vibration of the colon also may be combined with reflex effleurage. Place the right hand on the umbilicus, fingers spread and in firm skin contact, and exert a little pressure on the abdomen while the patient is completely relaxed. Grasp your right wrist with your left hand and exert evenly a fairly strong trembling movement. Repeat the maneuver in each of the four abdominal quadrants. The patient must be relaxed; therefore, it is essential to perform this stroke during the period of exhalation. Instruct the patient to breathe deeply then exhale during the trembling action.

Adrenal Stimulation Massage

Adrenal stimulation encourages production of beneficial hormones. Follow these procedures to massage the adrenal.

- Locate the position of the adrenals by putting the right hand on the waist while standing behind the patient. Put the fingertips of your left hand on the lower angle of the right shoulder blade. Then place the thumb of your right hand on a point approximately halfway between the two hands. Then slide the thumb close to the spine. That is the location of the upper pole of the kidney. One fingerbreadth above that is the location of the adrenals. Tap fast and firmly, drumming over the adrenals with the fingertips of alternating hands, like a hammer mill. This small treatment can also banish drowsiness for awhile in meetings or when you are at work in your office.
- Administer alternating very hot water applications and very cold water applications, one minute of cold for each six minutes of hot, ending with cold. Repeat one or both treatments daily.
- Use a cold spray from the shower to the adrenal areas followed by tapotement (tapping with fingertips) over the area immediately beneath the shoulder blades to reflexively stimulate the adrenals, which will indirectly stimulate the thyroid. Forcefully tap your fingers, hand over hand, your wrists being like a hinge, to throw your fingertips onto the selected area. Follow the tapping with rubbing, as your fingertips should have caused a bit of smarting.

Aroma Massage

This can be any style of massage with the addition of scented oils, which have been reported to have a stimulating, calming, or relaxing effect. A few studies show that peppermint scent can perk a person up (*Health*, October 1995, 59).

Citrus fragrance has restored stress-induced suppression of the immune system and has led to calmer behavior in mice. The use of massage with citrus fragrance has been found to reduce the need for high doses of anti-depressants in depressed patients (*Nihon Shinkei Seihin Yakurigaku Zasshi* 15, no. 1 [1995]: 39).

Dry Brush Massage

The brush massage can be given by a helper or self-administered. Use a circular motion over all portions of the body with a medium stiff brush, keeping the brush in contact with the skin and manipulating it with a circular and creeping movement, varying the speed and pressure of the movements—faster over the large skin areas, and slower and with lighter pressure over the fingers or neck. This type of massage can be used for neurological problems, anxiety, general physical conditioning, convalescence, and aches and pains, especially in the neck and back.

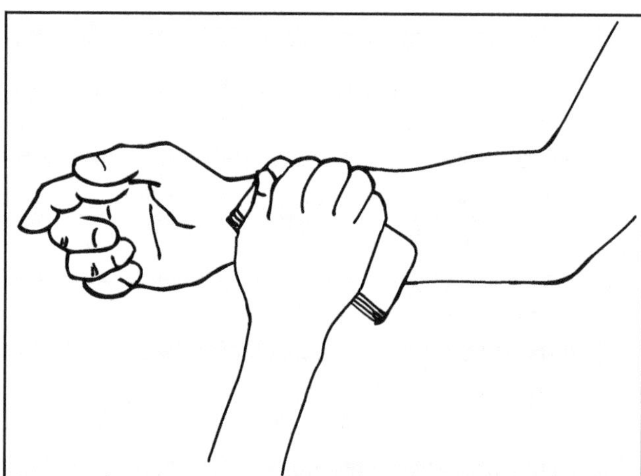

Ice Massage

The ice rub is best used for acute back strain. Take a 10- to 16-ounce disposable cup that can be torn with the fingers or cut with scissors as the ice melts. Fill the cup with water and freeze.

The area of pain is blocked off with towels to catch the runoff water from the melting ice. At least six inches of skin need to be exposed—preferably the area of pain and about two inches beyond in all directions. Tear off the bottom end of the cup to expose the ice about one inch. Hold the top of the cup and rub the ice on the exposed skin, keeping the ice constantly moving to prevent over cooling. The patient at first feels unpleasantly cold, then painful, then burning in the area being rubbed, then a pleasant numbness in the previously painful area. Often a single treatment is curative for an acute back strain. Repeat as often as every two hours.

Special Massage Strokes

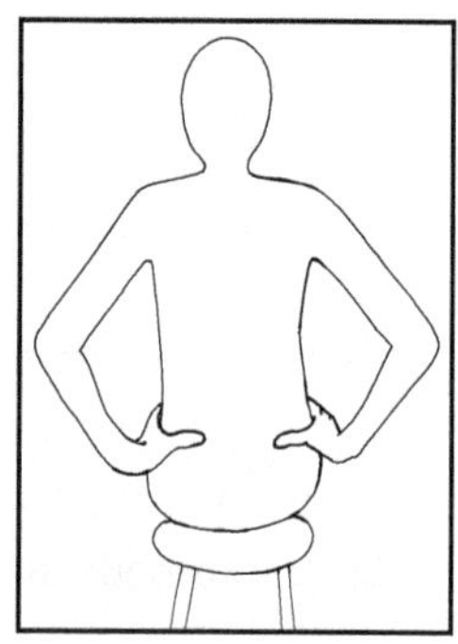

- *To relax the tired back.* Put your hands on your waist, fingers toward the front, and thumbs in the back. Feel with the thumbs for rope-like muscles on either side of the spine. Put firm pressure with the thumbs on the outer edges of these muscles, aiming the pressure toward the spine.
- *To open up the nasal passages* place your index and middle finger beside the nostrils at the base of the cheekbones directly below the eye. Press upward to relieve sinus pain and congestion and to open up the nasal passage.
- *Headache.* With one hand, press the hollow at the back of your head at the very base of the skull. At the same time, put your thumb and forefinger of the other hand in the upper hollows of the eye sockets just beneath the ridge for the eyebrows on either side of the bridge of the nose. Press firmly in these points.
- *Constipation.* While lying on your back, knees bent, put three fingers on the spot three finger-widths below your navel. Using your fingertips press downward toward the spine, breathing deeply. If you do this exercise regularly, it will help to prevent constipation.

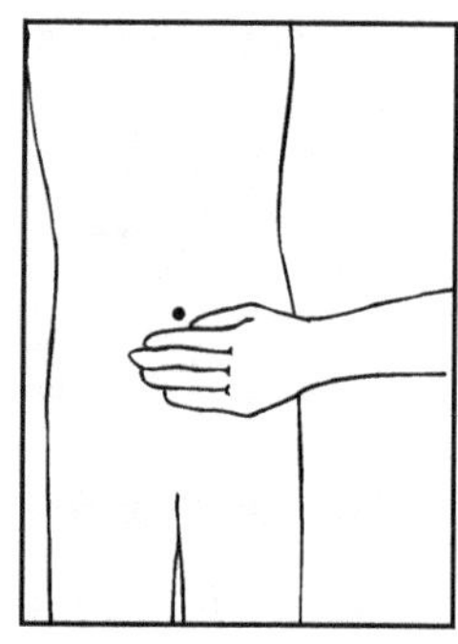

- *Menstrual Pain.* While lying face down with your arms underneath your body, place each fist against your groin on the crease where the front of the torso meets the thigh. Stimulate this spot by slowly raising one leg at a time straight up behind you.
- *Insomnia.* Lie on your back and place two tennis balls between your shoulder blades on the spine at about the level of your heart. The tennis balls should be enclosed in a sock to keep them from rolling away. With the knees bent, roll around on the balls so that they press into the area between the shoulder blades. Continue the treatment for 20 minutes.

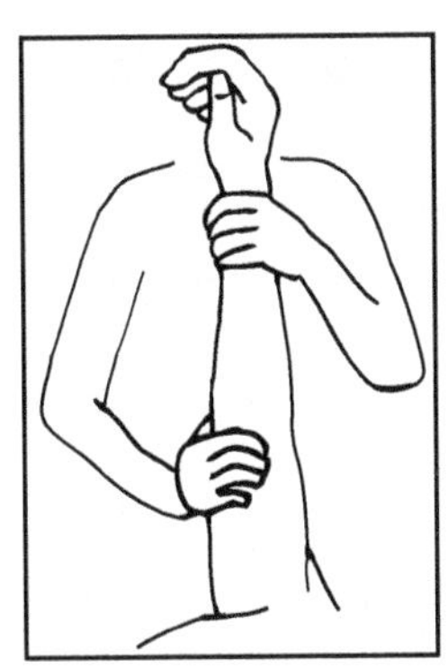

- *Nausea.* Rub the tissues between the two bones of the forearm about three fingerbreadths above the most prominent crease between the wrist and the hand. By rubbing this area you will forget the nausea. Repeat on the other arm.

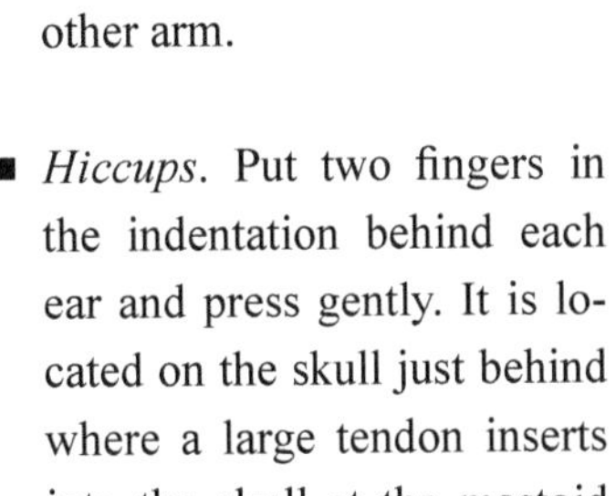

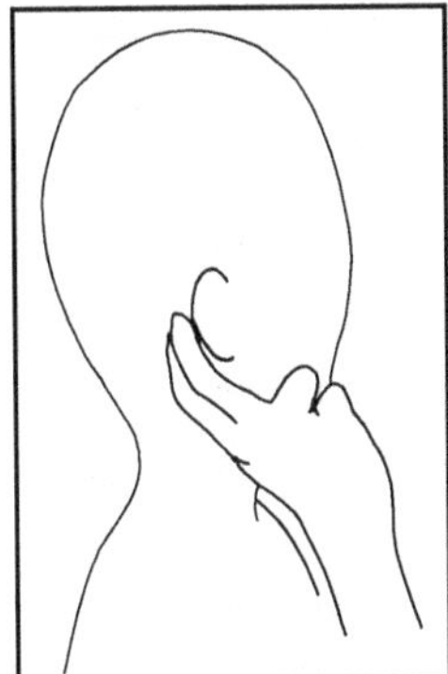

- *Hiccups.* Put two fingers in the indentation behind each ear and press gently. It is located on the skull just behind where a large tendon inserts into the skull at the mastoid bone.

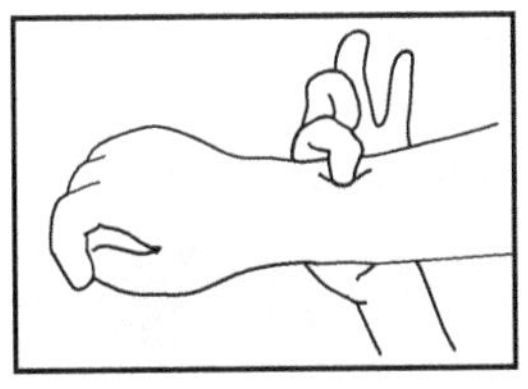

- *Carpal Tunnel Syndrome.* Lay your painful arm in the palm of the non-painful hand. Press the area between the two bones of the forearm, on the top of the hand, two fingerbreadths above the crease between the hand and the wrist. Put the thumb on the smooth side of the arm and the forefinger on the hairy side of the arm and press together firmly in a pincher action. If pressing these points hurts the non-tender hand, then press the areas one side at a time, using the knuckles instead of the fingers.
- *In diabetic neuropathy,* a continuous stroking of the back and lower extremities, shoulders, and backs of the arms, taking between 25 and 30 minutes merely continuing the stroking, and then 10 to 15 minutes of the rubbing of the front of the legs and arms, is helpful. The treatment should be done at least twice a week for 10 to 12 treatments and then every 10 to 14 days for two to three months. The circulation can often be improved to the point that the severely compromised circulation can come back into service (*Massage* #20, March-April 1996, 102).
- *Improve immune system.* A massage can help you sleep, can improve your immune system, and can even help to fight off colds and flu. It may take a massage every week for 10 to 12 weeks, or several massages a week for several weeks to make the natural killer cells increase in number and vigor.

Thymus Stimulation Massage

Stimulate the thymus, the source of T-cells, by tapping on the middle of the chest, gently but firmly pounding rapidly with one fist after the other just below the middle of the breastbone. Do not bruise the tissue. This treatment should be pleasant, not jolting.

Music Therapy

"When rightly used music is a precious gift of God, designed to uplift the thoughts to high and noble themes, to inspire and elevate the soul" (Ellen G. White, *Education,* 167).

Music can relieve pain in recovery rooms or operating suites. Within minutes of listening to soothing music a 32-year-old cancer patient who had been racked with pain that could not be relieved by drugs felt relaxed, and her respiration deepened and became regular. Her hands relaxed, and she fell into a deep sleep. Playing soothing music in the coronary care unit promotes rest and reduces elevated blood pressure and heart rate. The need for narcotics and sedatives can be reduced by playing soothing music (*National Enquirer*, January 22, 1991).

A Pennsylvania state university report showed that students who listened the most to rock music had the highest levels of depression scores on psychological tests (*USA Today*, April 12, 1994).

Oatmeal Bath

To administer an oatmeal bath, loosely tie one pound of uncooked oatmeal in a large piece of gauze, a pillowcase, or kitchen towel, and hang it or hold it under the bathtub spigot in such a way that the water runs through the oatmeal, using the hot water first to soften the oatmeal and encourage the dissolving of the starch. After the tub has been filled, the bag of oatmeal should be left in the bath water, and the patient may use the bag to sponge the surface of the body.

One heaping cup of uncooked rolled oats, ground fine in a blender, can be substituted for the one pound bag. It is stirred into the bathtub. The patient should remain in the tub for 20 to 30 minutes or longer and finish by patting the skin dry with the bare hands. Use for poison ivy, eczema, hives, and any itching affliction.

Petroleum Milk

The most effective treatment we have found for eczema, dermatitis, dry skin, or winter itch for hands is petroleum milk. It has helped many to heal. While the hands are still wet from washing or from the bath, an amount about the size of a large bean of petroleum jelly is taken between the palms and rubbed vigorously to mix with the water still on the hands. We call the resulting emulsion "Petroleum Milk."

Sun Bath

Exposure to the sun is critical to good health. A sun bath consists of exposing the skin to the sun once a day for 15 to 20 minutes on each side.

Wounds

For fresh wounds that are dirty, use plain running water to flush out particles of dirt. If you have not been successful with plain water, try water and soap, or water and vinegar as a cleansing agent. While flooding the wound, use your clean hands and tweezers to lift particles of trash and attempt to clear dirt particles, oil, debris, or various chemicals from the wound.

Plain petroleum jelly from a pharmacy or department store can also be cleansing and healing. In a study done by Major David Phillips at Fort Bragg, North Carolina, on 34 patients having 38 surgical wounds, half were treated with bacitracin ointment and half were treated with petroleum jelly. He found there was no significant difference in infection rates between patients treated with one or the other. He estimated that between 8 and 10 million dollars could be saved annually in healthcare costs if dermatologists and surgeons switched from antibiotic ointment to petroleum jelly (*Reuters Health Information Services*, Inc., July 29, 1996). It is our opinion that even more could be saved if the wound were simply dressed with a clean dressing and no petroleum. The petroleum serves only to prevent sticking of the dressing, which may or may not be desirable. Dressing removal is one way of removing crusts and debriding or cleaning up the wound.

Aloe vera significantly decreased wound healing time, both when applied topically, as well as when taken internally as juice.

Dressing a fresh wound with ordinary honey from the kitchen is one of the most effective remedies for preventing wound infections you can find. Simply pour it on the wound or on the dressing and apply directly to the wound. Change the dressing twice every day.

Alternating hot and cold compresses can be used to good advantage for wounds having traumatic nerve damage and slow healing. In the water for the hot compresses, use comfrey tea as a healing herb. In the cold water, use St. John's wort tea. With these two herbs, make a strong solution and pour the tea into the water used for wetting the compresses. On the first day apply the compresses six times a day; the second day four times; and from day three and onward three times a day or more as needed by the severity of the case.

A witch hazel wash or poultice made from strong witch hazel tea can be stimulating for healing in slow healing cases. Dip a gauze, or clean cloth or square of paper toweling, in the tea and make a cold compress. Simply lay the wet piece over the wound and allow it to dry for 10 to 15 minutes. Repeat every 10 to 15 minutes for 30 to 90 minutes.

To make an antibiotic tincture, take one cup of grain alcohol (get this kind from a liquor store) and add one ounce of each of the following herbs: echinacea, gotu kola, chaparral, and astragalus. Swirl twice daily for three weeks. The tincture has strong antimicrobial properties. If you cannot find one or two of the herbs, use what you can find.

Herbal Remedies

Introduction

When compared to drugs—street drugs, prescription drugs, or even over-the-counter drugs—herbs are incredibly safe. In spite of millions of doses of herbs used every day, it is rare to hear of anyone being hurt by an herb. If an adverse reaction does occur, no matter how minor, it is front page news, not only in medical journals, but in the local newspapers. On the other hand, the diseases, disabilities, and deaths caused by drugs are ignored as if they are a natural part of life. This is unfortunate, as herbs have been safely and very effectively used for thousands of years by persons having much less general knowledge than we have today.

Most herbs work in a nutritive way. Most drugs work, by contrast, in a pharmacologic (toxic) way. We can look at their actions as intoxicating one system to capture its energy for another system. In the process, much damage is done. So, I recommend herbs to you as being safe and effective when used knowledgeably and moderately.

Many common herbs contain medicinal factors at a nontoxic level when used in the form of teas. Every family should have the knowledge of these properties, knowing how to identify the herbs in the woods and fields and having certain herbs fresh and available for use. Dried herbs should be stored in an airtight, dark container to prevent loss of strength. Herbs are best taken as tea, but capsules, pills, tablets, tinctures and other concentrated forms of herbs can be taken also. Allowing herbs to steep longer than 30 minutes can extract from a few herbs toxic or undesirable properties. Read the instructions and information in this section for more information about safely using herbs.

Herbs can be divided into four categories:

- **Adaptogens** (like ginseng, ashwaganda, licorice) have the ability to normalize the function of a tissue or organ, have a regulatory effect on the endocrine system, and can properly function to treat low or high activity in a hormone gland. These herbs can be used where there is stress, premature aging, and convalescence from sickness of any kind.
- **Bitters or aromatics** (like mint, gentian, angelica) are either bitter, or give off some kind of fragrance, as their names indicate. They stimulate digestion and help relieve constipation, nausea, motion sickness, and pain in the abdomen.
- **Nervines** (like kava kava, valerian, hops, passionflower, catnip) affect the nervous system, particularly the central nervous system, and help irritability, anxiety, insomnia, restlessness, and nervous tension.
- **Muscle relaxants** (like wood betony, black cohosh, cramp bark, kava kava) are excellent for muscle tension and tension headaches.

Herbs may be used internally by drinking them in the form of tea or using them in a enema. They may also be used externally in the form of tinctures, lotions, and liniment.

This section provides a list of the herbs to use for certain conditions and what conditions or disorder each herb fights. It also contains helpful information about precautions for some herbs.

Aloe Vera

Biostymin, a substance found in aloe vera acts as a biologic stimulator in allergic and infectious diseases. Investigators believe the beneficial effects are due to a stimulatory reaction in the adrenals, spleen, and reticuloendothelial tissues. The increased production of antibodies and disease fighting proteins, as well as the increased hormonal activity of the adrenals, appear to be the means of benefit in such diseases as asthma, chronic leg ulcers, burns, digestive tract disorders, shingles, baldness (both spot baldness and falling hair), acne, and a host of other diseases and physical problems.

Anti-inflammatory Herbs

Anti-inflammatory herbs include angelica, arnica, basil, boswellia, bromelain (found in pineapples), cardamom, chamomile, chaparral, chives, cilantro, devil's claw, echinacea, flax seed oil, garlic, hawthorn, licorice root, meadowsweet, parsley, papaya, rosemary, St. John's wort, turmeric, white willow bark, wild lettuce tea, and wild yam.

Antimicrobial Herbs

Antimicrobial herbs include alfalfa, aloe vera, barberry, bayberry, blue cohosh, burdock, catnip, chamomile, chaparral, comfrey, coriander, dandelion, elderberry, echinacea, garlic, golden seal, hops, licorice, the mints, Pau d'Arco, sage, St. John's wort, tarragon, thyme, turmeric (sprinkle dry powder on infected wounds), uva-ursi, and others. These herbs have antimicrobial qualities including antiviral, antifungal, and antibacterial properties. Witch hazel has antimicrobial actions when used externally on boils, infected eczema or athlete's foot, impetigo, or infected wounds.

Antiseptic Herbs

Chaparral, charcoal powder, cinnamon, cloves, eucalyptus, garlic powder, onions, thyme, turmeric, and uva-ursi are all used as antiseptic herbs. The herbs may be made up for external use by mixing a little water with the powdered herb at the time of need.

Arnica Liniment

Mix one pint of sweet oil with two tablespoons of tincture of arnica. Another way to make a liniment is to heat the leaves or flowers of arnica in olive oil over low heat. Fill a double boiler with dried arnica flowers, cover the flowers with olive oil, boil the water in the bottom of the double boiler for two to three hours. While still warm, strain and add to the mixture a small lump of beeswax or paraffin, which will melt in the hot oil. This is to give body to the liniment. Use for skin infections, muscle aches and pains, arthritis, rheumatism, and stiff joints.

Aromatherapy

Aromatherapy can be quite helpful for a variety of disorders.

- The fragrance of fir, pine, and cedar is good for pulmonary disorders.
- Headaches can be helped by peppermint essential oil, chamomile, or true lavender.
- Hot flashes can be helped by sage, fennel, geranium, or rose.
- Insomnia can be helped by ylang-ylang, neroli, or rose. Also make a strong aroma of lavender on your pillow for sleeplessness.
- Low back pain can be helped by lemon grass, rosemary, or lavender (its perillyl alcohol is the active substance).
- For menstrual cramps use geranium; for muscle spasms, sage, or lavender.
- For osteoarthritis use frankincense, rosemary, or lavender. Rosemary contains an antioxidant called carnosol. It also functions as an anticarcinogen (*Carcinogenesis* 23, no. 6 [June 2002]: 983).

Castor Oil Compress

Make the compress by wetting a cotton cloth with castor oil, laying it on the skin over the area, and covering with a piece of plastic or wool. Castor oil increases the number of T-cells in the area. It may be helpful for suspected appendicitis, abdominal pain, tennis elbow, or sprained ankles.

Castor oil has been used for anointing the upper and lower eyelids for cataracts and conjunctivitis. It could be rubbed on the eyelids at night in much the same way a lotion is applied. It could also be applied to a small piece of cloth and laid on the eyelids as a poultice or compress. We have had no experience with castor oil in cataracts, but applying the oil should do no harm.

Comfrey Compress

The fresh leaves, or dry leaves moistened with hot water, may be whizzed in a blender with a little water. Take a paper towel and spread the material completely over a paper towel. It may be laid directly on the skin of the affected area. Cover completely with a piece of plastic, allowing the plastic to extend over the edges an inch on all sides. Hold the compress in place with a roller bandage, an ace bandage, or a 50- to 60-inch strip of cloth specially prepared for this purpose, cutting a strip from a bed sheet or other long piece, wrapping it around the entire body or an extremity, and pinning it in place. Make a neat, snug bandage. Leave the compress on for 30 minutes to eight hours. At the end of the time, remove the compress, sponge the surface clean with a damp washcloth, and rub the area with a cold mitten friction. Dry thoroughly and replace clothing. Comfrey has very powerful healing properties.

Fungus Herbal Formula

For toenail fungus, mix the following herbs together:

1 pint vinegar, any kind
2 oz calendula flowers, dry
2 oz myrrh crystals or powder

For fingernails, mix:

1 cup vinegar
1 cup DMSO
2 oz calendula
2 oz myrrh

Put the ingredients together in a container large enough to allow you to shake it or stir it daily for two or three weeks. After two or three weeks of mixing, the formula will have reached its strongest concentration. At that time, strain and pour it into a dark bottle. Store in a cool, dark place.

Apply it at least twice a day to toenails, and more frequently to fingernails as they are more difficult to cure. Apply at least six times daily to fingernails and allow to air dry. The treatment must be kept up until the nail grows out normal, which may take longer for toenails than for fingernails—up to a year or more. When you are dressing and when you are undressing are the most favorable times for the application to the toenails. While on long drives, air trips, sitting in seminars, etc. are the best times for fingernails, as they need frequent application.

Garlic

To use fresh garlic, blenderize one cup of tomato juice with one to three cloves of fresh garlic. Drink this cocktail three to five times daily. If tomato juice cannot be used, substitute any vegetable broth or juice tolerated or use plain water. Sip or drink slowly to avoid excessive burning of the mouth or nausea, which comes from drinking it too fast. Use when fighting a bacterial or fungal infection, high cholesterol, atherosclerosis, or cancer. As late as World War II, garlic was used as an effective replacement for antibiotics.

To use garlic as an anticoagulant, steam or bake the garlic until the hot quality has barely disappeared. This develops ajoene and diallylsulfide, which are both strong anticoagulants.

Garlic has been shown to have a significant protective action in many conditions. Onions also help in most of the same conditions.

There are a wide variety of reported uses for garlic, such as:

- Decelerating aging
- Taking care of colic in both infants and adults. Use a small dose for babies—one-fourth teaspoon minced, fresh, or dry granules in three ounces of water
- Helping clotting inside veins
- Combats infection. Use three large cloves three times daily for five days
- Reduces blood sugar and combats the complications of diabetes
- Combats asthma, whooping cough, and bronchitis
- Prevents heart attacks, reduces swelling
- Increases the excretion of heavy metals
- Dilates blood vessels and reduces high blood pressure
- Prevents and treats hypertension
- Attacks intestinal, skin, and blood parasites
- Reduces high hemoglobin (14.0 grams or above in women, and 15.5 in men)
- Treats colds and sore throats (by taking garlic, symptoms often disappear in a few hours)

Lotion

This entry contains a variety of lotion recipes.

Acid Mantle Cream

9.6 oz of oil mixture
19.2 oz of distilled water
1.6 oz emulsifying wax
1.6 oz vegetable glycerin
½ oz essential oil of your choice for fragrance
16 drops vitamin E oil as a preservative
1 tsp citric acid crystals as a stabilizer

Anti-itch Lotion

Shake or blenderize all of the following ingredients.

1 tbsp Tradescantia extract
¼ cup hand lotion
1 tbsp aloe vera gel
1 tsp oil of cloves
2 tbsp water

For a simplified version for minor itching, add the following ingredients and shake or blenderize.

¼ cup hand lotion
1 tsp clove oil

Janitza's Lotion Recipe

The following recipe will produce a wonderful above-average lotion, but you must have a very accurate scale to accomplish good results. You will also need a handheld stick blender. This recipe makes four eight-ounce bottles of lotion. You may divide the recipe to make smaller amounts.

Pitcher # 1
9.6 oz oil mixture
1.6 oz emulsifying wax
16 drops of vitamin E oil

Pitcher # 2
19.2 oz distilled water
1.6 oz glycerin
½ oz essential oil

In pitcher #1 weigh out the oil mixture, which could be any one kind of oils or combinations of oils. For example you could use oil of avocado, sweet almond, and jojoba, as long as all of them combined total the amount needed for the formula, which is 9.6 oz. Weigh out the emulsifying wax and add to pitcher #1, along with the vitamin E oil.

Have the essential oil ready. You may use any kind by itself or a combination of blends. Lavender, lemongrass, peppermint, tea tree, pine tree, etc,. are some favorites. You must consider and choose what you are trying to accomplish since each one has different benefits on the body.

Put the oil and the wax pitcher into a pot of hot water, or double boiler, on the stove to melt the wax.

While the wax is melting, in pitcher #2 weigh out the distilled water and glycerin.

Once the wax is all liquid in pitcher #1, bring it out of the hot water. Slowly pour the ingredients from pitcher #2 into pitcher #1 while using the stick blender on low to blend. (If you mix on high, you will incorporate a lot of air or bubbles into the lotion). As you are mixing, the lotion will cool down and will become more viscous or thick.

As the lotion thickens, add the essential oil, which will help to prevent spoilage for a long time. Now quickly pour the lotion into bottles and wait until it is completely cooled before you put the cap on. Refrigerate unused lotion to preserve it longer.

Precautions to Take with Some Herbs

With the medicinal use of herbs coming more and more into vogue in today's society, it behooves everyone who uses herbs to give careful study to their proper selection. A few herbs in common use today have toxic properties that the home remedies user should know. But when compared with over-the-counter drugs, herbs are still extremely safe to use.

1. **Devil's Claw Root** – Recently introduced from South Africa, this herb stimulates contraction of the uterine smooth muscle and should not be used during pregnancy. The seeds, leaves, and bark of many plants contain a cyanoglycoside, amygdalin, which liberates hydrogen cyanide. This substance has anticancer properties.Eating large amounts of these substances, or small amounts for long periods, can result in chronic cyanide poisoning or mutagenesis in cells, leading to possible birth defects or cancer. Amygdalin is found in the seeds of apricots, bitter almonds, cassava, cherries, choke cherries, millet, peaches, pears, apples and plums. The symptoms of poisoning are goiter, loss of ability to walk steadily,

and blurring of vision, leading sometimes to blindness. Apparently a fairly large quantity of the food item is needed to produce toxic symptoms. In the usual quantities no ill effects can be sensed.

2. **Ginseng** is a most common herbs that a lot of people use. It has been used for thousands of years by the Orientals as a stimulant and tonic. Those who advocate its use claim that it helps the body adapt to stress, corrects thyroid and adrenal malfunction, stimulates the nervous system, and produces a sense of well-being and even euphoria. Ginseng contains a number of pharmacologically active ingredients, mainly glycosides. It contains small amounts of plant estrogens that may cause swollen and painful breasts.
3. **Licorice root** can cause sodium retention if used for long periods of time, which could raise blood pressure and lead to potassium loss. However, it may be very desirable in adrenal exhaustion or malfunction.
4. **Pennyroyal** oil has been used to induce menstruation and abortion. It contains the ketone pugelone, which is toxic to the liver and kidneys and may cause death. As little as one teaspoonful of the concentrated oil can cause seizures.

To avoid problems with overusing herbs, we recommend that medicinal herbs be taken preferably as teas, and that the tea leaves or powder be steeped for only 30 minutes, never boiled or allowed to stand overnight, before straining.

Remedies for Certain Conditions

Asthma	Garlic
Boils	Charcoal, hops, yellow dock (as a poultice)
Bronchitis	Mullein, white oak bark
Burns	Aloe vera, comfrey
Cancer	Blue violet, chamomile, chaparral, flaxseed, garlic, graviola, red clover
Childbirth	Angelica (to expel afterbirth), black cherry, black cohosh (for pain), buckwheat plant, cotton root bark, partridgeberry, red raspberry leaf, squaw vine
Colds	Basil tea, red clover tea, woodruff tea
Colic	Carob paste, catnip, charcoal
Constipation	American senna, aloe vera, chamomile (cleansing the intestines), flaxseed (one tablespoon blended with three prunes in water), wheat bran (one to four tablespoons)
Cystitis	Bearberry (uva ursi), buchu, burdock, corn silk, watermelon seed
Dandruff	Corn oil (rubbed into scalp), soap root powder solution
Diarrhea	Carob powder (make a thin paste with water, take up to one-fourth cup), catnip tea, charcoal (one heaping tablespoon in water with each loose stool), comfrey tea
Dietary need of sterols	Alfalfa leaf tea, apples, black cohosh, cherries, ginseng, hops, licorice root tea, peaches, red raspberry leaf
Diuresis	Alfalfa, buchu, burdock, corn silk, dandelion
Edema	Charcoal, strong pekoe tea used as a poultice (three bags per cup of water), strong solution of water and salt or water and Epsom salts (one-fourth cup in four gallons)
Emetic	Garlic clove (blended in water, drink quickly)
Epilepsy	Catnip, cow parsnip, hops, any sedative herb, valerian root
Fever	Bayberry, meadowsweet, joe-pye weed, white willow bark
Fever blisters, lips, and genitals	Golden seal (used internally or externally)
Gallbladder	Aloe vera

Headache	Celery (several stalks eaten raw), lemon (the juice of one lemon or orange blended with 2 tablespoons of sesame seed), skunk cabbage
Hiccups	Dill (weed or seed, taken as a tea)
Insect repellent	Basil, citronella, golden seal, melissa, pennyroyal (place a little of the herb in the corner of a handkerchief and pin to the clothing)
Insomnia	Catnip, dill weed tea, hops, partridge berry, sage, skullcap, valerian
Kidney stones	Gravel root, lemon (one teaspoon olive oil and half lemon every morning), marshmallow root, stone root, trailing arbutus
Laxative	Flaxseed, licorice, psyllium, senna
Lactation	Catnip, chamomile, spurge
Measles	Ginger tea, red clover
Menstrual cycle regulation	Calendula flowers, cotton thistle, iceland moss, lady's mantle, marigold blossoms, mugwort, shepherd's purse, silverweed, St. John's wort
Menstrual pain	False Solomon's seal (half cup per day), red raspberry leaf, skullcap, tansy, white cedar bark
Mental stimulant, memory	Ginkgo, rosemary tea
Nephritis	Buchu, soybeans (cooked, one-fourth cup daily)
Nervousness	Catnip, hops, skullcap
Nipples	Strong golden seal tea as a wet dressing for 20 minutes daily
Pain	Mullein flowers and mullein root tea mixed with catnip, chamomile, mint, nettle, skullcap, or Solomon's seal (use one or several). Also white willow bark or geranium oil for shingles
Parasites	Aloe vera, artemisia annua (wormwood), black walnut hulls, fennel seed, garlic, golden seal, psyllium seed, pumpkin seed, thyme
Peptic ulcers	Aloe vera, cabbage juice (taken fresh, the first three to five minutes after juicing), catnip, charcoal, comfrey tea, echinacea, golden seal, myrrh, violet leaf tea
Poison ivy	Aloe vera, charcoal, jewel weed leaves (crushed and rubbed over the exposed area), onion slices (cut and laid on the itchy areas)
Ringworm	Mulberry leaves
Sedative	Black cherry root bark, catnip, celery (several stalks eaten raw), chamomile, hops, lavender, lemon verbena, passion flower, peppermint, sage, skullcap, St. John's wort, valerian root
Sunburn	Aloe vera
Tonic	Chaparral, red clover
Tonsillitis	Golden seal (make tea and gargle), pekoe tea (three bags to one cup water, gargle every half hour)
Toothache	Charcoal (make into a thick paste), clove bud or clove oil (apply directly), plantain root powder and myrrh heated in olive oil
Ulcers of skin	Charcoal (poultice), comfrey (poultice), hot water soaks
Vaginitis	Buchu, comfrey root tea, golden seal (douche), slippery elm suppository (see "Women's Conditions and Diseases" in the *Conditions and Diseases* section)
Vomiting	Carob paste (see "Diarrhea" above for recipe), catnip, charcoal, wild mint leaves

Tea

Infusion

Where instructions are not stated with the remedy, use the standard of one teaspoon of dried (leaf and stem) herb to one cup of water. Boil the water, add the herb, cover tightly, and set away from the fire to steep for 15 minutes. Boiling the herb can destroy the active elements. Strain. Drink two to three cups per day for one week unless otherwise directed.

Decoction

Boil the water, add the herb, cover, and simmer gently for 5 to 30 minutes depending on the hardness of the outer portion (root or bark) of the herb. Boiling tea vigorously can damage the active elements. Strain. Drink two to four cups per day for one week unless otherwise directed. Some herbs may be taken long term—months or years.

Tincture, Extract

Alcoholic Tinctures

Each herb has a specific percentage of alcohol most perfectly dissolving the active principle of that herb. Unless specified, assume that a 30 percent alcoholic solution with water is the most favorable. Generally it is a proportion of one to two ounces of the herb to one pint of 30 percent alcoholic solution. Allow the mixture to set for two weeks, agitating daily. Strain and store in a glass container in a dark, cool place. An alcoholic tincture lasts several years.

Cayenne Extract Tincture

Extract of cayenne is an alcoholic extract made from one teaspoon of red pepper to eight ounces of rubbing alcohol. Soak for two weeks, swirling it once daily. You may start using the tincture immediately; however, the tincture is most effective after two weeks. Apply it to the areas where pain is felt six times a day for the first six days, then twice a day thereafter. As long as you keep using it, the pain will stay away.

Vinegar Tinctures

Generally one ounce of the dried herb to one pint of vinegar is the correct proportion. If a fresh herb is used, generally about five ounces per pint is the correct proportion.

Uses for Certain Herbs

Aloe vera	Abscesses, acne, alopecia, arthritis, asthma, baldness, burns, callouses, colitis, constipation, dandruff (use as a shampoo), dermatitis, diaper rash, digestive tract disorders, diverticulitis, dry skin, fever blisters, fungus diseases, impetigo, infected wounds, insect stings, itching, liver diseases, mouth ulcers, peptic ulcers (esophagus, stomach, pylorus, duodenum), poison ivy, psoriasis, pyorrhea, rashes, shingles, skin problems, sore throat (gargle and swallow), sunburn, warts, X-ray burns
Ashwaganda root	Anti-inflammatory, antioxidant, antistress, antitumor, cardioprotective, central nervous system, heart, irritability, insomnia, lungs
Black cherry, root or bark	childbirth pain, cough, diarrhea, hemorrhoids, ringworm
Boswellia	Fibromyalgia
Buchu	Bladder, diuresis, diaphoresis (produce sweating), kidney, and prostate problems
Catnip	Colds, coughs, daytime tranquilizer, diarrhea, headache, nausea and vomiting, sleep
Charcoal	Colds, diarrhea, gas, poisoning, sinusitis, sore throat, venomous bites and stings
Comfrey	Chronic skin ulcers
Dill	Bad breath (chew some), insomnia
Echinacea	Finest immune system stimulant available

Garlic	Acne, allergies, anemia, angina, antibacterial agent, anticoagulation, antifungal agent, antioxidant, antispasmodic, antiviral, arteriosclerosis, arthritis, asthma, athlete's foot, bad breath, blood clots, bronchitis, cancer, candida albicans, childbirth infections, childbirth afterpains, cholesterol elevation, colds, colitis, concentration (poor), constipation, coughs, cystitis, diabetes, digestive disorders, diuretic, dizziness, dysentery, eczema, edema, emphysema, expectorant, fats high in the blood, gas (intestinal), headache, heart disease, heavy metal poisoning, hemolysis prevention, hemorrhoids, high blood pressure, hoof and mouth disease, hypoglycemia, immunity stimulation, influenza and colds, insect repellent, insomnia, intestinal gas, intestinal parasites in dogs and man, laxative, leprosy, lupus erythematosus, malaria, menstrual pain, menopause syndrome, parasites, plague (cholera, typhus), plantar warts, polio, polycythemia, poultices, pyorrhea, respiratory disorders, sciatica, sore throat, swellings, thyroid supplement, tooth whitener, triglyceride elevation, tuberculosis, tumor growth inhibition, whooping cough
Ginkgo Biloba	Macular degeneration, memory loss, stress
Ginseng	Aging, stress (all varieties contain high amounts of plant estrogens and progesterone)
Golden seal	Colds, colitis, conjunctivitis, dermatitis, fever blisters on lips or genitals, insect repellent (place leaves in an open container), sores in mouth or on tongue
Hops	Inflamed bowel (place poultice on abdomen), sedative, skin abscesses
Hawthorn	Lowers blood pressure, increases strength of the heart, normalizes rhythm
Horse Chestnut	Arthritis pain, coughs, deep vein thrombosis, diarrhea, edema, rheumatic pain, thrombophlebitis, varicose veins
Juniper	Bladder or kidney problems, diuretic, flatulence
Kava-kava	Anxiety, arthritis, asthma, insomnia, weight loss
Lemon Balm	Pain, sedative, sleep, viruses
Licorice	Antioxidant and antitumor activity, colds, coughs, hepatitis B, menopause, protects the endocrine system by preventing overproduction of hormones (used for almost any hormone problem), regulates hormones, respiratory infections, skin inflammations, ulcers. Licorice does cause sodium retention in some people, so do not use if someone has hypertension. Very good for adrenal exhaustion
Milk Thistle	Hepatitis, liver and gallbladder problems
Oregano	Digestion, phlegm
Oregon Grape (Barberry)	Diarrhea, digestion, gallblader, heartburn, high blood pressure, liver, pinkeye, ulcers
Pycnogenol	Anticancer, anti-inflammatory, asthma
Red clover	Antitumor, general tonic, menopause
Rosemary	Acne, blemishes and dry skin, decongestant, digestion, infection prevention, mix leaves into foods to retard spoiling
Sage	Antiperspirant, digestion, labor pain, reduce blood sugar, sore throat, wound treatment
Sarsaparilla	Congestive heart failure, high blood pressure, anticancer properties
Slippery Elm	Aching joints, bruises, cough, cuts, sore throat
Stinging Nettle	Bladder, kidney stones, mild diuretic, urinary tract problems
Stevia	High blood pressure

Turmeric Acne, antibacterial, arthritis, autoimmune disorders, liver, minor cuts and scrapes, oily skin, parasites, liver problems, tendonitis, tooth abscesses

Tradescantia virginiana (Spiderwort) Cancer, insect bites, itching, kidneys, laxative, stings, stomach

Uva Ursi Bloating caused by PMS, congestive heart failure, high blood pressure, minor wounds, urinary tract infections

Valerian Anxiety, bronchial spasms, calming, cough, epilepsy, insomnia, mild tranquilizer, tension headaches

White willow bark Anti-inflammatory, pain

Anticoagulation Herbs

Herb	Mechanism of Action
Alfalfa	Contains coumarin constituents
Angelica	Contains coumarin constituents
Aniseed	Contains coumarin constituents
Asafoetida	Contains coumarin constituents
Celery	Contains coumarin constituents
Chamomile	Contains coumarin constituents
Clove	Inhibits platelet activity
Dong Quai	Inhibits platelet activity
Echinacea	Inhibits platelet activity
Evening Primrose Oil	Inhibits platelet aggregation
Fenugreek	Contains coumarin constituents
Fever Few	Inhibits platelet aggregation
Garlic	Inhibits platelet aggregation
Ginger	Inhibits platelet aggregation
Gingko biloba	Inhibits platelet aggregation
Ginseng, Panax	Inhibits platelet aggregation
Goldenseal	Inhibits platelet aggregation
Horse Chestnut	Contains coumarin constituents
Kava Kava	Inhibits platelet aggregation
Licorice	Inhibits platelet aggregation
Meadowsweet	Contains salicylate constituents
Parsley	Contains coumarin constituents
Poplar	Contains salicylate constituents
Prickly Ash, Northern	Contains salicylate constituents
Quassia	Contains coumarin constituents
Red Clover	Contains coumarin constituents
White Willow/Willow bark	Contains salicylate constituents

Dietary Information

Introduction

Diet is a vital component of maintaining one's health. Various foods contain a variety of vitamins and minerals that promote health and fight disease. This section contains useful information regarding nutrients, diets, food sensitivites, and other dietary information.

Disease-Fighting Foods

Following are a handful of diseases and specific foods that help to fight the disease. Some entries also contain foods that should be avoided.

Angina –	Vegan diet, low protein diet, and no free fats of any kind
Antibiotic functions –	Licorice root, elderberry, raw garlic and raw onion
Anti-inflammatory activity (lupus, arthritis, multiple sclerosis, peptic ulcers, ulcerative colitis, Crohn's disease) –	Cabbage juice, olives, pineapples, apples, hawthorn berry tea, flaxseed and flaxseed oil (one to three teaspoons, one to three times daily), celery (three stalks pureed once or twice a day). Omit for three months tomatoes, potatoes, eggplant, peppers, pimento, paprika; also omit these gluten grains: wheat, rye, and barley.
Asthma –	Garlic (sautéed in oil and take one tablespoon every 10 minutes in acute attack), garlic tea (one clove blenderized with one cup of hot water and strained)
Blood clots –	Garlic (lightly steamed and take six to ten cloves a day), all kinds of greens, especially parsley, and pineapple
Cancer prevention –	Garlic, soybeans, all fruits, especially citrus and grapes, vegetables, especially members of the cabbage family, and onions
Cancer treatment –	Garlic, citrus, grapes soybeans, flaxseed, parsley, celery, broccoli carrots, asparagus, and licorice root
Cataracts –	Vegetables and pineapples. Omit milk (known to promote cataracts)

Cystitis –	Omit all of these foods: eggs (greatest offender), citrus, nectarines, apple juice, red and green apples, guava, peaches, tomatoes, chilies, spicy food, strawberries, avocados, lima beans, figs, nuts, rye bread, bananas, mayonnaise, onions, pineapple, brewer's yeast, fava beans, prunes, chicken livers, dairy products, cheeses, meat, corned beef, vitamins buffered with aspartate, Nutrasweet (aspartame), saccharine, vinegar, alcoholic beverages, champagne, beer, carbonated drinks, coffee, tea, colas, and chocolate
Detoxification –	Garlic, citrus, cilantro, and spirulina
Diabetic neuropathy –	Peanuts, cantaloupes, grapefruit, whole grains, beans, and all citrus
Gout –	Omit these purines: animal products, beans, yeast, and asparagus
Heart disease –	Flaxseed, wheat, oats, rye, rice, barley, corn, peanuts, carob, greens, beets, squash, celery (three stalks pureed once or twice a day), and salt-free diet
Macular degeneration –	Blueberries, bilberry tea, and Pycnogenol (pine extract)
Ovarian cancer –	Omit these ova injuring foods - all dairy products, especially yogurt, and cream
Stomach –	Olives (4 to 20 with each meal), aloe, angelica, and bayberry root bark
Warts –	Savoy cabbage juice (four to six ounces daily)

Elimination and Challenge Diet

If a person experiences any of the following symptoms, he or she may be allergic to a certain food and should try the elimination and challenge diet:

- Learning disabilities, poor concentration, difficulty keeping organized or focused on a task, overeating, and other neurologic disorders (fatigue, sleepiness)
- Pallor, flushing, dark circles or bags under eyes, acne, eczema, and other types of skin problems or dermatitis
- Respiratory tract symptoms, such as coughing, sneezing, colds, sore throats, sinusitis, asthma, high pitched or unclear sounding voice, or fever
- cystitis, bladder pain, or bed wetting (adult and children)
- Leg aches, growing pains, or restless legs
- Backache, painful muscles or other musculoskeletal symptoms (cramps, arthritis, or joint pains)
- Headache, tinnitus (ringing in the ears), dizziness, blurred vision, or stuttering
- Mouth ulcers (canker sores or aphthous ulcers)
- Indigestion, gas, constipation, food cravings, or nausea

Foods to Avoid

Animal Proteins

- Beef
- Dairy products (over 60 percent of all food allergies are from dairy products)
- Eggs
- Fish
- Pork

Beverages

- Beer, alcohol
- Citrus fruits/juices
- Colas, coffee, tea

Fruits

- Apples
- Bananas
- Strawberries

Grains and Nuts

- Nuts (all kinds)
- Oatmeal
- Rice
- Seeds
- Wheat

Legumes

- Legumes, including peanuts and soybean products

Miscellaneous

- Artificial food colors
- Cane sugar
- Chocolate
- Garlic
- Yeast

Vegetables

- Corn (cornstarch and corn products)
- Lettuce
- Onion
- Tomatoes, potatoes, eggplant, and peppers

When testing to discover foods to which one is sensitive, omit all of the "foods to avoid" for one to six weeks. When the sensitivity symptoms have disappeared, start adding back foods one at a time every five to seven days until symptoms reappear. Then you know that the last food you added back to your diet may be one causing sensitivity, and you must eliminate it from your diet. Wait again until symptoms disappear and continue adding back one food every five to seven days. Several foods may be at fault so continue the test until all foods have been added back that you desire to test.

Foods Allowed

Dried Fruits

- Currants
- Dates
- Figs
- Pineapple
- Prunes
- Raisins

Fruits

- Apricots
- Avocado
- Blackberries
- Blueberries
- Cantaloupe
- Figs
- Grapes
- Honeydew
- Kiwi
- Mango
- Nectarine
- Papaya
- Peach
- Pear
- Persimmon
- Pineapple
- Plums
- Pomegranate
- Raspberries
- Watermelon

Grains

- Grains (barley, buckwheat, millet, rye)

Herbs

- Basil
- Bay leaf
- Dill
- Parsley
- Sage
- Thyme

Thickener

- Arrowroot
- Tapioca

Vegetables

- Artichoke
- Asparagus
- Avocado
- Beets
- Broccoli
- Cabbage
- Carrots
- Cauliflower
- Celery
- Collards
- Cucumber
- Kale
- Melons
- Okra

- Olives
- Rhubarb
- Rutabaga
- Spinach
- Squash (acorn, butternut, hubbard, summer)
- Sweet potatoes
- Swiss chard
- Turnip
- Zucchini

Fasting

Twenty Reasons to Fast

1. To lose weight fast or kick off a weight control program
2. To feel better physically
3. To look and feel more energetic
4. To save money and share with the needy
5. To give the whole system a rest
6. To cleanse the body
7. To lower blood pressure and cholesterol levels
8. To assist in quitting smoking, drinking, and drugs
9. To get rid of phobias and other mental illnesses
10. To let the body heal itself: allergies, ulcers, psoriasis, injuries, ulcerative colitis, arthritis, and mental strain
11. To relieve tension and develop calmness
12. To sleep better
13. To digest food better
14. To regulate bowels
15. To sharpen the senses and quicken mental processes
16. To obtain better self-control and restraint in eating
17. To seek spiritual strength
18. To slow the aging process
19. To regulate menstrual periods
20. To encourage milk production in young mothers

Short-term Fasting

Short-term fasting, from two to five days, profoundly suppresses certain hormones such as LH (luteinizing hormone), GH (growth hormone), and TSH (thyroid stimulating hormone)—all three are from the pituitary. This may be one of the reasons making dietary changes, such as becoming a vegetarian, may cause a loss of menstrual periods for several months. It is regarded as favorable for the overall health of the woman to have this hormone response to fasting (*Journal of Clinical Endocrinological Metabolism* 85 [2000]: 207).

Sometimes missing one to three meals can help to control colds, flu, asthma, skin problems (acne, eczema, rosacea, etc.), arthritis, indigestion, constipation, high blood sugar and hypertension, and many more problems. Fasting for even one day may also help to clear the liver, kidneys, and colon; remove toxins and impurities from the blood, make the eyes clear, and freshen the breath. You can also calm your mind, sharpen your senses, and provide a feeling of greater energy. Following the fast, for those who have a poor appetite or never feel hungry, you will have an increased appreciation for food and a keener appetite.

Daily Fast of 16-18 Hours

A daily fast of 16 to 18 hours is the most favorable type of meal pattern for most individuals. The two meals of the day are taken during a six-hour period early in the day, and the other 18 hours are spent fasting. Take nothing between meals. This pattern is shown to have many advantages. If you adopt this meal pattern, you will be in a fasting state for approximately half your life. This pattern has been shown to result in less asthma, arthritis, allergies, cancer, diabetes, and hypertension.

Fasting for Longer Than Five Days

Fasting from all food for longer than five days straight might result in nutrient deficiencies and wasting of internal organs with loss of muscle and organ mass. You should always continue to drink plenty of water while fasting, 8 to 12 or more eight-ounce glasses per day. One should not fast for the purpose of losing weight unless a fast is used to kick off a new commitment to eating better and more healthfully. Another exception is for individuals who are extremely overweight and need to take off some substantial poundage right away.

Rheumatoid arthritis is helped by selected fasting up to five days. This may or may not include certain fruit juices, melons, or fruits. The fasting rejuvenates the body and helps to prevent or control such diseases as cancer, allergies, arthritis, diabetes, obesity, heart disease, and a host of other problems.

Certain individuals should not fast—those who have Type I diabetes or are insulin-dependent, those who have gout, eating disorders, epilepsy (unless it is to test for food sensitivities), certain types of kidney disease, malnutrition, pregnancy, and sometimes in lactation, severe bronchial asthma, terminal illness, or far advanced tuberculosis.

Children probably should not fast, unless for short periods and of their own choosing. They might not be able to understand the purpose of the fast, and feel deprived or abused.

Juice Fasting

Juice fasting is very simple and can be maintained for as long as one month. Have two or three large glasses of juice (only enough to make you feel you have had a meal without feeling stuffed) sipped during the meal and mixed with saliva before swallowing. Fruit juices can be used in the morning and vegetable juices for later meals if you prefer.

If the fast is to be maintained for longer than five days, a "mono-fresh-vegetable" fast may be the wisest course. With this method only one vegetable is eaten at a meal, such as a fast of carrots, beets, or other juices. You may alternate a vegetable meal with a fruit meal, such as grapes or any grape product. Total food fasts longer than five days should not be attempted without professional supervision, as sudden death (although rare) has been reported.

Hunger does not constitute a serious problem in fasting. It is a minor inconvenience after the first day or so, and usually after the third day the person may feel as if he or she could fast forever.

The Lemon and Grapefruit Juice Fast

The lemon and grapefruit juice fast is another form of fasting. First thing in the morning, take the juice from one lemon and add a pint of cold or very, very warm water. If there is any nausea, cold water will taste better. The water should be sipped slowly. About half an hour after the first beverage, the person may have an urge to have a bowel movement. Some may wish to take a plain hot water enema at this time.

At breakfast time, drink a quart of warm or cold water to which has been added the juice of one grapefruit. Again the beverage is sipped slowly, allowing each mouthful to warm or cool in the mouth. At lunchtime another quart of water is taken after eating one grapefruit. Eating the grapefruit instead of squeezing it will exercise the muscles of the face and jaw. This increases the production of dopamine, a neurohormone. At supper drink a pint of water into which has been squeezed the juice of one lemon or one-half grapefruit.

Breaking the Fast

While fasting energy should be conserved as much as possible, and if a vacation from work can be planned at that time, it is often to the person's advantage.

This program may be continued for one to seven days. After each drink, the mouth should be rinsed and the teeth brushed to prevent citric acid damage to the teeth. The fast should be broken with fresh raw fruit such as oranges, peaches, berries, grapes, etc., beginning with the equivalent of about one-half to one orange; then increase slowly to one orange and two almonds at the next meal. At each meal increase the quantity of food taken, adding a small amount (one-quarter to one-half a slice) of plain bread or plain cereal until full meals are again taken after the number of days the fast was maintained.

Fat-Free Diet

To maintain a fat-free diet, do not eat items from this list: meat, beef, chicken, veal, pork, cheeses, salad oil, butter/margarine, milk, dairy products, bullion, ice cream, pastries, chocolate, nuts, peanuts, soybeans, fried foods, mayonnaise, peanut butter, coconut, olives, avocado, or any food you know has free fats in it.

There are plenty of foods you can eat, such as wheat bread, whole grains, cereal grains (rice, macaroni, oats and oatmeal, millet, rye, corn, barley, wheat, buckwheat, and other pastas), vegetables, fruits, no-oil salad dressing, popcorn (hot air, microwave, covered kettle without oil), pudding (made with nut milk), kidney beans, sauces and butters made from cereals, and cheeses and milks made without oils. For drinks, you can have fruit juices of fruits not on the avoid list, water, herb teas, coffee substitutes. For seasonings, salt, garlic salt or powder, onion salt or powder, lemon juice, herbs (no spices), chopped onion, celery, parsley, cucumber, or tomato.

Flaxseed

We are often asked if there is any toxicity in flaxseed, especially since one author has mentioned the possibility of cyanide as an ingredient of flaxseed. We have the following to report after our investigation:

Flaxseed has been used for centuries in the Middle East, where the seeds have been pressed and the oil used fresh; then the remaining husks were ground up and used in the black bread so common and nutritious in that area. Wayne Martin, a research chemist who lived and worked in the Middle East for many years, told me that until World War II the people there were some of the most healthy in the world. After the war, commercial vegetable oils were introduced, and flaxseed is little used now, with a steady deterioration in their health. I asked him if there were any toxic substances such as cyanide present, and he replied that there was none.

I also reviewed available literature, and, except for reference in one book that is no longer in print, I found nothing to indicate toxicity of flaxseed. Just to be certain, however, I called a professor of nutrition at Loma Linda School of Health who is a recognized authority on fats and oils. He knew nothing of any toxicity other than rancidity, which very easily occurs since the omega-3 fatty acids in flaxseed and the other oils oxidize readily when exposed to air.

Food Sources High in Certain Nutrients

Amino Acids

Beans, peas, lentils, whole wheat bread, oatmeal, rice, cereals, almonds, Brazil nuts, walnuts, pecans, pumpkin seeds, flaxseed, chia, sunflower seed, avocados, bananas, dates, figs, cherries, apricots, and grapes.

Anticoagulation and Anti-blood Clotting Capabilities

Red or purple grape juice, garlic, carrots (or other deep yellow fruits and vegetables), parsley (or other dark green fruits and vegetables), flaxseed, flaxseed oil, peanuts, soy, turmeric, and ginger.

Antioxidants

See "Oxygen Radical Absorbent Capacity (ORAC)" in this section.

Beta-carotene

Carrots, spinach, peaches, pumpkin, cantaloupe, squash, sweet potato, kale, turnip greens, collard greens, broccoli, romaine lettuce, cilantro, and thyme.

Biotin

Most of the biotin the body needs is actually produced in the intestines, but additional biotin can be found in a variety of foods including romaine lettuce, carrots, tomatoes, Swiss chard, whole wheat bread, avocado, raspberries, raw cauliflower, beans, bran cereals, brown rice, oatmeal, molasses, wheat germ, peas, currants, rice bran, rice germ, rice polishing, and peanut butter.

Boron

Boron is one of the minerals essential for strong bones. Thus, it is especially good for osteoporosis. It is found in kelp, alfalfa, snap beans, apples, pears, and grapes.

Calcium

Studies in Western countries indicate that calcium supplements have little, if any, effect on bone loss (*British Medical Journal* 298 [1989]: 137–140).

We recommend a totally vegetarian diet to prevent fractures from osteoporosis, as there are plenty of non-dairy sources that provide as much or more calcium than milk. One of those foods is kale, which has been found to raise calcium levels in the blood higher than milk (*American Journal of Clinical Nutrition* 51 [1990]: 656, 657).

Following is the milligrams of calcium found in a one cup serving of a variety of vegetables. For comparison, a one cup serving of whole cow's milk contains 288 mg of calcium.

Source	Calcium (mg/serving)
Seaweed	**1,000–3,500**
Sesame seed	**2,100**
Turnip greens	**450**
Collards	**360**
Bok choy	**330**
Almonds	**330**
Tofu	**290**
Chinese cabbage	**250**
Spinach	**250**
Kale	**200**
Parsley	**200**
Mustard	**180**
Dandelion greens, raw	**150**
Okra	**150**

Continued on next page

Continued from previous page

Source	Calcium (mg/serving)
Figs	78
Bread	50–90
Soy sprouts, raw	50
Lettuce, raw Romaine	40
Strawberries	31
Alfalfa sprouts, raw	25
Beans and peas	20 for split peas to 130 for soybeans
Lettuce, raw head	10

Eicosopentanoic Acid, Omega-3

Walnuts and flaxseed. Take two tablespoons of each daily. The flax can be ground in a seed mill or blender and sprinkled on cereal or stirred into juice.

Essential Fatty Acids

Whole grains, nuts, avocado, olives, seeds, and legumes.

Flavonoids, Bioflavonoids

Flavonoids, also known as bioflavonoids, give plants their pigment color. Purple grapes, citrus fruits, dark vegetables like broccoli, red beans, pinto beans, black beans, cranberries, blueberries, artichokes, blackberries, prunes, raspberries, strawberries, red delicious apples, Granny Smith apples, pecans, sweet cherries, plums, russet potatoes, spinach, Brussels sprouts, onions, and garlic. Herbs such as parsley, thyme, and peppermint also contain flavonoids.

Iodine

Seaweed, kelp, strawberries, asparagus, garlic, lima beans, dulse, sesame seeds, soybeans, spinach, summer squash, Swiss chard, turnip greens, vegetables grown near the ocean, and iodized table salt.

Iron

Pure tahini, sesame halva, oat flakes, almonds, dried figs, cooked spinach, humus, cooked garbanzo beans, cooked dry beans, cooked lentils, dried dates, whole wheat bread, cooked green peas, cooked potato, collard greens, kale, mustard, beets, turnip greens, dried apricots, dried peaches, prunes, raisins, whole grains cereals, whole wheat pasta, and blackstrap molasses.

Lithium

Seaweed, potatoes, lemons, and sugarcane.

Lysine

Hemp seeds, watercress, soybeans, carob, black beans, green beans, kidney beans, navy beans, snap beans, string beans, wax beans, lentils, asparagus peas, black caraway, fennel flower, spinach, amaranth, quinoa, and buckwheat.

Magnesium

Magnesium supplementation has been found to be beneficial in a number of different kinds of problems. A listing of these includes rhythm disturbances of the heart, such as atrial fibrillation, chronic constipation, diabetes, hypertension, toxemia in pregnancy, and many other conditions.

Other conditions known to improve with magnesium supplementation include asthma, angina, acute myocardial infarction, high blood pressure, cardiomyopathy, congestive heart failure, low HDL, mitral valve prolapse, eosinophilia-myalgia syndrome, fatigue, glaucoma, fibromyalgia, migraine and tension headaches, restless leg syndrome, kidney stones (use magnesium citrate as it is the most beneficial form in kidney stones), noise-induced hearing loss, and premenstrual syndrome.

Foods high in magnesium include whole grains, all nuts, seeds, soy and black beans, fresh green leafy vegetables, corn, avocados, okra, butternut squash, carob flour, figs, cantaloupe, and bananas. Following is a chart with additional natural foods and portion sizes:

Food	Portion	Mg
Cottonseed flour	½ cup	650
Wheat bran	½ cup	490
Brewer's Yeast	½ cup	231
Buckwheat	½ cup	229
Filberts	½ cup	184
Sesame seed, whole	½ cup	181
Pistachios	½ cup	158
Corn, field	½ cup	147
Pecans	½ cup	142
Malt extract, dry	½ cup	140
Soy beans, cooked	½ cup	138
Black-eyed peas, dried, cooked	¼ cup	98

Continued on next page

Continued from previous page

Food	Portion	Mg
Almonds, whole	¼ cup	**96**
Tofu	3 oz.	**95**
Cashews	¼ cup	**94**
Kidney beans, dried, cooked	¼ cup	**82**
Brazil nuts	¼ cup	**79**
Shredded wheat	1 cup	**67**
Peanuts, roasted, chopped	¼ cup	**63**
Walnuts, black, chopped	¼ cup	**60**
Banana	1 medium	**58**
Avocado	½ medium	**56**
Peanut butter	2 tbsp.	**56**
Cowpeas (black-eyed)	½ cup	**55**
Blackstrap molasses	1 tbsp.	**52**
Potato	1 medium	**51**
Oatmeal	1 cup	**50**
Corn, sweet	½ cup	**48**
Chestnuts	½ cup	**41**
Celery, raw	½ cup	**22**

Manganese

Avocado, berries, nuts, seeds, whole grains, green leafy vegetables, and legumes (such as peanuts, peas, and beans).

Myoinositol

Beans, cantaloupe, peanuts and nuts, grapefruit and other citrus, legumes, yeast, wheat germ, blackstrap molasses, collard greens, kale, mustard greens, raw parsley, and all whole grains. This nutrient is very good to treat diabetic neuropathy or other forms of neuropathy.

Oxalates

Citrus fruits, apples, grapes, cranberries, beans, rhubarb, beet greens, poke weed, chard, endive, spinach, almonds, cashews, sweet potatoes, tomatoes, okra, figs, gooseberries, plums, currants, and raspberries.

Phenylalanine

Sesame seeds, sunflower seeds, peanuts, almonds, avocado, and lima beans.

Phosphorus (Phosphate)

Phosphorus is essential in the development of bones and teeth. Foods high in phosphorus are whole grain cereals, cooked beans, peanuts, peanut butter, cauliflower, cooked dandelion greens, cooked plantains, raspberries, cooked peaches, turnip greens, strawberries, winter squash, cooked celery, cooked plums, scallions, cooked kale, cooked carrots, and nectarines.

Potassium

The following foods are high in potassium. This milligrams listed are per one-half cup portion.

Food	Mg
"Blackstrap" Molasses (3 oz. only)	**2,927**
Yeast, Torula	**2,046**
Yeast, Bakers'–dry	**1,998**
Soya Grits	**1,942**
Brewers' Yeast,	**1,894**
Soy Beans–dry, raw	**1,677**
Soy Milk–dry powder	**1,640**
Apricots–dried	**1,561**
Lima Beans–dry	**1,499**
Rice Bran–dry	**1,495**
Bananas–dehydrated	**1,477**
Peaches–dried	**1,191**
Wheat Bran–dry	**1,050**
Mung Beans–dry	**1,028**
Wheat Germ–dry	**1,020**
Pistachio Nuts	**972**
Sunflower Seeds	**920**
Parsley–raw	**903**
Figs–dried	**900**
Chestnuts–dried	**875**
Raisins	**840**
Garbanzos–dry	**797**
Almonds	**773**
Lentils–dry	**757**
Sesame Seeds–whole	**725**
Peanuts–with skins	**720**
Currants–dried	**719**
Brazil Nuts	**715**
Peanuts–without skins	**700**
Spinach, raw	**700**
Prunes	**694**

Proanthocyanidins

Apples, grapes, blueberries, elderberries, and other fruits.

Salicylates

Potatoes, cucumbers, peppers, tomatoes, apples, apricots, blackberries, boysenberries, cherries, currants, dewberries, gooseberries, grapefruit, lemons, melons, nectarines, oranges, peaches, plums, prunes, raisins, raspberries, strawberries, almonds, and grapes.

Selenium

Brazil nuts (other nuts), asparagus, cream of wheat, whole wheat products (such as crackers, pasta, cereals, and English muffins).

Taurine

Legumes, particularly beans and carob, also in food yeast, nuts, and seeds, virtually all plant foods high in protein.

Tryptophan

Wheat, bran flakes, shredded wheat, bananas, oats, mangoes, dried dates, sesame, chickpeas, sunflower seeds, pumpkin seeds, spirulina, most nuts, peanuts, brown rice, soybeans and soy products, and all animal products.

Tyrosine

Spirulina, sesame seeds, almonds, pumpkins seeds, peanut flour, soy protein, tofu, lupins, lima beans, avocados, bananas, pumpkin leaves, mustard greens, spinach, turnip greens, watercress, whole wheat, whole oats, legumes, and whole grains.

Vitamin B3, Niacin

Avocados, brewer's yeast, dates, collards, lima beans, roasted peanuts, prunes, wheat germ, and whole wheat products.

Vitamin B6

Brewer's yeast, sunflower seeds, wheat germ, soybeans, lentils, brown rice, chickpeas, and green vegetables.

Vitamin C

Broccoli, Brussels sprouts, orange juice, snow peas, kiwi, oranges, green peppers, cantaloupe, strawberries, baked potatoes, sweet potatoes, and tomatoes.

Vitamin E

Wheat, rye, oats, fortified cereals, corn, peas, parsley, spinach, carrots, onion, garlic, avocados, hazelnuts, sunflower seeds, almonds, Brazil nuts, safflower nuts, pumpkin seeds, flaxseeds, flaxseed oil, walnuts, olive oil, sunflower oil, and soybean oil.

Zinc

Asparagus, banana, beans (common, mature, dry), beets, nuts, breads (rye, whole wheat), pop corn, pumpkin seed, cabbage, carrots, chickpeas, corn, corn meal, lentils, lettuce, oatmeal, peanuts (raw or roasted), peanut butter, tofu, soybeans wheat germ, and shredded wheat.

Gluten-Free Diet

Gluten is found in wheat, barley, rye, malt, and in many prepared products. If a person is found to be gluten intolerant, labels must be carefully read. Gluten is not found in millet, rice, corn, amaranth, popcorn, quinoa, teff, wild rice or buckwheat.

Grape Diet, "Grape Cure"

The grape diet was especially designed by a woman doctor in Europe for life-threatening diseases such as cancer, schizophrenia, rheumatoid arthritis, and lupus.

It is a good idea to fast (water only) for one to two days if possible before starting this diet.

Then, for one month, eat three meals a day of only grapes, raisins, grape juice, and grapes in any other form.

After that, adopt a vegan diet low in natural sugar with no free-fats and no textured vegetable proteins (TVP). Be sure not to overeat as this complicates internal biochemistry and inhibits healing.

Greens Diet

This diet is beneficial for life-threatening diseases such as cancer, diabetes, schizophrenia, rheumatoid arthritis, lupus, and pancreas diseases. It stimulates natural insulin in the body, regulates sugar in the cells and blood, feeds the glands, builds resistance to disease, helps restore function of the pancreas, contains antimicrobial and anticoagulant properties, nourishes the body, calms the nerves, soothes and heals the body, and stimulates cell growth and activity. In addition to diet and teas, one should also engage in exercise that complements the diet.

Diet

- *Stage I* – Fast one day each week. You may include lemons, garlic and onions.
- *Stage II* – For two days eat the following for breakfast and lunch: a green salad including some raw and/or steamed vegetables (Romaine lettuce, kale, mustard, collards, turnip greens, asparagus, broccoli, string beans, green peas, okra, spinach, chard, beet greens, etc.).
- *Stage III* – For three days eat the following for breakfast and lunch: include the foods from stage II plus legumes (no soybeans or peanuts), flaxseed and other vegetables, including tomatoes, cucumbers, celery, radishes, green peas, asparagus, etc. (no avocado, carrots, beets, potatoes).

Repeat this diet for the next four weeks or until your blood sugar or blood pressure is under control—consistently below 90, or below 120/80—or your cancer is under control.

The following natural supplements may be included on your fast days and/or with your meals:

- 5-6 steamed garlic cloves
- 2 tablespoons flaxseed
- 1 tablespoon fenugreek
- Lemon wedges (one-fourth of the lemon)
- Aloe vera (2 to 4 ounces) with each meal (use the fresh plant when possible)
- Chromium picolinate, 600 mcg. daily for diabetics only
- One-half teaspoon turmeric at each meal up to 2 teaspoons

Teas

- Alfalfa – 1 tablespoon in 1 cup of boiled water, steep 20 minutes, cool, and drink.
- Dandelion (leaf) – 1 teaspoon in 1 cup of boiled water, steep 20 minutes, cool, and drink.
- Buckthorn (leaf) – 1 teaspoon in 1 cup of boiled water, steep 20 minutes, cool, and drink.
- Echinacea (root) – 1 tablespoon in 1 cup of water, simmer 20 minutes, cool, and drink.
- Spirulina (powder) – 1 teaspoon in approximately 4 ounces distilled water, stir, and drink.

You may drink one as a single tea or mix into a combination of three or four at once.

Exercise

- Walk a minimum of three miles at least five days weekly.
- Sun bath about 15 to 20 minutes three times a week.
- Do breathing exercises: Inhale to the count of four; hold the breath to the count of seven; exhale to the count of nine, blowing out all the stale, trapped air, through pursed lips; and repeat four times at least three times each day.
- Take a neutral bath at least three times weekly (sitting in a tub of warm water, not much warmer than your body's temperature, for at least one hour). The important thing is to relax.

Omega-3 Fatty Acids

Omega-3 fatty acids are present in the following oils: walnut, flaxseed, soybean, pumpkin seed, evening primrose; canola (rapeseed), perilla. It is also present in the following nuts and seeds: walnuts, flaxseeds, soybeans, and pumpkin seeds.

Oxygen Radical Absorbent Capacity (ORAC)

Because the following foods absorb free radicals produced by the environment and the body's own metabolic processes, they are known as antioxidants. The daily needs of an adult are 3,000 to 5,000 ORAC units. The following ORAC units are based on just under a one-half cup serving.

Fruits	
Prunes	5,770
Raisins	2,830
Blueberries	2,400
Blackberries	2,036
Cranberries	1,750
Strawberries	1,540
Raspberries	1,220

Continued on next page

Continued from previous page

Plums	949
Oranges	750
Grapes, red	739
Cherries	670
Kiwi	602
Cantaloupe	252
Banana	221
Apple	218
Apricots	164
Peach	158
Pear	134
Watermelon	104
Herbs	
Oregano	200,129
Turmeric	159,277
Sorghum	100,800
Cumin	76,800
Parsley, dry	74,349
Basil, dry	67,553
Cinnamon	67,536
Vegetables	
Kale	1,770
Spinach, raw	1,260
Brussels sprouts	980
Alfalfa sprouts	930
Spinach, steam	909
Broccoli florets	890
Beets	841
Bell peppers	713
Onion	450
Corn	400
Eggplant	390
Cauliflower	377
Peas, frozen	364
White potatoes	313
Sweet potatoes	301
Carrots	207
String beans	201
Tomato	189
Zucchini	176
Yellow squash	150

Source: *Agriculture Research,* February 1999

Potassium Broth

Potassium broth is a high source of minerals and electrolytes. It brings nourishment to the cells. To make a basic potassium broth, boil two potatoes in two to four cups of water until potato peelings are well cooked. Strain and give liquid to the patient unsalted.

To make a potassium broth with other nutrients, combine the following ingredients in a pot, cover with water (about 8 cups) and simmer for 60 minutes: 3 potatoes, 1 onion, 6 garlic cloves, 4 stalks of celery, 4 carrots, and 1 teaspoon salt (or to taste).

Strain the broth and store in a large glass jar in the refrigerator. Throughout the day, warm a cup and sip on it to regain the nutrients your body needs.

Signs of Nutrient Deficiencies

Boron

Symptoms of deficiency include osteoporosis, loss of energy, and reduced efficiency in producing heat and manufacturing raw products for good muscle and bone strength.

Dietary sources include legumes, apples, pears, grapes, and their juices.

Choline

Symptoms of deficiency include liver dysfunction and low serum cholesterol.

Dietary sources are whole grains, potatoes, cauliflower, tomatoes, soy products, peanuts and other legumes, and leaf lettuce.

Copper

Symptoms of deficiency include anemia, slow clot lysis (twice the length of time necessary to dissolve small blood clots inside the blood vessels) and increased arterial constriction leading to an increase in blood pressure. Muscle cramps, poor coordination and balance are more common. Copper deficiency appears to increase the potential for oxidative damage to tissues, especially when combined with high intake of free fructose (confectioners sugar, frosting on commercial cakes and pies, and somewhat from table sugar and other concentrated sugars). Low copper levels are associated with an increased sensitivity to aches and pains. Individuals who have chronic pain should ensure an adequate copper intake.

The elderly are more susceptible to copper deficiencies than younger individuals.

Wilson's disease is a genetic disorder that results in excessive accumulation of copper in many parts of the body, particularly the liver. This condition is readily treatable, but if Wilson's disease is left untreated, it can be fatal. (See also "Wilson's Disease, Copper Overload" in the *Conditions and Diseases* section.)

Foods containing copper include whole grains, beans, peas, and green leafy vegetables.

Folic Acid

Symptoms of deficiency include birth defects if deficiency is present during pregnancy, fatigue, loss of appetite, constipation, sore tongue, headaches, sleeplessness, restless legs, paranoia, memory impairment, and neurologic signs.

Dietary sources are whole grains, legumes, green leafy vegetables, seeds, and nuts.

Vitamin B1 (thiamin)

Symptoms of deficiency include loss of appetite, irritability, tiredness, constipation, depression, nausea, and neuropathy.

Dietary sources are legumes and whole grains.

Vitamin B2 (riboflavin)

Cracks and dermatitis at the edges of the mouth are classic signs of riboflavin deficiency.

Vitamin B3 (niacin)

Dermatitis, diarrhea, and dementia (the three D's) are the classic signs of B3 deficiency, which are caused by the three M's (meat, meal, and molasses). Simply adding collards to the diet could fix the problem, because these large green leaves are laden with plenty of niacin.

Dietary sources are collards, avocados, brewer's yeast, dates, lima beans, roasted peanuts, prunes, wheat germ, and whole wheat products.

Zinc

Symptoms of deficiency include fatigue, dermatitis, acne, loss of taste, poor wound healing, loss of appetite, reduced immune system functioning, delayed growth, reduced development of sex glands, diarrhea, skeletal abnormalities, loss of hair, behavioral disturbances, white spots on fingernails, infertility, and night blindness.

Dietary sources are pumpkin seeds and other kinds of seeds, soybeans, potatoes, whole grains, nuts, popcorn, and legumes.

Signs of Vitamin Overload

There are many nutrients in the body that have a tendency to go up or down in relationship to some other nutrient. Following is a table showing these kinds of relationships. If one of these nutrients goes up, the one on the other side will go down like a see-saw, and conversely as well. Because of the interrelationship of nutrients, it can be hazardous to take supplements.

Phosphorus	Calcium
Sodium	Calcium
Protein	Calcium
Copper	Calcium
Vitamin C	Calcium
Zinc	Copper
Calcium	Iron
Protein	B12
Vitamins C and E	A
Vitamin C	B12
Sugar	B vitamins
Sugar	B12

Notice that if nutrients are taken in doses greater than the recommended daily allowance (RDA), harmful effects can occur.

Iron

In elderly people and menstruating women, iron supplements may often be taken for years. Daily doses higher than 100 milligrams (six times the RDA) can interfere with the absorption of zinc, the utilization of calcium, and the regulation of the immune system. Zinc helps speed wound healing and regulates the immune system, as well as strengthens bones and assists in regulating the production of many substances in the body such as encouraging histidine production from histamine.

Vitamin A, Beta-Carotene

Doses of more than 25,000 IU (five times the RDA) can lead to liver damage, hair loss, blurred vision, and headaches. Beta- carotene may also encourage some types of cancer when given in over-dosage for a long time.

Vitamin B3 (Niacin)

Doses of 2,000 milligrams (100 times the RDA) are used to help lower cholesterol. Patients who take this much should be monitored for jaundice and liver damage.

This nutrient source is found in potatoes, whole wheat, collards, and tomatoes. In one study of three adult males, given large doses of nicotinic acid to treat high blood cholesterol, there was a loss of central vision. The nicotinic acid can cause retention of fluid and swelling in the retina, which could lead to a loss of vision. After the vitamin was discontinued, some improvement of vision occurred.

Vitamin B6

More than 400 milligrams a day (200 times the RDA) can cause numbness in the mouth and hands and difficulty walking.

However, vitamin B6 supplementation reduces serum norepinephrine as well as systolic and diastolic blood pressure (*American Journal of Natural Medicine* 3, no. 4 [May 1996]: 16). Nutrient sources of vitamin B6 include potatoes, spinach, peanuts, brewer's yeast, peas, sunflower seeds, and wheat germ.

Vitamin B12

The small intestine of healthy humans can contain bacteria that are capable of producing vitamin B12. There are at least two groups of germs normally in the small bowel, *pseudomonas* and *klebsiella*. These may synthesize significant amounts of the vitamin, high enough in the intestinal tract to be absorbed in the terminal ileum, the B12 absorption section of the small bowel (*Nature* 283 [February 21, 1980]: 781). Both of these germs can overgrow, however, and cause an unhealthy small bowel.

Factors that affect vitamin B12 needs:

- Meat and other animal products and refined carbohydrates (sugars) when used generously may more than double the amount of B12 you must have from all your sources to stay healthy.
- Persons who use drugs, tobacco, chemicals, or beverages (alcohol, caffeine, etc.) that destroy B12 will require more B12 to stay healthy.
- Mega-doses of vitamin C may produce B12 deficiency by destroying the cobalamins during the time both B12 and vitamin C are in the intestinal tract together. More than 500 mg of vitamin C can destroy 50 to 95 percent of B12 in the intestinal tract. If both vitamin C and B12 must be taken for some condition, B12 should be taken at the beginning or before the meal, and vitamin C should be taken after meals.
- Alcohol affects B12 similarly to mega-doses of vitamin C.
- Oral contraceptives increase the need for vitamin B12.
- Cooked eggs decrease B12 absorption.
- Intestinal parasites, especially tapeworms, and explosively growing bacteria in the intestinal tract such as from infected or inflamed intestines, can effectively compete with the host for B12 and make the requirements higher. *Helicobacter pylori* infection can cause malabsorption of vitamin B12.
- Almost 90 percent of older people with serum B12 levels less than 150 show evidence of tissue vitamin B12 deficiency. Older people are more subject to disability from low B12 than younger individuals (*Journal of the American Geriatric Society* 44 [1996]: 1355). We can see wisdom for persons over age 60 with low B12 levels taking a supplement. About 100 mcg daily chewed for two minutes before swallowing (to get the "salivary factor") will probably be enough to supply the system with all its needs. However, if the person has some symptom ascribed to B12 deficiency such as anemia, numbness, tingling, poor memory, etc., 1000 mcg should probably be taken until the symptoms disappear. Only a small fraction of the B12 taken in is actually absorbed, less than 1 percent. Fortunately, the RDA for B12 is only about .17 to .20 mcg.

Vitamin C

Overdoses can cause stomachaches and diarrhea, and it is suspected of causing kidney stones in some people. It can change blood sugar readings, giving false low readings and making insulin regulation difficult. Large doses of vitamin C may cause iron deficiency anemia by blocking the functions of copper, a mineral essential for iron transport in the blood (*Science News* 124 [October 29, 1983]: 281).

Vitamin D

Sunning will never create an overdose, but too many supplements (daily doses of 50,000 IU, 125 times the RDA) can cause buildup of calcium deposits that interfere with the functioning of muscles, including heart tissues.

Vitamin E

Anyone prone to easy bruising or bleeding, any woman with heavy periods, and any person with a tendency toward having hemorrhagic strokes should not take more than the maximum recommended daily amount of vitamin E.

Since vitamin E has been considered an anti-aging vitamin, it has become very fashionable to use quite a large dosage. An overdose could cause oozing of blood into the retina that can result in vision loss. Macular degeneration could result from excessive use of vitamin E (*Medical Tribune* 37, no. 16 [1996]: 17). For the same reason, the small doses of aspirin recommended to avoid a second heart attack can cause an advance of macular degeneration. Aspirin can promote small hemorrhagic oozing in the retina, resulting in vision loss.

Vitamin E can also become a powerful blood-thinner if taken in large doses, and it has dangerous, additive hemorrhage-promoting effects when taken with other blood-thinners such as aspirin, heparin, or warfarin. Even when taken by itself in large doses, vitamin E has caused life-threatening bleeding within the brain and blindness from retinal bleeding in people who sustained skull trauma during falls or collisions. Worse yet, the studies showed that long-term, large daily doses of vitamin E raise the blood level of cholesterol and make atherosclerosis worse (*Journal of the American Medical Association* 293 [2005]: 1368, 1389).

Soybeans

These legumes are America's most neglected nutritional treasure. They are certainly an all-American crop, since this country produces the largest soybean crop in the world. We even ship to the Orient where the population eats them whole in a variety of dishes, which protect against prostate and breast cancer, as well as many other cancers, heart disease, symptoms of menopause, and osteoporosis. Ten to 12 ounces of tofu per day can assist a woman to actually gain bone density.

Following is a list of some of the beneficial effects of soybeans:

- Provides a rich supply of antioxidants that assist in slowing down aging and protecting against free-radicals, which can lead to heart disease, cancer, stroke, and cataracts
- Controls cholesterol
- Protects against osteoporosis, which results in less hip, wrist, and ankle fractures and humpback in women
- Suppresses symptoms of menopause, most specifically hot flashes
- Boosts the immune system
- Puts less strain on the kidneys and protects them
- Lowers the risk of contracting lung cancer, prostate cancer, breast cancer, and most other cancers
- Hinders the activity of certain viruses, specifically HIV and Epstein Barr viruses, according to studies at Tokyo University
- Contains substances that normalize platelet aggregation, a factor involved in causing blood clotting; thus, inhibiting strokes and heart attacks
- Improves immune reactions at a cellular level
- Helps to emulsify bile and fats in the intestinal tract

Are all soy products equally rich in these beneficial nutrients? The answer to that question is no. The following is a list of foods and their calcium and isoflavone content that appeared in the August/September 1997 issue of *Health Counselor*, page 58.

Amount	Calories	Calcium	Isoflavones
½ cup tofu	120	120–300 mg	31 mg
1 cup TVP	120	170	very small quantity or none
½ cup soy flour	163	200	55–90
½ cup tempeh	204	80	50–70
½ cup cooked soybeans	149	88	55–90
1 cup soy milk	80	200–300	negligible to none unless homemade
2 oz. isolated soy protein	50–90	50	negligible to none

Soybeans are available as whole soybeans, which may be used in stir fries or haystacks; tofu, which can be used in anything from stir fries to cheesecake; soy milk; cracked soybeans, which can be used similarly to grits to thicken and enrich soups, stews, or other dishes.

Soybeans have an anti-estrogen effect in male mice, which may be the important regulator nutrient that retards cancer growth in the prostate and in the breast.

Soybeans may slow down the too-rapid development of young girls, which is causing quite an epidemic in the United States. Many young girls are starting their menstrual periods at age nine or ten. Soybeans may slow down this process of precocious puberty.

It has also become obvious that many people are becoming iron-overloaded in the United States. Soybean products tend to help maintain a normal iron balance in both men and women. One piece of research showed that diets restricted in animal foods were likely to cause both men and women to take up less iron (*Journal of Nutrition* 125 [1995]: 212). Far from regarding this as a negative factor for soybeans, it is a very positive one. Some felt earlier that the effect of plant estrogens found in soy was potentially adverse, but experience proves quite the reverse (*Journal of Nutrition* 125 [1995]: 771S).

Vegetarianism

There are serious scientific reasons why we recommend a vegetarian diet to our patients. Since time is required to get new menus and learn new recipes, as well as to allow the tastes to change, you may want to wade in slowly rather than dive in as some do. The important thing is to get started. Some items you should begin to omit are discussed below.

The foods and herbs with the highest anti-cancer activity include garlic, soybeans, cabbage, ginger, licorice, and vegetables of the cabbage family. Citrus fruits contain a host of active phytochemicals. The phytochemicals in grains reduce the risk of heart and artery disease as well as cancer.

For years there had been the question as to whether a vegetarian diet supplies all nutrients needed for human nutrition. In 1996 officials of the Department of Agriculture (USDA) and the Department of Health and Human Services (HHS) endorsed vegetarian diets and the guidelines for the first time (*Science News* 149 [January 6, 1996]: 6).

A vegetarian diet gives a person greater endurance. A study done by Dr. Per-Olaf Astrand using nine highly trained athletes demonstrated clearly the increased endurance produced by a vegetarian diet. The athletes had their diets changed every three days. At the end of every three-day period the athletes pedaled a stationary bicycle at a high speed until they were exhausted. Those on a high protein, high-fat diet, very high in meat became exhausted in 57 minutes. Those taking a mixed diet lower in meat, fat, and protein than the first diet became exhausted after one hour and 54 minutes. Those on a vegetarian diet with high unrefined carbohydrate content became exhausted after 2.78 hours.

Not only are plant based food preparations digested and handled in the body more healthfully than any animal food products, but the likelihood of encountering food poisoning is much less. While plant foods are not wholly without problems, they are a small fraction of the problems encountered in the meat, poultry, and dairy industry in regards to food safety.

Several studies have reported a substantial increase in healthcare costs in individuals who eat meat. The annual costs are measurable and include hypertension, heart disease, cancer, diabetes, gallbladder disease, obesity, musculoskeletal disorders, and food-borne illnesses.

- Heart Disease $24 Billion
- Hypertension $8.7 Billion
- Cancer $18.8 Billion
- Diabetes $4.6 Billion
- Gallstones $4.8 Billion
- Total $60.9 Billion

Research indicates that excessive protein in the diet, especially animal protein, increases the risk of osteoporosis. Eating meat can cause a loss of calcium from the body. One explanation is that meat tends to be rich in amino acids that contain sulfur, such as methionine. The higher the animal protein intake, the lower the density of bones and the greater the risk for fractures. Interestingly, higher consumption of vegetable protein does not appear to be related to osteoporosis or bone fractures.

Soybeans and greens are good natural sources of calcium. Greens also have properties that help prevent cancer. One possible reason for the favorable absorption of calcium from plant products like green leafy vegetables is their low phosphorus content. Dark green leafy vegetables can have three to five times as much calcium as phosphorous.

Cancer is another problem linked to excess animal protein. In countries where animal protein consumption is high, there is a greater incidence of lymphoma, a deadly cancer of the lymph glands. It is also said that the high uses of animal protein increases the risk of cancers of the breast, colon, prostate, kidney and womb (endometrium). However, soy protein products such as soy flour and textured vegetable protein have cancer-fighting abilities. Studies of human populations that consume soy suggest that soy has a role in preventing a variety of cancers, including colon, rectal, prostate, stomach, lung, and breast.

With our growing understanding of diet in relation to health, a plant-based diet has emerged as the optimal way to maximize longevity and the quality of living.

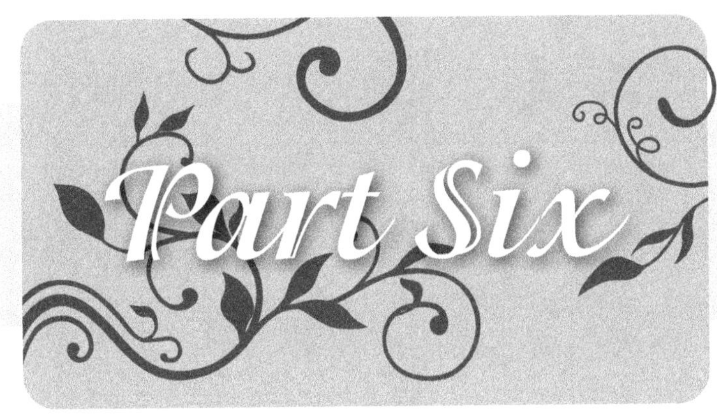

Supplemental Information

Introduction

This section contains additional information about a variety of conditions and diseases as well as helpful tips on how to maintain one's health.

12-Step Program

To correct any unwanted obsessive, compulsive, or habitual behavior, one can follow these steps. The first thing to realize is that in order to receive God's help I must realize my weakness and deficiency and apply my mind to the great change to be done in me. I must arouse to earnest and persevering prayer and effort. Wrong habits and customs must be shaken off. It is only by determined endeavor to correct these errors and to conform to right principles that the victory can be gained.

1. I recognize my helpless and hopeless condition, and that my life is out of control in regard to addictive behavior such as sex, hurt feelings, temper, gossip, food, alcohol, tobacco, caffeine, drugs, etc.
2. If there is help for me it can come only through You who can give me a balanced Christian life.
3. Therefore, I throw myself on Your mercy to take my will and my life. Take my will for I am willing to be changed.
4. Help me, loving Father, to search my mind for any sin that will separate me from You. Help me to have the revelation by Your Holy Spirit of all my hidden sins and defects.
5. Help me to call my sins fearlessly by their exact names.
6. Make me entirely ready to have You remove all these defects of character and the sins and compulsions that I do from habit.
7. Help me, Father, to work tirelessly with You to remove my shortcomings and mold my life according to Your will.
8. I cannot remember everyone I have harmed, and I am asking You to make me remember and be willing to make amends to them all.
9. I shall, with Your help, courageously go to meet such people wherever possible and confess my wrong dealing with them and repair that damage, except when to do so would injure them or others.
10. I am continuing to take personal inventory, and when I am wrong promptly admit it.
11. I am seeking through prayer, Bible study, and meditation to improve my conscious contact with You. I am praying only for knowledge of Your will and for my ability to take hold of Your grace to carry it out.
12. I am praying for a spiritual awakening as the result of these steps. I am trying to carry this message to others and to practice these principles in all my situations and relationships.

Abdominal Pain

How to tell What it Means

The following can cause abdonimal pain: a muscle spasm, any drug, colitis, gas, overeating, food sensitivity, smoking or drinking, an arthritic spine, pneumonia, a bulging or "slipped" disk, shingles, an abscess, a bruise, or a viral infection.

Always think of the simplest and least life-threatening problem first, and treat for that condition to see if that eliminates the problem. Furthermore, if you treat any acute abdominal pain lasting more than half an hour as appendicitis and treat it vigorously, you can usually stop even serious problems without professional help.

To give you an idea of what may be the cause of the pain, we will list the various afflictions by location of the pain.

- Pain in the right upper quadrant of the abdomen: hepatitis, swollen liver because of heart failure, gallbladder disease, pancreatic cancer, pancreatitis, diverticulitis, and kidney problems.
- Pain in the left upper quadrant of the abdomen: enlarged spleen, diverticulitis, gastritis, stomach ulcer, stomach cancer, hiatus hernia, pancreatitis, pancreatic cancer, and pleurisy.
- Pain in the right lower quadrant of the abdomen: appendicitis, bowel cancer, Crohn's disease, infectious diarrhea, ectopic pregnancy, endometriosis, irritable bowel disease, kidney stones, overeating, ovarian cysts, ovulation, pelvic inflammatory disease, and tumors.
- Pain in the left lower quadrant of the abdomen: all of those in the right lower quadrant except appendicitis; diverticulitis is a common cause.
- Pain in the upper middle abdomen: stomach ulcer, duodenal ulcer, stomach cancer, gastritis, eating fresh yeast bread, stomach irritants, and food sensitivities.
- Pain in the lower middle abdomen: bladder infection, kidney stones, endometriosis, pelvic inflammatory disease, degenerating uterine fibroids, uterine cancer, ovarian cancer, ovulation, irritable bowel disease, arteriosclerosis, and abdominal aneurysm.

Adverse Effects of Cortisone or Prednisone

After taking corticosteroid medication, most people have an immediate sense of well-being, following by a sense of uneasiness, unhappiness, and insomnia. In some, the emotional problem progresses to deep depression and the person may become suicidal (*British Medical Association* 316 [1998]: 244).

Cortisone, stanozolol, and prednisone are all members of the steroid group of drugs. They are famous for weakening the immune system and causing infections. Using this family of drugs in any form (shots, pills, sprays, or ointments) can cause acne, blood sugar changes, cataracts, diabetes, weight gain with fat distribution changes in "buffalo hump," glaucoma, growth retardation, hair growth on face and hands, increased bone fractures, irregular menstrual cycles, severely reduced immunity, mental and emotional changes, moon face, muscle wasting, osteoporosis, reduced resistance to infection, salt retention and edema, hypertension, stomach and duodenal ulcers, suppression of the adrenal glands, and stretch marks and thinning of the skin.

Aging

Psychological Factors of Aging

How conscientious a person is in studies, chores, handling money, etc., in childhood correlates with how long a person lives according to a study conducted by H. S. Friedman in 1993. The mindset of conscientiousness may have more wide-range effects on health-related activities than has yet been recognized.

Predictors to Impair Health:

- Deliberate, conscience-violating actions
- Impulsive, under-controlled personalities
- Any criminal activity
- Major family stresses that persist long-term

Risks for Premature Death:

- Parental divorce during childhood
- Unstable marriage patterns in adulthood
- Childhood personality disorders remaining uncorrected into adulthood
- Adult maladjustment to job, family, home
- Psychosocial factors not resolved

Nutritional Factors of Aging

The following foods and nutrients help combat the aging process and are good for the body:

Folic Acid

- Prevents clotting, supports the nervous system

Soybeans

- Guards against maladies of aging
- Reduces heart disease
- Inhibits cancer
- Slows and heals (when already present) osteoporosis
- Soothes menopause syndrome
- Resolves hypercholesterolemia
- Heals kidneys

Acetyl-L-Carnitine

(found in whole grains and vegetables like asparagus)

- Reduces aging
- May also reduce blood pressure
- May reduce the likelihood to have diabetes (lowers the sugar level)

Red Peppers

- An experimental diet used for testing learning performance on aging mice contained 20 percent red peppers. The mice that were fed peppers showed much better acquisition of knowledge and avoidance of injury than did a control group of mice given a common diet (*Journal of Nutritional Science and Vitaminology* 45 [1999]: 143–149).
- One cup per day in humans has been shown to reverse age-related effects such as loss of balance and a lack of coordination (*Clinical Pearls News* 10, no. 2 [February 2000]: 21).

Antioxidants

(Aging Acceleration and Deceleration)

- There are certain foods that increase the rate at which oxidation occurs in the body, oxidation being a factor that causes aging. Those foods and diets favoring oxidation are as follows: high-fat diet, high protein diet, abundant refined sugar, high salt diet, high grains intake, the use of alcohol, the ingestion of margarine, whipped creams, and commercial peanut butter, B-vitamins in pills (particularly high doses of B1, B3, pantothenic acid and B6), and vitamin D.
- An antioxidant is a food that has the ability to neutralize free radicals. Antioxidants such as vitamins C, E, A, beta-carotene, and nutrients such as selenium, and many others coming from fruits, vegetables, whole grains, nuts, and seeds, reduce the aging effects on the brain.

Fruits High in Antioxidant Capacity per 100 g					
Prunes	5,770	Raspberries	1,220	White grapes	446
Raisins	2,830	Plums	949	Bananas	251
Blueberries	2,400	Oranges	750	Apple	218
Blackberries	2,036	Red grapes	739	Apricot	164
Cranberries	1,750	Cherries	670	Peach	158
Strawberries	1,540	Kiwi fruit	602	Pear	134
Vegetables High in Antioxidant Capacity per 100 g					
Kale	1,770	Beets	841	Peas, frozen	364
Spinach, raw	1,260	Red bell peppers	713	Carrots	207
Brussels sprouts	980	Onion	450	String beans	201
Alfalfa sprouts	930	Eggplant	390	Tomato	189
Spinach steamed	909	Corn	377	Zucchini	176
Broccoli florets	890	Cauliflower	377		

At 60 percent less table sugar than is average, persons can be expected to live about 35 percent longer. Even when eating lots of calories, if these calories come from starchy carbohydrates rather than heavy table sugars, one can expect about 20 percent longer life span. Apparently excessive sugar generates free radicals that accelerate aging.

Studies show oxidized protein accumulates with age. Further, there is a decrease of an enzyme (glutamine synthetase) activity in the frontal lobe, especially in a person with Alzheimer's disease, where there is an accumulation of an abnormal protein named amyloid (*Annals of New York Academy of Sciences* 738 [November 17, 1994]: 44).

There is already evidence that animal protein is not handled as well as plant protein and is more likely to become oxidized before consumption than plant protein. Various excitotoxins from the environment such as chemicals used on foods in transport or during production can be a cause of the death of certain nerve cells in the central nervous system (*Toxicology and Applied Pharmacology* 134 [1995]: 1).

A study done by the National Institutes of Health showed that reducing calories by 30 percent lowered cholesterol, blood pressure, and the risk of heart disease. Restricting calorie intake may also reduce the risk of cancer, and diabetes.

Calorie restriction is the "only [uncontroverted health] manipulation we currently know that increases life span," said Dr. Richard Sprott of the National Institute of Aging. Simply restricting one's total calories can increase survival. Reducing total calorie intake is one of the most important methods to reducing the accelerated rate of aging.

A 15-year study from Loma Linda University revealed that elderly individuals with high caloric intake had lower cognitive function than did those who consumed a diet lower in calories. Low educational attainment and the use of psychotropic drugs, including coffee and its relatives, were also associated with poorer mental function (*American Journal of Epidemiology* 143, no. 12 [June 15, 1996]: 1181–1190).

Predictors of Accelerated Aging

Poor pulmonary function is associated with a lower mental functioning in later life.

Joint impairment and weak thigh muscles contribute significantly to reduction in vigorous exercise.

The earlier in life you begin strength training and physical exercise, the less likely you are to become frail in old age.

Diabetes has been linked to a 30 percent increased risk of getting Alzheimer's disease.

Reduce your exposure all through life to certain solvent groups such as benzene, toluene, phenols, and alcohols, ketones, and other organic solvents.

If you do not chew well, you may lose brain cells. Nobody knows why, but the following research study indicates that chewing is important. The upper molars of laboratory mice were cut off. At the end of the test period, memory for space was evaluated, and numbers of hippocampal neurons were counted. Molarless mice showed a decrease in both learning ability in a water maze and neuron density in the hippocampus area of the brain compared with control mice. These changes increased the longer the molarless condition persisted. The data suggest a possible link between reduced chewing and brain cell loss, and may be one risk factor for senile impairment (*Brain Research* 826, no. 1 [April 24, 1999]: 148–153).

Water Intake and Aging

One-third of Americans over the age of 50 are likely to be dehydrated, from mild to severe.

The concerns of dehydration include:

- Increased risk of stroke
- Increased risk of heart attack
- Increased incidence of bladder cancer
- Increased allergies and dermatitis
- Skeletal signs and symptoms increase
- Backache
- Development of kidney stones (At least eight cups of water per day can prevent most stones, even in people prone to forming stones.)
- Reduction in endurance in physical activities
- An increased risk of some cancers, particularly urinary tract cancer
- Deep vein clots (probably the disease to be feared most from chronic dehydration)

The more calories burned each day, the more water one needs. Coffee, alcohol, soda, tea, and hot chocolate should not be counted as liquids meeting the fluid needs of the body as they actually encourage loss of water through the kidneys.

BMI (Body Mass Index) and Aging

Government guidelines recommend a BMI of 25 or less. When the body mass index reaches 27 or higher, weight becomes a serious health concern. It has also been determined that people with a BMI of 17 to 22 live longer than those with a higher BMI.

To check your Body Mass Index (BMI):

- Multiply your weight in pounds by 0.45 to get kilograms.
- Convert your height to inches.
- Multiply the number of inches by .0254 to get meters.
- Square that number (multiply it by itself).
- Divide this into your weight in kilograms.

Exercise and Aging

A study on aging done by the National Institute on Aging showed that people over the age of 70 who had difficulty performing daily activities (climbing stairs, ability to walk half a mile, ability to get up easily from a chair, and had difficulty with balance) were all indicators of becoming disabled in the next four years.

The number of times in 30 seconds an elderly person can rise from a straight-backed chair without using their hands or arms indicates lower body strength. As an example, an 80-year-old woman who can stand up 10 times in 30 seconds is about normal for that age. But doing only 10 of these chair stands at age 60 is below average. While people at that level may function all right now, they are at risk of losing mobility by age 75. At 60 a woman should be able to do 20 in 30 seconds; at 70, 15; and at 80, 10.

Elderly people, even up to 96 years of age, have been shown to benefit from a high-intensity exercise program. A group of ten elderly persons in a nursing home were given an exercise program and demonstrated marked improvement in strength, walking speed, and mobility. This group demonstrated greater stability on their feet, were less likely to suffer falls, and increased leg strength ranging up to 374 percent (*Journal of the American Medical Association* 263 [June 13, 1990]: 3029–3034).

Blood Chemistry Factors in Aging

Elevated non-fasting plasma homocysteine levels are associated with increased rates of mortality from all causes, especialy from heart disease, Alzheimer's, and cancer in the elderly (*Archives of Internal Medicine* 159 [1999]: 1077).

A five-year study done by the National Institutes of Health showed that high iron levels are an increased risk of coronary heart disease deaths, as well as total number of deaths from all causes. Four thousand men and women aged 71 and over were studied. The higher their iron levels, the higher their risk of death, especially from coronary heart disease. There is also growing research indicating that high iron levels specifically result in an increased risk of heart attacks and cancer. These studies reveal that the picture is not entirely simple and other factors may be involved (*American Journal of Cardiology* 79 [1997]: 120).

Insulin resistance is a strong marker for the aging process. The condition is inherited but requires an unhealthful lifestyle for it to fully develop. Measures should be taken at once, as soon as the diagnosis is made, to correct the lifestyle in order that the aging process can be retarded (*Internal Medicine World Report,* January 15–31, 1995, 30).

If insulin resistance is not treated, it leads to diabetes, as well as an increased risk of hypertension, heart disease, and cancer.

Growth Hormone, Sleep, and Aging

Adequate quantities of growth hormone promote a long life and stimulate muscle growth and strength. Mental acuity is also improved. To increase growth hormone naturally, adults need sleep, especially before midnight. The pituitary produces about twice as much before midnight as after midnight. So, go to bed three or more hours before midnight. Even if you sleep only three hours after midnight, it will give you about twice as much growth hormone as you would get if you slept six hours after midnight, but only if one is asleep. There are none of the unwanted side effects from this program that one gets from hormone supplements, and it doesn't cost anything.

Growth hormone naturally decreases as we age. Researchers from London discovered that physical exercise also stimulates the production of growth hormone, thus slowing down the aging process (*Clinical Endocrinology,* Oxford, 51 [1999]: 687).

Anti-aging Herbs

Schizandra chinensis, gotu cola, ashwagandha, CoQ-10, and ginseng are beneficial herbs that delay aging. Ginseng is said to retard aging and lengthen the life span. It is said to improve muscular motility and stretching.

Antacids, Contraindications

Antacids may actually increase acid production. The calcium carbonate nearly doubles the amount of gastric acid in people who suffer from duodenal ulcers.

Side-effects of magnesium antacids include diarrhea, potassium deficiency, abnormally high magnesium levels, and iron deficiency. Aluminum-based antacids may cause constipation, weakness, anemia, delayed gastric emptying, and perforation of the colon. Calcium-containing antacids may cause milk-alkali syndrome, rebound acidity, and calcium phosphate deposits in the kidney tubules. Sodium in antacids may induce salt and water retention, worsening edema and ascites, hypertension, and cardiac failure. Bicarbonate antacids may induce alkalosis. Antacids containing sodium bicarbonate could be harmful to the kidneys.

Other adverse effects of antacids include osteomalacia induced by lack of phosphorus. Aluminum-containing antacids block the absorption of phosphorus, and phosphorus is required for strong bones. While consuming antacids, patients absorb up to 20 times less fluoride. Aluminum is currently under scrutiny as a cause of premature senile dementia. Aluminum is retained in the brain and other organs, and scientists believe that excess levels of aluminum are possibly responsible for some of the increasing incidence of Alzheimer's disease (premature senile dementia).

Blood Viscosity

Blood viscosity refers to the thickness of blood caused by the levels of cells, minerals, proteins, various chemicals, nutrients, supplements, and waste products, as well as water intake. The viscosity can be high or low. Results of high blood viscosity include clumping of red cells, rigidity of red cells, thickening of plasma, and increased risk of clotting. The size of red blood cell clusters or clumps fluctuates depending on the flow, speed, and friction qualities of the blood and blood vessels. The lower the rate of flow, the larger the aggregates formed. Just after meals, especially if the meal is high in fats, sugars, and salt, the flow is retarded. This accounts in part for the desirability of remaining active following meals when the blood is heaviest and least likely to flow briskly.

Heart and cancer patients usually show higher degrees of aggregation than persons in good health. The more clumps or aggregates, the greater the viscosity. An increase in blood viscosity usually comes before the appearance of symptoms of stroke or heart attack. Cigarette smoking increases blood viscosity as does chronic anxiety (L. Dintenfass and G. V. F. Seaman, ed., *Blood Viscosity in Heart Disease and Cancer* [Pergamon Press, 1981]).

It has been discovered that in persons with intermittent claudication (lameness on walking), the blood is quite thick and has a slow-flow condition somewhat like honey on a cold morning. Too many red blood cells, and plasma containing too many nutrients and wastes, promotes the development of intermittent claudication (L. Dintenfass and G. V. F. Seaman, ed., *Blood Viscosity in Heart Disease and Cancer* [Pergamon Press, 1981]).

If your hemoglobin is above 15 grams, donate blood if you are an eligible donor. Also drink plenty of water to thin your blood. Thick blood flows with greater difficulty.

Cilantro is believed to be effective for normalizing the hematocrit, as is garlic, and also spirulina.

Caffeine

Caffeine is the most commonly used psychoactive substance. Caffeine has been found to carry an increased risk of heart attacks, osteoporosis, breast cancer, fibrocystic breast disease, endometriosis, peptic ulcer, GERD (gastroesophageal reflux disease), bladder disease, anxiety and nervousness, infertility, hypertension, poor job performance, headaches, serious depression, severe insomnia, overweight, strokes, low levels of iron, copper, and zinc, and many other problems (*Science News* 145 [January 22, 1994]: 61). In 1996 it was reported that caffeine is also responsible for reducing estrogen and/or testosterone levels, in both instances the amount of available hormone was reduced. Apparently caffeine works to bind sex hormones (*American Journal of Epidemiology* 144 [1996]: 642).

Quitting a coffee habit of just one cup a day can bring on headaches, fatigue, sleepiness, nervousness, restlessness, and difficulty concentrating. These symptoms of caffeine withdrawal peak at about 20–48 hours after the last cup, creating the "weekend headache" suffered by many workday caffeine drinkers who don't partake on Saturday or Sunday morning. The less you drink, the less likely that occasional abstinence will cause withdrawal symptoms. Rest assured that after you have completely quit, your energy and concentration will return to the levels you enjoyed as a caffeine user (*Journal of Pharmacology and Experimental Therapeutics* 255 [1990]: 1123–1132).

Caffeine intake in pregnancy has also been associated with low birth weight, miscarriage, and withdrawal symptoms in the baby, including breathing difficulties.

To minimize withdrawal symptoms for someone trying to stop caffeine, keep a cup of coffee in the refrigerator. If a headache, nervousness, or any other symptom begins, take a tablespoonful of the coffee. This will often be adequate to stop the symptom in its tracks. If the headache or other symptom threatens again, even 10–20 minutes later, take another tablespoonful. Usually all symptoms will cease by five days.

Cholesterol

In addition to the total fat contained in animal meat and eggs, eating these foods introduces still another harmful substance—cholesterol. Other factors such as smoking, poor posture, low vital capacity, lack of exercise, irregular schedule, underactive thyroid, blood pressure elevation, tension, overwork, and overweight may cause one's cholesterol to be elevated.

While the body needs some cholesterol, it can produce all it requires. Stress hormones and sex hormones both have cholesterol as a part of their raw materials, and those who are under emotional tension will find this to be a cause of elevated blood cholesterol.

The normal body can handle (although not so easily) the amount of cholesterol present in about three ounces of animal protein (meat, fish, etc.) daily. Any more than that gets stored in the blood and tissues. The excess stored cholesterol forms plaques inside the blood vessels, and in time these turn into ulcers or ruptured plaques resembling abscesses in some way. The products from theses ruptures are carried to more distant locations, causing serious problems like strokes and heart attacks. This condition is known as atherosclerosis. In some countries atherosclerosis is almost unheard of and cholesterol levels run 60–90, whereas in America our high animal diet causes cholesterol levels to run up to 250 or more.

The ideal for an American should probably run no more than around 100 plus the person's age. The heart attack rate is four times higher if cholesterol is over 260, than if it is below 200. A mere 10 percent reduction in cholesterol reduces by 25 percent the likelihood of a heart attack. Therefore, reducing the cholesterol from 200 to 180 (10 percent reduction), would reduce that person's risk of heart attack by 25 percent, calculated by age and other risk factors.

On our usual high-fat refined diet, these plaques begin to form even in very young people, gradually building up over a period of time and narrowing the channels in the blood vessels. This narrowing reduces the amount of blood flow to the tissues. The heart compensates by elevating the blood pressure more and more, eventually producing high blood pressure.

If the coronary vessels that serve the heart become sufficiently clogged by plaque, any circumstance that further reduces the already diminished oxygen supply to the heart muscle will cause the heart to "cry out" in pain—the pain of angina. A slight exertion such as running a short distance, an emotional episode, or even a single big, salty or fatty meal, can bring on an angina attack.

To understand how fat does this, we need to observe what happens after fat is eaten. It enters the blood as tiny fat balls called chylomicrons. When these balls stick onto red blood cells, there is blockage of blood flow to the tiniest blood vessels, the capillaries. The red blood cells then clump together in formation resembling rows of coins, and they have lost much of their efficiency in picking up and transporting oxygen.

It is this process of depriving the body cells of oxygen that causes cholesterol to form the atherosclerotic plaques. The artery walls become much more easily penetrated by fats and cholesterol when the blood that bathes them is deficient in oxygen, thus encouraging the plaques to form. The plaques cause a gradual deterioration in hearing, vision, joint function (with backaches, ankle, knee and hip pain), digestion, and finally, brain function leading to senility.

There is much sobering evidence that the average Western diet produces diseased arteries and other problems even in young children. Changing to a proper diet and lifestyle, the plaques will quickly shrink and gradually begin to disappear so that near normal circulation will be restored. By lowering the blood fats by a diet low in fats of all kinds, as well as low in refined carbohydrates like sugar, honey, and molasses, which become converted to triglycerides (a common fat in the blood), diabetes can also be corrected. Every member of the family—from the youngest child on—will have better health if the following foods are eliminated: meat, milk, eggs, cheese, high-fat foods, sugar, refined foods, salt, coffee, tea, colas, chocolate, and alcohol.

Cholesterol is also caused by a lack of vitamin E, C, B12, fiber (especially whole grains), and fruits and vegetables (especially legumes).

Vitamin E in supplements is found in the form of alpha-tocopherol, while vitamin E in foods comes as a different compound, gamma-tocopherol. Alpha-tocopherol displaces gamma-tocopherol in our tissues, but it is gamma-tocopherol that offers the protection from artery disease. Therefore, getting vitamin E naturally in our food is the best method, since it is unclear if vitamin E from pills is safe and effective.

Cleansing Program

Sluggish elimination systems in the liver, skin, bowel, lungs, and kidneys can be caused by chronic dehydration. The first objective of any cleansing program is good hydration. The next objective is repairing damaged tissues.

After completing a cleansing program, you should expect to have more energy and be lighter on your feet. If your blood pressure is high, it should come down. If it is low, it should come up. Cholesterol and triglycerides should be reduced on this program, and many chronic health problems should disappear.

Ten-day detoxification program

Days one to three

- Take no food or drink except that mentioned.
- Take a rounded to heaping teaspoon of activated charcoal stirred in water four times daily.
- Drink eight to ten additional glasses of pure water throughout the day.
- Start each day by drinking 16 ounces of warm water with the juice of one fresh lemon first thing for ten days. Also drink eight ounces of freshly made apple juice for breakfast, and eight ounces of freshly made carrot juice for lunch, and either of these juices at about 6:00 p.m.
- A herbal mix should be taken on the first day of the cleansing program consisting of the following formula:
    - 1 tablespoon of Artemisia annua
    - 1 tablespoon of licorice root powder
    - 1 tablespoon of freshly ground hawthorn berries
    - 1 tablespoon of silymarin (milk thistle)
    - 1 quart of gently boiling water.

  Add the first three herbs to the water and simmer for 20 minutes. Turn off the heat and add the silymarin. Cover and steep for 30 minutes. Strain and drink one cup every four hours until it is all gone.

A mistake that many people make on a cleansing program is that they do not take enough charcoal. While we suggest a certain amount, this is a minimum, and more can be taken if it is desired. The second thing to recognize is that if you have a chronic disease for which you are taking a medicine on a daily basis, you should not use charcoal, as charcoal will take up your medicine along with any other toxin in the body. Children taking charcoal on a daily basis must be watched to be certain they are having a daily bowel movement.

Days four to ten

Continue drinking the fresh apple juice (may substitute freshly made grape juice or watermelon juice) and fresh carrot juice. You may now drink more than eight ounces of the freshly made juice if you desire.

Add a large handful of fresh spinach, three stalks of celery, and a small handful of parsley to a serving of carrot juice each day. These vegetables may be eaten, or may be pureed, or juiced as you desire. You may also have a large fresh salad for lunch (no head lettuce, use leaf lettuce, spinach, cabbage, broccoli, etc.), and two raw vegetables such as sliced radishes, carrots, celery, onion, green peas, baby okra pods, summer squash, etc., but only two of these.

For dressing use one to two tablespoons of freshly ground flaxseed sprinkled over the salad. Garlic powder or onion powder (avoid salted varieties) and lemon juice may be added as desired.

At supper you may have two or more pieces of a single fruit, such as two apples, two bunches of grapes, two peaches or more, but not a mixture of several kinds of fruits. Do not eat between meals, and never eat the last meal of the day closer to bedtime than four hours.

Days four and five only

Prepare a stimulus for the liver and gallbladder as follows:

- 4 ounces of fresh orange juice
- 4 ounces of fresh lemon juice
- 8 ounces of pure water
- 3 to 5 cloves of fresh garlic
- 1 inch of fresh ginger root

Blend these together until smooth, and slowly sip four ounces in the morning and four ounces in the evening for these two days only.

After day ten

Begin breaking the program, but continue to eat raw fruits and vegetables as before. However, now you may add some cooked brown rice, oatmeal, legumes, nuts, seeds, whole grain breads, and potatoes, starting with a very small serving of only one of these items and gradually increasing the amount until you are eating a regular amount that is appropriate for you.

Starting on day five of breaking the fast, cooked vegetables can also be added, but in very small quantities. Use no foods that come from an animal.

After the ten days, eat a plant-based diet with 50 to 75 percent of it consisting of raw foods for at least one month.

Exercise

A study found that regardless of how out of shape a person is, the risk of death from all causes could be reduced by merely becoming fit through a regular exercise program.

Regular exercise increases the number of natural killer cells in both humans and animals and assists them with certain blood proteins to destroy bacteria, viruses, and tumor cells. Competitive exercise reduces natural killer cells and increases the prevalence of infection. The stress of intense exercise lowers resistance to disease, pointing out the need to describe exercise as "vigorous but not violent." Regular moderate exercise is most notably beneficial in persons over the age of 50 (*Physician and Sports Medicine* 27, no. 6 [1999]: 47).

Exercise improves brain function apparently through the action of calcium and certain amines such as dopamine (*Physiology and Behavior* 60 [1996]: 177).

Increased levels of physical activity correlate with a reduced incidence of blood clots and emboli that can cause heart attacks, thrombosis, as well as hemorrhage into the brain (*The Physician and Sports Medicine* 21 [1993]: 14).

About 75 percent of morning exercisers will still be exercising a year later compared to 50 percent of people who exercise at midday, and 25 percent of those who exercise in the evening.

Marathon competitors were found to be six times more likely to catch some kind of respiratory infection the week following a marathon competition. Blood tests showed a 60 percent rise in stress hormones. Competitive exercise is not good for most people's health.

After especially heavy physical exercise, a rest day or two is quite beneficial. It should be kept in mind that, beyond a certain level, additional exercise carries no added benefits to the health, but may weaken the immune system.

Exercise at a moderate level reduces blood sugar and helps diabetics keep good control.

A single bout of prolonged exercise, which is quite vigorous and lasting several hours, can reduce cholesterol and triglyceride levels as well as other blood fats (*Journal of the American Medical Association* 276 [1996]: 221).

Average men have a heart rate (pulse) from 72 to 76 beats per minute, while women average 75 to 80. In general, the lower your resting pulse rate, the more efficient your heart, and the healthier you are. In general, the higher the resting pulse rate, the heavier load your heart is working under, and the higher your risk for coronary heart disease.

Your exercising pulse rate can be determined by jogging in place for two minutes, raising your feet four to five inches from the floor. You should jog at the rate of 70 to 80 steps a minute. Each time you lift your left foot, that counts as one step. Immediately after exercising, count the number of pulse beats for six seconds. Add a zero to get your exercise pulse rate per minute. Try to exercise at a level that you perceive to be moderate, noticing your breathing. If you can breathe easily and maintain a conversation, your exercise is not too strenuous. If your breathing is interfering somewhat with the ease of talking but you can still maintain conversation, you are probably still within your target zone, but if you can only say a word or two occasionally, your exercise is too strenuous. If you are not in good physical condition, with regular vigorous exercise, you can reduce your heart rate at rest by 5 to 10 beats per minute in a month's time.

Target Zone for Pulse

Age	Minimum/Maximum
16–20	142–171
21–25	138–167
26–30	134–163
31–35	131–159
36–40	127–155
41–45	124–151
46–50	120–146
51–55	117–142
56–60	113–138
61–65	110–134
66–70	106–130
71–75	103–126

You can tell if you are working too strenuously if your pulse rate is over 120 after five minutes of quitting exercise. After 10 minutes, your pulse rate should always be below 100. When you start an exercise program, your pulse rate will rise rapidly to a high level. After some weeks of exercising, it will take more exercise to bring the heart rate up to a minimum, which you should aim for in your workout. You should not work so strenuously as to get your pulse rate above the maximum, nor so leisurely as to fail to get it up to the minimum.

Seven Easy Exercises in Seven Minutes

Do these exercises **slowly** three times.

1. *Neck* – Turn the head all the way to the left and to the right. Then, chin up and back, down and forward.
2. *Arms*
   a. Biceps – Place a bottle filled partly with water or dumbbells in each hand and flex the arm toward the shoulders, elbows down by your side. Do not make the bottle too heavy. Do 3 to 10 repetitions.
   b. Triceps – Bend forward at the hips so that the trunk makes a 90-degree angle with the thighs and lift the water bottles backwards at arms length, arms extended, elevating the water bottles behind the back, straight up toward the ceiling. Do 3 to 10 repetitions.
3. *Abdominal Crunch*
   a. Lie on the floor, knees bent slightly with your feet flat on the floor, hands folded over your chest. Lift head and chest up from the floor, hold three to ten seconds and repeat 3 to 10 times depending on your strength.
   b. From a sitting position, lean back 45 degrees, hold for one to three seconds and repeat 3 to 10 times.
4. *Glutei* – Contract buttocks while sitting, standing, waiting, answering the phone, etc. Hold the contraction as long as possible. Repeat as many times per day as you can think of it.
5. *Quadriceps*
   a. Cycling and running strengthen the quadriceps.
   b. Run or walk slowly in place, pulling the knees as high as possible into the air.
   c. Walk up long steps or repeatedly up and down on a low, very steady stool. Repeat 10 to 50 times.
6. *Calves* – Stand up on your toes, holding it one to three seconds, and repeat 3 to 10 times. Then stand on one foot at a time, holding the other knee high in the air.
7. *Thighs* (Back and Lateral)
   a. Half squats strengthen the hamstrings. Keep toes pointing straight ahead to prevent knee strain.
   b. Leg to the side, rising on the toes of the opposite foot, repeat 3 to 10 times for each leg.

How to Handle Shin Splints

Athletes whose sports activities involve repeated jarring impact to the legs often result in pain beside the shins. One treatment is to stop the activity until pain subsides and then gradually work back up to the desired level. This will often prevent recurrence.

To prevent shin splints or help heal existing ones, do the following two stretches.

1. Stand facing a wall with your toes about two feet from the wall. Place your hands in front of you on the wall at shoulder height and lean your chest into the wall while keeping your heels flat on the floor. Hold that position for ten seconds, push away from the wall for five seconds, then lean in again for ten more seconds. Do this 3 times.
2. Stand up on your toes and hold it for one to three seconds. Repeat 3 to 10 times.

Exercise in Older Persons

As a person gets older, exercise is the key to continued independence. There are eight basic guidelines to follow in developing an exercise program for older persons:

1. Decide how much time you are willing to spend, starting with 30 minutes to two hours daily, at least four days a week.
2. Choose an exercise partner, if at all possible. This helps insure the continuance of the exercise program. Purposeful labor, such as gardening, also has a coercive factor that helps ensure continuance.
3. Precede each workout with a two or three minute warm-up. Don't stretch yet, wait until you begin warming up.
4. Pay attention to safety.
5. Do exercises that give a full range of motion of every joint in the body.
6. Work by the principle of gradually placing a greater and greater demand on your strength until your muscles are in good shape.

7. Learn the amount of daily workout that gives you the desired health benefits without either over exercising or falling short of your need. You should be able to completely recover from exercise strain by a 20 to 30 minute nap or a night of sleep. If you cannot recover in that length of time, you are over exercising.
8. Cool-down gradually.

Muscle Stretches

Both a warm-up and a cool-down phase of vigorous exercise are necessary. The warm-up is to protect joints, the back, knees, feet, etc. The cool-down is to protect the heart, lungs, and blood vessels. In the warm-up period, one should start off walking slowly for five to ten minutes, then do a good stretch. To stretch earlier may result in soreness and stiffness, whereas after muscles are warmed up, they are more efficiently and safely stretched. This pays off in speed and comfort.

Muscles make up about 40 percent of body weight. The psoas muscle and quadratus lumborum (under the spine) are large muscles that can get very tense, tight, shortened, overworked, strained, or weakened.

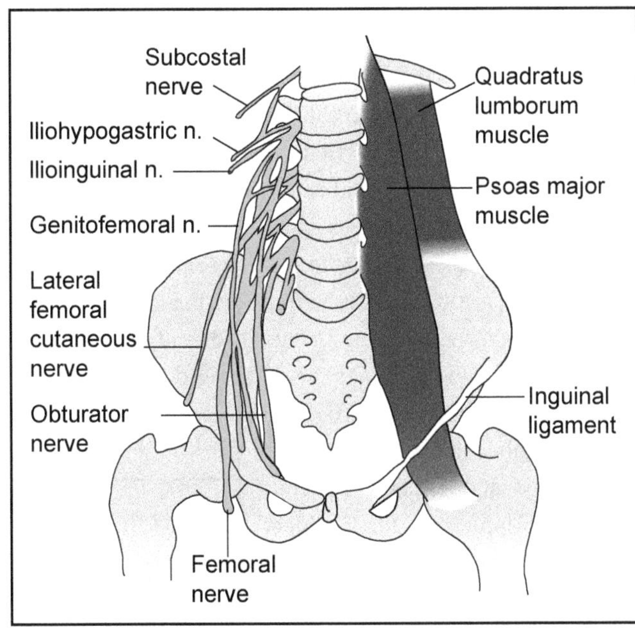

They can develop trigger points that telegraph pain to other parts of the body. Headaches, increased blood pressure, numbness in the hands, sciatica, TMJ, and backaches may result from this contracture of muscles. A group of stretches and postures can have both a preventive as well as a healing virtue. Do the stretches slowly, gently, and with concentration on proper form. Do not hold the breath, but breathe regularly. Only 1 to 3 repetitions of each posture should be done, unless otherwise directed, taking only a few minutes to go through the routine.

Stretch at least three times a week to maintain flexibility. A stretching session should last 10 to 20 minutes. Each stationary stretch should be held 10 seconds or more, working up to 30 seconds. Usually a stretch is repeated about 4 times. Do not stretch until it hurts. If there's any pain, stop. Don't bounce. Stretching should be gradual and relaxed. Focus on the muscle groups you want to stretch, and don't hold your breath.

Stretches for Common Muscles

- Pelvic tilt – For abdominal and buttock muscles, lie on the floor with the knees bent and feet flat on the floor, arms relaxed by your sides. Exhale, tightening your buttocks and pulling in your abdomen. This will tighten your abdomen and decrease the curve in your lower back. Hold for three seconds. Start with 3 repetitions and work up to 6 repetitions of six seconds each.

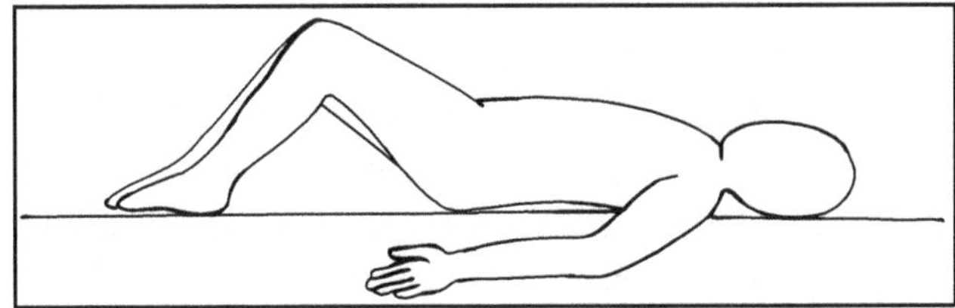

- Knee to chest – For hip muscles, assume the same starting position as for the pelvic tilt. Bring your right knee toward your chest as far as you can, breathing deeply and evenly. Hold for five seconds. Return to start, then extend the right leg straight. Wobble it a bit to keep the muscles relaxed and return to the starting position. Repeat with the other leg. Start with 3 repetitions and work up to 10.

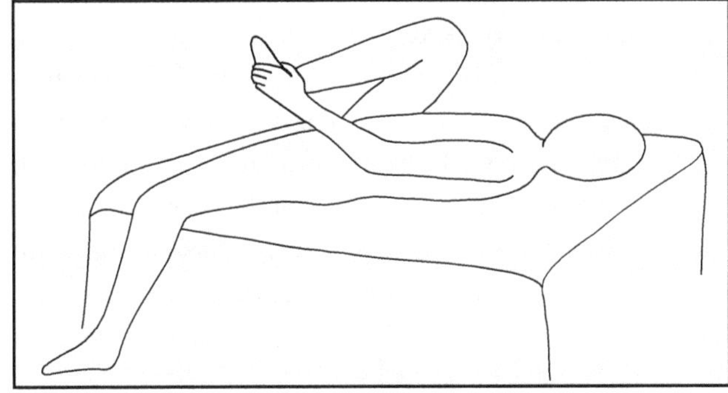

- Double knee to chest – For hip and abdominal muscles, from the pelvic tilt starting position, pull both knees to your chest, one at a time and clasp your arms around them. Curl your head and shoulders forward and rock gently back and forth several times. Do 3 to 5 repetitions.

- Bent knee partial sit-ups – For abdominal and hip muscles, use the pelvic tilt starting position. Exhale, and leading with your outstretched arms, pull in your abdominal muscles, raising the upper part of your body toward your knees until your shoulder blades are barely off the floor. Don't sit up all the way. Hold the position for five seconds, breathing evenly, then inhale and slowly lower your head and shoulders to the floor. Do 3 to 5 repetitions and work up to 15.

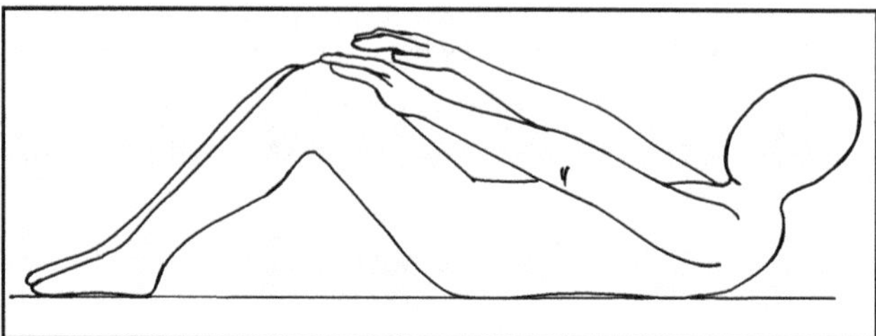

- Standing pelvic tilt – This is for abdominal and buttock muscles. Stand erect and tighten your abdominal muscles, squeezing the buttocks at the same time. This will decrease the curve in your lower back and help strengthen critical supporting muscles. Do 5 repetitions.
- Cat stretch – For abdominal muscles and back extensor muscles, get down on all fours on the floor with your back straight. Drop your head and pull in your abdominal muscles, curving your back like a cat. Hold for five seconds, relax your abdominal muscles and roll your head straight back, arching your spine until you feel a stretch in your extensors. Do 3 to 5 repetitions.
- Ear to knee stretch – This is the most valuable stretch because it relaxes the quadratus lumborum, probably the most overlooked source of pain in the low back. Sit in a chair, spread the legs wide apart, place the palms on the ankles, and let the trunk sink between the knees to loosen up the back. Then slowly bend the trunk to the left until the ear touches the left knee. Rotate the head slightly to the right, slowly raise the right arm until it is hanging over the head. Hold for ten seconds, then slowly raise the trunk. Repeat with the opposite side, right ear to right knee.
- The psoas stretch – The psoas muscles extend from the thighs and hip joint where they insert, up to their origin in the mid and lower spine. They tighten up from too much sitting and cause pain in the mid back. To stretch the psoas muscles, stand with the feet together, toes pointed straight ahead, put the left foot back and the right foot forward, keeping toes pointed straight ahead. Raise the left arm directly overhead, right arm at side. Bend knees slightly and tip trunk backward slightly. A stretching sensation will be felt under the belt on the left side. Hold for ten seconds, breathing deeply. Repeat on the other side. Perform this stretch before and after long bouts of sitting.
- Splenius stretch – Do not hold a tilt of the head or stretch of the neck for a long time. The splenii arise in the upper back and insert into the side of the head and top of the neck. To stretch these muscles, tuck the chin in, grasp the crown of the head and gently exert forward pressure.

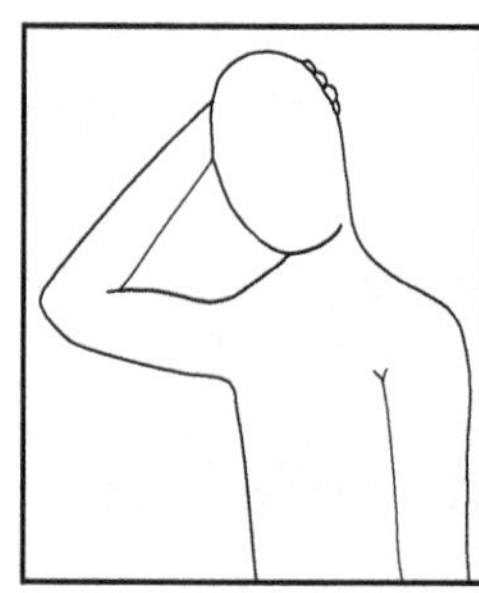

- Trapezius stretches – While sitting in a chair, grasp the seat with the left hand to stabilize shoulders. With the right hand pull the head slowly to the right and forward, slightly turning the face to the left, giving it a little stretch. Breathe deeply and repeat on the other side.
- Scalene stretches – Located just above the collar bone, deep inside, when irritated it can mimic a pinched nerve, a whiplash, and cause pain or numbness in the thumb, forefinger, back of the arm, or shoulder blade. This stretch is similar to the trapezius stretch. While sitting, grasp the chair bottom with the left hand, place the right hand on top of the head, and pull the head gently to the right. As this is being done, guide your head slightly backward. Breathe deeply and repeat on the other side.
- Wrist and forearm stretches – Gripping a small object with intensity can overwork the wrist extensor on top of the forearm. Wrist pain and tennis elbow symptoms may appear after a single strain, such as trying to open a jar. Typists can overwork these muscles. Stretch the arm straight in front, bending the wrists down with the fingers firmly extended, pointing straight down to the floor. Twist the hand to the outside

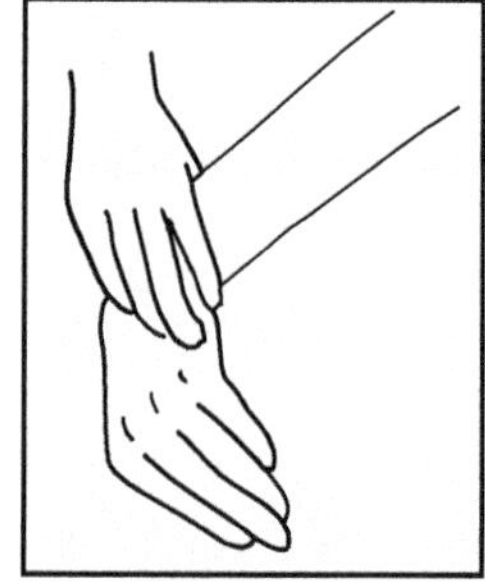

while pressing down and inward with the other hand. Breathe deeply and repeat with the other hand.

- The Indian squat – This stretch can ease calf pain, stretch the hips, and deep tendons of the back. With the feet one foot apart, squat as deeply as possible, keeping the feet turned slightly outward and flat on the floor. Fold the arms and rest them on the knees to maintain balance. Indians squat in this position for hours.

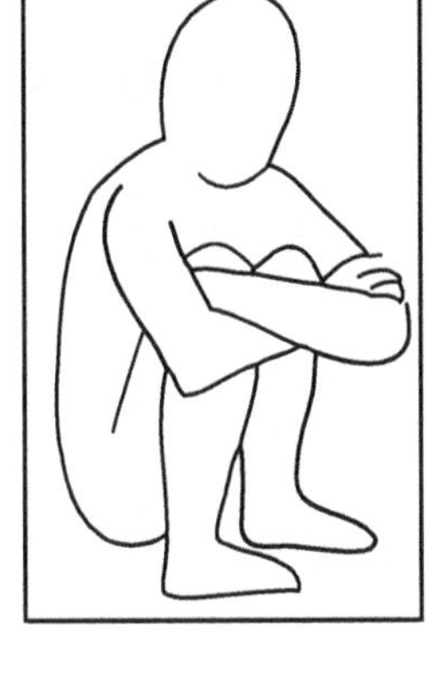

- Gluteal stretch I – The work of the glutei extends and rotates the thigh and supports the back. If irritated the pain resembles sciatica. A twist is the best stretch for the glutei. While sitting in a chair put the left leg over the right and hook the right arm around the left knee to stabilize the legs. Hold onto the chair with the left hand and slowly turn to the left while exhaling. A stretch should be felt in the left buttock. Repeat on the other side while breathing deeply.

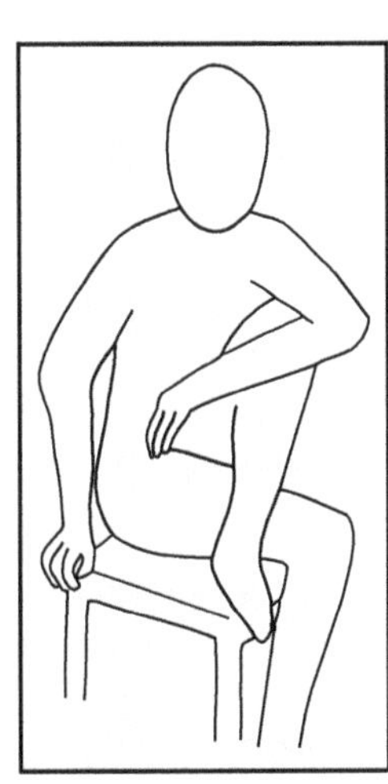

- Gluteal stretch II – Prop your right foot on a stool and bend the right knee. Slowly move the left shoulder toward the right knee. Breathe out and enjoy the twist, which stretches the right buttock. Repeat on the opposite side.

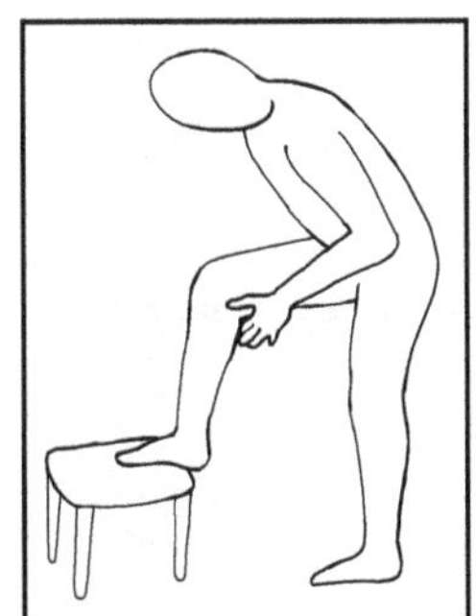

- Chest and arm stretches – Overworking the pectorals, biceps, or coracobrachialis muscles causes one to be round shouldered and have a forward head.
- Jaw stretching – Twenty-two percent of Americans are known to clinch their jaws. Teeth grinding may be a part of their syndrome. Slowly open the mouth as widely as can be comfortably done 10 times. Next, make a fist and put it beneath the chin and open the mouth against some mild resistance from your fist 3 times. Repeat this sequence 12 or so times a day. This may gradually improve or remove TMJ.

Correcting Forward Head, Humpback

To correct this posture, the chest should be stretched. Try to touch your fingertips together behind your upper back in this way: Reach the right hand back up over the right shoulder toward the left shoulder while curling the left hand up under the left shoulder blade to try to reach the right hand and make a hand clasp. Repeat with the opposite direction, breathing deeply periodically.

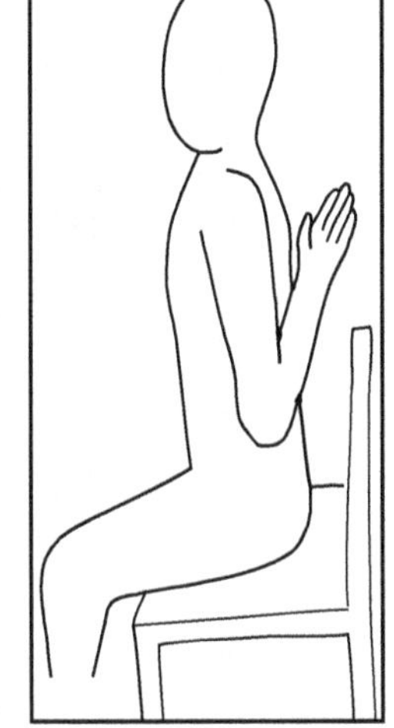

Second version: Stand with hands at shoulder height and place one hand on each side of a doorway. The feet should be in a position so that you can lean forward into the space while grasping the sides of the door. You should feel a good stretch in the pectoral muscles.

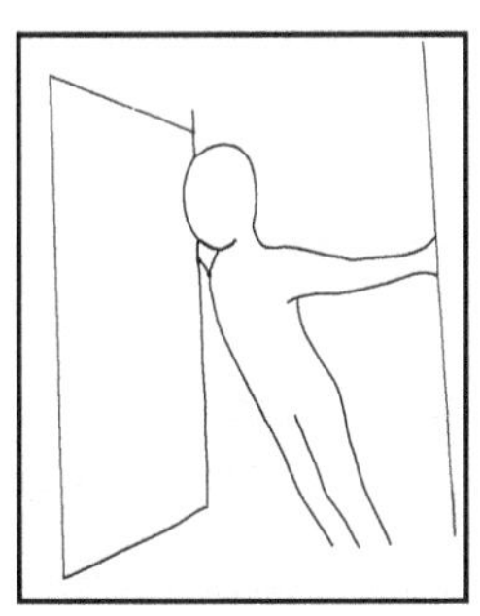

Third version: Place the hands at a higher level on the doorway and lean again to get a stretch in a different place. To stretch the coracobrachialis muscles (long thin fibers that help move the arm), reach straight ahead with right hand and grip the side of the doorway, thumb pointed toward floor. Straighten the elbow. Next, turn your body 180 degrees so the right arm is extended directly behind. Repeat with the left arm. This also stretches the biceps fully.

Health Recovery Program

Eighty percent of overweight adults develop diabetes. Probably 75 percent or more of these could be cured simply by following the Health Recovery Program. Use the program if you have had premature aging signs such as adult acne, allergies, an appendectomy, arthritis, boils, cataracts, diabetes, frequent colds or sore throats, a heart rate over 80, overweight, nail problems, peptic ulcers, skin problems, slow healing, or a tonsillectomy.

The Health Recovery Program is also beneficial if you have a metabolic problem such as compulsive eating,

One-Mile Walk Test						
Find your fitness rating and fitness level by completing this test. Spend five minutes in gentle stretching and walking slowly, gradually increasing your pace until you have built up a brisk walking pace. Walk on a measured track such as the quarter-mile track, which some high schools and many parks have. Then while using a stopwatch, walk as briskly as possible and try to maintain a steady pace. Time your walk in minutes and seconds. Find your age and then read down until you find your finishing time for one mile.						
Age	**Sex**	**Level 1**	**Level 2**	**Level 3**	**Level 4**	**Level 5**
40-49	Female	under 14.1	14.2-15.0	15.1-16.0	16.1-17.3	over 17.3
	Men	under 12.5	12.6-13.9	14.0-14.4	14.5-15.3	over 15.3
50-59	Female	under 14.4	14.5-15.4	15.5-16.9	17.0-18.1	over 18.1
	Men	under 13.2	13.3-14.2	14.3-15.1	15.2-16.3	over 16.3
60-69	Female	under 15.1	15.2-16.2	16.3-17.3	17.4-19.1	over 19.1
	Men	under 14.1	14.2-15.1	15.2-16.2	16.3-17.2	over 17.2
70-79	Female	under 18.2	18.3-19.9	20.0-21.4	21.5-24.1	over 24.1
	Men	under 15.1	15.2-15.4	15.5-18.5	18.6-20.2	over 20.2

constipation, cravings, depression, diarrhea, dizziness, fatigue, hay fever, headaches, heart palpitations, impatience or irritability, loss of ability to organize your work or concentrate, indigestion, intestinal gas, involuntary jumping or jerking, nervousness, ringing in the ears, sensation of pressure in (or band around) the head, sense of frustration, sleeplessness, or unsteadiness on the feet.

What to Eat

Breakfast is simply fruits and whole grains with nuts or seeds. Lunch is simply vegetables and whole grains with nuts or seeds. Following is a suggested meal plan:

Breakfast

- Main Dishes (choose one)
  - Whole grain cereals (boiled, baked, dry)
  - Fruit crisps
  - Whole grain waffles
  - Whole grain alternates
  - Quinoa
  - Amaranth
  - Buckwheat
  - Breakfast beans
  - Scrambled soy
  - Baked beans
  - Nut casseroles
- Hot Fruit Dishes without sugar or honey (choose one)
  - Steamed prunes or other dried fruit
  - Cooked apples, pears, crushed pineapple, etc.
  - Applesauce or any fruit sauce
  - Fruit puddings, fruit leather or jerky, purees
- Raw Fruit (choose one kind, but have as many pieces of that kind as you like)
  - Any fruit of your choosing, preferably choosing one of the kind in the hot dish, to keep the meal simple
- Whole Grain Bread, preferably of the same grain as the main grain cereal
- Spreads and milks (choose one of each if desired)
  - Nut or soy milk
  - Nut butter or fruit spread

Lunch

- Main Dishes (choose one)
  - Legumes
  - Potatoes or potato dishes
  - Whole grain roasts, casseroles, stews, dumplings, etc.
  - Sweet potatoes, or any root vegetable
  - Whole grain pastas, baked or boiled
- Hot vegetable dish (your choice)
- Raw vegetable or salad. Keep the salad simple, one or two items, nicely prepared.
- Whole grain breads, crackers, rice, etc.
- Olives or avocado, nut or vegetable spread, gravies, sauces (nut cream sauce, onion-lemon puree, bean puree, tomato-pepper puree, etc.)

Foods to Use Sparingly

Dried fruits (like raisins, dates, figs), sweet fruits (like bananas, mangoes, watermelon, grapes), sweet vegetables (like sweet potatoes, yams, acorn squash), and nuts and seeds, as well as their butters (like peanut butter, almond butter, tahini.)

Foods to Avoid

Sugar; pastries; dairy cheeses; dairy products (like milk, ice cream, buttermilk, yogurt, cottage cheese, sour cream, butter); refined grains (like white bread, white buns, white crackers, white cakes, white cookies, white noodles, white rice); cereals and granolas made with sugar, honey, or oil; free fats; spices; vinegar and commercial condiments made with vinegar or spices (like pickles, relish, mustard, mayonnaise, ketchup, hot pepper sauce); caffeine drinks; soft drinks; meat in any form (high probability of containing hormones, cancer, viruses, and germs of other diseases); fish (high probability of containing mercury and other harmful toxins); and high protein meat substitutes.

When and How to Eat

There should be at least five hours between meals. Do not vary mealtime.

Take no fluids with meals. Eat well. Chew well. Blood sugar levels in rapid eaters fluctuate more widely than in those who eat slowly, chewing their food well.

What to Drink

Drink enough water between meals to keep the urine almost colorless. For most people, this will be an average of six to eight glasses a day. Drink water no closer than about 15 minutes before meals, and wait about 30 minutes or more after meals. Generally the less fluid taken with meals the better. Much weakness and fatigue are because of compensatory water shifts, and the person is actually "wilted" even if no thirst is experienced.

What Activity to Do

Exercise is your best friend. The minimal amount is 20 minutes per day. One hour daily is better, but on certain days three to five hours may be needed. Do not get sunburned and do not make your muscles sore with too much exercise. Both of these are unhealthful. Gradually build to a good exercise level without ever developing sore muscles. Exercise helps keep your appetite under control, neutralizes stress, lowers blood cholesterol, promotes digestion, and normalizes blood sugar. Make it your companion. Breathe deeply while exercising and meditate on nature as you workout.

Lab Tests

The following brief discussion of the significance of each blood test is intended to help you learn more about your body and to detect possible problems in early stages when treatment or changes in habits will be most effective. Abnormal test results may indicate a disorder needing medical attention, but they may also result from heavy exercise immediately before the blood was drawn, eating prior to having your blood drawn, or some processing error. If you feel that there was an error, you may choose to have the lab test conducted again.

- **URIC ACID** is a waste product that is normally excreted in urine. Elevated levels are found in gout, arthritis, kidney diseases, prolonged fasting in an overweight person, and following the use of some diuretics. Evaluation by your doctor is indicated if you have an elevated level.
- **UREA NITROGEN (BUN)** is a waste product of the liver that is excreted by the kidneys. High values may suggest that the kidneys are not adequately working. BUN is also elevated by high protein diets and strenuous exercise. Abundant water drinking, moderation in exercise, a totally vegetarian diet, and pregnancy all lower the BUN.
- **CALCIUM AND PHOSPHORUS** levels in the blood are regulated by the parathyroid glands and the kidneys. Most of the calcium and phosphorus in the body is found in bone; however, these minerals are necessary for proper blood clotting and nerve and muscle cell activity. Because of a relationship between the lifestyle and the control of these minerals, high or low levels in the blood may have no connection with the levels in the bone.
- **CREATININE** is a waste product removed from the blood by the kidneys. Low levels are insignificant; elevated levels, however, indicate that the kidneys are not working properly, and a change in the lifestyle to protect the kidneys is urgent, as failure to act when the level first begins to go up could result in developing kidney failure and an irreversible need for dialysis.
- **BUN/CREATININE RATIO** is the mathematical relationship between BUN and creatinine. Values outside the expected range are not significant if both BUN and creatinine are normal. When BUN and creatinine are abnormal, this ratio aids the doctor in determining more specifically what is wrong.

- **CPK** is an enzyme located primarily in the heart muscle, skeletal muscle, and brain. Elevated values are encountered in primary muscle disease and following a heart attack; however, any brain or muscle damage, such as a bruise, injection of medicines into muscles, or vigorous activity, may result in elevated values.
- **GLUCOSE** is the term used for blood sugar. Elevated levels are caused by eating prior to your blood test and by diabetes. If you have a blood glucose level greater than 175, even if you had eaten shortly before the blood test, you should consult your doctor. Even known diabetics should report an elevated glucose level (greater than 200) to their doctor.
- **CHOLESTEROL** is a fat in the blood that has been associated with heart and artery disease. If it is above the ideal range, you should take measures to bring it down. Low values of this fat are not important. The level is not affected by eating recently.
- **TRIGLYCERIDES** are another form of fat found in the blood. They, however, are markedly affected by what you have eaten. The triglycerides in your blood may remain at a high level for up to 12 hours after a meal. However, even if you have just eaten and your triglyceride value is higher than 300, take measures to bring it down. Again, low values are not important.
- **HIGH DENSITY LIPOPROTEIN (HDL)** is one of several types of fats that together are measured as cholesterol. It has been shown that higher levels of this HDL cholesterol lower the risk of developing heart disease. Approximately 45 to 90 is an ideal range.
- **PERCENT HDL CHOLESTEROL** calculates the amount of the total cholesterol made up of the high-density type. Studies have shown that the higher the number (the percentage) the lower the risk of developing heart disease.
- **CHOLESTEROL/HDL CHOLESTEROL RATIO** is another calculation used to define the relative amounts of cholesterol and the HDL cholesterol. In this calculation, the lower the number (the ratio), the lower the risk of developing heart disease. A table or a reference range will be given on your laboratory report.
- **TOTAL PROTEIN, ALBUMIN, and GLOBULIN** are tests that measure the amount and type of protein in your blood. These measurements provide a general index of overall health and nutrition. Globulin is the antibody protein important for fighting disease. A low globulin value or a very high globulin value could mean disease. If one of these tests is slightly abnormal, but all other tests are within normal limits, it is probably not significant. Large deviations from normal warrant further evaluation by your doctor. We prefer seeing total protein on the low side of normal, but still in the reference range, as high blood protein encourages loss of calcium from bones.
- **A/G RATIO** is the mathematical relationship between albumin and globulin. High or low values are not important in the screening situation if both albumin and globulin fall within expected ranges.
- **THYROXINE (T4)** is a thyroid hormone that helps your body regulate its metabolism or ability to use the food that you eat. Elevated levels may be caused by hormone medications or birth control pills. Any value outside the reference range is an indication for further evaluation.
- **BILIRUBIN** is a breakdown product of hemoglobin. It is produced in the liver and excreted in bile. Elevated levels may indicate liver disease or a blood disorder causing red blood cells to be broken down at an increased rate.
- **SGPT, SGOT and GGT** are abbreviations for proteins called enzymes that aid various chemical activities within cells. These enzymes are found in the muscles, liver, and heart. Injuries to cells release these enzymes into the blood. Liver damage from alcohol and a number of diseases are reflected in elevated values and should be evaluated. Low values are not significant.
- **ALKALINE PHOSPHATASE** is an enzyme primarily found in the bones and liver. An abnormally high value could mean liver disease or bone disease. Expected values are high for those who are growing (children, pregnant women, etc.). Low values are not significant. Elevated levels appear in people with osteoporosis, those one have been sedentary for a long time, and in people with liver disease.
- **LDH** is an enzyme present in all the cells of the body. Any condition that damages cells will raise the amounts in the blood. If the blood is not processed promptly and properly by the laboratory, high levels may occur from breakdown of red blood cells. If all values except LDH are within expected ranges, there is probably a processing damage to the red blood cells and further evaluation is not required.
- **POTASSIUM** is controlled by the kidneys. It is important for the proper functioning of the nerves and muscles, particularly in the heart and blood vessels.

Any value outside the expected range, high or low, requires medical evaluation. This is especially important if you are taking a diuretic or heart medication.

- **SODIUM and CHLORIDE** values relate to your body's salt and water concentration. The kidneys and the adrenal glands regulate blood levels. Minor changes may result from food intake and/or changes in fluid balance (i.e. dehydration after exercise). Large variations outside normal limits may indicate a variety of disorders. Abnormal results should be rechecked and discussed with your physician.
- **IRON** helps to make new red blood cells. It is not the same as the anemia-screening test, although low levels may help to explain anemia. High levels may also indicate disease and increase risks for strokes, cancer, and heart attacks, as iron is a pro-oxidant in high levels. Any value outside expected ranges should be evaluated. Ideal values range between 20 and 90.

Magnets

Beginning about 1990 the idea of using magnetic fields to enhance healing or control pain captured the general public's attention and thousands of persons in the United States have been treated using magnets instead of drugs for disorders such as arthritis, migraines, carpal tunnel syndrome, back pain, muscle spasms, and many other disorders.

Magnets have also been used for lung infections; pelvic disorders, including pelvic inflammatory disease and painful menstruation; prostatic hypertrophy; pigmented skin lesions; pain control; wound healing; schizophrenia; heart irregularities; swelling; inflammation; sore muscles; sleep enhancing; multiple sclerosis; Parkinson's; and epilepsy.

Roughly 80 percent of chronic pain sufferers get benefit from magnetic therapy. In 1998 a report was published by Baylor University researchers in *Archives of Physical Medicine and Rehabilitation* about magnets controlling pain in 76 percent of patients with post-polio syndrome. Tufts University researchers found benefit for patients suffering with fibromyalgia. New York Medical College researchers of Valhalla found magnetic foot pads to relieve numbness, tingling, and pain associated with diabetic neuropathy.

There are several theories as to how the magnets work, but the explanations that seem the most probable are that magnets attract particles in the blood, which creates some heat and circulation within the blood vessels, causing them to dilate, which allows more blood to flow into an injured area and thereby speeds the healing process. Another theory holds that magnets interact with the iron in red blood cells, improving their ability to carry oxygen.

Both simple magnets and electromagnetic devices, some of which are pulsating and some of which have steady current, have been used to good advantage in reduction of pain medication. Slow-healing bone fractures, pain syndromes of all kinds, and inflammatory conditions have all been treated with magnets with varying degrees of results, some outstanding and some only mild or moderate.

When the negative pole of a magnet is held against the skin, the capillary walls dilate slightly, boosting the blood flow to painful areas and relaxing muscle spasms. They diminish the transmission of electrochemical reactions at the junction between two nerves. One of the nicest things about magnets is that there are no side effects. Another good feature is their low cost, much less expensive than medications, and they are a one-time expense. They last for years without reduction in effectiveness.

The neodymium-boron magnets, called "neo magnets" for short, work as well as the more expensive magnets. A typical refrigerator magnet is about 10 gauss (unit of measure of magnetism), but medical magnets range from 45–10,000 gauss. Fix the magnet to the skin with adhesive tape over the area of pain or with snug fitting clothing over the painful area. If you do not have pain relief in a day or so, reposition the magnet a few inches away. If you have no pain relief in 30 days, magnets are probably not going to be effective in your case.

The permanent or Pharaoh magnets such as the material used on flexible magnetic signs attached temporarily to vehicle doors, can generate only a few hundred gauss. The pads need to be placed directly on the skin for it to be effective, as even one inch away from the skin reduces the intensity so much as to be probably ineffectual.

If you decide to try magnets as a home remedy, you will need to experiment with the little disks. Put the pole next to your skin and hold it in place with tape or by attaching two disks to each other with a layer of clothing between them.

Nerve Cell Damage

Nearly a thousand new chemicals are introduced every year into the environment. Many of these are neurotoxins, but it may be decades before they are recognized as such. A listing of some of these neurotoxins is as follows: glutamate, aspartate, phenylalanine, and cystine, which is added to bread dough. These are found in products such as toddler foods; salad dressings; puddings; sugarless gum, candy, and drinks; sodium caseinate; hydrolyzed vegetable protein; soy protein extract; TVP; yeast extracts; and almost all diet foods and foods containing "natural flavors."

Caffeine, as found in colas, coffee, tea, and chocolate, is a neuroexciter, made much worse by low magnesium.

A variety of problems may arise because of a long-term intake of neurotoxins, which may affect learning, behavior, and function of neurotransmitters; adversely affect the development of certain diseases of the nervous system, including seizures, migraine headaches, strokes, Alzheimer's, AIDS, and dementia; and may determine how extensive the damage will be after one has trauma. Attention deficit disorder and hyperactivity disorder may also have a link with these neurotoxins. Not only personality expression may be altered, but also violence control and the ability to reproduce. The taking of neurotoxins by pregnant women may cause their offspring to have learning disorders and all the problems mentioned above. As individuals age the blood-brain barrier lets down, especially after middle age, so that older persons are at even greater risk.

In animals, an 80 percent reduction in the neurotransmitter acetylcholine in the brain of unborn animals occurred with glutamate exposure. Glutamate is the most toxic amino acid in the development of the brain of the unborn. Some people are resistant to damage, others only moderately so, but some are extremely sensitive. Glutamate is normally the most common excitatory neurotransmitter in the brain. Because of this it must be kept inside the cell, but in trauma or strokes it gets outside the cell and adds more damage than the original problem. Since we take it in with food, glutamate gets outside the cell from the bloodstream where it is available to do damage. A low level of magnesium increases the excitability of glutamate and increases damage.

MSG increases the stress reaction in humans. Stress increases the production of free radicals. Mood swings are caused by MSG and other excitotoxins. If there is a reduction in glucose, such as in the hypoglycemia syndrome, there is a marked increased sensitivity of brain cells to excitotoxins.

Cheeses are all high in excitotoxins. It has been shown that excitotoxins cause weight gain in animals. It may be that much of the weight gain in the United States is caused by the excitotoxins (neurotoxins).

It has been observed by some neurosurgeons that strokes and brain trauma, Alzheimer's, ALS, and Parkinson's disease are all made worse by MSG and aspartame.

Blood Chemistry and CBC Report (The meaning of certain reports)

Test	Condition Increasing	Condition Decreasing
Blood Enzymes		
Alkaline Phosphatase Ideal: 20–115	Conditions reflecting increased osteoblastic activity of bone	
	Cancer may be the cause	
	Paget's disease (metabolic disease of the bone)	
	Rickets	
	Liver disease	
	Hyperparathyroidism	
CPK – Creatinine Phosphokinase Ideal: 25–235	Myocardial infarction	
	Skeletal muscle disease	
	Overuse of muscles	
GGT – Gamma-glutamyl transpeptidase Ideal: 0–65	Obstructive jaundice	
	Liver disease	
	Cancer of prostate with bone metastases	
	Sarcoidosis	
Hepatic congestion	Myocardial infarction	
	Acute pancreatatitis	
LDH – Lactic dehydrogenase Ideal: 100–225	Appears in blood serum in elevated concentrations when liver and muscle cells are injured. It rises later and persists longer than other enzymes.	
	Untreated pernicious anemia	
	Myocardial infarction	
	Pulmonary infarction	
	Liver disease	
SGOT – Transaminase Ideal: 5–40	Myocardial infarction	
	Skeletal muscle disease or damage	
	Liver disease, mostly acute	
	Fatty liver	
SGPT – Serum glutamic pyruvic transaminase Ideal: 5–50	Hepatitis	
	Infectious mononucleosis	
	Cirrhosis	
	Obstructive jaundice	
	Metastatic cancer	

Test	Condition Increasing	Condition Decreasing
Complete Blood Count (CBC)		
Hemoglobin Ideal: 13–15 (male) / 10.5–13 (female)	Normal in people living in high altitudes	Viral infections may cause bone marrow to decrease function for a few days
	Stress polycythemia	Increase in fluid intake
	Congenital heart disease	Erythrocytosis
		Pregnancy
Hematocrit Ideal: Roughly three times the hemoglobin	Normal in people living in high altitudes	Viral infections may cause bone marrow to decrease function for a few days
	Stress polycythemia	Increase in fluid intake
MCV (mean corpuscular volume) Ideal: 80–99	Macrocytic anemia	Microcytic anemias
	(Pernicious anemia, folic acid deficiency, sprue, liver disease.)	(iron deficiency, chronic blood loss, vitamin B6 deficiency)
MCH (mean corpuscular hemoglobin) Ideal: 27-36	Macrocytic (large cell) anemia	Microcytic (small cell) anemia
MCHC (mean corpuscular hemoglobin concentration) Ideal: 32–39	Polycythemia anemia	Hypochromic
Platelets Ideal: 80–300,000	Chronic granulocytic leukemia	Thrombocytopenic purpura (Idiopathic or due to drugs)
	Hemoconcentration	Acute leukemia
	Myelofibrosis	Aplastic anemia
	Splenectomy	Cancer chemo- therapy
		Myelofibrosis
		Hypersplenism
		Multiple myeloma
		Metastic cancer
		Pernicious anemia
RBC Ideal: 4.2–5.4 (male) / 4–5 (female)	Diarrheas, dehydration	Drug toxicities
	Polycythemia	Anemias
	Poisoning	Leukemias
	Pulmonary fibrosis and emphysema	Hemorrhage
	Hypoxia (heart or lung disease)	Iron deficiency
		B12 or folic acid deficiency
		Lead poisoning
WBC (white blood count) Ideal: 2.8–5.5	Acute and chronic infections	Aplastic anemia
	Leukemia	Agranulocytosis
	Following menstruation	Toxic agents
	Following trauma	Viral diseases
	Dehydration	Systemic lupus
	Exercise	Some phases of leukemia

Test	Condition Increasing	Condition Decreasing
WBC Differential		
Bands (immature neutrophils) / Ideal: 1–2		
Basophils / Ideal: 0–1	Increased in neoplasms	
Eosinophils / Ideal: 0–4	Allergies	
Lymphocytes / Ideal: 20–40	Chronic infections, viruses, cancer, and tuberculosis	Excessive adrenal activity
Monocytes / Ideal: 1–5	Chronic infections, clean-up jobs and several days after trauma, surgery and other inflammations	
Neutrophils, Polys / Ideal: 40–60	Increased in response infection, to acute bacterial trauma or surgery.	Toxicities
	Fight acute inflammation.	
Plasma cells / Ideal: 0	Chronic disease, cancer, multiple myeloma	
Electrolytes		
Calcium Ideal: 8.5–10.5	Tumor or hyperplasia of parathyroid	Hypoparathyroidism
	Hypervitaminosis D	Diarrhea
	Multiple myeloma	Celiac disease
	Nephritis	Rickets
	Cancer metastatic to bone	Osteomalacia
	After parathyroidectomy	Malnutrition
	Malabsorption after heavy exercise	Nephrosis
Chloride Ideal: 95–102	Nephritis	Diabetes
	Urinary obstruction	Diarrhea
	Cardiac decompensation	Vomiting
	Anemia	Pneumonia
	Ether anesthesia	Heavy metal poisoning
	Dehydration	
	Cushing's syndrome	
	Burns	
	Intestinal obstruction	
	Febrile conditions	
	Diuretics	
Creatinine Ideal: 0.5–1.4	Nephritis	
	Chronic renal disease	
Phosphorus Ideal: 2.5–4.5	Excessive intake of phosphates (grains)	Hyperparathyroidism
	Hypoparathyroidism	
Potassium Below 8	Addison's disease	Diabetic acidosis
	Oliguria (tubular necrosis)	Diarrhea
	Tissue breakdown or hemolysis	Vomiting
	Heart becomes susceptible to rhythm disturbance	Diuretics

Test	Condition Increasing	Condition Decreasing
Sodium Ideal: 135–140	Dehydration	Chronic nephritis
	Nephritis	Alkali deficit
	Pyloric obstruction	Addison's disease
	Myxedema (low Thyroid)	
	Diuretics	
Urea (BUN) Ideal: 6–12	Acute or chronic renal disease	Severe liver failure
	Obstructive uropathy	Pregnancy
	Mercury poisoning	Starvation
	Nephrotic syndrome	
	Sluggish kidney	
	Dehydration	
Uric Acid Ideal: 6 and under (male) / 5 and under (female)	Acute leukemia (because of the destruction of nuclei in the RBC, uric acid crystals form and stop up the kidneys)	
	Lymphomas treated by chemotherapy	
	Toxemia of pregnancy	
	Fasting	
	Too much protein	
	Familial hypleruricemia	
Gastrointestinal function		
A/G ratio Ideal: 1.0–2.2	Low globulin or elevated albumin	High globulin or low albumin
Albumin Ideal: 3.5–5.5	Multiple myeloma	Chronic liver disease
	Cirrhosis	Loss of protein
	Chronic hepatitis from burns	Proteinuria
		Nephritis
		Nephrosis
Bilirubin Ideal: 0.1–0.5	Hemolytic anemia (indirect)	
	Biliary obstruction	
	Hepatocellular damage	
	Pernicious anemia	
	Hemolytic disease of newborn	
	Eclampsia	
	High protein diet including meat substitutes	
	Congenital enzymatic liver cell defect	
Globulin, total Ideal: 1.5–4.5	Chronic infections	
	Liver disease	
	Collagen disease	
	Hyperimmune states	
	Hypo or agammaglobulinemia	

Test	Condition Increasing	Condition Decreasing
Protein, total Ideal: 6.0–8.0	Hemoconcentration	Malnutrition
	Shock	Hemorrhage
	See under "globulin"	
Glucose		
Glucose Tolerance Test Ideal Fasting: 70–85 Half an hour: 105 1 hour: 135–145 2 hours: 70–85 3 hours: 70–85 4 hours: 70–85 5 hours: 70–85	Nephritis	Hypoglycemia
	Diabetes	Hyperinsulinism
	Hyperthyroidism	Hypothyroidism
	Early hyperpituitarism	Late hyperpituitarism
	Cerebral lesions-stroke	Pernicious vomiting
	Infections	Addison's disease
	Pregnancy	Extensive hepatic damage
	Fasting before glucose loading for lab tests	
Hormones		
Thyroid (T4) Ideal: 4–12	Hyperthyroidism	Hypothyroidism
	Drugs such as ACTH	
	"The pill" can make it high or low	
Lipids		
Cholesterol (HDL, LDL) Ideal: 100 + age of person	Familial hyperlipemia	Pernicious anemia
	Obstructive jaundice	Hemolytic jaundice
	Diabetes	Hyperthyroidism
	Hypothyroidism	Severe infection
	Increased fats and cholesterol in diet	Terminal states of debilitating disease
	Not enough raw foods	
	Overweight	
	Lack of exercise	
	Stress	
Triglycerides Ideal: same as age of person or <110	Refined carbohydrates	Starvation
	Concentrated foods	
	Dairy products	
Miscellaneous		
RA latex test (Rheumatoid Arthritis factor)	Rheumatoid arthritis (non-specific)	
	Collagen diseases (non-specific)	
RPR (rapid plasma reagin) Ideal: negative	Screening test for non-specific antibodies associated with syphilis	

Toxic Heavy Metals

Aluminum

There are approximately four or more times the amount of aluminum in the brain cells in Alzheimer's with neurofibrillary tangles than in nerve cells not having these tangles. Sources for aluminum range from aluminum cans, aluminum foil, any baked goods containing baking powder made with aluminum, nondairy creamers, processed meat and cheese, antiperspirants, aluminum cookware, antacids, and contaminants in certain things such as dolomite and bone meal. Aluminum interferes with certain metabolic enzymes including those having to do with metabolizing sugar. Aluminum also weakens the blood-brain barrier, allowing toxins and drugs to get through the barrier into the brain.

Forty-six residents of a geriatric center having Alzheimer's disease were studied for their past consumption of foods containing large amounts of aluminum additives. It was found that the dietary intake of aluminum may affect the risk of developing this disease. The intake of the following foods was significant for Alzheimer's patients: commercial packages of pancakes, waffles, biscuits, muffins, cornbread, corn tortillas (containing some form of aluminum or baking powder containing aluminum), American cheese, chocolate pudding, beverages, salt, and chewing gum (*Age and Aging* 28 [1999]: 205–209).

There have been several studies showing an increased risk in population groups for Alzheimer's disease when there were elevated aluminum concentrations in public drinking water supplies (*Neurology* 46 [1996]: 401).

Many factors increase the absorption of aluminum, especially the use of excessive supplements of vitamin C, kidney failure, and low levels of calcium and magnesium. Aluminum is transported in the blood by a protein called transferrin that also transports iron. The highest concentration of transferrin receptors in the brain is in the hippocampus and in the grey matter, the same areas that degenerate in Alzheimer's disease.

Cadmium

Cadmium is a contaminant in refined carbohydrate foods and in tobacco smoke. It is high in organ meats, fish, and shellfish. In the human body, adverse effects of cadmium may be found in the kidneys and liver, especially, but also in the bones, lungs, and stomach. It can also decrease the birth weight of infants and result in birth defects and growth retardation in children.

Iron Overload

While iron is an essential nutrient, when it accumulates in the blood or tissues in too great a quantity, it becomes toxic or hazardous in various ways. Too much iron may lead to liver disease, malignancies or chronic infections, chronic renal failure, hemochromatosis, and stroke.

Lead, Tin Intoxication

Water is now allowed to contain 20 PPB of lead. However, tests show that there is 10 to 15 percent absorption in adults and 50 percent in children! Learning difficulties and hyperactivity occur in children having high lead levels. Decreased concentration occurs in adults. Avoid drinking softened water, as you will get more cadmium and lead.

It is important to note that lead absorption is greater if one is fasting. And zinc, iron, copper, calcium, and magnesium deficiencies all cause a greater absorption of lead. Lead in one's food or the atmosphere goes to the bones, blood, soft tissue, brain, and neural mitochondria.

Lead decreases myelin-synthesizing enzymes, the enzymes that help form a sleeve around nerve cells to improve function. Kidney tubules and blood vessels are damaged. Hypertension is likely. Lead damages the internal structure of the cells' mitochondria.

Household sources of lead include moonshine, paint, house dust, soil in the yard and street, newsprint, lead pipes, three-piece cans used for canned foods, drinking water, milk, toothpaste, kettles, and painted glassware.

Traces of both lead and tin may be found in canned foods, depending on the kind of can-making technology used in production of the food. Nonsoldered cans produce lower lead levels in foods compared to soldered cans (*Food Additives and Contaminants* 8 [1991]: 485).

Mercury Poisoning

A Canadian study revealed infants whose mothers consumed mercury-containing fish during pregnancy are at risk of delayed lung development. Fish in many areas of the United States are known to be contaminated with mercury.

Thallium Excess

"Burning" feet has been associated with thallium excess. Other symptoms are muscle cramps, numbness in fingers and toes, intestinal problems, heart rhythm problems, and hair loss. Any or all of these symptoms may be attributed to thallium excess. Sources of thallium have been found in toxic waste dumps, near cement plants, smelting plants, and wherever thallium compounds are processed. Food grown on these soils even years after the contamination has been removed or cleaned up may represent a major source of exposure. Water and inhalation are other sources. Smokers have twice as much thallium as nonsmokers. Colloidal minerals may indicate levels of thallium on the label. A hair analysis is a reliable indicator for thallium excess.

Treatment of thallium excess can be with activated charcoal or Prussian blue, which interrupts the enterohepatic cycling of thallium, encouraging fecal elimination of the metal. Brewer's yeast and foods high in potassium are also very helpful to prevent thallium-induced toxicity and to increase renal excretion of thallium. Garlic and selenium increase excretion of heavy metals and may help with thallium.

Treatment of Heavy Metal Poisoning

If you know you have been exposed to heavy metals, attempts should be made to excrete lead, mercury, silver, and other heavy metals that may have deposited in the tissues or circulated for some time in the blood.

It has been suggested since the 1700s that emersion in mineral water would help to increase the secretion of lead from the body. Significant lead levels can cause fatigue, headaches, and a vague sense of not being well. Those more seriously affected become weak and may become paralyzed with anemia as a complicating factor. The mineral water can be made by putting a cup of salt and a cup of Epsom salts in a bathtub full of water and immersing the patient in it up to the neck. The bath temperature should be at a comfortable level, enabling the patient to stay in the bath for two to four hours at a time. In a study reported in 1990, lead was excreted in the urine in all patients treated in this manner, the major lead being excreted during the second hour of immersion, but continuing into the third and fourth hours (*British Journal of Industrial Medicine* 43 [1986]: 713; *Medical History* 82, no. 10 [1990]: S101).

Another method for eliminating heavy metals from the body is eating one globe (entire head) of garlic two times per day. Cook for one minute and ten seconds in a microwave; ten minutes in a 350-degree oven; or seven to nine minutes in a stove-top steamer. Eat with meals starting at the beginning of the meal and eating along with the meal. One may also eat a small handful of cilantro, perhaps half to one cup of the chopped fresh herb, daily.

Heavy metals can be excreted to some degree, and this excretion can be encouraged by eating garlic and/or cilantro and drinking plenty of water. Large doses of each should be given over a period of one to six months, depending on the severity of the heavy metal intoxication. The use of charcoal helps slightly to excrete heavy metals. Use one tablespoon mixed in water four times per day for four to six months.

Absorption of lead and its retention may be blocked by generous use of tofu in the diet (*American Journal of Epidemiology* 153, no. 12 [June 15, 2001]: 1206).

Cadmium poisoning may be helped by chlorella, which is said to bind strongly to cadmium. If it binds to cadmium, it is possible that it will bind to other heavy metals. In cases of lead, mercury, aluminum, pesticides, copper, gold, nickel, or PCB intoxication or exposure, chlorella should probably be taken along with other methods to assist in the excretion of these toxic substances. In addition to protein, fats, and celluloses, chlorella has a 3.3 percent glucosamine level, which may be helpful in the leaky gut syndrome or in joint and tendon problems. Chlorella might be of help in Alzheimer's disease as both aluminum and zinc are implicated in its development. Use the maximum dose instructions on the bottle.

Spirulina may also be helpful in heavy metal intoxications as many other sea weeds. Silica is necessary for the control of cholesterol, to protect against aluminum poisoning, and to insure healthiness of collagen, an intercellular connective tissue.

Water

Your body needs about one milliliter of water for every calorie you burn. If you are quite active and burn 4,000 calories a day, you will need about four quarts of water. If you are very inactive, burn only 1,000 calories, you will need one quart each day.

The marvels of water continue to be understood better. Water as a remedial agent is unsurpassed, approaching that of a universal remedy in its various applications of steam, hot water, cold water, and ice.

The plastic used to store water and soft drinks imparts dimethylterephthalate to the water, which is carcinogenic. Chlorine is known to damage the thyroid gland and can cause cardiovascular problems. Other contaminants in drinking water may be arsenic, fluoride, industrial pollutants, lead, pesticides, herbicides, and radioactive particles.

Almost all drinking water in the municipal water systems in the United States contains toxic contaminants. The degree of intoxication the person experiences depends on how much tap water is drunk, as well as how much of the water vapor the person breathes while bathing, cleaning, or showering. Persons who work in the water industry, and those who have long skin contact with water may be just as vulnerable, or more, than persons who drink a lot of tap water every day (*Science News* 149 [February 10, 1996]: 84).

Water is a simple and free cure or treatment for various ailments. Some of the following disorders can be cured and others helped by the free use of water, enough to keep the urine pale: lower back pain, many canker sores, chronic fatigue syndrome, diabetes, headaches, asthma, allergies, colitis, rheumatoid arthritis, depression, high blood pressure, high blood cholesterol, alcohol dependency, neck pain, various stones and calcifications, and many others.

The American College of Sports Medicine reminds all athletes that they will have fewer injuries if they replace fluid lost during exercising. Drink plenty of fluids both before and after exercising. Two eight-ounce glasses are recommended to be taken two hours before an exercise event and repeated as needed.

As many as one-third of Americans over the age of 50 are likely to have chronic, mild dehydration, if not moderate or severe. The concerns of dehydration include the risk it poses for kidney stones (at least eight cups of water per day can prevent most stones, even in people prone to forming stones), reduction in strength and endurance in physical activities, and an increased risk of some cancers, particularly urinary tract cancer. But the disease to be feared most from chronic dehydration is strokes. The more calories burned each day, the more water one needs. Coffee and alcoholic drinks, soda, tea, and chocolate should not be counted as liquids meeting the fluid needs of the body as they actually encourage loss of water through the kidneys.

Interesting Facts about Water

- Drink sufficient water to urinate every two to four hours while awake and to keep your urine clear and light in color.
- If you are feeling cranky, irritable, or having muscular cramps, there is a chance you are dehydrated. Drink one to two cups of water before engaging in strenuous activities and take a water break about every fifteen minutes. Don't wait until you feel you need to drink.
- Get a good source of drinking water, not your city water from the tap. There have been several different studies to support the hypothesis that public drinking water and wells having a lot of surface run-off water can increase the likelihood of getting cancer and developing a mineral imbalance (*Journal of Environmental Pathology Tox. and Onc.* 13, no. 1 [1994]: 39).
- If you are having distress or weakness, or almost any kind of symptom, drink a glassful of water every ten minutes for an hour. Persons taking chemotherapy for cancer should watch their symptoms and, if distress begins to develop, start the drinking routine. It may keep you from having hours of misery.
- In hydrotherapy, if mechanical stimulation is given to the skin along with the temperature changes, a greater impression can be made on the nervous system. With mechanical stimulation, such as percussion from streams of water or rubbing or brushing of the skin during the application of hot or cold water more decided changing of the skin temperature occurs. At the same time, the mechanical stimulation, apart from the temperature change, evokes a blood vessel, nervous, or muscular response.

Weight Control

Obesity is defined as 10 percent or more above ideal weight, morbid obesity is 20 percent or more above ideal weight. Although ideal weight is not precisely known, use the following guidelines to calculate your weight: allow yourself 100 pounds for your first five feet in height. Allow five pounds for each inch thereafter if you are a woman, six to seven if you are a man, depending on how muscular you are.

If you measure over 0.5 cm in skin fold thickness over the triceps (back of upper arm), you are probably overweight if you are a man, or 0.8 cm if you are a woman. Do not allow an accumulation of fat in specific areas such as the abdomen, bust, or hips.

For some people, they are driven to eat. They are considered impulsive or compulsive eaters or food-addicts. To determine whether you are an impulsive or compulsive overeater, answer these questions:

1. Do you eat when you're not hungry?
2. Do you go on eating binges for no apparent reason?
3. Do you have feelings of guilt and remorse after overeating?
4. Do you give too much time and thought to food?
5. Do you look forward with pleasure and anticipation to the moments when you can eat alone?
6. Do you plan these secret binges ahead of time?

7. Do you eat sensibly before others and make up for it alone?
8. Is your weight affecting the way you live your life?
9. Have you tried to diet for a week (or longer) only to fall short of your goal?
10. Do you resent the advice of others who tell you to "use a little will power" to stop overeating?
11. Despite evidence to the contrary, have you continued to assert that you could diet "on your own" whenever you wish?
12. Do you crave to eat at a definite time, day or night, other than meal time?
13. Do you eat to escape from worries or trouble?
14. Has a physician ever treated you for being overweight?
15. Does your food obsession make you or others unhappy?

How did you score? If you answered yes to three or more of these questions, we believe you have a compulsive eating problem or are well on the way to having one. For compulsive overeaters, and for certain other persons, a support group may be used to great advantage. If there is not a support group in your area, organize your own weight control club.

Six Ways to Burn Fat

1. Do not have long fasts, but eat moderately as a routine. If you cut back too much on calories, the body perceives that as starvation and reduces the rate at which it burns calories. Slower weight loss results. However, a day or two of fasting per week, separated by at least one day, will have a good effect.
2. Don't drink alcohol. It suppresses the body's ability to burn fat.
3. Eat breakfast or you will have more difficulty losing weight. Breakfast gets the metabolism going for the day with calories burned right away. Omit supper, as food eaten after about 3:00 p.m. is more likely to be stored than burned.
4. Do not do the most vigorous exercise you can, but do more moderate exercise. Very vigorous exercise burns carbohydrates rather than fat, at least in the initial part of exercise. Moderate exercise, on the other hand, burns fat from the beginning. Get one to two hours of exercise and/or vigorous useful labor in a day.
5. Tone up your muscles, as muscle tissue burns more calories and makes metabolism higher. Some moderate strengthening exercises are quite sufficient.
6. Exercise after eating as this practice helps burn more calories during the exercise session.

Helpful Tips for Overweight People

Get up from the table at the end of 35 to 45 minutes, after a leisurely meal in which you have taken small bites, thoroughly chewed, and eaten slowly. The enjoyment from and much of the benefit of food comes from the length of time the food spends in the mouth.

Drink sixteen ounces or more of water 30 to 60 minutes before each meal and before a party. The cause of much stuffing is really thirst. If you must be present where others are eating at a time you do not have a meal regularly scheduled, drink water or plain herbal tea. Take tea bags with you for just such occasions. Regularity in all things is essential.

Eat more complex carbohydrates. Some consider potatoes and pasta to be an enemy to a weight reduction program. Far from it, as these foods will actually suppress the appetite and carry far fewer calories than those containing free fats or heavy quantities of protein. Use whole grain pastas.

Although you may be faced with a smorgasbord of choices at a meal, confine your choices to two or three simple foods such as beans over rice plus one vegetable. When these are served with a simple salad (sliced tomatoes as contrasted to a tossed salad containing five to ten items), and bread, they make a nourishing meal.

Don't even look at the serving bowls or other peoples' food during the meal. Determine that your first plateful is your only food for that meal, even if you are still hungry. Quickly stand up after the meal and excuse yourself to the bathroom to brush your teeth. Brushing your teeth will discourage you from nibbling while clearing the table.

Be entirely honest in everything you do, talking or eating. Never misrepresent the quantity you have eaten. Bear in mind that as a general rule people eat more food than they believe they have.

Train yourself to think of something higher than physical satisfaction when eating, such as "This good bread will give me steady nerves"; "chewing longer will make my stomach healthy." Make the mealtimes social events for the family. Plan some small item to share. This is an ideal time to speak of spiritual subjects, to train the children in attitudes about life. Do not watch TV or listen to radio or read the newspaper during meals if you have a problem with appetite control. There is too much encouragement to improper eating from the media. Furthermore, you will become distracted and eat more than you intended.

Rewards for perfect behavior and weight loss should be in such areas as exercise outings, household items, clothing purchased, or persons visited, rather than rewards in eating or food binges. There are no vacations from your commitment anymore than from a commitment to the marriage contract. This is for real, and it is a spiritual commitment.

When you talk to friends or a counselor, talk about the solutions to your problems rather than about your longing for food, hunger, or your difficulty in staying on the program.

Divine aid in appetite control, thought control, and performance control should be sought every day.

Get a trusted friend who will be willing to give you encouragement and help you to stay committed to maintaining your resolve to become healthier. This friend is very important when temptations are strong. The giving of daily weight loss reports to members of the family may put an emphasis on weight loss that can be discouraging. The emphasis should always be on sticking to the program, obtaining better health, doing one's duty in setting a good example, and other things of this nature, rather than on weight loss. Your part is working the program. God's part is rectifying your weight issue in accordance with His promise. He will give you strength to work it out. Focus on His strength.

Practical Suggestions for Those Who Want to Lose Weight

- Weigh and record your weight on a chart or card.
- Understand that this is a long-term program (lifetime).
- Follow these guidelines during the first week:
    - Eat a good breakfast, large lunch, and light supper.
    - Do not eat between-meals or snack at bedtime.
    - Do not eat rich desserts or fried foods (any pungent or strong stimulant to the taste buds invites compulsive eating).
    - Begin to take smaller lunch and supper helpings, toward the end of the week, but be realistic (serve your plate with what is known to be needed and allow no seconds and no changes of mind except to eat less, and no taking of food you decided against earlier). Eat regularly.
    - Take smaller bites. Learn to chew thoroughly and eat slowly.
    - Don't use table salt on your food since salty food invites loss of control.
- Exercise
    - Walk a minimum of one mile a day if you are not disabled. If you cannot walk, design a set of arm and body movements into a 15 to 20 minute exercise program. You should recognize you have had a "workout" when you have finished. Try to engage in one to two hours of exercise and/or useful labor a day.
    - Use leg and arm swings for a warm-up, along with gentle stretches.
    - A small trampoline, stationary bike, or other indoor equipment can be used for additional exercise after dark, while making phone calls, or when the weather keeps you indoors.

Weight Control Club or Support Group

You will find a whole new life open up to you if you start your own weight control club. Print up a small leaflet giving the time, day, and length of the weekly programs, or simply promote your club by word of mouth and announcements in church or school meetings. It is best to commit to conducting the program for at least a year.

You may choose to charge a small amount like $5.00 per session if you need to purchase materials, rent facilities, or ensure that persons understand that the club means business. Have a monthly meeting for families, and invite a guest to speak on health. Show films on general health, not on weight control, as people get tired of hearing about losing weight and need to retrain their brains to think about good health and not just weight loss.

Every three months plan an outing to some type of recreation area. You may rent bicycles at a nearby park and cycle around it, go canoeing, or plan a hike.

At the meetings, serve nothing but hot or iced herbal teas or water. Demonstrate that people can have a good time socializing and going on outings without food.

The focus of the meetings should be on general health principles and increasing the overall health of everyone in the group. However, weight loss should still be an overall goal of the group. Make exercise sheets available to track everyone's exercise progress. Also, plan on keeping track of everyone's weight loss on a chart or personal weight cards.

There are lots of existing weight loss clubs and groups. Gather ideas from other clubs and adapt what will work for your group. The most important thing is to develop a support system of individuals who all desire the same outcome: learning how to live healthier lives.

Spiritual Steps in Appetite Control

Since being overweight has many spiritual implications, no program is complete without special attention to spiritual matters. We believe that there are several steps that can assist one in recovery from being overweight.

- You must admit that you are powerless over appetite and that your food has become unmanageable. Admission of powerlessness is the first step of liberation; you must perceive that only through utter defeat are you able to make the first step toward strength.
- You must come to believe that only God can restore you to complete physical, mental, and spiritual health.
- You must make the decision to cause your will and life to coincide with the will and way of your heavenly Father.
- You must take a fearless moral inventory.
- You must daily admit to your heavenly Father the exact nature of your wrongs. Actually call yourself an overeater or a glutton in your private prayers. Do not fail to confess the full truth of the matter. Do not miss a single instance in which you have misjudged or indulged.
- You must seek through prayer and meditation to improve your ability to picture heavenly themes in the imagination, praying for the knowledge of our Father's will for you and the power to carry that out.
- Having had a spiritual awakening as a result of these steps, you should try to carry this message to others who have similar needs.

Index

Symbols

A

B

E

F

M

Q

R

S

We invite you to view the complete
selection of titles we publish at:

www.TEACHServices.com

Scan with your mobile
device to go directly
to our website.

Please write or email us your praises, reactions, or
thoughts about this or any other book we publish at:

P.O. Box 954
Ringgold, GA 30736

info@TEACHServices.com

TEACH Services, Inc., titles may be purchased in bulk for
educational, business, fund-raising, or sales promotional use.
For information, please e-mail:

BulkSales@TEACHServices.com

Finally, if you are interested in seeing
your own book in print, please contact us at

publishing@TEACHServices.com

We would be happy to review your manuscript for free.

CPSIA information can be obtained
at www.ICGtesting.com
Printed in the USA
LVHW022255170623
750084LV00007B/528

9 781572 587151